Aug 2023

Welcome

SATRD

MW00837262

The American Psychiatric Association Publishing

TEXTBOOK of
ANXIETY, TRAUMA,
AND OCD-RELATED
DISORDERS

THIRD EDITION

The American Psychiatric Association Publishing

TEXTBOOK of
ANXIETY, TRAUMA, AND OCD-RELATED DISORDERS

THIRD EDITION

EDITED BY

Naomi M. Simon, M.D., M.Sc.
Eric Hollander, M.D.
Barbara O. Rothbaum, Ph.D., ABPP
Dan J. Stein, M.D., Ph.D.

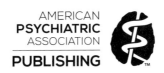

AMERICAN
PSYCHIATRIC
ASSOCIATION
PUBLISHING

If you wish to buy 50 or more copies of the same title, please go to www.appi.org/specialdiscounts for more information.

Copyright © 2020 American Psychiatric Association Publishing

ALL RIGHTS RESERVED

Third Edition

Manufactured in the United States of America on acid-free paper
24   23   22   21   20   5   4   3   2   1

American Psychiatric Association Publishing
800 Maine Avenue SW
Suite 900
Washington, DC 20024-2812
www.appi.org

Library of Congress Cataloging-in-Publication Data
Names: Simon, Naomi M., editor. | Hollander, Eric, 1957- editor. | Rothbaum, Barbara O., editor. | Stein, Dan J., editor. | American Psychiatric Association Publishing, issuing body.
Title: The American Psychiatric Association Publishing textbook of anxiety, trauma, and OCD-related disorders / edited by Naomi Simon, Eric Hollander, Barbara O. Rothbaum, Dan J. Stein.
Other titles: Textbook of anxiety, trauma, and OCD-related disorders | Textbook of anxiety disorders.
Description: Third edition. | Washington, DC : American Psychiatric Association Publishing, [2020] | Preceded by: Textbook of anxiety disorders / edited by Dan J. Stein, Eric Hollander, Barbara O. Rothbaum. 2nd ed. c2010. | Includes bibliographical references and index. |
Identifiers: LCCN 2019057573 (print) | LCCN 2019057574 (ebook) | ISBN 9781615372324 (hardcover ; alk. paper) | ISBN 9781615372928 (ebook)
Subjects: MESH: Anxiety Disorders | Stress Disorders, Traumatic | Obsessive-Compulsive Disorder
Classification: LCC RC531 (print) | LCC RC531 (ebook) | NLM WM 172 | DDC 616.85/22—dc23
LC record available at https://lccn.loc.gov/2019057573
LC ebook record available at https://lccn.loc.gov/2019057574

British Library Cataloguing in Publication Data
A CIP record is available from the British Library.

We dedicate this volume to the memory of Donald F. Klein;
his pioneering contributions to the field inspired us,
and he generously mentored several generations of
anxiety disorder researchers, including many of our
contributing authors.

Contents

PART I
Approaching Anxiety Disorders

PART II
Core Principles for Treating Anxiety Disorders

PART III
Generalized Anxiety Disorder

PART IV
Obsessive-Compulsive and Related Disorders

PART V
Panic Disorder and Agoraphobia

PART VI
Social Anxiety Disorder (Social Phobia)

PART VII
Specific Phobia

PART VIII
Trauma- and Stressor-Related Disorders

PART IX
Anxiety Disorders and Comorbidity

PART X
Anxiety Disorders in Special Populations

Contributors

Jonathan S. Abramowitz, Ph.D.
Professor of Clinical Psychology, Department of Psychology and Neuroscience, University of North Carolina–Chapel Hill, Chapel Hill, North Carolina

Anne Marie Albano, Ph.D., ABPP
Professor of Medical Psychology in Psychiatry, Columbia University Vagelos College of Physicians and Surgeons, New York, New York

Andrea R. Ashbaugh, Ph.D.
Associate Professor, School of Psychology, University of Ottawa, Ontario, Canada

Sudie E. Back, Ph.D.
Associate Professor, Clinical Neuroscience Division, Department of Psychiatry and Behavioral Sciences, The Medical University of South Carolina, Charleston, South Carolina

Amanda Waters Baker, Ph.D.
Assistant Professor, Department of Psychiatry, Massachusetts General Hospital/Harvard Medical School, Boston, Massachusetts

David S. Baldwin, M.A., D.M., FRCPsych
Professor of Psychiatry, Clinical and Experimental Sciences, Faculty of Medicine, University of Southampton, Southampton, United Kingdom

Borwin Bandelow, M.D., Ph.D.
Department of Psychiatry and Psychotherapy, University Medical Center, Göttingen, Germany

David H. Barlow, Ph.D., ABPP
Professor Emeritus of Psychology and Psychiatry, Center for Anxiety and Related Disorders, Boston University, Massachusetts

Abigail L. Barthel, M.A.
Graduate student, Department of Psychological and Brain Sciences, Boston University, Boston, Massachusetts

Janna Marie Bas-Hoogendam, M.Sc.
Doctoral student, Department of Psychiatry, Leiden University Medical Center; Developmental and Educational Psychology, Institute of Psychology, Leiden University; Leiden Institute for Brain and Cognition, Leiden, Netherlands

Katja Beesdo-Baum, Ph.D.
Professor, Technische Universität Dresden, Institute of Clinical Psychology and Psychotherapy, Behavioral Epidemiology, Center for Clinical Epidemiology and Longitudinal Studies, Dresden, Germany

Colleen Gribbin Bloom, M.S.W.
Program Manager, Field Instructor, Columbia School of Social Work, Center for Complicated Grief, New York

Christina L. Boisseau, Ph.D.
Associate Professor, Department of Psychiatry and Behavioral Sciences, Northwestern University Feinberg School of Medicine, Chicago, Illinois

Kathleen T. Brady, M.D., Ph.D.
Professor and Director, Clinical Neuroscience Division, The Medical University of South Carolina, Charleston, South Carolina

J. Douglas Bremner, M.D.
Professor of Psychiatry and Behavioral Sciences and Professor of Radiology, Emory University School of Medicine, Atlanta; Staff Physician, Atlanta Veterans Clinic General Mental Health (AVC GMH), Atlanta VA Medical Center, Decatur, Georgia

Lily A. Brown, Ph.D.
Assistant Professor, Department of Psychiatry, University of Pennsylvania, Philadelphia, Pennsylvania

Richard A. Bryant, Ph.D.
Professor, School of Psychology, University of New South Wales, Sydney, Australia

Jennifer L. Buchholz, M.A.
Graduate student in Clinical Psychology, University of North Carolina–Chapel Hill, Chapel Hill, North Carolina

Elisabetta Burchi, M.D.
Research Fellow, Autism and Obsessive Compulsive Spectrum Program, Albert Einstein College of Medicine, Psychiatric Research Institute at Montefiore-Einstein (PRIME), Bronx, New York

Mark Burton, Ph.D.
Postdoctoral Fellow, Emory University School of Medicine, Department of Psychiatry and Behavioral Sciences, Atlanta, Georgia

Fredric N. Busch, M.D.
Professor of Psychiatry, Weill Cornell Medical College; Faculty, Columbia University Center for Psychoanalytic Training and Research, New York, New York

Rebecca P. Cameron, Ph.D.
Interim Department Chair and Professor, Department of Psychology, Sacramento State University, Sacramento, California

Craig Campbell, M.D.
Health Sciences Clinical Professor of Psychiatry and Program Director, UCSF Fresno, Fresno, California

Denise April Chavira, Ph.D.
Professor, Department of Psychology, UCLA, Los Angeles, California

Eduardo Cinosi, M.B.B.S., MRCPsych
Hertfordshire Partnership University NHS Foundation Trust, St. Albans, United Kingdom

Jeremy D. Coplan, M.D.
Professor of Psychiatry, SUNY Downstate Medical Center, Brooklyn, New York

Bernadette M. Cortese, Ph.D.
Postdoctoral Scholar and Assistant Professor, Department of Psychiatry and Behavioral Sciences, Medical University of South Carolina, Charleston, South Carolina

Stephen J. Cozza, M.D.
Associate Director, Center for the Study of Traumatic Stress, Uniformed Services University for the Health Sciences, Bethesda, Maryland

Kevin J. Craig, M.B.B.Ch., M.Phil., MRCPsych
Medical Director, P1vital Limited; University of Oxford Department of Psychiatry, Warneford Hospital, Oxford, United Kingdom

Michelle G. Craske, Ph.D.
Distinguished Professor and Vice Chair, Department of Psychology, University of California, Los Angeles, California

Andrew J. Curreri, M.A.
Doctoral student, Center for Anxiety and Related Disorders, Boston University, Boston, Massachusetts

Grishma Dabas, B.Sc.
Ph.D. candidate, MacAnxiety Research Centre and Department of Psychiatry and Behavioural Neurosciences, McMaster University, Hamilton, Ontario, Canada

Jonathan R.T. Davidson, M.D.
Emeritus Professor, Department of Psychiatry and Behavioral Sciences, Duke University School of Medicine, Durham, North Carolina

Jürgen Deckert, M.D.
Professor of Psychiatry, Department of Psychiatry, Psychosomatics and Psychotherapy, Center of Mental Health, University Hospital of Würzburg, Würzburg, Germany

Michael Diamond, M.D.
Research Fellow, Autism and Obsessive Compulsive Spectrum Program, Albert Einstein College of Medicine, Psychiatric Research Institute at Montefiore-Einstein (PRIME), Bronx, New York

Darin D. Dougherty, M.D.
Associate Professor of Psychiatry, Harvard Medical School; Director of Medical Education, Obsessive Compulsive Disorder Institute, Department of Psychiatry, Massachusetts General Hospital, Boston, Massachusetts

Boadie W. Dunlop, M.D.
Associate Professor, Department of Psychiatry and Behavioral Sciences, Emory University School of Medicine, Atlanta, Georgia

Jane L. Eisen, M.D.
Clinical Director, Division of Depression and Anxiety Disorders, McLean Hospital, Belmont, Massachusetts

Thalia C. Eley, Ph.D.
Professor of Developmental Behavioural Genetics, and Lab Director, Emotional Development Intervention and Treatment (EDIT), SGDP Centre, Institute of Psychiatry, Psychology and Neuroscience, King's College, London, United Kingdom

Todd J. Farchione, Ph.D.
Research Associate Professor, Center for Anxiety and Related Disorders, Boston University, Boston, Massachusetts

Jan Fawcett, M.D.
Professor of Psychiatry, University of New Mexico School of Medicine, Albuquerque, New Mexico

Naomi A. Fineberg, M.B.B.S., M.A., MRCPsych
Professor of Psychiatry, University of Hertfordshire and Consultant Psychiatrist, Highly Specialised Obsessive Compulsive Disorders Service, Hertfordshire Partnership University NHS Foundation Trust, Welwyn Garden City; Senior Clinical Research Fellow, Department of Psychiatry, University of Cambridge School of Clinical Medicine, Addenbrooke's Hospital, Cambridge, United Kingdom

Edna B. Foa, Ph.D.
Professor, Department of Psychiatry, University of Pennsylvania, Philadelphia, Pennsylvania

Andrew W. Goddard, M.D.
Professor, Department of Psychiatry, UCSF Fresno, Fresno, California

Benedetta Grancini, M.D.
Department of Biomedical and Clinical Sciences, University of Milan; Psychiatry Unit, ASST Fatebenefratelli-Sacco, Milan, Italy

Benjamin D. Greenberg, M.D., Ph.D.
Associate Professor of Psychiatry and Human Behavior, Butler Hospital, Warren Alpert Medical School of Brown University, Providence, Rhode Island

Richard G. Heimberg, Ph.D.
Professor of Psychology, Department of Psychology, Temple University, Philadelphia, Pennsylvania

Gert-Jan Hendriks, Ph.D., M.D.
Appointed Professor of the Treatment of Anxiety Disorders and Depression in Older Adults, Overwaal Centre of Expertise for Anxiety Disorders, OCD and PTSD, Institution for Integrated Mental Health Care Pro Persona, Nijmegen, Netherlands

John M. Hettema, M.D., Ph.D.
Professor, Department of Psychiatry, Texas A&M Health Science Center, Bryan, Texas; Associate Professor of Psychiatry, Virginia Institute for Psychiatric and Behavioral Genetics, Virginia Commonwealth University, Richmond, Virginia

Stefan G. Hofmann, Ph.D.
Professor, Department of Psychological and Brain Sciences, Boston University, Boston, Massachusetts

Elizabeth Hoge, M.D.
Director, Anxiety Disorders Research Program, and Associate Professor of Psychiatry, Georgetown University School of Medicine, Washington, DC

Eric Hollander, M.D.
Director, Autism and Obsessive Compulsive Spectrum Program and Anxiety and Depression Program, Montefiore Medical Center and Albert Einstein College of Medicine; Professor of Psychiatry and Behavioral Sciences, Albert Einstein College of Medicine, Bronx, New York

Arielle Horenstein, M.A.
Doctoral student, Department of Psychology, Temple University, Philadelphia, Pennsylvania

Jonathan D. Huppert, Ph.D.
Professor and Sam and Helen Beber Chair of Clinical Psychology, Department of Psychology, The Hebrew University of Jerusalem, Mt. Scopus, Jerusalem, Israel

Simona C. Kaplan, M.A.
Doctoral student, Department of Psychology, Temple University, Philadelphia, Pennsylvania

Cary S. Kogan, Ph.D.
Professor, School of Psychology, University of Ottawa, Ontario, Canada

Karen Kraus, M.D.
Health Sciences Clinical Associate Professor of Psychiatry, Director of Child Psychiatry, UCSF Fresno, Fresno, California

Barry Lebowitz, Ph.D.
Professor, Department of Psychiatry, University of California San Diego, La Jolla, California

Roberto Lewis-Fernández, M.D.
Professor and Director, New York State Center of Excellence for Cultural Competence, Hispanic Treatment Program, and Anxiety Disorders Clinic, New York State Psychiatric Institute; Department of Psychiatry, Columbia University Vagelos College of Physicians and Surgeons, New York, New York

Betty Liao, Ph.D.
Clinical Psychologist, Director of Wellness and Mental Health Support Services, UCSF Fresno, Fresno, California

Olivia Losiewicz, B.A.
Clinical Research Coordinator, Department of Psychiatry, Massachusetts General Hospital, Boston, Massachusetts

Jessica L. Maples-Keller, Ph.D.
Assistant Professor, Department of Psychiatry and Behavioral Sciences, Emory University School of Medicine, Atlanta, Georgia

Zoya Marinova, M.D., Ph.D.
Hertfordshire Partnership University NHS Foundation Trust, St. Albans, United Kingdom

Daniel Marrello, B.Sc.
M.Sc. candidate, MacAnxiety Research Centre and Department of Psychiatry and Behavioural Neurosciences, McMaster University; Neuroscience Graduate Program, McMaster University, Hamilton, Ontario, Canada

Alexander C. McFarlane, M.D.
Professor, Centre for Traumatic Stress Studies, The University of Adelaide, Adelaide, Australia

Sandra Meier, Ph.D.
Associate Professor of Psychiatry, Department of Psychiatry, Dalhousie University, Halifax, Nova Scotia

Emily Mellen, B.A.
Research Assistant, McLean Hospital, Harvard Medical School, Belmont, Massachusetts

Julia Merker, B.S.
Research Assistant, McLean Hospital, Harvard Medical School, Belmont, Massachusetts

Barbara L. Milrod, M.D.
Professor of Psychiatry, Weill Cornell Medical College; Faculty, New York Psychoanalytic Institute, New York, New York

Charles B. Nemeroff, M.D., Ph.D.
Professor and Acting Chair, Associate Chair for Research, Department of Psychiatry; Director, Institute for Early Life Adversity Research, Dell Medical School, University of Texas at Austin, Austin, Texas

Ella L. Oar, Ph.D.
Doctor, Centre for Emotional Health, Department of Psychology, Macquarie University, Sydney, New South Wales, Australia

Miranda Olff, Ph.D.
Professor, Amsterdam UMC, Department of Psychiatry, Amsterdam Neuroscience, Amsterdam; Arq Psychotrauma Expert Group, Diemen, Netherlands

Michael W. Otto, Ph.D.
Director, Center for Anxiety and Related Disorders; Professor of Psychology, Boston University, Boston, Massachusetts

Beth Patterson, B.Sc.N., B.Ed., M.Sc.
MacAnxiety Research Centre, McMaster University; Department of Psychiatry and Behavioural Neurosciences, McMaster University, Hamilton, Ontario, Canada

Sandra S. Pimentel, Ph.D.
Associate Professor, Department of Psychiatry and Behavioral Sciences, Montefiore Medical Center/Albert Einstein College of Medicine, Bronx, New York

Mark H. Pollack, M.D.
Chairperson and Professor, Rush University Medical Center, Chicago, Illinois

Carolyn Ponting, M.A.
Doctoral student, Department of Psychology, UCLA, Los Angeles, California

Brianna Prichett, B.S.
Research Assistant, Department of Psychiatry and Human Behavior, Brown Medical School, Providence, Rhode Island

Ronald M. Rapee, Ph.D.
Distinguished Professor, Centre for Emotional Health, Department of Psychology, Macquarie University, Sydney, New South Wales, Australia

Steven A. Rasmussen, M.D.
Mary E. Zucker Professor and Chairman, Department of Psychiatry and Human Behavior, Brown Medical School, Providence, Rhode Island

Scott L. Rauch, M.D.
President and Psychiatrist in Chief, McLean Hospital, Belmont; Chair, Partners Psychiatry and Mental Health; Professor of Psychiatry, Harvard Medical School, Boston, Massachusetts

Jemma Reid, M.B.B.S., MRCPsych
Hertfordshire Partnership University NHS Foundation Trust, St. Albans, United Kingdom

Kerry J. Ressler, M.D., Ph.D.
Professor, McLean Hospital, Harvard Medical School, Belmont, Massachusetts

Charles Reynolds, M.D.
Professor of Geriatric Psychiatry, Department of Psychiatry, University of Pittsburgh, Pittsburgh, Pennsylvania

Eline F. Roelofs, M.D.
Doctoral student, Department of Child and Adolescent Psychiatry, Curium, Leiden University Medical Center; Department of Psychiatry, Leiden University Medical Center; Leiden Institute for Brain and Cognition, Leiden, Netherlands

Valerie Rosen, M.D.
Associate Professor of Psychiatry, Department of Psychiatry, Dell Medical School, University of Texas at Austin, Ascension Seton Family of Hospitals, Austin, Texas

Barbara O. Rothbaum, Ph.D.
Professor, Department of Psychiatry and Behavioral Sciences, Emory University School of Medicine, Atlanta, Georgia

William C. Sanderson, Ph.D.
Professor of Psychology; Director, Ph.D. Program in Clinical Psychology; and Director, Anxiety and Depression Clinic, Hofstra University, Hempstead, New York

Alan F. Schatzberg, M.D.
Professor, Department of Psychiatry and Behavioral Sciences, Stanford University School of Medicine, Stanford, California

Franklin R. Schneier, M.D.
Co-Director, Anxiety Disorders Clinic, New York State Psychiatric Institute; Special Lecturer, Department of Psychiatry, Columbia University, New York, New York

Josien Schuurmans, Ph.D.
Senior Researcher, Amsterdam University Medical Center, Vrije Universiteit, Psychiatry, Amsterdam Public Health Research Institute, Amsterdam, Netherlands

Erin Shanahan, B.S.
Clinical Research Coordinator, Autism and Obsessive Compulsive Spectrum Program, Albert Einstein College of Medicine, Psychiatric Research Institute at Montefiore-Einstein (PRIME), Bronx, New York

Isobel Sharpe, B.Sc.
M.P.H. candidate, MacAnxiety Research Centre, McMaster University, Hamilton, Ontario, Canada

M. Katherine Shear, M.D.
Marion E. Kenworthy Professor of Psychiatry, Columbia University School of Social Work, Columbia University Vagelos College of Physicians and Surgeons; Director, Center for Complicated Grief, New York

Ayotunde Shodunke, M.B.B.S., M.Sc., MRCPsych
Hertfordshire Partnership University NHS Foundation Trust, St. Albans, United Kingdom

Nicole A. Short, Ph.D.
Assistant Professor, Department of Anesthesiology, University of North Carolina at Chapel Hill, Chapel Hill, North Carolina

Naomi M. Simon, M.D., M.Sc.
Director, Anxiety and Complicated Grief Program, Department of Psychiatry, New York University Langone Health; Professor of Psychiatry, NYU School of Medicine, New York, New York

Natalia Skritskaya, Ph.D.
Adjunct Associate Research Scientist, Columbia School of Social Work, Center for Complicated Grief, New York

Jordan W. Smoller, M.D., Sc.D.
Director, Center for Human Genetic Research, Massachusetts General Hospital; Associate Professor of Psychiatry, Harvard Medical School, Boston, Massachusetts

Carolyn Spiro-Levitt, Ph.D.
Clinical Assistant Professor, Department of Child and Adolescent Psychiatry, Hassenfeld Children's Hospital at New York University Langone, New York

Stephanie Jarvi Steele, Ph.D.
Visiting Assistant Professor, Psychology Department, Williams College, Williamstown, Massachusetts

Simona Stefan, Ph.D.
Visiting Scholar, Department of Psychological and Brain Sciences, Boston University, Boston, Massachusetts; Assistant Professor, Department of Clinical Psychology and Psychotherapy, Babes-Bolyai University, Cluj-Napoca, Romania

Dan J. Stein, M.D.
Professor and Chair, Department of Psychiatry and Mental Health, University of Cape Town, South Africa; Director, South African Medical Research Council Unit on Anxiety and Stress Disorders; Visiting Professor, Mt. Sinai Medical School, New York, New York

Murray B. Stein M.D., M.P.H.
Professor, Department of Psychiatry and Department of Family and Preventive Medicine, and Director, Anxiety and Traumatic Stress Disorders Program, University of California, San Diego, California

Amina Sutherland-Stolting, M.D.
Chief Resident in Psychiatry, UCSF Fresno, Fresno, California

Michaela B. Swee, M.A.
Doctoral student, Department of Psychology, Temple University, Philadelphia, Pennsylvania

Ilanit R. Tal, Ph.D.
Department of Psychiatry, University of California San Diego, La Jolla, California

Alexandra S. Tanner, M.A.
Doctoral student in Clinical Psychology, UCLA, Los Angeles, California

Charles T. Taylor, Ph.D.
Associate Professor, Department of Psychiatry, University of California San Diego, La Jolla, California

David F. Tolin, Ph.D.
Director of the Anxiety Disorders Center and Adjunct Associate Professor of Psychiatry, Institute of Living and Yale University School of Medicine, Hartford, Connecticut

Antolin Trinidad, M.D., Ph.D.
Associate Clinical Professor of Psychiatry, Yale University School of Medicine, New Haven, Connecticut

Thomas W. Uhde, M.D.
Professor and Chair, Department of Psychiatry and Behavioral Sciences, Medical University of South Carolina, Charleston, South Carolina

Michael Van Ameringen, M.D., FRCPC
Professor, MacAnxiety Research Centre, Department of Psychiatry and Behavioural Neurosciences, and Neuroscience Graduate Program, McMaster University, Hamilton, Ontario, Canada

Nic J.A. van der Wee, M.D., Ph.D.
Professor of Biological Psychiatry, Department of Psychiatry, Leiden University Medical Center; Leiden Institute for Brain and Cognition, Leiden, Netherlands

Claire Van Genugten, M.Sc.
Doctoral student, Amsterdam University Medical Center, Vrije Universiteit, Psychiatry, Amsterdam Public Health Research Institute, Amsterdam, Netherlands

Richard Oude Voshaar, Ph.D., M.D.
Professor of Geriatric Psychiatry, University Medical Center Groningen, Department of Psychiatry, Groningen, Netherlands

Rushi H. Vyas, M.D.
Assistant Director of Consult Liaison Medicine, Department of Psychiatry, Inova Fairfax Hospital, Fairfax, Virginia

Mengxing Wang, M.A.
Doctoral student, Department of Psychology, Stony Brook University, Stony Brook, New York

Ryan D. Webler, B.A.
Doctoral student, Clinical Psychology, University of Minnesota, Minneapolis

P. Michiel Westenberg, Ph.D.
Professor, Institute of Psychology, Leiden University; Leiden Institute for Brain and Cognition, Leiden, Netherlands

Monnica T. Williams, Ph.D.
Associate Professor, Department of Psychological Sciences, University of Connecticut, Storrs, Connecticut

Thomas N. Wise, M.D.
Professor of Psychiatry, Johns Hopkins University School of Medicine, Baltimore, Maryland; Professor of Psychiatry, George Washington University School of Medicine, Washington, DC; Psychiatrist, Inova Fairfax Hospital, Fairfax, Virginia

Brittany K. Woods, M.A.
Doctoral student, Center for Anxiety and Related Disorders, Boston University, Boston, Massachusetts

Sidney Zisook, M.D.
Professor, Department of Psychiatry, University of California San Diego, La Jolla, California

Disclosure of Interests

David S. Baldwin, M.A., D.M., FRCPsych: *Attendee:* Advisory boards hosted by LivaNova and Mundipharma; *Lecture Fees:* Janssen.

Borwin Bandelow, M.D., Ph.D.: *Speakers Board:* Hexal, Janssen, Lilly, and Lundbeck; *Advisory Board:* Mundipharma and Lundbeck.

Kevin J. Craig, M.B.B.Ch., M.Phil., MRCPsych: *Employee and Stockholder:* GW Pharmaceuticals Plc.

Jürgen Deckert, M.D.: *Research/Grants:* European Union, in cooperation with P1Vital; Government of Bavaria, in cooperation with BioVariance.

Naomi A. Fineberg, M.B.B.S., M.A., MRCPsych: *Research/Grants:* European College of Neuropsychopharmacology, National Institute for Health Research, Horizon 2020; *Speaker:* Abbott, Sun Pharma; *Travel and Expenses:* British Association for Psychopharmacology, European College of Neuropsychopharmacology, Royal College of Psychiatrists, The International College of Neuropsychopharmacology; *Income:* Taylor & Francis; *Leadership:* National Health Service OCD treatment service; *Board Membership:* various registered charities linked to OCD.

Andrew W. Goddard, M.D.: *Royalties:* UptoDate; *Research/Grants:* National Network of Depression, University of California–San Francisco; *Advisory Board:* HWP, Almatica Pharma Inc. (August 2018).

Richard G. Heimberg, Ph.D.: *Royalties:* Oxford University Press; *Advisor and Stockholder:* Joyable, Inc.

Eric Hollander, M.D.: *Research/Grant:* Takeda.

Charles B. Nemeroff, M.D., Ph.D.: *Research/Grants:* National Institutes of Health, Stanley Medical Research Institute; *Consulting* (past 3 years): Xhale, Takeda, Taisho Pharmaceutical Inc., Bracket (Clintara), Fortress Biotech, Sunovion Pharmaceuticals Inc., Sumitomo Dainippon Pharma, Janssen Research and Development LLC, Magstim Inc., Navitor Pharmaceuticals Inc., TC MSO Inc., Intra-Cellular Therapies Inc.; *Stockholder:* Xhale, Celgene, Seattle Genetics, Abbvie, OPKO Health Inc., Antares, BI Gen Holdings Inc., Corcept Therapeutics Pharmaceuticals, TC MSO Inc.; *Scientific Advisory Boards:* American Foundation for Suicide Prevention, Brain and Behavior Research Foundation, Xhale, Anxiety Disorders Association of America, Skyland Trail, Bracket (Clintara), Laureate Institute for Brain Research Inc.; *Board of Directors:* American Foundation for Suicide Prevention, Gratitude America, Anxiety Disorders Association of America. *Income Sources or Equity of $10,000 or More:* American Psychiatric Publishing, Xhale, Bracket (Clintara), CME Outfitters, Takeda, Intra-Cellular Therapies Inc., Magstim; *Patents:* Method and devices for transdermal delivery of lithium (US 6,375,990B1); method of assessing antidepressant drug therapy via transport inhibition of monoamine neurotransmitters by ex vivo assay (US 7,148,027B2); Compounds, Compositions, Methods of Synthesis, and Methods of Treatment (CRF Receptor Binding Ligand) (US 8,551, 996 B2).

Josien Schuurmans, Ph.D.: *Speaker:* Pfizer conferences, 2011.

Naomi Simon, M.D., M.Sc.: *Spousal Equity:* GI Therapeutics; *Research/Grants:* National Institutes of Health, Department of Defense, Highland Street Foundation.

Dan J. Stein, M.D., Ph.D.: *Research/Honoraria:* Biocodex, Lundbeck, Servier, Sun.

David F. Tolin, Ph.D.: *Research/Grants:* Biohaven Pharmaceuticals, Pfizer, Palo Alto Health Sciences.

Thomas W. Uhde, M.D.: *Speaker's Bureau:* Jazz Pharmaceuticals.

Michael Van Ameringen, M.D., FRCPC: *Advisory Board:* Allergan, Lundbeck, Purdue; *Clinical Trials/Studies:* Janssen Ortho Inc.; *Research/Grants:* Hamilton Academic Health Sciences Organization (HAHSO) Innovation Grant (AFP Innovation Grant); *Speaker's Bureau:* Allergan, Lundbeck, Pfizer, Purdue.

The following authors have no competing interests to report: Andrea R. Ashbaugh, Ph.D.; Amanda Waters Baker, Ph.D.; Christina L. Boisseau, Ph.D.; Frederic N. Busch, M.D.; Denise April Chavira, Ph.D.; Eduardo Cinosi, M.B.B.S., MRCPsych; Michelle G. Craske, Ph.D.; Thalia C. Eley, Ph.D.; Benedetta Grancini, M.D.; John M. Hettema, M.D., Ph.D.; Arielle Horenstein, M.A.; Simona C. Kaplan, M.A.; Cary S. Kogan, Ph.D.; Roberto Lewis-Fernández, M.D.; Jessica Maples-Keller, Ph.D.; Zoya Marinova, M.D., Ph.D.; Sandra Meier, Ph.D.; Barbara L. Milrod, M.D.; Ella L. Oar, Ph.D.; Sandra S. Pimentel, Ph.D.; Carolyn Ponting, M.A.; Ronald M. Rapee, Ph.D.; Jemma Reid, M.B.B.S., MRCPsych; Valerie Rosen, M.D.; Barbara O. Rothbaum, Ph.D.; Franklin Schneier, M.D.; Ayotunde Shodunke, M.B.B.S., M.Sc., MRCPsych; Carolyn Spiro-Levitt, Ph.D.; Michaela B. Swee, M.A.; Alexandra S. Tanner, M.A.; Rushi H. Vyas, M.D.

Foreword

Consider anxiety and the biological systems through which it operates to be analogous to the immune system. Hardwired by evolution and varying genetic risk profiles but given greater precision and specificity by exposure to threats in the environment, it evolved to keep us safe and well. Like the immune system, even when responding to relevant targets, appropriate activation can have unwanted consequences (e.g., pain, swelling, fever). For some, the consequences of even an appropriate or excessive immune response can be harsher than the actual microbial threat or injury. More unfortunately a common scenario, the immune system, rather than reacting to an external threat, targets the self in autoimmune disease. Adding insult to injury, each of these systems can activate the other, because inflammation is both a risk factor and a response in mood and anxiety disorders. As with the approaches available to diminish inflammation, we clinicians can minimize anxiety with avoidance of the threat, suppression with pharmacotherapy, or better yet, retraining or desensitization so that benign challenges are no longer triggers or the response is made more homeostatic. This immune metaphor is not intended to be clever but rather to explain by analogy to those who misunderstand or might trivialize the neurobiological and experiential underpinnings of these often-disabling disorders.

We've come a long way in our understanding, classification, and treatment of anxiety and anxiety-related disorders. As a medical student in 1971, I presented a case of "phobic anxiety depersonalization syndrome," a condition described by the eminent British psychiatrist Sir Martin Roth. A few years later, as a newly minted psychiatrist unashamed to manifest interest in the medication treatment of psychiatric disorders, I was quite taken with the early observational studies reported by Don Klein, employing what he called "pharmacological dissection," and with the subsequent randomized antidepressant trials of "phobic anxiety" by residents just ahead of me in the Massachusetts General Hospital psychiatry residency program, Jim Ballenger and Dave Sheehan. Those moments were pivotal in the emergence of the modern conceptualization of panic disorder as distinct from other anxiety syndromes.

As has been the neo-Kraepelinian tradition in psychiatry, efforts to accomplish greater differentiation of phenotypes as represented by evolving classification and diagnostic criteria led to increased recognition and acceptance of anxiety syndromes by those who experience them, to the evolution of greater understanding of risk and vulnerability, and to the emergence of new and enhanced therapies. These essential elements of the story are critically reviewed and presented in the first part of this impressive volume, "Approaching Anxiety Disorders," which describes the foundational elements of classification, inherited risk, neurobiology of fear circuitry, other environmental contributors, and enormous societal burden.

As with the immune analogy, many points of therapeutic intervention are evidence based; we are moving closer to a time when we will have precision in knowing to whom which approach or combination of approaches should be offered. The current tools of treatment are detailed in the section on "Core Principles for Treating Anxiety Disorders." The volume then turns its focus to specific diagnostic categories and clinical issues, comprehensively presented in state-of-the-art reviews that bring us to the brink of the future. The textbook itself, now in its third edition, evolved from discussion at the Scientific Council of the Anxiety Disorders Association of America, now the Anxiety and Depression Association of America (ADAA), and its publication by American Psychiatric Association Publishing underscores the centrality of anxiety and its disorders to the field.

A word about the ADAA, which was established nearly 40 years ago as the Phobia Society of America: when the Phobia Society of America was formed in 1979 by a small group of psychiatrists, psychologists, social workers, patients, and family members, its purpose was to convene those who wanted answers to these questions: How can we better understand these disorders? What can we do to help those who experience them? By 1990, several years after DSM-III (American Psychiatric Association 1980) published criteria for diagnosing distinct anxiety disorders, the organization had changed its name to the Anxiety Disorders Association of America to reflect the breadth of conditions the organization represents. During the past few decades, research into the phenomenology, pathophysiology, and neurobiology of anxiety disorders has expanded, and the neurobiology of fear and anxiety remains the best understood area of psychiatric neuroscience. Kudos to Naomi Simon, Barbara Rothbaum, Eric Hollander, and Dan Stein for, as editors, making a resource such as this extraordinary textbook available to clinicians and students.

Jerrold F. Rosenbaum, M.D.
Chief of Psychiatry
Massachusetts General Hospital
Stanley Cobb Professor of Psychiatry
Harvard Medical School

Reference

American Psychiatric Association: Diagnostic and Statistical Manual of Mental Disorders, 3rd Edition. Washington, DC, American Psychiatric Association, 1980

On behalf of the Anxiety and Depression Association of America (ADAA), I am honored to comment on the 2020 updated edition of the textbook, *The American Psychiatric Association Publishing Textbook of Anxiety, Trauma, and OCD-Related Disorders.*

When the ADAA was established nearly 40 years ago (as the Phobia Society of America), no "anxiety disorders field" existed. Everything was labeled as a phobia. People who had anxiety felt misunderstood and misdiagnosed. They often felt alone and marginalized.

This resource will make a difference not only for the professionals who will use the textbook during their course of studies but also for the millions of people who are suffering and hoping for improved treatment options. This textbook will inform the current professionals in the field and, more importantly, will foster interest and understanding in the field's early career professionals. This new edition will also promote evidence-based communications with other critical stakeholders, such as legislators, patient-centered organizations, and other health care professionals.

Although we have made tremendous strides in the field, more needs to be done. Unfortunately, what Jerilyn Ross, one of the founders of the Phobia Society of America, wrote in 2010 still stands today: "We have a long way to go, especially with regard to understanding the onset of the disorders and their impact on special populations—women, children, adolescents, and the elderly. Posttraumatic stress disorder, common to all populations, presents an ongoing—and growing—global challenge." I would now add that we also need to do more to address the specific mental health issues of a multicultural society.

The contributors to this edition are renowned experts in the field who spend both their intellect and passion to help change patient outcomes. Their research changes people's lives. The authors and those who have collaborated with them are the ones who help support the ADAA's promise to find new treatments and one day prevent and cure these disorders.

Susan K. Gurley, J.D.
Executive Director
Anxiety and Depression Association of America

Preface

As long as humans have been humans, we have experienced anxiety. Stress, fear, and anxiety are ubiquitous experiences. When is anxiety a disorder? When is professional intervention indicated? Key considerations include the intensity, severity, and clustering of associated symptoms, their persistence, and, as with all psychiatric disorders, their level of associated distress and impairment. Patients with anxiety and related disorders often do not realize they have a treatable condition and may not present with a chief complaint aligned with DSM-5 gateway symptoms (American Psychiatric Association 2013). Although great research advances have been made in neuroscience, genetics, and understanding biological responses to stress as well as the development of experimental models of phenomena, such as fear conditioning and extinction, we still do not have diagnostic biomarkers and depend on patient self-awareness of symptoms and clinical assessment. These and other factors, including structural barriers (e.g., lack of sufficient providers) and attitudinal barriers (e.g., stigmatization of seeking psychiatric care), continue to contribute to the underdiagnosis of patients with anxiety, despite the very high prevalence of anxiety disorders globally and their well-documented substantial global burden of disability and associated socioeconomic costs. Educators and advocacy groups have done a tremendous amount in the past decades to increase awareness, and the explosion of the internet has made information readily available to patients and clinicians (when one can sort through it to find evidence-based information), but more work needs to be done.

Anxiety disorders are treatable conditions. As a field, we have made great strides in building a broad armamentarium of evidence-based treatment approaches and tools. Efforts in the dissemination and implementation of evidence-based interventions, such as cognitive-behavioral therapies, as well as the development of novel approaches of delivery to overcome barriers to access are ongoing. Digital phenotyping as a clinical tool to support diagnosis and intervention is in its infancy. As our understanding of the pathophysiology of anxiety and stress-related disorders grows, we are learning a tremendous amount about how and why our interventions may work for some patients and not others, offering future promise for a personalized medicine approach to the treatment of anxiety disorders as well as strategies for targeted prevention and early intervention. Perhaps precisely because of the long evolutionary history of anxiety, and cross-species similarity in the phenomenology and psychobiology of stress responses, preclinical and translational neuroscience and genetics are beginning to help identify targets for novel treatments to help address the need for even more effective first-line and next-step interventions for anxiety disorders. This exciting time promises continued discovery and translation into clinical practice. As we move forward as a field, we also return to core principles of identifying and treating patients in practice.

This third edition of the *Textbook of Anxiety Disorders*, now entitled *The American Psychiatric Association Publishing Textbook of Anxiety, Trauma, and OCD-Related Disorders* to reflect the updated categories of DSM-5, provides a review and update on the relevant science and core transdiagnostic and disease-specific principles as well as state-of-the-art reviews of psychotherapy and pharmacotherapy treatment approaches and their combinations. The organization of the volume and individual chapters has been retooled for DSM-5. Some chapters have been updated, and some have been completely rewritten. The contributors are a who's who of experts on anxiety, trauma, and OCD-related disorders. For specific conditions, including generalized anxiety disorder, social anxiety disorder, panic and agoraphobia, specific phobia, OCD, and trauma- and stressor-related conditions such as PTSD and persistent forms of grief, we include sections on phenomenology, pathogenesis, and treatment. Special sections focus on the issues of comorbidity, as well as specific issues for children and older adults. Transdiagnostic interventions, such as Barlow's Unified Protocol, are included as new chapters. The National Institute of Mental Health focuses on Research Domain Criteria (RDoC) with cross-cutting core features that may not form clear boundaries by conditions, so we need to be supple in our ability to think both diagnostically and transdiagnostically in our assessment, treatment, and research. Anxiety disorders, with many overlapping biological features, such as fear neurocircuitry and inflammatory stress responses, and symptom expressions, such as panic attacks, worry, and avoidance, offer both challenge and opportunity to collaborate across professions, continue to expand our knowledge, improve the personalization and effectiveness of our treatments, and ensure delivery of those treatments to those who need them. It is our hope you will find this book a useful tool in your own work.

We are extremely grateful to the scores of authors who have contributed outstanding scholarly updates or new chapters to this state-of-the-art book. We also wish to express our gratitude to our colleagues and patients who have each taught and inspired us and to our families who have supported us.

Naomi M. Simon, M.D., M.Sc.
Eric Hollander, M.D.
Barbara O. Rothbaum, Ph.D., ABPP
Dan J. Stein, M.D., Ph.D.

Reference

American Psychiatric Association: Diagnostic and Statistical Manual of Mental Disorders, 5th Edition. Arlington, VA, American Psychiatric Association, 2013

PART I

Approaching Anxiety Disorders

CHAPTER 1

Classification of Anxiety and Related Disorders

Cary S. Kogan, Ph.D.
Andrea R. Ashbaugh, Ph.D.

In 2013, DSM-5 (American Psychiatric Association 2013) was published. With respect to anxiety and related disorders, systematic reviews were conducted to guide proposed changes to structure and content. Whereas DSM-IV-TR (American Psychiatric Association 2000) included 12 anxiety disorder categories comprising various disorders with fear as a common characteristic, grouping not only disorders such as generalized anxiety disorder (GAD) and specific phobias together but also OCD and PTSD, DSM-5 reconfigures major groupings of fear-based disorders into three more-narrowly focused groups meant to better reflect common diagnostic validators: *anxiety disorders* (comprising 12 disorders), *obsessive-compulsive and related disorders* (OCRD; comprising 9 disorders), and *trauma- and stressor-related disorders* (TSRD; comprising 7 disorders). Although some have raised concerns about the lack of integration of neuroscientific findings, perpetuation of categorical rather than dimensional conceptualizations, expansion of disorder entities, and mixed field trial results (Frances 2014; Regier et al. 2013), these criticisms are tempered when one considers that the DSM-5 developers worked within the limitations of the current state of evidence to produce a clinically useful classification. Tables 1–1 through 1–3 summarize the changes to DSM-5, providing a brief description of the important diagnostic features of each disorder.

Given the concerns raised by experts about DSM-5, we review challenges faced by any categorical nosology of psychopathology, explore alternative approaches, and provide justifications for maintaining the status quo. We then review the rationale for the current DSM-5 classifications of anxiety disorders, OCRD, and TSRD and research on the reliability and validity of DSM-5.

TABLE 1–1. Overview of key features and changes in the classification and definitions of DSM-5 obsessive-compulsive and related disorders

Disorder	DSM-IV category	Key features	Changes to diagnostic criteria*
OCD	Anxiety disorders	Obsessions (recurrent, intrusive thoughts, images, or impulses) or compulsions (repetitive behaviors or mental acts aimed at reducing distress)	Individual no longer needs to recognize obsessions as being a product of the mind; Obsessions can be related to real-life problems; Person no longer required to recognize that obsessions or compulsions are excessive or unreasonable; Specifiers concerning insight expanded (specify if with good or fair insight, with poor insight, or with absent insight/delusional beliefs); Can specify if tic related
Body dysmorphic disorder	Somatoform disorders	Persistent preoccupation with perceived physical flaw that is minimally or not observable to others; Repetitive behaviors or mental acts in response to appearance concerns	Person must have engaged in repetitive behaviors or mental acts in response to appearance concerns; Can specify if with muscle dysmorphia; Can specify degree of insight (see OCD)
Hoarding disorder	—	Persistent difficulty discarding possessions resulting in excessive clutter that compromises intended use of space	New DSM-5 disorder
Trichotillomania (hair-pulling disorder)	Impulse-control disorders not elsewhere classified	Recurrent hair pulling; Recurrent attempts to stop hair pulling	Removal of requirement that hair pulling be associated with tension before pulling or when resisting pulling; Removal of requirement that hair pulling be associated with pleasure, gratification, relief
Excoriation (skin-picking) disorder	—	Recurrent skin picking resulting in skin lesions; Repeated attempts to stop skin picking	New DSM-5 disorder

Note. *Criteria listed in this column are *not* the complete diagnostic criteria but reflect major changes to the criteria from DSM-IV-TR to DSM-5.

Challenges of Psychiatric Classification

A coherent framework for organizing concepts according to current evidence is essential for the utility and viability of any scientific discipline. In the case of psychopathology, a framework can be found in widely used classifications such as DSM-5 and the World Health Organization's (WHO's) *International Statistical Classification of Diseases and Related Health Problems*, 11th Revision (ICD-11; World Health Organization 2019). Ideally, classifications establish the boundaries of psychopathology through reliable and valid definitions for disease entities. They offer a common language for precise communication, hypothesis testing, and theory generation. Psychiatric classifications should be clinically useful, providing an efficient means for clinicians to access knowledge and to ensure effective communication with professionals and patients. Classifications serve a role in public health by helping governments monitor the prevalence of disorders, appropriately allocate resources, and develop evidence-based policies.

DSM-III (American Psychiatric Association 1980) introduced a major shift in psychiatric classification, emphasizing narrowly defined symptom-based criteria sets without pronouncing on etiology (Kendler 1990). Under this framework, mental illnesses were defined according to a descriptive phenomenology, grouping commonly co-occurring signs and symptoms together into categories best understood as syndromes rather than diseases (Blashfield and Keeley 2010). Syndromes are conceptually and clinically useful rather than reflecting any true "carving of nature at its joints" (Plato 1952). Disorders that appeared to have fear or anxiety as a core feature were grouped together under anxiety disorders, including agoraphobia with panic attacks, agoraphobia without panic attacks, social phobia, simple phobia, panic disorder, GAD, OCD, and PTSD. Subsequent revisions of DSM were based on similar principles, and the structure and content of the "Anxiety Disorders" section were mostly similar. This approach to classification improved the reliability and, to some degree, the validity of psychiatric diagnoses over earlier schemes and led to important advances in the understanding of mental illness.

However, several limitations of categorical classification persist, including high rates of comorbidity, challenges in demarcating boundaries between normality and pathology, inadequate differentiation of severity within categories, and lack of integration of evidence of underlying causal mechanisms of psychopathology. Dimensional models of psychopathology were advanced as a solution to these shortcomings, and although they were considered by the DSM-5 Task Force, categories were maintained, but with the integration of dimensional assessment tools (American Psychiatric Association 2013).

Comorbidity

Comorbidity presents a problem for categorical classifications when multiple diagnoses arise as an artifact of arbitrarily imposed boundaries better understood as reflecting the variation in severity of latent (unobservable) constructs. For example, the National Comorbidity Survey Replication (Kessler et al. 2005), a population-level study of the prevalence of DSM-IV (American Psychiatric Association 1994) disorders, found that 40% of cases evidenced comorbidity, which was associated with greater lev-

TABLE 1–2. Overview of key features and changes in the classification and definitions of DSM-5 trauma and stressor-related disorders

Disorder	DSM-IV category	Key features	Changes to diagnostic criteria*
Reactive attachment disorder	Other disorders of infancy, childhood, or adolescence	Persistent and consistent emotionally withdrawn behavior toward caregiver Socioemotional disturbances Evidence of extremes of insufficient care given by caregivers	Formerly reactive attachment disorder of infancy or early childhood, inhibited type Must be developmental age ≥ 9 months Clearer and stricter criteria with regard to number of required criteria to describe socially inhibited behavior Must exhibit both withdrawn behavior toward caregiver *and* socioemotional disturbance Cannot meet criteria for autism spectrum disorder Can specify as persistent if symptoms are present for >12 months Can specify as severe if all diagnostic criteria are met
Disinhibited social engagement disorder	Other disorders of infancy, childhood, or adolescence	A pattern of actively approaching unfamiliar adults Evidence of extremes of insufficient care by caregivers	Formerly reactive attachment disorder of infancy or early childhood, disinhibited type Behaviors are not limited to impulsivity Must be developmental age ≥ 9 months Clearer and stricter criteria with regard to number of required criteria to describe socially disinhibited behavior Can specify as persistent if symptoms present for > 12 months Can specify as severe if all diagnostic criteria are met
PTSD	Anxiety disorders	Exposure to traumatic event Symptoms persist > 1 month	Traumatic event no longer needs to provoke intense fear, helplessness, or horror

TABLE 1–2. Overview of key features and changes in the classification and definitions of DSM-5 trauma and stressor-related disorders *(continued)*

Disorder	DSM-IV category	Key features	Changes to diagnostic criteria*
		Symptoms of reexperiencing (e.g., nightmares, flashbacks), avoidance of reminders of the event, changes in cognition and mood (e.g., exaggerated negative beliefs about self, others, world; inability to experience positive emotions), and alterations in arousal and reactivity (e.g., exaggerated startle response, sleep disturbances)	Repeated exposure via electronic media, television, movies, and pictures (unless work related) does not constitute traumatic event; Reexperiencing symptoms relabeled as intrusions; Avoidance now limited to avoidance of internal or external reminders; Alterations in arousal and reactivity now include reckless or self-destructive behavior; Can now specify if dissociative symptoms present; Separate diagnostic criteria for children age ≤ 6 years
Acute stress disorder	Anxiety disorders	Exposure to traumatic event; Symptoms of intrusions, negative mood, dissociation, avoidance, or arousal; Symptoms occur from 3 days up to 1 month after the event	Traumatic event no longer needs to provoke intense fear, helplessness, or horror; Repeated exposure via electronic media, television, movies, and pictures (unless work related) does not constitute a traumatic event; Intrusions, avoidance, and arousal remain potential symptoms but are no longer required symptoms; Symptoms must persist at least 3 days instead of 2 days
Adjustment disorder	Adjustment disorder	Development of behavioral or emotional symptoms after stressful event; Symptoms do not meet criteria for another mental disorder	Chronic and acute specifiers removed

Note. *Criteria listed in this column are *not* the complete diagnostic criteria but reflect major changes to the criteria from DSM-IV-TR to DSM-5.

els of severity. Furthermore, latent class analysis of these data suggested the existence of several classes in which certain internalizing disorders (i.e., mood and anxiety disorders) were highly comorbid, such that different latent classes represented increasing levels of severity (Kessler et al. 2005). These findings are consistent with other sources of evidence that indicate high rates of co-occurrence of depression and anxiety clinically (e.g., Regier et al. 1998). Therefore, a significant challenge for any categorical classification is optimizing the divisions of disorders to minimize comorbidity. Developers of DSM-5 were aware of these problems and, within the limits of a categorical framework, sequenced disorder groupings into separate internalizing and externalizing clusters (American Psychiatric Association 2013) reflecting evidence supporting a dimensional operationalization of psychopathology (Kotov et al. 2017).

Boundaries With Normality

Categorical classifications must establish thresholds between normality and pathology. This is challenging when dealing with symptoms of anxiety disorders, OCRD, and TSRD that are often continuous with normality (Smith et al. 2018) and that fluctuate over time. Absent a definitive definition of what constitutes a mental disorder, thresholds used to determine whether an individual warrants a diagnosis are typically set according to the presence of a minimum constellation of symptoms alongside other features of "pathosuggestiveness," including persistence of sufficient duration, intensity of symptoms, frequency of symptoms, significant distress, and impairment (First and Wakefield 2013). Despite this criterion-based, objective approach, a values-based clinical judgment often remains necessary, contributing to the unreliability of diagnoses.

A pragmatic view of classification asserts that the classification system should help determine eligibility for health care services. Thus, decisions of where to place thresholds as well as how easily clinicians can ascertain whether a threshold is met have consequences to patient care. A detrimental consequence of applying thresholds is the overreliance on the *unspecified* or *other specified* categories when patients need care but do not meet the threshold for a disorder. DSM-5 attempted to address this by providing guidance on differentiating disorders from normality. In DSM-5, this information is often included in the "Differential Diagnosis" sections.

Severity of Disorders

DSM-5 developers recognized that categorical classification limits the ability to characterize the range of severity, particularly for disorders with broad dimensionality (reviewed in Kotov et al. 2017). Because treatment selection is often predicated on disorder severity, with interventions ranging from watchful waiting to psychotherapy to somatic treatments, a binary diagnosis (present or absent) does not provide sufficient information for clinical staging. Considerations of severity are also important from a population health point of view. For example, Kessler et al. (2005) found that although rates of mental disorders are high within the general population (26.2%), 40.4% of those disorders are mild, suggesting that many cases may not require specialist attention. DSM-5 addresses this limitation by adopting a spectrum approach within diagnostic grouping when possible (Clark et al. 2017). For example, DSM-5 includes anxiety disorder–specific scales that allow clinicians to characterize behavioral, cogni-

TABLE 1–3. Overview of key features and changes in the classification and definitions of DSM-5 major anxiety disorders

Disorder	DSM-IV category	Key features	Changes to diagnostic criteria*
Separation anxiety disorder	Other disorders of infancy, childhood, or adolescence	Persistent, developmentally inappropriate, and excessive fear of separation from important attachment figures	Elimination of requirement that symptoms start before age 18 In adults, symptoms should persist ≥ 6 months
Selective mutism	Other disorders of infancy, childhood, or adolescence	Persistent and consistent failure to speak in social situations in which speaking is expected	None
Specific phobia	Anxiety disorders	Persistent and excessive fear of specific objects or situations (e.g., animals, heights, receiving injections)	All individuals regardless of age must report symptoms for ≥ 6 months Individual no longer needs to recognize that fear is excessive or unreasonable, but fear must be out of proportion to actual danger
Social anxiety disorder (social phobia)	Anxiety disorders	Persistent and excessive fear of social situations in which one might be scrutinized, embarrassed, or humiliated	Individual no longer needs to recognize that fear is excessive or unreasonable, but fear must be out of proportion to actual threat All individuals regardless of age must report symptoms for ≥ 6 months Social fears may not be related to general medical condition (e.g., Parkinson's disease), or fear, anxiety, and avoidance must be excessive *Generalized* specifier removed and replaced by *performance only* specifier
Panic disorder	Anxiety disorders	Recurrent, unexpected panic attacks Persistent worry about additional panic attacks and consequences of panic attacks	No longer specified with and without agoraphobia

TABLE 1–3.	Overview of key features and changes in the classification and definitions of DSM-5 major anxiety disorders *(continued)*		
Disorder	**DSM-IV category**	**Key features**	**Changes to diagnostic criteria***
Agoraphobia	Anxiety disorders	Persistent and excessive fear or avoidance of situations in which escape or help may be difficult to obtain if panic attack or other embarrassing symptom occurs	Now an independent disorder Symptoms must persist for ≥ 6 months Multiple situations (at least two of five categories) must be feared Fear can be of having not only panic-like symptoms but also other embarrassing symptoms (e.g., incontinence) If another medical condition is present, fear, anxiety, or avoidance related to medical symptoms must be excessive
Generalized anxiety disorder	Anxiety disorders	Persistent, excessive, uncontrollable worry Physical symptoms (e.g., muscle tension, restlessness) when worrying	None

Note.   *Criteria listed in this column are *not* the complete diagnostic criteria but reflect major changes to the criteria from DSM-IV-TR to DSM-5.

tive ideation, and physical symptoms. Dimensional measurement of anxiety disorders with self-report scales has adequate psychometric properties for distinguishing clinical from nonclinical samples as well as for characterizing severity (Lebeau et al. 2012).

Etiology of Psychopathology

Psychopathology arises from multiple factors, including genetic, behavioral, and environmental sources and their interactions. Validated stress-diathesis models of mood and anxiety disorders (Barlow 2000) posit the contribution of three factors: a generalized biological vulnerability, a generalized psychological vulnerability, and disorder-specific psychological vulnerabilities. These factors, in combination with specific life experiences, determine the expression of symptoms classified as mood and anxiety disorders.

More recently, updated stress-diathesis models reflect findings suggesting that some generalized biological vulnerability factors (i.e., genetic polymorphisms) are better understood as conferring individuals with greater responsivity to environmental influences, including positive, negative, and neutral influences (e.g., Leighton et al. 2017). These "differential susceptibility" models emphasize that those with more responsive variants of genes can show various trajectories depending on their environmental exposures.

Although information about etiology can be found in ancillary sections of DSM-5, it is rarely incorporated into criteria sets. Initially, DSM-5 developers intended to integrate diagnostic validators emerging from neuroscientific, genetic, neuroimaging, and cognitive science into the classification, but they determined during the process that the evidence was insufficient to dispense with a descriptive taxonomy (Kupfer and Regier 2011). However, knowledge about shared genetic risk, familiality, common neural circuitry, and other biomarkers informed the overall organization of groupings. For example, examination of 11 validators according to validation approaches introduced by Robins and Guze (1970) led to the introduction of the OCRD grouping (Stein et al. 2014, 2016). Future revisions may well succeed in incorporating underlying biological and psychological mechanisms alongside clinical phenomenology.

Evidence for Dimensionality of Anxiety Disorders, Obsessive-Compulsive and Related Disorders, and Trauma- and Stressor-Related Disorders

Most mental disorders are best understood as expressions of extremes along one or more continuous latent variables rather than as qualitatively distinct taxa (Meehl 1992). Rates of comorbidity, as well as of those of unspecified or other specified diagnoses among anxiety disorders, TSRD, and OCRD, suggest that these disorders are not taxonomic but rather emerge as a result of extremes along several hierarchically organized shared latent variables (Clark and Watson 1991; Watson 2005). Many question the utility of segregating anxiety and mood disorders into discrete entities when psychosocial (i.e., transdiagnostic cognitive-behavioral therapy exemplified by the

Unified Protocol for emotional disorders; Andrews 2018; Barlow et al. 2011) and psychopharmacological treatments are largely nonspecific for internalizing disorders (Clark et al. 2017; Kotov et al. 2017).

Application of statistical methodologies to self-report measures indicates that latent variables (e.g., negative affectivity, positive affectivity, and autonomic hyperarousal; Clark and Watson 1991) better explain patterns of expressed psychopathology. In particular, elevated neuroticism (negative affectivity) is consistently found to confer increased risk for the development of mood and anxiety-related disorders (Forbes et al. 2016). Other subordinate latent variables vary across studies, but the strongest support exists for a "fear" factor (specific phobia, social anxiety disorder, panic disorder, agoraphobia, separation anxiety disorder, and OCD) and a "distress" or "anxious-misery" factor (major depressive disorder, persistent depressive disorder, GAD, and PTSD) (Prenoveau et al. 2010; Watson 2005). Interestingly, latent variables such as negative affectivity show high heritability, with specific individual disorder manifestation being related to distinct early psychosocial stressors (Barlow et al. 2014). However, evidence also indicates that some facets of anxiety disorders and related constructs have taxonicity (Kotov et al. 2005; Woodward et al. 2000).

In summary, evidence suggests that mood and anxiety symptoms vary over time, show diagnostic comorbidity and subthreshold expression, and may be better explained by a limited number of dimensionally defined variables. Critics of categorical classifications assert that dimensional classifications built around latent variables offer a more direct characterization of psychopathology based on etiological mechanisms. Furthermore, dimensional models are more comprehensive, allowing for subthreshold phenomena to be codified and targeted for treatment. Finally, dimensional models are expected to reduce diagnostic disagreement because they reduce measurement error inherent to binary clinical categorizations.

Alternative Models of Classification

To address limitations of categorical classifications, several research groups have proposed alternative models. The two models that have received greatest attention are the National Institute of Mental Health's (NIMH's) Research Domain Criteria (RDoC; Cuthbert and Insel 2013) and the Hierarchical Taxonomy of Psychopathology model (HiTOP; Kotov et al. 2017).

Research Domain Criteria

The RDoC was conceptualized as a research-oriented nosology intended to liberate researchers from having to submit NIMH grant applications tied to specific diagnostic categories (Cuthbert and Insel 2013). Rather than organizing mental disorders according to a descriptive phenomenology, RDoC focuses on a set of mechanisms based on empirically validated neural circuitry–behavior relationships that are proposed to undergird and cut across many mental health problems as well as normative behavior (Cuthbert and Insel 2013). Research projects based on this model are expected over time to improve our understanding of the pathophysiology of mental illness and to move the field away from reified categories. Because the RDoC is used primarily at this time for generating basic research rather than as a nosology, we do not discuss it further here.

HiTOP

HiTOP is the product of a consortium of clinical researchers interested in addressing the limitations of traditional categorical classifications of mental illness by applying statistical techniques (e.g., factor analysis) to identify syndromes according to empirically determined covariation of symptoms (Kotov et al. 2017). Commonly co-occurring symptoms are grouped together under homogeneous classificatory entities defined dimensionally. The hierarchical component refers to the further clustering of syndromes into subfactors and then into the broader constructs of spectra. This structure allows for shared and distinct aspects of psychopathology to be represented simultaneously without artificially segregating disorders into discrete, mutually exclusive groups with overlapping symptoms. HiTOP is expressed as a "work in progress" espousing an empirical approach devoid of a priori assumptions regarding which aspects of psychopathology are discrete and which are continuous. Nonetheless, HiTOP developers assert that evidence supports the "continuity of psychopathological phenotypes" (Krueger et al. 2018).

HiTOP developers argue that a data-driven approach provides a more veridical mapping between causal variables and observable variability in psychopathology, thus offering the potential of disambiguating the complex interactions between latent and other intervening (e.g., epigenomic) variables across development. This approach is expected to better explicate etiology, addressing the thorny issues of equifinality (the tendency for similar manifestations to reflect differing etiologies) and multifinality (the tendency for the same etiologies to result in different expressions of psychopathology) (Cicchetti and Rogosch 1996). Moreover, HiTOP spectra, such as the internalizing spectrum, are found to have greater predictive power (Kim and Eaton 2015) and greater stability over time (Markon et al. 2011) than disorder-specific categories.

Although HiTOP may be useful in redefining our understanding of psychopathology, its implementation has limitations. First, not all symptoms have been included in analyses used to develop HiTOP. Additional research is needed to provide a comprehensive model of psychopathology for classification purposes. Second, dispensing with categorical classifications creates disjunctions in health data sets used by policymakers (Reed 2018). Third, although HiTOP may reduce comorbidity that arises as an artifact of imposing categories on dimensional constructs, comorbidity can reflect meaningful information for clinical decision making (Fava et al. 2014). Fourth, most clinical decisions are binary, requiring thresholds to be imposed on any dimensional system used in clinical practice (Kraemer et al. 2004). Finally, evidence is currently insufficient that clinicians can easily and reliably use dimensional classifications in clinical decision making to improve treatment outcomes (Tyrer 2018).

Maintaining Categorical Classifications

Alternative models of classification such as HiTOP offer conceptual advantages over categorical classifications but are not yet ready for clinical use. In addition to the limitations noted, other important functions of psychiatric classifications must be addressed before DSM or ICD can be replaced by or integrated with a dimensional scheme.

With respect to health system data, which countries report to the WHO using ICD codes, mental disorder coding must align with established classification conventions applicable to all health conditions. DSM and ICD are organized as hierarchical categorical systems such that each entry is a mutually exclusive label used to collect and track morbidity and mortality data (Kessler 2002).

Second, categorical classifications are more amenable to clinical and public policy decision making, which often requires binary decisions related to eligibility for reimbursement and treatment selection (Kessler 2002). Disease constructs are often extremes on dimensionally defined biological processes (Kessler 2002). Thus, clinically useful categorical constructs, such as panic disorder, can be complemented with dimensional approaches, such as the anxiety severity scales in DSM-5, to capture the breadth of illness severity.

Finally, notwithstanding evidence for latent variables, inclusion of discrete anxiety disorders in explanatory models accounts for additional variance (Clark and Beck 1988), supporting their validity as separable psychopathological constructs. This is further reinforced by epidemiological studies that report the existence of a significant number of single-disorder cases in 12-month and lifetime prevalence estimates (Kessler et al. 2005).

ICD-11, an Alternative to DSM-5

Although dimensional classifications are not yet viable for clinical use, ICD is a widely used alternative to DSM-5. Both are intended primarily for clinical use but differ with respect to their mandates, audience, applications, and development. ICD is the WHO classification system covering all health conditions for health authorities of its 194 member states, including the United States and Canada, as part of its core constitutional responsibility. In May 2019, ICD-11 (statistical version) was approved by the World Health Assembly, with the *ICD-11 Clinical Descriptions and Diagnostic Guidelines for Mental, Behavioural and Neurodevelopmental Disorders* (CDDG) expected to be published in 2020. The CDDG is a mental health specialist version of the ICD-11 that contains information akin to that found in DSM-5 (Reed et al. 2019). Countries relay health information to the WHO in ICD codes despite regional differences in use of DSM and ICD at the clinical encounter level. ICD is used by approximately 75% of the world's psychiatrists, and the remainder primarily use DSM-5 in clinical practice, particularly in the United States and Canada. DSM-5 is used by psychiatrists, other physicians, and mental health professionals primarily for diagnostic formulation and also for research.

Despite structural and conceptual differences, the developers of DSM-5 and ICD-11 engaged in a process of harmonization to avoid disjunctions in health statistics internationally, facilitate universality of research findings, and avoid unintentional inconsistencies of concepts leading to differential labeling of cases across the classifications (American Psychiatric Association 2013; First 2009). Harmonization is most evident at the meta-structure level of disorder groupings. However, important differences remain that reflect meaningful differences in interpretation of research findings and, in the case of ICD-11, the importance placed on global applicability and clinical utility, particularly in low-resource settings (International Advisory Group for the Revision of ICD-10 Mental and Behavioural Disorders 2011). Table 1–4 presents the conceptual differences between DSM-5 and ICD-11 for the disorders covered in this volume.

A critical distinction between ICD-11 and DSM-5 is the approach to case definitions. Whereas in DSM-5, *caseness* often requires a minimum number of criteria be met for a specified time, ICD-11 defines *caseness* according to the presence of essential features that are operationally defined, with greater flexibility if unequivocal evidence for minimal symptom counts or strict time frames do not exist (First et al. 2015). This better reflects how practitioners assign diagnoses in practice. Developers of both classifications emphasized the importance of clinical utility (First et al. 2004; Keeley et al. 2016a), although only the WHO explicitly evaluated this in field trials (Reed et al. 2018a).

Given the different approaches to case definitions, a key question is whether the classifications meet minimal psychometric standards. Field trials were conducted to address this question but were implemented quite differently. DSM-5 conducted evaluative field trials at 11 sites across the United States and Canada to determine primarily the test-retest reliability of diagnoses (Regier et al. 2013). ICD-11 developers took a multistepped developmental approach to their field trials such that the data collected informed iterative revisions of the classification before publication (Evans et al. 2015; Keeley et al. 2016a; Reed et al. 2018a, 2018b). Initially, the WHO conducted internet-based trials to test hypotheses about proposed changes to the classification, comparing ICD-10 with ICD-11 directly (Keeley et al. 2016b). A second wave of field trials examined joint-rater performance of high-disease-burden disorders for the revised guidelines in 13 clinical settings worldwide (Reed et al. 2018b).

Results of the DSM-5 field trials identified a broad range of reliability estimates, depending on the diagnostic category (Regier et al. 2013). Only two categories relevant to this volume were examined; very good reliability was found for PTSD ($\kappa=0.67$) and questionable reliability for GAD ($\kappa=0.20$). Without further information on the source of unreliability for GAD, DSM-5 developers could not make further revisions, and the American Psychiatric Association decided to revert to DSM-IV-TR criteria. ICD-11 field trials examined high-disease-burden disorders, and results relevant to this volume included reliability estimates for PTSD ($\kappa=0.49$), complex PTSD ($\kappa=0.56$), panic disorder ($\kappa=0.57$), agoraphobia ($\kappa=0.62$), GAD ($\kappa=0.62$), and social anxiety disorder ($\kappa=0.88$). Importantly, the WHO is making further revisions to guidelines for categories in which reliability was found to be suboptimal ($\kappa<0.70$). The methodology used allowed the developers to identify specific aspects of the guidelines that give rise to poorer reliability, which will be the basis for further revision or educational efforts (Reed et al. 2018b). Finally, ICD-11 developers explicitly assessed facets of clinical utility of diagnostic categories according to the operational definition provided in First et al. (2004). Generally, clinicians participating in the ICD-11 field trials rated guidelines as easy to use, possessing good fit with patient presentations, clear and understandable, adequately detailed, efficient to use, and useful for differential diagnosis (Reed et al. 2018a). Despite the more flexible guideline approach of ICD-11, field trials supported its reliability and clinical utility.

TABLE 1–4.   Comparison of DSM-5 and ICD-11ª conceptualizations of anxiety, obsessive-compulsive, and stress-related disorders

DSM-5/ICD-11 category	DSM-5 disorder	ICD-11 disorder	Key differences
Anxiety disorders/ Anxiety and fear-related disorders	Separation anxiety disorder	Separation anxiety disorder	DSM-5 requires the presence of three of eight specific symptoms, whereas ICD-11 provides six examples of symptom types without a specified count.
			DSM-5 requires a minimum of 4 weeks of symptoms for children and adolescents (typically 6 months for adults), whereas ICD-11 requires the persistence of symptoms and suggests several months.
	Selective mutism	Selective mutism	None
	Specific phobia	Specific phobia	ICD-11 does not include phobic stimulus specifiers, which have little clinical utility.
	Social anxiety disorder (social phobia)	Social anxiety disorder	ICD-11 has no "performance only" specifier because data suggest that social anxiety disorder symptoms exist on a continuum of severity.
	Panic disorder	Panic disorder	DSM-5 requires 4 or more of a list of 13 possible symptoms to qualify as a panic attack, whereas ICD-11 requires several of 13 symptoms but is not limited to these symptoms.
			DSM-5 specifies that culture-specific symptoms cannot count toward the minimum of four symptoms. ICD-11 has no such requirement.
			Note: In both systems, the specifier (qualifier in ICD-11) "with panic attacks" can be applied to other disorders when panic attacks are a manifestation of extreme anxiety states wholly consistent with that disorder and not panic disorder. ICD-11 qualifier can be applied only to current (past month) disorders and is applicable only to certain specified disorders.
	Agoraphobia	Agoraphobia	DSM-5 requires symptoms be present in two or more of five specified situations, whereas ICD-11 provides examples rather than a definitive list.
			DSM-5 criterion that fear is out of proportion to actual danger is not specified in ICD-11 essential features.
			Both systems allow for co-occurring diagnosis of panic disorder.

TABLE 1–4. **Comparison of DSM-5 and ICD-11ª conceptualizations of anxiety, obsessive-compulsive, and stress-related disorders** (*continued*)

DSM-5/ICD-11 category	DSM-5 disorder	ICD-11 disorder	Key differences
Anxiety disorders/Anxiety and fear-related disorders (*continued*)	Generalized anxiety disorder	Generalized anxiety disorder	ICD-11 differentiates between general apprehensiveness and excessive worry, either of which may fulfill the requirement for diagnosis. It does not require that the individual find it difficult to control worry. DSM-5 requires ≥ 6 months of anxiety and worry, whereas ICD-11 indicates symptoms must persist for at least several months. DSM-5 requires presence of three or more of six specified symptoms. Five of six symptoms listed in ICD-11 are the same as in DSM-5 but allow for others (sympathetic autonomic overactivity listed in ICD-11 rather than fatigue). Fatigue is omitted from ICD-11 to improve differentiation from depression.
Obsessive-compulsive and related disorders (OCRD)	OCD	OCD	Criteria and essential features are conceptually equivalent. However, "sense of incompleteness" can count for an obsession in ICD-11, reflecting data supporting sensory phenomena in OCD. Insight specifiers in DSM-5 cover three levels of insight, whereas ICD-11 qualifier has two levels. ICD-11 does not include a tic-related specifier because classification covers all health conditions, including tic disorders, classified in "Diseases of the Nervous System" chapter.
	Body dysmorphic disorder	Body dysmorphic disorder	In addition to preoccupation with one or more perceived defects or flaws, ICD-11 includes "general ugliness" as a possible source of preoccupation. Furthermore, ICD-11 includes the concept of excessive self-consciousness about perceived defects or flaws.

TABLE 1–4. Comparison of DSM-5 and ICD-11[a] conceptualizations of anxiety, obsessive-compulsive, and stress-related disorders (continued)

DSM-5/ICD-11 category	DSM-5 disorder	ICD-11 disorder	Key differences
Obsessive-compulsive and related disorders (OCRD) (continued)			In ICD-11, repetitive behaviors are one of three possible manifestations of preoccupation. Others include camouflaging the defect and marked avoidance of social situations.
			Although muscle dysmorphia is subsumed under this category, ICD-11 does not include a "with muscle dysmorphia" qualifier, unlike DSM-5. Insight specifiers/qualifiers are as described for OCD.
	No DSM-5 equivalent	Olfactory reference disorder	Not included in DSM-5, disorder is defined by persistent preoccupations with perceived foul or offensive body odor and associated behaviors that occur in response.
	Illness anxiety disorder (not classified here)	Hypochondriasis (health anxiety disorder)	Classified in DSM-5 "Somatic Symptom and Related Disorders" as illness anxiety disorder; this condition is conceptualized in ICD-11 as an OCRD/anxiety and fear-related disorder rather than as a somatoform disorder.
			ICD-11 includes a separate grouping titled "bodily distress disorder" that is phenomenologically distinct from hypochondriasis, capturing who are patients distressed by symptoms and seeking a medical diagnosis to explain symptoms rather than those who are fearful of a medical diagnosis.
			ICD-11 allows for the presence of somatic symptoms, whereas DSM-5 excludes the diagnosis if such symptoms are more than mild in severity.
	Hoarding disorder	Hoarding disorder	In ICD-11, excessive acquisition is specifically related to repetitive urges and behaviors related to amassing or buying items. ICD-11 does not include "with excessive acquisition" specifier.
	Trichotillomania (hair-pulling disorder)	Trichotillomania (hair-pulling disorder)	Classified in ICD-11 under subcategory within OCRD of body-focused repetitive behavior disorders.
	Excoriation (skin-picking) disorder	Excoriation (skin-picking) disorder	Classified in ICD-11 under subcategory within OCRD of body-focused repetitive behavior disorders.

TABLE 1–4. Comparison of DSM-5 and ICD-11[a] conceptualizations of anxiety, obsessive-compulsive, and stress-related disorders (*continued*)

DSM-5/ICD-11 category	DSM-5 disorder	ICD-11 disorder	Key differences
Trauma- and stressor-related disorders/ Disorders specifically associated with stress	Reactive attachment disorder	Reactive attachment disorder	Conceptually similar between DSM-5 and ICD-11.[b]
	Disinhibited social engagement disorder	Disinhibited social engagement disorder	Conceptually similar between DSM-5 and ICD-11.[b]
	PTSD	PTSD	DSM-5 PTSD is a polythetic disorder requiring exposure to trauma in one of four ways, one or more of five intrusive symptoms, one or more of two avoidance symptoms, two or more of seven changes in cognition and mood, and two or more of six symptoms of alterations in arousal and reactivity. Symptoms must have persisted for > 1 month. ICD-11 PTSD requires exposure to trauma with emergence of a characteristic syndrome that lasts for at least several weeks and consists of three core features—reexperiencing, deliberate avoidance, and persistent perceptions of heightened and current threat. In contrast to DSM-5, changes in cognition and mood are part of a separate disorder, ICD-11 complex PTSD (see next row). ICD-11 does not include "with dissociative symptoms" or "with delayed expression" specifiers.
	No equivalent category in DSM-5	Complex PTSD	In ICD-11, complex PTSD is conceptualized as requiring exposure to extremely threatening or horrific trauma, typically prolonged or repeatedly, accompanied by the same three core features as ICD-11 PTSD, with additional symptoms of severe and pervasive problems in mood regulation, persistent changes in cognition and mood, and persistent difficulties in sustaining relationships and feeling close to others.
	Persistent complex bereavement disorder (not classified here)	Prolonged grief disorder	Classified in DSM-5 Section III, "Conditions for Further Study."

TABLE 1–4.   Comparison of DSM-5 and ICD-11[a] conceptualizations of anxiety, obsessive-compulsive, and stress-related disorders (*continued*)

DSM-5/ICD-11 category	DSM-5 disorder	ICD-11 disorder	Key differences
Trauma- and stressor-related disorders/ Disorders specifically associated with stress (*continued*)	Acute stress disorder	Acute stress reaction (not classified as a mental, behavioral, or neurodevelopmental disorder [see "Key Differences"])	DSM-5 requires exposure to a traumatic event and nine or more symptoms of intrusion, negative mood, dissociation, avoidance, or arousal. Symptoms occur 3 days–1 month after event. Equivalent category in ICD-11 is conceptualized as a normal reaction to exposure to trauma that may nonetheless necessitate health care services. It is classified in the chapter "Factors Influencing Health Status or Contact With Health Services," not as a mental or behavioral disorder.
	Adjustment disorders	Adjustment disorder	DSM-5 concept of distress must be out of proportion to the severity or intensity of the stressor, whereas ICD-11 refers to a maladaptive reaction evidenced by preoccupation with an identifiable psychosocial stressor. ICD-11 does not include specifiers for the type of emotional or behavioral disturbance or to indicate whether the condition is acute or persistent (chronic).

Note. [a]Comparisons made based on published information about essential features of these ICD-11 categories at the time of writing, not on ICD-11 guidelines, which are scheduled to be published in 2020 (Kogan et al. 2016; Maercker et al. 2013; Stein et al. 2016).
[b]Based on definitions provided by World Health Organization on ICD-11 for Mortality and Morbidity Statistics; complete ICD-11 guidelines not available at the time of writing.

Reorganization of Anxiety Disorders in DSM-5

A major change in DSM-5 from previous versions is the separation of the OCRD and TSRD from the anxiety disorders. Although seemingly cosmetic, this reorganization represents an important shift in the way these disorders are conceptualized.

To align DSM-5's meta-structure more closely with our understanding of mental disorders (Regier et al. 2013), DSM-5 working groups reviewed the scientific literature to examine evidence for common validators, which for the anxiety disorders included 1) structural analysis of self-report data; 2) research on fear conditioning, stress reactivity, and information processing; 3) brain circuitry related to fear processing; 4) similarities in symptom presentation and comorbidity; and 5) genetics (Craske et al. 2009; Friedman et al. 2011a, 2011b). Although these reviews emphasized the preliminary nature and inconsistencies of research, the investigators decided to separate anxiety disorders from OCRD and TSRD.

The decision to separate OCRD from other anxiety disorders was based on evidence that 1) not all subtypes of OCD are characterized by anxiety (e.g., symmetry-related rituals often satisfy a need for "just rightness" rather than functioning to reduce anxiety); 2) changes in frontostriatal functioning are implicated in OCD but not in other anxiety disorders; and 3) OCD is characterized by deficits in executive function not found in other anxiety disorders (Hollander et al. 2008; Stein et al. 2010). However, support for separating OCD from other anxiety disorders was not universal (Stein et al. 2010), highlighting that meta-structure decisions are often a compromise, with advantages and disadvantages to each solution.

Several DSM-IV-TR disorders were moved from other sections to the OCRD section. OCRD are characterized by 1) obsessions and compulsions, 2) similar underlying etiology, and 3) either comorbidity with or similar treatment response as OCD (Hollander et al. 2008). However, the strength of evidence required to classify disorders as OCRD is inconsistent. For example, illness anxiety disorder (e.g., hypochondriasis) remained with the somatic symptom and related disorders because of insufficient evidence of similarity to other OCRD (Phillips et al. 2010), but it is placed among the OCRD in ICD-11.

Similarly, although TSRD share many features with anxiety disorders, several findings suggest that they are distinct. Anxiety disorders and PTSD share similar information-processing biases, elevated anxiety in response to direct and contextual threat, and hyperactivity of the amygdala (Craske et al. 2009). However, even though a stressor can precipitate the onset of other anxiety disorders, most cases have no identifiable precipitating stressor, whereas by very definition, symptoms of PTSD develop after a traumatic event(s). PTSD also shares several symptoms with other disorders, such as lack of concentration and anhedonia with depression, and intense externalizing emotions, such as anger, and can be characterized by dissociation (Friedman et al. 2011a). In summary, no clear consensus exists on how to classify anxiety disorders, but the decision to separate OCRD and TSRD into separate groupings was based on key nonoverlapping features to enhance clinical utility and encourage further research into the validity of these groupings.

Changes to Symptom Criteria

Changes from DSM-II (American Psychiatric Association 1968) to DSM-III succeeded in increasing the reliability of DSM. Reliability has continued to be an important factor in assessing the utility of DSM-5 criteria, although variations in methodology sometimes make comparison across iterations of DSM difficult. However, many have argued that emphasizing reliability was detrimental to the validity of DSM, illustrated by the proliferative use of the not otherwise specified (NOS) categories. For example, according to DSM-IV-TR criteria for PTSD, a person who reports all symptom criteria consistent with PTSD but not fear, helplessness, or horror during the traumatic event (Criterion A2) should not be assigned a diagnosis of PTSD and would likely receive a diagnosis of either adjustment disorder or adjustment disorder NOS. This example highlights the reason that NOS disorders are frequently applied to patients with distressing symptoms.

In general, changes to the diagnostic criteria of most anxiety and related disorders have been nominal. The diagnostic criteria for PTSD are an exception, providing an excellent example of how diagnostic criteria have been refined in an attempt to improve reliability, validity, and precision. The evolution of the PTSD criteria also highlights the continued controversies surrounding these changes (Table 1–5).

The changes to DSM-5 PTSD criteria that now require four instead of three symptom clusters were based on factor analytic evidence. This is controversial for several reasons. First, several studies have identified alternative factor structures (Buckley et al. 1998; Foy et al. 1997; Taylor et al. 1998), and even when a four-factor structure was identified, no universal agreement could be found on the identified factors (e.g., Asmundson et al. 2000 vs. Simms et al. 2002). Finally, other changes were not made (e.g., moving GAD to the "Depressive Disorders" section) despite strong factor analytic and other evidence that supported such changes (Watson 2005). Some have argued that the changes to the PTSD diagnostic criteria have broadened the criteria to account for symptom heterogeneity to such an extent that clinical utility has been reduced (Galatzer-Levy and Bryant 2013). The continual shifting of symptom criteria for PTSD highlights the evolution of these constructs based on empirical data informing classification and the challenges of developing clinically useful categories from phenomena that are likely heterogeneous and dimensional in nature.

Conclusion

In this chapter, we examined the challenges of developing a single classification of mental illness that can accomplish all desired functions, including acting as an organizing scheme for the science of psychopathology, identifying homogeneous patient populations with similar treatment needs, and fulfilling public health monitoring needs. Limitations of categorical classifications, particularly for the mood and anxiety disorders, were highlighted, including artifactual comorbidity, arbitrary case thresholds, lack of severity staging, minimal integration of neuroscientific findings, and insufficient incorporation of pathophysiological mechanisms into disorder conceptualizations. The developers of DSM-5 and ICD-11 were aware of these limitations and

TABLE 1–5. **Evolution of PTSD: an example of criteria changes and challenges to the polythetic categories**

DSM-III

PTSD first appeared as a diagnosis (American Psychiatric Association 1980, p. 238).

Required existence of a "recognizable stressor," as well as at least one reexperiencing symptom, such as intrusive recollections of the event, dreams of the event, or flashbacks; at least one numbing symptom, such as diminished interest in significant activities, feelings of detachment, or reduced affect; and at least two other symptoms, such as hypervigilance, sleep problems, guilt relating to the event, memory impairment, avoidance of activities, or "intensification of symptoms by exposure to the event" (p. 238).

DSM-III-R

Narrowed the definition of *stressor* to define event as "outside the range of usual human experience and…would be markedly distressing to almost anyone" (American Psychiatric Association 1987), because the initial criteria for a stressor in DSM-III were considered too broad and subject to interpretation.

Significantly reorganized symptom criteria such that individuals were required to report at least one reexperiencing symptom (largely similar to those specified in DSM-III), three avoidance symptoms, and two symptoms of increased arousal.

Eliminated the requirement to exhibit at least one symptom of numbing, but subsumed symptoms of diminished interest, detachment, and restricted range of affect under the persistent avoidance criterion.

DSM-IV and DSM-IV-TR

Added a criterion requiring that individuals report experiencing fear, helplessness, or horror during event.

PTSD remained similar; shifted placement of certain symptoms somewhat. For example, physiological reactivity at exposure to reminders of the event fell under the increased arousal criterion in DSM-III-R and reexperiencing criterion in DSM-IV-TR.

DSM-5

Removed the requirement that individuals report experiencing fear, helplessness, or horror during the event; developers concluded that no incremental validity or clinical utility in this criterion could be found because PTSD symptoms do not differ in the presence or absence of experiencing fear, helplessness, and horror during the event (Friedman et al. 2011b).

Reconceptualized the definition of a traumatic event. How to define what constitutes a traumatic event, and even if an identifiable event is necessary, continues to be hotly debated.

Made major changes to the organization and symptoms that define PTSD. Individual must report at least one of five intrusion (formerly reexperiencing), one of two avoidance, and two of six hyperarousal symptoms as well as one of seven symptoms from a new group labeled "changes in cognition and mood." Decision to move from three to four symptom clusters was largely based on factor analytic studies (Friedman et al. 2011b), most of which supported a four-factor model.

attempted to address them to the extent possible (e.g., grouping internalizing disorders together), arguing that alternative models are not yet adequately validated for clinical use. We also discussed the HiTOP model as an alternative and concluded that although it shows promise for advancing the field, it is not yet ready for clinical implementation. Furthermore, we compared the development, use, and evaluation of DSM-5 and ICD-11 and highlighted the conceptual differences in the structure and content of these classifications. We reviewed the rationale for the separation of the OCRD and

TSRD from the anxiety disorders in DSM-5 and described examples of the evolution of criteria sets across versions of DSM to illustrate conceptual shifts for included disorders based on current evidence.

Despite concerns about perpetuating a categorical classification of mental illness, it is important to stress that a single nosology intended primarily for clinical use in no way obviates the ongoing development and validation of alternative models of psychopathology, particularly those that more directly reflect the pathophysiology of mental illnesses. Although the disorder categories in DSM-5 are practical rather than natural (Zacher 2000), they provide clinicians with a system that can be used effectively in clinical practice. No doubt, alternative models will continue to be refined and tested for use in diverse populations. We hope that convergence of knowledge across various research domains will be adequate to produce the paradigm shift anticipated for DSM-5. In the meantime, alternative models can, and do, serve a complementary role in informing clinicians' conceptualizations and understanding of psychopathology.

Key Points

- Psychiatric classifications serve multiple purposes, including assessing the need for mental health services, facilitating research, and serving public health functions. A priority for DSM-5 was to incorporate current evidence into a descriptive categorical classification to improve its reliability and validity in clinical settings.

- Although alternative psychopathology models have been proposed that address limitations of categorical classifications, these systems are not sufficiently comprehensive or adequately validated for clinical use. DSM-5 addresses some of the limitations of high comorbidity, thresholds with normality, disorder severity, and etiology to the extent possible given available evidence and the need to maintain a nosology with clinical utility.

- One goal of DSM-5 was to align the meta-structure of disorder categories more closely with our expanded understanding of mental disorders. Anxiety disorders are classified and organized as part of the broad spectrum of internalizing disorders that are often found to be comorbid and also include mood disorders.

- The most significant change to the DSM-IV-TR anxiety disorders was the introduction in DSM-5 of the obsessive-compulsive and related disorders and trauma- and stressor-related disorders as separate, but adjacent, groupings from anxiety disorders. This was based on empirical evidence suggesting that disorders within each grouping share key nonoverlapping validators. Although these groupings share some overlap with each other and with anxiety disorders, their separation also encourages further research into their unique phenomenology, etiology, and pathophysiology.

- DSM-5 takes a lifespan approach. Thus, disorders of childhood such as separation anxiety disorder and selective mutism are now incorporated into the "Anxiety Disorders" section, alongside specific phobia, social anxiety disorder (social phobia), panic disorder, agoraphobia, and generalized anxiety disorder.

- DSM-5 "Obsessive-Compulsive and Related Disorders" brings together OCD, body dysmorphic disorder, hoarding disorder, trichotillomania (hair-pulling disorder), and excoriation (skin-picking) disorder based on shared validators, including repetitive thoughts and associated behaviors.

- DSM-5 "Trauma- and Stressor-Related Disorders" brings together disorders in which a trauma or stressor is a necessary but not sufficient etiological factor in the development of the disorder, including disorders emerging in childhood (i.e., reactive attachment disorder and disinhibited social engagement disorder), PTSD, acute stress disorder, and adjustment disorders.

References

American Psychiatric Association: Diagnostic and Statistical Manual of Mental Disorders, 2nd Edition. Washington, DC, American Psychiatric Association, 1968

American Psychiatric Association: Diagnostic and Statistical Manual of Mental Disorders, 3rd Edition. Washington, DC, American Psychiatric Association, 1980

American Psychiatric Association: Diagnostic and Statistical Manual of Mental Disorders, 3rd Edition, Revised. Washington, DC, American Psychiatric Association, 1987

American Psychiatric Association: Diagnostic and Statistical Manual of Mental Disorders, 4th Edition. Washington, DC, American Psychiatric Association, 1994

American Psychiatric Association: Diagnostic and Statistical Manual of Mental Disorders, 4th Edition, Text Revision. Washington, DC, American Psychiatric Association, 2000

American Psychiatric Association: Diagnostic and Statistical Manual of Mental Disorders, 5th Edition. Arlington, VA, American Psychiatric Association, 2013

Andrews G: Internalizing disorders: the whole is greater than the sum of the parts. World Psychiatry 17(3):302–303, 2018 30192085

Asmundson GJG, Frombach I, McQuaid J, et al: Dimensionality of posttraumatic stress symptoms: a confirmatory factor analysis of DSM-IV symptom clusters and other symptom models. Behav Res Ther 38(2):203–214, 2000 10661004

Barlow DH: Unraveling the mysteries of anxiety and its disorders from the perspective of emotion theory. Am Psychol 55(11):1247–1263, 2000 11280938

Barlow DH, Farchione TJ, Fairholme CP, et al: Unified Protocol for Transdiagnostic Treatment of Emotional Disorders: Therapist Guide. New York, Oxford University Press, 2011

Barlow DH, Ellard KK, Sauer-Zavala S, et al: The origins of neuroticism. Perspect Psychol Sci 9(5):481–496, 2014 26186755

Blashfield RK, Keeley JW: A short history of a psychiatric diagnostic category that turned out to be a disease, in Contemporary Directions in Psychopathology. Edited by Millon T, Krueger R, Simonsen E. New York, Guilford, 2010, pp 324–336

Buckley TC, Blanchard EB, Hickling EJ: A confirmatory factor analysis of posttraumatic stress symptoms. Behav Res Ther 36(11):1091–1099, 1998 9737061

Cicchetti D, Rogosch FA: Equifinality and multifinality in developmental psychopathology (editorial). Dev Psychopathol 8(4):597–600, 1996

Clark DM, Beck AT: Cognitive approaches, in Handbook of Anxiety Disorders. Edited by Last CG, Michel H. Elmsford, NY, Pergamon, 1988, pp 362–385

Clark LA, Watson D: Tripartite model of anxiety and depression: psychometric evidence and taxonomic implications. J Abnorm Psychol 100(3):316–336, 1991 1918611

Clark LA, Cuthbert B, Lewis-Fernández R, et al: Three approaches to understanding and classifying mental disorder: ICD-11, DSM-5, and the National Institute of Mental Health's Research Domain Criteria (RDoC). Psychol Sci Public Interest 18(2):72–145, 2017 29211974

Craske MG, Rauch SL, Ursano R, et al: What is an anxiety disorder? Depress Anxiety 26(12):1066–1085, 2009 19957279

Cuthbert BN, Insel TR: Toward the future of psychiatric diagnosis: the seven pillars of RDoC. BMC Med 11:126, 2013 23672542

Evans SC, Roberts MC, Keeley JW, et al: Vignette methodologies for studying clinicians' decision-making: validity, utility, and application in ICD-11 field studies. Int J Clin Health Psychol 15(2):160–170, 2015 30487833

Fava GA, Tossani E, Bech P, et al: Emerging clinical trends and perspectives on comorbid patterns of mental disorders in research. Int J Methods Psychiatr Res 23(suppl 1):92–101, 2014 24375537

First MB: Harmonisation of ICD-11 and DSM-V: opportunities and challenges. Br J Psychiatry 195(5):382–390, 2009 19880924

First MB, Wakefield JC: Diagnostic criteria as dysfunction indicators: bridging the chasm between the definition of mental disorder and diagnostic criteria for specific disorders. Can J Psychiatry 58(12):663–669, 2013 24331285

First MB, Pincus HA, Levine JB, et al: Clinical utility as a criterion for revising psychiatric diagnoses. Am J Psychiatry 161(6):946–954, 2004 15169680

First MB, Reed GM, Hyman SE, et al: The development of the ICD-11 Clinical Descriptions and Diagnostic Guidelines for Mental and Behavioural Disorders. World Psychiatry 14(1):82–90, 2015 25655162

Forbes MK, Tackett JL, Markon KE, et al: Beyond comorbidity: toward a dimensional and hierarchical approach to understanding psychopathology across the life span. Dev Psychopathol 28(4 pt 1):971–986, 2016 27739384

Foy DW, Wood JL, King DW, et al: Los Angeles Symptom Checklist: psychometric evidence with an adolescent sample. Assessment 4(4):377–384, 1997

Frances A: Saving Normal: An Insider's Revolt Against Out-of-Control Psychiatric Diagnosis, DSM-5, Big Pharma, and the Medicalization of Ordinary Life. New York, William Morrow, 2014

Friedman MJ, Resick PA, Bryant RA, et al: Classification of trauma and stressor-related disorders in DSM-5. Depress Anxiety 28(9):737–749, 2011a 21681870

Friedman MJ, Resick PA, Bryant RA, et al: Considering PTSD for DSM-5. Depress Anxiety 28(9):750–769, 2011b 21910184

Galatzer-Levy IR, Bryant RA: 636,120 ways to have posttraumatic stress disorder. Perspect Psychol Sci 8(6):651–662, 2013 26173229

Hollander E, Braun A, Simeon D: Should OCD leave the anxiety disorders in DSM-V? The case for obsessive compulsive-related disorders. Depress Anxiety 25(4):317–329, 2008 18412058

International Advisory Group for the Revision of ICD-10 Mental and Behavioural Disorders: a conceptual framework for the revision of the ICD-10 classification of mental and behavioural disorders. World Psychiatry 10(2):86–92, 2011 21633677

Keeley JW, Reed GM, Roberts MC, et al: Developing a science of clinical utility in diagnostic classification systems field study strategies for ICD-11 mental and behavioral disorders. Am Psychol 71(1):3–16, 2016a 26766762

Keeley JW, Reed GM, Roberts MC, et al: Disorders specifically associated with stress: a case-controlled field study for ICD-11 mental and behavioural disorders. Int J Clin Health Psychol 16(2):109–127, 2016b 30487855

Kendler KS: Toward a scientific psychiatric nosology: strengths and limitations. Arch Gen Psychiatry 47(10):969–973, 1990 2222134

Kessler RC: The categorical versus dimensional assessment controversy in the sociology of mental illness. J Health Soc Behav 43(2):171–188, 2002 12096698

Kessler RC, Chiu WT, Demler O, et al: Prevalence, severity, and comorbidity of 12-month DSM-IV disorders in the National Comorbidity Survey Replication. Arch Gen Psychiatry 62(6):617–627, 2005 15939839

Kim H, Eaton NR: The hierarchical structure of common mental disorders: connecting multiple levels of comorbidity, bifactor models, and predictive validity. J Abnorm Psychol 124(4):1064–1078, 2015 26595482

Kogan CS, Stein DJ, Maj M, et al: The classification of anxiety and fear-related disorders in the ICD-11. Depress Anxiety 33(12):1141–1154, 2016 27411108

Kotov R, Schmidt NB, Lerew DR, et al: Latent structure of anxiety: taxometric exploration. Psychol Assess 17(3):369–374, 2005 16262462

Kotov R, Krueger RF, Watson D, et al: The Hierarchical Taxonomy of Psychopathology (HiTOP): a dimensional alternative to traditional nosologies. J Abnorm Psychol 126(4):454–477, 2017 28333488

Kraemer HC, Noda A, O'Hara R: Categorical versus dimensional approaches to diagnosis: methodological challenges. J Psychiatr Res 38(1):17–25, 2004 14690767

Krueger RF, Kotov R, Watson D, et al: Progress in achieving quantitative classification of psychopathology. World Psychiatry 17(3):282–293, 2018 30229571

Kupfer DJ, Regier DA: Neuroscience, clinical evidence, and the future of psychiatric classification in DSM-5. Am J Psychiatry 168(7):672–674, 2011 21724672

Lebeau RT, Glenn DE, Hanover LN, et al: A dimensional approach to measuring anxiety for DSM-5. Int J Methods Psychiatr Res 21(4):258–272, 2012 23148016

Leighton C, Botto A, Silva JR, et al: Vulnerability or sensitivity to the environment? Methodological issues, trends, and recommendations in gene-environment interactions research in human behavior. Front Psychiatry 8(8):106, 2017 28674505

Maercker A, Brewin CR, Bryant RA, et al: Diagnosis and classification of disorders specifically associated with stress: proposals for ICD-11. World Psych 12(3):198–206, 2013 24096776

Markon KE, Chmielewski M, Miller CJ: The reliability and validity of discrete and continuous measures of psychopathology: a quantitative review. Psychol Bull 137(5):856–879, 2011 21574681

Meehl PE: Factors and taxa, traits and types, differences of degree and differences in kind. J Pers 60(1):117–174, 1992

Phillips KA, Stein DJ, Rauch SL, et al: Should an obsessive-compulsive spectrum grouping of disorders be included in DSM-V? Depress Anxiety 27(6):528–555, 2010 20533367

Plato: Plato's Phaedrus. Translated by Hackforth R. New York, Cambridge University Press, 1952

Prenoveau JM, Zinbarg RE, Craske MG, et al: Testing a hierarchical model of anxiety and depression in adolescents: a tri-level model. J Anxiety Disord 24(3):334–344, 2010 20171054

Reed GM: HiTOP must meet the use requirements of the ICD before it can aspire to replace it. World Psychiatry 17(3):296–298, 2018 30192081

Reed GM, Keeley JW, Rebello TJ, et al: Clinical utility of ICD-11 diagnostic guidelines for high-burden mental disorders: results from mental health settings in 13 countries. World Psychiatry 17(3):306–315, 2018a 30192090

Reed GM, Sharan P, Rebello TJ, et al: The ICD-11 developmental field study of reliability of diagnoses of high-burden mental disorders: results among adult patients in mental health settings of 13 countries. World Psychiatry 17(2):174–186, 2018b 29856568

Reed GM, First MB, Kogan CS, et al: Innovations and changes in the ICD-11 classification of mental, behavioural and neurodevelopmental disorders. World Psychiatry 18(1):3–19, 2019 30600616

Regier DA, Rae DS, Narrow WE, et al: Prevalence of anxiety disorders and their comorbidity with mood and addictive disorders. Br J Psychiatry Suppl (34):24–28, 1998 9829013

Regier DA, Narrow WE, Clarke DE, et al: DSM-5 field trials in the United States and Canada, part II: test-retest reliability of selected categorical diagnoses. Am J Psychiatry 170(1):59–70, 2013 23111466

Robins E, Guze SB: Establishment of diagnostic validity in psychiatric illness: its application to schizophrenia. Am J Psychiatry 126(7):983–987, 1970 5409569

Simms LJ, Watson D, Doebbeling BN: Confirmatory factor analyses of posttraumatic stress symptoms in deployed and nondeployed veterans of the Gulf War. J Abnorm Psychol 111(4):637–647, 2002 12428777

Smith L, Reichenberg A, Rabinowitz J, et al: Psychiatric symptoms and related dysfunction in a general population sample. Schizophr Res Cogn 14:1–6, 2018 30112288

Stein DJ, Fineberg NA, Bienvenu OJ, et al: Should OCD be classified as an anxiety disorder in DSM-V? Depress Anxiety 27(6):495–506, 2010 20533366

Stein DJ, Craske MA, Friedman MJ, et al: Anxiety disorders, obsessive-compulsive and related disorders, trauma- and stressor-related disorders, and dissociative disorders in DSM-5. Am J Psychiatry 171(6):611–613, 2014 24880507

Stein DJ, Kogan CS, Atmaca M, et al: The classification of obsessive-compulsive and related disorders in the ICD-11. J Affect Disord 190:663–674, 2016 26590514

Taylor S, Kuch K, Koch WJ, et al: The structure of posttraumatic stress symptoms. J Abnorm Psychol 107(1):154–160, 1998 9505048

Tyrer P: Dimensions fit the data, but can clinicians fit the dimensions? World Psychiatry 17(3):295–296, 2018 30192102

Watson D: Rethinking the mood and anxiety disorders: a quantitative hierarchical model for DSM-V. J Abnorm Psychol 114(4):522–536, 2005 16351375

Woodward SA, Lenzenweger MF, Kagan J, et al: Taxonic structure of infant reactivity: evidence from a taxometric perspective. Psychol Sci 11(4):296–301, 2000 11273388

World Health Organization: International Classification of Diseases for Mortality and Morbidity Statistics. Geneva, World Health Organization, 2019

Zacher P: Psychiatric disorders are not natural kinds. Philosophy, Psychiatry, & Psychology 7(3):167–182, 2000

Recommended Readings

Clark LA, Cuthbert B, Lewis-Fernández R, et al: Three approaches to understanding and classifying mental disorder: ICD-11, DSM-5, and the National Institute of Mental Health's Research Domain Criteria (RDoC). Psychol Sci Public Interest 18(2):72–145, 2017 29211974

Craske MG, Rauch SL, Ursano R, et al: What is an anxiety disorder? Depress Anxiety 26(12):1066–1085, 2009 19957279

Friedman MJ, Resick PA, Bryant RA, et al: Classification of trauma and stressor-related disorders in DSM-5. Depress Anxiety 28(9):737–749, 2011a 21681870

Galatzer-Levy IR, Bryant RA: 636,120 ways to have posttraumatic stress disorder. Perspect Psychol Sci 8(6):651–662, 2013 26173229

Hollander E, Braun A, Simeon D: Should OCD leave the anxiety disorders in DSM-V? The case for obsessive compulsive-related disorders. Depress Anxiety 25(4):317–329, 2008 18412058

Kotov R, Krueger RF, Watson D, et al: The Hierarchical Taxonomy of Psychopathology (HiTOP): a dimensional alternative to traditional nosologies. J Abnorm Psychol 126(4):454–477, 2017 28333488

Regier DA, Rae DS, Narrow WE, et al: Prevalence of anxiety disorders and their comorbidity with mood and addictive disorders. Br J Psychiatry Suppl (34):24–28, 1998 9829013

Regier DA, Narrow WE, Clarke DE, et al: DSM-5 field trials in the United States and Canada, part II: test-retest reliability of selected categorical diagnoses. Am J Psychiatry 170(1):59–70, 2013 23111466

CHAPTER 2

Genetic Contributions to Anxiety and Related Disorders

John M. Hettema, M.D., Ph.D.

Jürgen Deckert, M.D.

Thalia C. Eley, Ph.D.

Sandra Meier, Ph.D.

Like most medical conditions, anxiety and related disorders are caused by a combination of genetic and environmental factors. We use the abbreviation ANX when referring to the five anxiety disorders in DSM-5: generalized anxiety disorder, panic disorder, agoraphobia, social phobia, and specific phobia (American Psychiatric Association 2013), whereas anxiety and related disorders (ARD) include OCD and PTSD. The genetic basis of ARD has been indirectly supported by well-established animal models of fear behaviors (Jacobson and Cryan 2010). Although animal models are considered a vital tool for advancing basic understanding of the biological basis of many human disorders, they are not considered here. Similarly, researchers continue to investigate the genetic basis of normal fear, anxiety symptoms, and anxious temperament, but we primarily address categorical adult clinical syndromes as defined in DSM. This chapter is divided into two main divisions of genetic research: 1) genetic epidemiology, including twin and family studies, and 2) molecular genetics, including linkage, genetic association, and epigenetic studies. We also review the extant literature of genetics of treatment response ("therapygenetics") for ARD. For more detailed overviews of the genetics of ARD, see Smoller (2016) and Shimada-Sugimoto et al. (2015).

Genetic Epidemiology

Genetic epidemiology seeks to understand how diseases and their risk factors are distributed in families. The "chain of evidence" for genetic investigations begins with family studies, which compare rates of illness in first-degree relatives of those who have the condition (case probands) with rates in relatives of healthy control participants. Higher rates in relatives of probands, as parameterized by a relative risk or odds ratio greater than 1.0, suggest familial aggregation. Next, either twin or adoption studies (not available for ANX) can differentiate genetic from within-family environment as the source of aggregation. Twin studies compare resemblance for a condition between members of a twin pair using the fact that identical (monozygotic) twins share 100% of their genes, whereas nonidentical (dizygotic) twins share only 50% of their segregating genes, on average. If resemblance for a trait or disorder is greater in monozygotic than in dizygotic pairs, then this is evidence for a genetic contribution to familial aggregation. With larger twin samples, one also may estimate the proportion of individual differences due to genetic effects (heritability). For conditions with substantial heritability, gene finding (linkage or association) studies are undertaken to identify which specific genes contribute to risk.

A 2001 meta-analysis summarized findings across extant family and twin studies for various adult ANX (Hettema et al. 2001). Those results suggested an overall moderate level of familial aggregation (OR 4–6) and heritability (30%–70%) across them. Thus, first-degree relatives of someone affected by an ARD are, on average, four to six times more likely to develop ARD than would a random individual. Fifty percent heritability means that genetic and environmental factors are approximately equally responsible for the etiology of ARD. Few family studies have been published since then, because it is now well established that all ARD aggregate in families. More twin studies have been conducted, however, with emphasis on the etiology of comorbidity or developmental risk. Table 2–1 summarizes the findings of that meta-analysis (Hettema et al. 2001), with additional information for OCD and PTSD.

Linkage Studies

As in other conditions, linkage studies were the first molecular genetic studies on ANX (reviewed by Smoller et al. 2008) and OCD (none were conducted for PTSD). Phenotypes studied were primarily panic disorder plus several for social phobia, specific phobias, and OCD. The number of families studied in each ranged from 1 to 120, making them considerably underpowered to detect linkage for common, genetically complex phenotypes such as ARD. Regions tentatively implicated were located on chromosome arms 1q, 2q, 3q, 4q, 7p, 9q, 12q, 13q, 14q, 15q, 16q, and 22q, with modest logarithm of the odds (LOD) scores ranging from 2.1 to 4.96. Some of these loci contained neurobiologically plausible genes such as *RGS* and *COMT* as well as genes for neuropeptide Y and GABA receptors. Reanalysis of panic disorder linkage studies found converging evidence for 4q21 and 7p in the Iowa and Yale family cohorts (Logue et al. 2012) and 15q11–13, including GABA receptor genes, in the Columbia University and Sardinian cohorts (Hodges et al. 2014). Meta-analysis across 162 ANX

TABLE 2–1. **Overview of findings from family and twin studies of anxiety and related disorders**

Disorder	Familial OR*	Twin heritability*
Panic disorder	3.4–15.6 (5.0; 3.0–8.2)	0.37–0.43 (0.43; 0.32–0.53)
Generalized anxiety disorder	5.0–6.6 (6.1; 2.5–14.9)	0.22–0.37 (0.32; 0.24–0.39)
Phobias	2.9–12.9 (4.1; 2.7–6.1)	0.20–0.39 (0.28)
OCD	1.0–5.9 (4.0; 2.2–7.1)	0.27–0.65
PTSD	None	0.23–0.71

Note. *Each cell provides the range of values from various studies followed by, where available, the summary statistic and its 95% CI.
Source. Browne et al. 2014; Duncan et al. 2018a; Hettema et al. 2001.

families found suggestive linkage on chromosomes 1, 5, 15, and 16 (Webb et al. 2012). Although early linkage studies in OCD were inconclusive, more recent studies in families with early onset OCD provided somewhat stronger evidence: 15q14, where the ryanodine receptor 3 (*RYR3*) gene is located (3 families, LOD 3.13; Ross et al. 2011), and 1p36 (33 families, LOD 3.77; Mathews et al. 2012).

Association Studies

ARD, like most common medical conditions, are not single-gene, Mendelian disorders but are highly polygenic in etiology. Association studies thus replaced linkage as the method of choice to study their genetic basis.

Candidate Gene Association Studies

In contrast to linkage studies, association studies make it possible to evaluate the contribution of individual genes or variants within genes to the heritability of ARD. Like other complex psychiatric phenotypes, most ANX association studies performed thus far have focused on candidate genes, which are chosen based on limited a priori hypotheses such as position under a linkage peak, mouse quantitative trait loci, or putative biological function. Most studies focused on monoaminergic neurotransmitter systems (mechanisms of pharmacological agents) and hypothalamic-pituitary-adrenal axis function (stress response). The most frequently studied variants among these include the serotonin transporter–linked promoter region (5HTTLPR) polymorphism of *SLC6A4*, the Val158Met polymorphism of *COMT* (rs4680), *RGS2* variant rs4606, and *FKBP5* polymorphisms.

Although findings are still mixed, low-expression 5HTTLPR genotypes are the variants most consistently associated with OCD (Sinopoli et al. 2017), as supported by meta-analysis across 10 studies (Taylor 2016). A meta-analysis comprising the 23 most widely studied variants in panic disorder indicated significant association of *COMT* rs4680, whereas results for other candidate genes remained inconsistent or negative or did not clearly replicate (Howe et al. 2016). Sex-specific effects of *COMT* variant rs4680 in OCD are supported by a meta-analysis of 11 studies in which the Met allele was associated with significantly higher risk in males (Taylor 2016). *RGS2* was initially implicated in the etiology of ANX by rodent studies (Yalcin et al. 2004). Independent and meta-analytic analyses of patients with panic disorder and healthy control participants supported the potential role of *RGS2* (Hohoff et al. 2015). Functional *FKBP5* polymorphisms reportedly increase risk for PTSD in interaction with negative life events (Binder et al. 2008; Mehta et al. 2011). Similar observations were reported for *ADCYAP1R1* (Mercer et al. 2016; Ressler et al. 2011).

Undeniably, candidate gene studies have opened the door to understanding the genetic architecture of ARD. However, our knowledge of their pathogenesis is limited; thus, the likelihood of selected candidate genes being causally related to ARD can be assumed to be very low, and any observed association in a single study is likely to be a false positive (Sullivan 2007). Moreover, the genetic architecture of ARD is known to be highly polygenic, with individual common variants expected to have very modest effects, so that small sets of candidate genes cannot be considered valid models explaining the etiology of these conditions. Much larger studies covering extensive variation over the genome are therefore required to obtain meaningful results.

Genome-Wide Association Studies

Unlike candidate gene studies, which rely on a priori knowledge for gene selection, technological advances have allowed genome-wide association studies (GWASs) to provide an unbiased and hypothesis-free approach to test for associations of common genetic variants across the whole genome. GWAS testing of hundreds of thousands to several million variants requires large samples to secure adequate statistical power. The level of probability needed to reach genome-wide significance (GWS) in a standard GWAS is the standard $\alpha=0.05$ divided by the approximate number of tests (~1,000,000 single-nucleotide polymorphisms [SNPs]), for a derived multiple testing threshold of $P<5\times10^{-8}$. See Table 2–2 for a summary of extant GWASs of ARD.

The first ARD GWAS was attempted for panic disorder in a Japanese population followed by a meta-analysis including 1,147 panic case patients and 2,578 control participants, providing no GWS findings (Otowa et al. 2012). A three-stage discovery GWAS of 909 patients with panic disorder and 915 control participants identified a variant in *TMEM132D* on 12q24 (Erhardt et al. 2011), subsequently confirmed in a larger meta-analysis (Erhardt et al. 2012). Risk genotypes were associated with higher *TMEM132D* mRNA expression in human frontal cortex and Tmem132d mRNA expression in mouse anterior cingulate cortex. A recent GWAS conducted in almost 4,700 patients with panic disorder and 236,000 control participants did not identify any GWS loci. The most significant SNP ($P=3.1\times10^{-7}$) was located on chromosome 4 (A. Forstner, unpublished manuscript).

The first GWAS of childhood anxiety-related behaviors (negative cognition, negative affect, fear, social anxiety, and anxiety composite) in 2,810 children followed up by replication in 4,804 other children found no GWS loci. Although this analysis was underpowered, it provided the first estimates of the proportion of SNP-based heritability (10%) that could be captured genome-wide by common variants (Trzaskowski et al. 2013). SNP heritability estimates are typically limited to contributions from common variants and do not include other sources of heritability captured by twin studies such as rare variants, insertions or deletions, epigenetic effects, and gene-by-environment interactions. Accordingly, heritability estimates derived from twin studies as seen in

TABLE 2–2. **Genome-wide association findings for various anxiety, posttraumatic, and obsessive-compulsive symptoms and disorders**

Phenotype (by study)	Sample size, *n*	Most significant SNP	Nearest gene	*P*
Panic disorder	400	rs860554	*PKP1*	4.60×10^{-8}*
Panic disorder	438 (stage 1 of 3)	rs7309727	*TMEM132D*	5.10×10^{-7}
Panic disorder	2,435	rs10144552	*BDKRB2*	4.43×10^{-6}
Anxiety-related behaviors	2,810 (children)	rs16879771	*CAP2*	6.27×10^{-7}
		rs1952500	*STXBP6*	4.12×10^{-7}
Phobic anxiety	11,127	rs4911015	*LINC00351*	7.38×10^{-7}
Generalized anxiety	12,282 (Hispanic/ Latino)	rs78602344	*THBS2*	4.18×10^{-8}*
Social anxiety	14,592	rs708012	*MTCH1, FGD2*	1.55×10^{-8}*
		rs78924501	*PKN2-AS1*	3.58×10^{-8}*
Anxiety sensitivity	730	rs13334105	*RBFOX1*	4.39×10^{-8}*
Agoraphobic symptoms	1,370	rs78726293	*GLRB*	3.30×10^{-8}*
Composite anxiety disorders	2,294	rs4692589	*MFAP3L*	8.63×10^{-7}
Composite anxiety disorders (case-control)	18,186	rs1709393	*LOC152225*	1.65×10^{-8}*
Composite anxiety disorders (factor score)		rs1067327	*CAMKMT*	2.86×10^{-9}*
Anxiety and stress disorders	31,880	rs7528604	*PDE4B*	5.39×10^{-11}*
Composite anxiety disorders	83,565	rs1187280	*NTRK2*	6.58×10^{-9}*
		rs4855559	*MYH15*	3.70×10^{-8}*
		rs2861139		2.61×10^{-9}*
		rs3807866	*TMEM106B*	4.80×10^{-8}*
		rs17189482		4.20×10^{-9}*
PTSD	1,091	rs8042149	*RORA*	2.50×10^{-8}*
PTSD	7,540	rs6812849	*TLL1*	3.10×10^{-9}*
PTSD	413	rs10170218	*LINC01090*	5.09×10^{-8}
PTSD	3,494	rs6482463	*PRTFDC1*	2.03×10^{-9}
PTSD	147	rs717947	*BC036345*	1.28×10^{-8}*
PTSD	759	rs7866350	*TBC1D2*	1.10×10^{-6}
PTSD	5,049 (European ancestry)	rs159572	*ANKRD55*	2.34×10^{-8}*
	1,312 (African American)	rs11085374	*ZNF626*	4.59×10^{-8}*
PTSD	3,678	Gene-based	*NLGN1*	1.00×10^{-6}
PTSD	254	rs6681483	*OR11L1*	1.83×10^{-6}

TABLE 2–2.   **Genome-wide association findings for various anxiety, posttraumatic, and obsessive-compulsive symptoms and disorders (continued)**

Phenotype (by study)	Sample size, n	Most significant SNP	Nearest gene	P
PTSD	9,691 (African American)	rs139558732	KLHL1	3.33×10^{-8}*
	9,954 (European ancestry)	chr8_125827954_I		1.3×10^{-7}
	20,730 (European ancestry + African American)	rs7400289	MZT1	5.49×10^{-8}
OCD	7,022	rs11081062	DLGAP1	2.49×10^{-6}
OCD	5,061	rs4401971	PTPRD	4.13×10^{-7}
OCD	9,725	rs4733767	CASC8/ CASC11	7.10×10^{-7}
OCD	813	rs12151009	EML2	1.34×10^{-5}
Obsessive-compulsive symptoms	6,931	rs8100480	MEF2BNB	2.56×10^{-8}*

Note. Study participants were adults of European ancestry except where indicated.
SNP=single-nucleotide polymorphism.
*Genome-wide significant association: $P < 5 \times 10^{-8}$.

Table 2–1 tend to be substantially higher than those derived from most large-scale GWASs (Manolio et al. 2009). A GWAS of generalized anxiety symptoms (Dunn et al. 2017) reported a significant association with a variant intronic to *THBS2* in an adult sample ($N = 12,282$) of Hispanic/Latino ancestry that was not supported by replication (SNP heritability 7%). A GWAS for social anxiety symptoms reported separate GWS associations in African and European ancestry subgroups but not in the transethnic meta-analyses (SNP heritability 12%) (Stein et al. 2017).

Important considerations in the genetic research of ARD are the fuzzy boundaries among these syndromes, their high comorbidity, and the degree to which they share genetic risk factors. ARD have extensive lifetime comorbidity with one another as well as with mood and other disorders. Many of these disorders coaggregate in families, and twin studies suggest that this is a result of shared genetic and environmental risk factors (Chantarujikapong et al. 2001; Hettema et al. 2005). Furthermore, genetic factors underlying individual differences in dimensions of anxious temperament also overlap with genetic risk for these disorders (Bienvenu et al. 2007; Hettema et al. 2006). This suggests that the gene networks underlying the dysregulation of emotional processes that produces a progression of anxiety-related traits, ANX, and possibly mood disorders partially overlap with genes for OCD and PTSD. It has therefore been hypothesized that focusing on clusters of ARD might be far more efficient than examining individual disorders.

A GWAS meta-analysis that assembled data from seven independent samples ($N = 18,186$) used both case-control and dimensional indicators to capture all five ANX. For both indicators, GWS associations were observed. Any ANX case-control analyses identified an uncharacterized noncoding RNA locus on chromosomal band 3q12.3, and analyses using a dimensional factor score identified a significant association with variants located in a block containing *CAMKMT* and two other genes on chromosomal band 2p21. The SNP heritability estimates were 14% and 11%, respectively (Otowa et al. 2016). The 2p21 locus was recently replicated in an independent study conducted in approximately 16,000 U.S. soldiers (Hettema et al., in press).

The largest GWAS of ANX conducted so far also made use of composite case-control and dimensional measures, including data from more than 80,000 individuals from the U.K. Biobank (Purves et al., in press). Five GWS loci could be identified, and SNP heritability for these phenotypes was estimated in the range of 25%–30%. Two of the GWS variants were located within intergenic regions and underscore the potential significance of the noncoding genome in the etiology of ANX. Additional novel loci were *NTRK2*, a receptor for brain-derived neurotrophic factor (BDNF) involved in stress response; *TMEM106B*, recently associated with major depression (Wray et al. 2018); and *MYH15*, which is highly expressed in the human brain and was previously associated with nonsyndromal deafness. A GWAS exploring the genetic underpinnings of anxiety and stress-related disorders in iPSYCH included 12,655 case patients with either grouping and 19,225 population-based control subjects and indicated consistent GWS association with *PDE4B*, a gene involved with signal transduction (Meier et al. 2019). Strikingly, mice displaying anxious behavior after exposure to chronic stress showed alterations in the expression of Pde4b in the hippocampus and prefrontal cortex.

Several genome-wide associations have been reported for PTSD (for review, see Daskalakis et al. 2018; Duncan et al. 2018a). These included the genes *RORA*, *TLL1*, *LINC01090*, *PRTFDC1*, *BC036345*, *ANKRD55*, and *ZNF626*. GWS associations are unexpected in studies with such limited sample sizes (all <10,000), and none of these loci has yet been confirmed. The first wave of meta-analyses by the Psychiatric Genomic Consortium (PGC)-PTSD in more than 20,000 subjects across four ancestry groups estimated substantial SNP heritability (29% of females; 7% of males). They identified a GWS locus in African American subjects that did not extend to the rest of the sample (Duncan et al. 2018b). However, their next wave of analyses in 30,000 patients with PTSD and 170,000 control subjects detected three genome-wide significant loci plus several others that were sex specific (Nievergelt et al. 2019).

Two independent GWASs for OCD were initially conducted, neither of which produced GWS findings (Mattheisen et al. 2015; Stewart et al. 2013). Meta-analysis of these samples totaling 2,688 case patients and 7,037 control participants again produced no GWS results; however, the distribution of *P* values shifted toward significance (International Obsessive Compulsive Disorder Foundation Genetics Collaborative and OCD Collaborative Genetics Association Studies 2018). This indicates that with growing sample size, some currently suggestive findings are likely to reach GWS. In addition, a GWAS of obsessive-compulsive symptoms (den Braber et al. 2016) and an exome-focused GWAS of OCD (Costas et al. 2016) have been published without GWS findings as yet. For most variants identified by GWASs, replications in larger studies are warranted to determine whether these or other novel genes truly play a critical role in susceptibility to ARD.

Epigenetic Studies

Epigenetic research has been expanding rapidly in psychiatry and other medical fields (Kular and Kular 2018). It has been suggested that epigenetic mechanisms are responsible for the biological encoding of environmental influences, thereby representing the linking point between genes and environment. Epigenetic modifications can be of long-lasting nature but also are temporally dynamic and responsive to environmental factors altering gene regulation and expression. Epigenetic processes include DNA methylation (mDNA) at cytosine sites, which can result in alterations in affinity of DNA binding sites to regulatory proteins as well as histone acetylation and methylation of specific amino acids that shift chromatin availability for transcriptional activity. Epigenetics processes therefore have been postulated to play a key role in the etiology of ARD (Nieto et al. 2016). Like association studies, early studies targeting methylation alterations largely focused on candidate genes putatively involved in stress response, neurotransmission, and neuroplasticity. Perhaps most studied is the *FKBP5* gene in PTSD (Klengel et al. 2013). Unfortunately, the sample sizes of most candidate methylation studies were limited, thereby lacking the statistical power to detect signals that would survive multiple testing corrections.

Recent advancements in technology, however, now render it possible to examine mDNA patterns at a genome-wide level. The first epigenome-wide association study (EWAS) assessing more than 480,000 cytosine residues observed significant differential mDNA at 40 CpG sites. For most of these sites, relatively lower methylation levels were found in the patients with panic disorder than in the control subjects (Shimada-Sugimoto et al. 2017). In a cohort of 1,522 subjects, significantly increased mDNA at a CpG site in the promoter of the *ASB1* gene correlated with higher levels of generalized anxiety symptoms (Emeny et al. 2018). Finally, sex-stratified analyses in an EWAS including 89 patients with panic disorder and 76 healthy control subjects identified a GWS association at a CpG site regulating HECA expression in females. The same site, located in the enhancer region of the *HECA* gene, also was found to be hypermethylated in a female replication sample (Iurato et al. 2017).

The first EWAS of 65 patients with OCD and 97 healthy control subjects found several differentially methylated genes, suggesting an important role for methylation in the etiology of OCD (Yue et al. 2016). Because of the seminal role of traumatic life events in its pathogenesis, epigenetic mechanisms are possibly of greater relevance in PTSD than is direct genetic variation. Several EWASs with a few hundred individuals have been performed thus far but have not achieved GWS (Daskalakis et al. 2018).

Of note, the sample sizes of EWASs conducted to date have been much smaller than those of GWASs. Thus, increased sample sizes and an optimization of study designs, including longitudinal and genetically sensitive approaches, are required to advance this promising field.

Therapygenetic Studies

A fair number of studies have investigated the genetics of therapeutic response in treatment studies of depression, but the field is still relatively new for ARD. Despite inconsistent disease association findings, interest in serotonin genes persists because of their potential for predicting treatment response. The low-expression 5HTTLPR genotype predicted a better treatment outcome in children with various ANX (Eley et al. 2012) and similarly improved response to 1 week of in vivo exposure therapy in adult panic patients (Knuts et al. 2014). However, the association between 5HTTLPR genotype and cognitive-behavioral therapy (CBT) outcomes in children was not replicated in another cohort. Consistent with previous studies, short-allele homozygotes showed more positive treatment outcomes, but the effects were smaller and nonsignificant (Lester et al. 2016). Similarly, effects of 5HTTLPR, 5HTR2A, and 5HTR1B genotypes on treatment response to antidepressants in OCD have been inconsistent (Zai et al. 2014).

No effects of *COMT* variants have been found for outcomes of CBT in social anxiety (Andersson et al. 2013), but the rs4680 variant has been reported to be associated with a favorable response to pharmacological treatment with venlafaxine in generalized anxiety disorder (Narasimhan et al. 2012). Consistent with the direction of disease association findings, panic disorder patients with long *MAOA* risk alleles benefit less from CBT (Reif et al. 2014). *RGS2* variants were reported to indicate how likely patients with social phobia were to benefit from sertraline treatment (Stein et al. 2014). Further replication is needed for preliminary observations that the Met/Met genotype of the *COMT* gene predicted better response to citalopram (Vulink et al. 2012) and the *BDNF* Met allele predicted worse outcome to CBT (Fullana et al. 2012). In PTSD, 5HTTLPR (Mushtaq et al. 2012), the functional BDNF polymorphism (Felmingham et al. 2013), an *FKBP5* polymorphism (Wilker et al. 2014), and an FAAH polymorphism (Spagnolo et al. 2016) were reported to modulate response to different psychotherapeutic interventions or sertraline pharmacotherapy. Like other candidate gene studies, consistent independent replication is needed to confirm these tentative findings.

In the first therapygenetic GWAS of children with various ANX (Coleman et al. 2016), no GWS association was found with treatment response to CBT. However, a polygenic score for differential susceptibility to the environment was found to be associated with differential outcome following treatment with three different modes of CBT delivery in this sample (Keers et al. 2016). Specifically, those with high polygenic scores for susceptibility to the environment had the best outcome following individual CBT with a therapist and the least good outcome following parent-led guided CBT. Those receiving group CBT had outcomes between these two. Similarly, no GWS associations were reported in treatment outcome for exposure-based CBT in adult patients with panic or phobia (Coleman et al. 2017). For pharmacotherapy in generalized anxiety disorder, no GWS effect on response to venlafaxine could be identified (Jung et al. 2017). The first GWAS in OCD exploring treatment response to serotonin reuptake inhibitors found a significant association near *DISP1* (Qin et al. 2016), a microdeletion region previously implicated in neurological development. No GWASs for PTSD therapy have yet been published.

Perspectives

Genetics of ARD has entered the era of genome-wide analyses. Cohort numbers are still far smaller than those for some other disorders such as schizophrenia. Consortia such as the Anxiety Neuro Genetics Study, UK Biobank, iPsych, PGC-ANX, PGC-

PTSD, and PGC-OCD will vigorously pursue the identification of genes for anxiety and related phenotypes. Given the hypotheses generated by twin studies, some of the genes identified will be pleiotropic (i.e., cross-disorder genes likely underlying the broader affective disorder spectrum). Other genes may more specifically relate to individual endophenotypes involved in the pathogenesis of fear, anxiety, trauma, and obsessive-compulsive phenotypes, ranging from threat-response behaviors such as startle to fear network connectivity in the brain.

Environment plays a major role in the pathogenesis of ARD; thus, epigenetic mechanisms likely will play an important role in mediating gene–environment interactions. This approach is still in its infancy. Although not reviewed here, a major advantage of the study of the genetic basis of ARD is the availability of valid animal models. They will contribute to a better understanding of mechanistic pathways at the neuronal level and more complex processes such as gene–gene and gene–environment interactions. Finally, genome-wide studies provide estimation of polygenic risk scores, which, together with clinical and fear network information, might allow tailoring of therapies at the individual level for an envisioned future of precision medicine.

Key Points

- Anxiety and related disorders (ARD) run in families, with moderate heritability (30%–70%).

- ARD do not "breed true"; rather, they share etiological risk factors among themselves and with comorbid conditions, such as mood disorders.

- As for other mental illnesses, linkage and candidate gene studies have provided little insight into the genetic mechanisms underlying anxiety disorders.

- Upcoming large-scale genome-wide association studies for ARD are poised to discover many novel susceptibility loci.

References

American Psychiatric Association: Diagnostic and Statistical Manual of Mental Disorders, 5th Edition. Arlington, VA, American Psychiatric Association, 2013

Andersson E, Rück C, Lavebratt C, et al: Genetic polymorphisms in monoamine systems and outcome of cognitive behavior therapy for social anxiety disorder. PLoS One 8(11):e79015, 2013 24260145

Bienvenu OJ, Hettema JM, Neale MC, et al: Low extraversion and high neuroticism as indices of genetic and environmental risk for social phobia, agoraphobia, and animal phobia. Am J Psychiatry 164(11):1714–1721, 2007 17974937

Binder EB, Bradley RG, Liu W, et al: Association of FKBP5 polymorphisms and childhood abuse with risk of posttraumatic stress disorder symptoms in adults. JAMA 299(11):1291–1305, 2008 18349090

Browne HA, Gair SL, Scharf JM, et al: Genetics of obsessive-compulsive disorder and related disorders. Psychiatr Clin North Am 37(3):319–335, 2014 25150565

Chantarujikapong SI, Scherrer JF, Xian H, et al: A twin study of generalized anxiety disorder symptoms, panic disorder symptoms and post-traumatic stress disorder in men. Psychiatry Res 103(2–3):133–145, 2001 11549402

Coleman JR, Lester KJ, Keers R, et al: Genome-wide association study of response to cognitive-behavioural therapy in children with anxiety disorders. Br J Psychiatry 209(3):236–243, 2016 26989097

Coleman JR, Lester KJ, Roberts S, et al: Separate and combined effects of genetic variants and pre-treatment whole blood gene expression on response to exposure-based cognitive behavioural therapy for anxiety disorders. World J Biol Psychiatry 18(3):215–226, 2017 27376411

Costas J, Carrera N, Alonso P, et al: Exon-focused genome-wide association study of obsessive-compulsive disorder and shared polygenic risk with schizophrenia. Transl Psychiatry 6:e768, 2016 27023174

Daskalakis NP, Rijal CM, King C, et al: Recent genetics and epigenetics approaches to PTSD. Curr Psychiatry Rep 20(5):30, 2018 29623448

den Braber A, Zilhão NR, Fedko IO, et al: Obsessive-compulsive symptoms in a large population-based twin-family sample are predicted by clinically based polygenic scores and by genome-wide SNPs. Transl Psychiatry 6:e731, 2016 26859814

Duncan LE, Cooper BN, Shen H: Robust findings from 25 years of PTSD genetics research. Curr Psychiatry Rep 20(12):115, 2018a 30350223

Duncan LE, Ratanatharathorn A, Aiello AE, et al: Largest GWAS of PTSD (N=20 070) yields genetic overlap with schizophrenia and sex differences in heritability. Mol Psychiatry 23(3):666–673, 2018b 28439101

Dunn EC, Sofer T, Gallo LC, et al: Genome-wide association study of generalized anxiety symptoms in the Hispanic Community Health Study/Study of Latinos. Am J Med Genet B Neuropsychiatr Genet 174(2):132–143, 2017 27159506

Eley TC, Hudson JL, Creswell C, et al: Therapygenetics: the 5HTTLPR and response to psychological therapy. Mol Psychiatry 17(3):236–237, 2012 22024766

Emeny RT, Baumert J, Zannas AS, et al: Anxiety associated increased CpG methylation in the promoter of Asb1: a translational approach evidenced by epidemiological and clinical studies and a murine model. Neuropsychopharmacology 43(2):342–353, 2018 28540928

Erhardt A, Czibere L, Roeske D, et al: TMEM132D, a new candidate for anxiety phenotypes: evidence from human and mouse studies. Mol Psychiatry 16(6):647–663, 2011 20368705

Erhardt A, Akula N, Schumacher J, et al: Replication and meta-analysis of TMEM132D gene variants in panic disorder. Transl Psychiatry 2:e156, 2012 22948381

Felmingham KL, Dobson-Stone C, Schofield PR, et al: The brain-derived neurotrophic factor Val66Met polymorphism predicts response to exposure therapy in posttraumatic stress disorder. Biol Psychiatry 73(11):1059–1063, 2013 23312562

Fullana MA, Alonso P, Gratacòs M, et al: Variation in the BDNF Val66Met polymorphism and response to cognitive-behavior therapy in obsessive-compulsive disorder. Eur Psychiatry 27(5):386–390, 2012 22153732

Hettema JM, Neale MC, Kendler KS: A review and meta-analysis of the genetic epidemiology of anxiety disorders. Am J Psychiatry 158(10):1568–1578, 2001 11578982

Hettema JM, Prescott CA, Myers JM, et al: The structure of genetic and environmental risk factors for anxiety disorders in men and women. Arch Gen Psychiatry 62(2):182–189, 2005 15699295

Hettema JM, Neale MC, Myers JM, et al: A population-based twin study of the relationship between neuroticism and internalizing disorders. Am J Psychiatry 163(5):857–864, 2006 16648327

Hettema JM, Verhulst B, Chatzinakos C, et al: Genome-wide association study of shared liability to anxiety disorders in Army STARRS. Am J Med Genet B Neuropsychiatr Genet, in press

Hodges LM, Fyer AJ, Weissman MM, et al: Evidence for linkage and association of GABRB3 and GABRA5 to panic disorder. Neuropsychopharmacology 39(10):2423–2431, 2014 24755890

Hohoff C, Weber H, Richter J, et al: RGS2 ggenetic variation: association analysis with panic disorder and dimensional as well as intermediate phenotypes of anxiety. Am J Med Genet B Neuropsychiatr Genet 168B(3):211–222, 2015 25740197

Howe AS, Buttenschøn HN, Bani-Fatemi A, et al: Candidate genes in panic disorder: meta-analyses of 23 common variants in major anxiogenic pathways. Mol Psychiatry 21(5):665–679, 2016 26390831

International Obsessive Compulsive Disorder Foundation Genetics Collaborative and OCD Collaborative Genetics Association Studies: Revealing the complex genetic architecture of obsessive-compulsive disorder using meta-analysis. Mol Psychiatry 23(5):1181–1188, 2018 28761083

Iurato S, Carrillo-Roa T, Arloth J, et al: DNA methylation signatures in panic disorder. Transl Psychiatry 7(12):1287, 2017 29249830

Jacobson LH, Cryan JF: Genetic approaches to modeling anxiety in animals. Curr Top Behav Neurosci 2:161–201, 2010 21309110

Jung J, Tawa EA, Muench C, et al: Genome-wide association study of treatment response to venlafaxine XR in generalized anxiety disorder. Psychiatry Res 254:8–11, 2017 28437668

Keers R, Coleman JR, Lester KJ, et al: A genome-wide test of the differential susceptibility hypothesis reveals a genetic predictor of differential response to psychological treatments for child anxiety disorders. Psychother Psychosom 85(3):146–158, 2016 27043157

Klengel T, Mehta D, Anacker C, et al: Allele-specific FKBP5 DNA demethylation mediates gene-childhood trauma interactions. Nat Neurosci 16(1):33–41, 2013 23201972

Knuts I, Esquivel G, Kenis G, et al: Therapygenetics: 5-HTTLPR genotype predicts the response to exposure therapy for agoraphobia. Eur Neuropsychopharmacol 24(8):1222–1228, 2014 24906789

Kular L, Kular S: Epigenetics applied to psychiatry: clinical opportunities and future challenges. Psychiatry Clin Neurosci 72(4):195–211, 2018 29292553

Lester KJ, Roberts S, Keers R, et al: Non-replication of the association between 5HTTLPR and response to psychological therapy for child anxiety disorders. Br J Psychiatry 208(2):182–188, 2016 26294368

Logue MW, Bauver SR, Knowles JA, et al: Multivariate analysis of anxiety disorders yields further evidence of linkage to chromosomes 4q21 and 7p in panic disorder families. Am J Med Genet B Neuropsychiatr Genet 159B(3):274–280, 2012 22253211

Manolio TA, Collins FS, Cox NJ, et al: Finding the missing heritability of complex diseases. Nature 461(7265):747–753, 2009 19812666

Mathews CA, Badner JA, Andresen JM, et al: Genome-wide linkage analysis of obsessive-compulsive disorder implicates chromosome 1p36. Biol Psychiatry 72(8):629–636, 2012 22633946

Mattheisen M, Samuels JF, Wang Y, et al: Genome-wide association study in obsessive-compulsive disorder: results from the OCGAS. Mol Psychiatry 20(3):337–344, 2015 24821223

Mehta D, Gonik M, Klengel T, et al: Using polymorphisms in FKBP5 to define biologically distinct subtypes of posttraumatic stress disorder: evidence from endocrine and gene expression studies. Arch Gen Psychiatry 68(9):901–910, 2011 21536970

Meier SM, Trontti K, Purves KL, et al: Genetic variants associated with anxiety and stress-related disorders: a genome-wide association study and mouse-model study. JAMA Psychiatry 2019 Epub ahead of print

Mercer KB, Dias B, Shafer D, et al: Functional evaluation of a PTSD-associated genetic variant: estradiol regulation and ADCYAP1R1. Transl Psychiatry 6(12):e978, 2016 27959335

Mushtaq D, Ali A, Margoob MA, et al: Association between serotonin transporter gene promoter-region polymorphism and 4- and 12-week treatment response to sertraline in posttraumatic stress disorder. J Affect Disord 136(3):955–962, 2012 21962566

Narasimhan S, Aquino TD, Multani PK, et al: Variation in the catechol-O-methyltransferase (COMT) gene and treatment response to venlafaxine XR in generalized anxiety disorder. Psychiatry Res 198(1):112–115, 2012 22417933

Nieto SJ, Patriquin MA, Nielsen DA, et al: Don't worry; be informed about the epigenetics of anxiety. Pharmacol Biochem Behav 146–147:60–72, 2016 27189589

Nievergelt CM, Maihofer AX, Klengel T, et al: International meta-analysis of PTSD genome-wide association studies identifies sex- and ancestry-specific genetic risk loci. Nat Commun 10(1):4558, 2019 31594949

Otowa T, Kawamura Y, Nishida N, et al: Meta-analysis of genome-wide association studies for panic disorder in the Japanese population. Transl Psychiatry 2:e186, 2012 23149450

Otowa T, Hek K, Lee M, et al: Meta-analysis of genome-wide association studies of anxiety disorders. Mol Psychiatry 21(10):1391–1399, 2016 26754954

Purves KL, Coleman JRI, Meier SM, et al: A major role for common genetic variation in anxiety disorders. Mol Psychiatry, in press

Qin H, Samuels JF, Wang Y, et al: Whole-genome association analysis of treatment response in obsessive-compulsive disorder. Mol Psychiatry 21(2):270–276, 2016 25824302

Reif A, Richter J, Straube B, et al: MAOA and mechanisms of panic disorder revisited: from bench to molecular psychotherapy. Mol Psychiatry 19(1):122–128, 2014 23319006

Ressler KJ, Mercer KB, Bradley B, et al: Post-traumatic stress disorder is associated with PACAP and the PAC1 receptor. Nature 470(7335):492–497, 2011 21350482

Ross J, Badner J, Garrido H, et al: Genomewide linkage analysis in Costa Rican families implicates chromosome 15q14 as a candidate region for OCD. Hum Genet 130(6):795–805, 2011 21691774

Shimada-Sugimoto M, Otowa T, Hettema JM: Genetics of anxiety disorders: genetic epidemiological and molecular studies in humans. Psychiatry Clin Neurosci 69(7):388–401, 2015 25762210

Shimada-Sugimoto M, Otowa T, Miyagawa T, et al: Epigenome-wide association study of DNA methylation in panic disorder. Clin Epigenetics 9:6, 2017 28149334

Sinopoli VM, Burton CL, Kronenberg S, et al: A review of the role of serotonin system genes in obsessive-compulsive disorder. Neurosci Biobehav Rev 80:372–381, 2017 28576508

Smoller JW: The genetics of stress-related disorders: PTSD, depression, and anxiety disorders. Neuropsychopharmacology 41(1):297–319, 2016 26321314

Smoller JW, Gardner-Schuster E, Covino J: The genetic basis of panic and phobic anxiety disorders. Am J Med Genet C Semin Med Genet 148C(2):118–126, 2008 18412108

Spagnolo PA, Ramchandani VA, Schwandt ML, et al: FAAH gene variation moderates stress response and symptom severity in patients with posttraumatic stress disorder and comorbid alcohol dependence. Alcohol Clin Exp Res 40(11):2426–2434, 2016 27716956

Stein MB, Keshaviah A, Haddad SA, et al: Influence of RGS2 on sertraline treatment for social anxiety disorder. Neuropsychopharmacology 39(6):1340–1346, 2014 24154666

Stein MB, Chen CY, Jain S, et al: Genetic risk variants for social anxiety. Am J Med Genet B Neuropsychiatr Genet 174(2):120–131, 2017 28224735

Stewart SE, Yu D, Scharf JM, et al: Genome-wide association study of obsessive-compulsive disorder. Mol Psychiatry 18(7):788–798, 2013 22889921

Sullivan PF: Spurious genetic associations. Biol Psychiatry 61(10):1121–1126, 2007 17346679

Taylor S: Disorder-specific genetic factors in obsessive-compulsive disorder: a comprehensive meta-analysis. Am J Med Genet B Neuropsychiatr Genet 171B(3):325–332, 2016 26616111

Trzaskowski M, Eley TC, Davis OS, et al: First genome-wide association study on anxiety-related behaviours in childhood. PLoS One 8(4):e58676, 2013 23565138

Vulink NC, Westenberg HG, van Nieuwerburgh F, et al: Catechol-O-methyltransferase gene expression is associated with response to citalopram in obsessive-compulsive disorder. Int J Psychiatry Clin Pract 16(4):277–283, 2012 22414277

Webb BT, Guo AY, Maher BS, et al: Meta-analyses of genome-wide linkage scans of anxiety-related phenotypes. Eur J Hum Genet 20(10):1078–1084, 2012 22473089

Wilker S, Pfeiffer A, Kolassa S, et al: The role of FKBP5 genotype in moderating long-term effectiveness of exposure-based psychotherapy for posttraumatic stress disorder. Transl Psychiatry 4:e403, 2014 24959896

Wray NR, Ripke S, Mattheisen M, et al: Genome-wide association analyses identify 44 risk variants and refine the genetic architecture of major depression. Nat Genet 50(5):668–681, 2018 29700475

Yalcin B, Willis-Owen SA, Fullerton J, et al: Genetic dissection of a behavioral quantitative trait locus shows that Rgs2 modulates anxiety in mice. Nat Genet 36(11):1197–1202, 2004 15489855

Yue W, Cheng W, Liu Z, et al: Genome-wide DNA methylation analysis in obsessive-compulsive disorder patients. Sci Rep 6:31333, 2016 27527274

Zai G, Brandl EJ, Müller DJ, et al: Pharmacogenetics of antidepressant treatment in obsessive-compulsive disorder: an update and implications for clinicians. Pharmacogenomics 15(8):1147–1157, 2014 25084207

Recommended Readings

Browne HA, Gair SL, Scharf JM, et al: Genetics of obsessive-compulsive disorder and related disorders. Psychiatr Clin North Am 37(3):319–335, 2014

Daskalakis NP, Rijal CM, King C, et al: Recent genetics and epigenetics approaches to PTSD. Curr Psychiatry Rep 20(5):30, 2018

Meier SM, Deckert J: Genetics of anxiety disorders. Curr Psychiatry Rep 21(3):16, 2019

CHAPTER 3

Neural Circuits in Fear and Anxiety

Research Domain Criteria: Preclinical to Clinical

J. Douglas Bremner, M.D.

In this chapter, we review neural correlates of fear and anxiety and the clinical neuroscience of human anxiety and trauma- and stressor-related disorders built on basic research. We make connections between neurobiology and functional neuroanatomy and the clinical and symptomatic presentation of patients with anxiety and trauma-related disorders based on DSM-5 (American Psychiatric Association 2013), as well as the Research Domain Criteria (RDoC)-based Negative Valence Systems Domain, including potential threat (anxiety), acute threat (fear), and sustained threat. This work is ongoing, and many of the models proposed may be subject to modification and revision as our knowledge base in this exciting area continues to expand.

Development of a Model for the Neural Circuitry of Fear and Anxiety

History of Biological Models for Anxiety

Hypotheses related to the neurobiology of human anxiety have a long history. Early neuroanatomical studies showed that removal of a cat's cerebral cortex—which left only subcortical regions including the amygdala, thalamus, hippocampus, and hypothalamus—resulted in accentuated fearful responses to potentially threatening or novel stimuli, accompanied by signs of diffuse sympathetic activation, such as increased blood pressure, sweating, piloerection, and increased secretion of epinephrine from the adrenal medulla (Cannon 1987). This behavioral response came to be referred to as *sham rage* and led to the original hypothesis that subcortical brain structures above the level of the midbrain, such as the hypothalamus, hippocampus, cingulate, entorhinal cortex, and thalamus, mediate human anxiety responses (Papez 1937; reviewed in LeDoux 1996). MacLean (reviewed in LeDoux 1996) later added the amygdala to the "Papez circuit" of "limbic" brain structures, so-called because of their evolutionary relationship to olfaction, which was hypothesized to play a role in fear and anxiety. Work by LeDoux (1993) and Davis (1992) confirmed the important role of the amygdala in animal models of fear and anxiety.

Neuroanatomical hypotheses have subsequently been developed related to specific anxiety disorders, including panic disorder, social anxiety disorder (social phobia), and generalized anxiety disorder (GAD; Charney et al. 2014), and trauma- and stressor-related disorders, including PTSD and acute stress disorder (Bremner and Pearce 2016; Campanella and Bremner 2016). These disorders were previously grouped under the anxiety disorders, but PTSD and acute stress disorder are now in a separate category of trauma- and stressor-related disorders in DSM-5. Nevertheless, it is useful to consider them together when evaluating neural circuits and systems that underlie their symptoms, because alterations in neurochemical and neurotransmitter systems that have been hypothesized to play a role in fear and anxiety—including norepinephrine, cortisol, benzodiazepines, and other neurochemical and neuropeptidal systems that mediate the stress response—also likely underlie the symptoms of all these disorders (Charney and Bremner 1999). Additionally, other psychiatric disorders linked to stress, including dissociative disorders and borderline personality disorder, have been characterized as part of the trauma spectrum disorders (Bremner 2002). They are not classified as trauma-related disorders, have not been the subject of extensive research, and are only lightly touched on here, although an understanding of the neural circuits involved in fear and anxiety will likely be informative to investigations of their neurobiology.

Animal models of fear and anxiety are directly translatable to the RDoC constructs of acute threat, potential threat, and sustained threat, all part of the Negative Valence Systems Domain. These three constructs all involve alerting, avoidance, and heightened attention behaviors with physiological arousal that are part of the body's fight-or-flight response but are activated by varying degrees of real or perceived threat. Their manifestations in psychiatry are seen as potential threat underlying the anxiety disorders (panic disorder, social phobia, GAD) and acute and sustained threats underlying PTSD and acute stress disorder.

Working Model for Fear and Anxiety

We have developed a working model for the neural circuitry of fear and anxiety based on data from animal studies, human brain lesion studies, and studies of the neurobiology of psychiatric disorders related to fear and anxiety (Bremner 2003, 2016; Bremner and Charney 2010). The model explains how information related to a threatening stimulus (e.g., being attacked by a tiger) enters the primary senses (smell, sight, touch, hearing, or the body's own visceral information), is integrated into a coherent image grounded in space and time, activates memory traces of previous similar experiences with the appropriate emotional valence (necessary to evaluate the true threat potential of the stimulus), and triggers an appropriate motor response. Specific brain circuits that mediate these responses make up the neural circuitry of fear and anxiety,

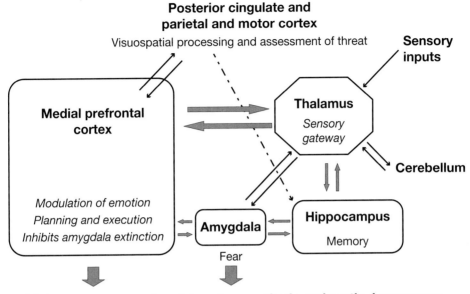

FIGURE 3–1. Neural circuits in fear and anxiety.

Brain areas involved in the circuit include the amygdala, hippocampus, and prefrontal cortex. Other brain areas are involved in processing sensory information, positioning in time and space, and making associations in memory and context as part of the response to threat, including the parietal cortex, insula, posterior cingulate, and cerebellum. The medial prefrontal cortex activates peripheral neurohormonal and autonomic responses to threat.

including the amygdala; hippocampus; frontal, temporal, and parietal cortices; insula; cerebellum; and visual association areas (Figure 3–1).

Primary sensory information enters through the primary sensory areas and is relayed from there to other parts of the brain. These sensory inputs are relayed through the dorsal thalamus to cortical brain areas, such as the primary visual (occipital), auditory (temporal), or tactile (postcentral gyrus) cortical areas. Olfactory sensory input, however, has direct inputs to the amygdala and entorhinal cortex. Input from peripheral visceral organs is relayed through the vagus nerve to the nucleus tractus solitarius and from there to the locus coeruleus, site of most of the brain's noradrenergic neurons, and other central brain areas. Information about peripheral inflammatory and autonomic function is also relayed through the vagus nerve to the brain. Primary association areas are adjacent to cortisol areas involved in processing the information (e.g., the primary occipital cortex [area 17] is medial and flanked by the visual association cortex [area 18]). More complex visual processes, such as facial recognition, are mediated by the adjacent lingual gyrus, fusiform gyrus, and inferior temporal gyrus.

Prefrontal and Parietal Cortex, Posterior Cingulate, Insula, and Cerebellum

Cognitive appraisal of potential threat is also an important aspect of the stress response. The parietal cortex, including the angular gyrus and inferior parietal lobule, is involved in placing an object in space and time and awareness of the self in space and time, which is critical in the response to a threat. The posterior cingulate, which has connections to the parietal cortex, hippocampus, and adjacent cortex, plays an important role in visuospatial processing, key to the evaluation of threat (Vogt et al. 1992). The prefrontal cortex also is involved in memory and cognition and, with the parietal cortex, has important dual reciprocal connections with all of the subcortical areas mentioned earlier as well as the insula (Selemon and Goldman-Rakic 1988). The dorsolateral prefrontal cortex is involved in declarative and working memory and action planning (Goldman-Rakic 1988). The prefrontal cortex and parietal cortex work in concert in the alerting and planning aspects of the stress response that are critical for survival. The anterior cingulate (Brodmann areas 24 and 32) is involved in selection of responses for action as well as emotion (Devinsky et al. 1995). This area and other medial portions of the prefrontal cortex, including the subgenual area (Brodmann area 25) and orbitofrontal cortex, modulate emotional and physiological responses to stress. Inhibition of the amygdala by the anterior cingulate/medial prefrontal cortex represents the neural correlate of extinction of fear responses (Quirk et al. 2006). Phineas Gage, in a famous case, had a railroad spike lesion his medial prefrontal cortex (including orbitofrontal cortex [Brodmann area 25], ventromedial prefrontal cortex, and anterior cingulate [Brodmann areas 24 and 32]) and experienced deficits in emotional intelligence and socially appropriate interactions (Damasio et al. 1994), showing its importance in human emotion. This area, together with the insula, also modulates peripheral cardiovascular and neurohormonal responses to stress, including heart rate, blood pressure, and cortisol response (Roth et al. 1988). Finally, the cerebellum, which is involved in motor coordination, also plays a role in the stress response (Adamaszek et al. 2017).

Hippocampus

The hippocampus, which is particularly vulnerable to stress, plays an important role in memory. The hippocampus and adjacent cortex mediate declarative memory function (e.g., recall of facts and lists) and play an important role in the integration of memory elements at the time of retrieval, as well as in assigning significance to events within space and time (Squire and Zola-Morgan 1991). The hippocampus also mediates memory for the context of events and, therefore, fear related to environments previously associated with threat (Phillips and LeDoux 1992). Stress is associated with decreased neurogenesis and loss of dendritic branching in the CA3 region of the hippocampus (Nibuya et al. 1995; Sapolsky 1996) and related memory deficits (Diamond et al. 1996). These effects are reversed by antidepressants (Duman et al. 2001; Santarelli et al. 2003) and enhancement of the environment, including running (van Praag et al. 1999). With long-term storage, memories shift from the hippocampus to the neocortical areas (Squire and Zola-Morgan 1991), at which time memories become indelible and resistant to modification. Following the development of indelible memories, *traumatic cues,* such as a particular sight or sound reminiscent of the original traumatic event, will trigger a cascade of anxiety- and fear-related symptoms with associated physiological responses, often without conscious recall of the original traumatic event. In patients with PTSD, however, the traumatic stimulus is always potentially identifiable. Symptoms of anxiety in patients with panic or phobic disorder, however, often are not related to an easily identifiable cue of a traumatic memory.

Amygdala

The amygdala plays a critical role in fear memory (Davis 1992; LeDoux 1993). *Conditioned fear*, in which pairing of a neutral (conditioned) stimulus with a fear-inducing (unconditioned) stimulus results in fear responses to the neutral stimulus alone, is mediated by the amygdala (Davis 1992; LeDoux et al. 1990). Lesions of the central nucleus of the amygdala block fear conditioning, whereas electrical stimulation of the central nucleus increases acoustic startle. The central nucleus of the amygdala projects to various brain structures involved in fear. It also has pathways through the lateral hypothalamus to the periphery, where it activates physiological responses to fear, including sympathetic autonomic function (Iwata et al. 1986). Electrical stimulation of the amygdala in cats resulted in peripheral signs of autonomic hyperactivity and fear-related behaviors that are seen in the wild when the animal is being attacked or is attacking, including alerting, chewing, salivation, piloerection, turning, facial twitching, arching of the back, hissing, and snarling, associated with an increase in catecholamine turnover (Hilton and Zbrozyna 1963). Electrical stimulation of the amygdala in human subjects resulted in signs and symptoms of fear and anxiety, including an increase in heart rate and blood pressure, increased muscle tension, subjective sensations of fear or anxiety (Chapman et al. 1954), and increases in peripheral catecholamines (Gunne and Reis 1963). These findings show that the amygdala plays an important role in fear and responses to threat. Increased activity of the amygdala and dysfunction of the anterior cingulate/medial prefrontal cortex in patients with PTSD likely underlie increased acquisition and failure of extinction, respectively, and represent the neural circuitry of anxiety disorders.

Neocortex

Ultimately, effective responses to threat require integration of multiple brain areas. The prefrontal cortex and anterior cingulate hold multiple pieces of information in working memory during the execution of a response (Goldman-Rakic 1988). The parietal cortex and posterior cingulate mediate visuospatial processing and awareness of self and the threat in space and time. The precentral gyrus (motor cortex) plans for action by executing potential movements (fight or flight) in thought before taking action. The cerebellum has a well-known role in motor movement and is involved in planning for action; however, studies consistently show a role in cognition and emotion as well (Adamaszek et al. 2017). Connections between these areas mediate response to threat and play a critical role in responses to threat that facilitate survival. The striatum (caudate and putamen) modulates motor responses to stress. The dense innervation of the striatum and prefrontal cortex by the amygdala indicates that the amygdala can regulate both of these systems. These interactions between the amygdala and the extrapyramidal motor system may be very important for generating motor responses to threatening stimuli, especially stimuli related to adverse experiences (McDonald 1991a, 1991b).

Neurohormonal Responses

Neurohormonal systems, including cortisol and the sympathetic and parasympathetic systems, are critical for the physiological responses that are necessary for survival in the face of threat. Activation of the sympathetic system results in increases in blood pressure and heart rate, increased respiration, sweating, piloerection, and pupil dilatation. Stress stimulates the release of corticotropin-releasing factor (CRF) from the paraventricular nucleus of the hypothalamus, which increases peripheral adreno-corticotropic hormone and cortisol levels. Norepinephrine cell bodies are located in the locus coeruleus in the midbrain, with axons releasing neurotransmitter through-out the cerebral cortex and fear network in response to stress (Bremner et al. 1996a, 1996b). The vagus nerve mediates the parasympathetic nervous system, which has opposite effects to the sympathetic system.

Function of the brain areas of the fear and anxiety network, including the prefrontal cortex, amygdala, and hippocampus, is mediated by specific neurochemical systems that mediate the stress response. Increased release of glucocorticoids, catecholamines (norepinephrine, epinephrine, and dopamine), serotonin, benzodiazepines, and en-dogenous opiates is associated with acute stress exposure. We have hypothesized that long-term dysregulation of these systems acting on brain areas outlined earlier in this chapter mediates the symptoms of pathological anxiety (Bremner and Charney 2010; Bremner and Pearce 2016; Bremner et al. 1999a).

Application of the Neural Circuitry Model of Anxiety and Fear to Anxiety Disorders

Clinical neuroscience research on PTSD and the anxiety disorders aims to apply find-ings related to the effects of stress on the brain in animals (which are used as models of both PTSD and anxiety) to patients with these disorders. Animal models have lim-itations and are not directly applicable to human anxiety disorders because different anxiety disorders are expressed in different ways (e.g., panic disorder has important symptomatic differences from PTSD). Animal models, however, can be very useful in guiding research in the trauma-related and anxiety disorders. We have posited that PTSD, panic disorder, and phobic disorders share many neurobiological and phe-nomenological characteristics and can benefit from the application of animal models of stress (Charney and Bremner 1999). OCD does not fit as easily with these disorders (and therefore is not discussed in depth in this chapter).

Neural circuits mediating symptoms of anxiety disorders can be studied by mea-suring neurotransmitter and hormone levels in blood, urine, and saliva; assessing behavioral and biochemical responses to pharmacological challenge to specific neu-rochemical systems; measuring brain structures with structural neuroimaging; pro-voking disease-specific symptoms in conjunction with functional neuroimaging; or using imaging to measure neuroreceptors.

Brain Imaging Studies in PTSD

Several replicated studies showed hippocampal atrophy with associated verbal mem-ory deficits in PTSD (Bremner and Vermetten 2012; Bremner et al. 1995; Kitayama et al. 2005; Smith 2005). Studies have also shown a reduction in N-acetyl aspartate, a marker of neuronal activity, in the hippocampus, as well as a failure of hippocampal activation during memory tasks as measured with functional neuroimaging (Bremner

2006). One study showed a genetic contribution to smaller hippocampal volume in PTSD (Gilbertson et al. 2002). Treatment with the selective serotonin reuptake inhibitor (SSRI) paroxetine resulted in an increase in hippocampal volume in patients with PTSD (Vermetten et al. 2003). Considering the role played by the hippocampus in the integration of memory elements stored in primary-sensory and secondary-association cortical areas at the time of retrieval, the findings suggest a possible neural correlate for symptoms of memory fragmentation and dysfunction in PTSD (Bremner 2006).

The anterior cingulate/medial prefrontal cortex is also implicated in PTSD. Studies in animals showed that early stress results in a decrease in neuronal branching in the medial prefrontal cortex (Radley et al. 2004). Researchers have used MRI to show smaller volume of the anterior cingulate in PTSD (Kitayama et al. 2006; Rauch et al. 2003; Woodward et al. 2006).

Researchers have used functional imaging, including functional MRI and PET, during provocation of PTSD symptom states to identify neural correlates of PTSD symptomatology and traumatic remembrance (Campanella and Bremner 2016). The most consistent finding from these studies was a decrease in medial prefrontal function (Bremner et al. 1999b; Shin et al. 2004), with some studies showing decreased hippocampal and parietal function and increased posterior cingulate function. Exposure to external threatening stimuli, such as exposure to fearful faces (Rauch et al. 2000) or fear conditioning (Bremner et al. 2005), was associated with increased amygdala function.

Several studies showed alterations in hippocampus and adjacent cortex (parahippocampus) function in panic disorder, with no change in hippocampal volume. Individuals with social phobia showed increased amygdala response to contemptuous faces (Stein et al. 2002). In simple phobias, altered amygdala function has not been consistently shown; instead, a circuit including increased visual association and decreased dorsolateral and hippocampal function has been associated with induction of phobic symptoms (Bremner 2005).

These findings point to a network of related regions as mediating symptoms of anxiety disorders. The anterior cingulate/medial prefrontal cortex, as reviewed here, plays an important role in the modulation of emotion and extinction of fear through inhibition of amygdala function. The amygdala is responsible for executing the fear response. The posterior cingulate plays an important role in visuospatial processing (Devinsky et al. 1995; Vogt et al. 1992) and is therefore an important component of preparation for coping with a physical threat. The posterior cingulate has functional connections with the hippocampus and adjacent cortex, which led to its original classification as part of the "limbic brain" (Gray 1982). The hippocampus is involved in declarative memory as well as contextual fear. We previously argued that anterior cingulate/medial prefrontal activation represents a "normal" brain response to traumatic stimuli that serves to inhibit feelings of fearfulness when no true threat is present. Failure of activation in this area or decreased blood flow in this region in individuals with PTSD may lead to increased fearfulness that is not appropriate for the context, a behavioral response highly characteristic of patients with PTSD, possibly through failure of inhibition of the amygdala.

Understanding neural circuits has clinical relevance for PTSD and anxiety disorders. According to our model, subcortical memory traces related to trauma may be indelible and account for repetitive memories specific to PTSD that are often resistant to treatment. Patients with anxiety disorders also have symptoms that reflect a continuous perception of threat. The inability to distinguish true threat from perceived threat in innocuous situations is, in fact, highly characteristic of the anxiety disorders. The animal model of contextual fear conditioning may represent a good model for these symptoms. Preclinical data reviewed earlier suggest that the hippocampus plays an important role in the mediation of contextual fear and that increased responding to a conditioned stimulus is due to hippocampal dysfunction. Hippocampal atrophy in PTSD, as described earlier in this chapter, therefore provides a possible neuroanatomical substrate for abnormal contextual fear conditioning and chronic feelings of threat and anxiety in PTSD.

Alterations in Neurochemical Stress Response Systems in Patients With Anxiety Disorders

Patients with trauma-related and anxiety disorders have long-term alterations in neurochemical systems that mediate the stress response and have been shown to be sensitive to chronic stress (Tables 3–1, 3–2, and 3–3).

Hypothalamic-Pituitary-Adrenal Axis Function in PTSD

Studies on the effects of stress on neurohormonal systems in animals have been applied to PTSD, with several studies reporting alterations in hypothalamic-pituitary-adrenal (HPA) axis function in PTSD (reviewed in Yehuda 2006). In general, studies show decreased or normal resting cortisol levels, and studies that used assessment in plasma at multiple time points over a 24-hour period showed decreased resting cortisol levels (Bremner et al. 2007; Yehuda 2006; Yehuda et al. 1994, 1996). Other studies showed heightened cortisol response to stress, including traumatic reminders (Elzinga et al. 2003). Other findings in PTSD include enhanced cortisol negative feedback inhibition that seems to result from increased responsiveness of glucocorticoid receptors (Yehuda et al. 1993) and elevated levels of CRF in cerebrospinal fluid (Baker et al. 2005; Bremner et al. 1997b). The neuroendocrine alterations observed in PTSD suggest an increased sympathetic and central CRF activation in the face of reduced cortisol signaling.

Norepinephrine in PTSD

Studies have documented alterations in other stress-responsive neurochemical systems in PTSD. Animal studies show norepinephrine plays a key role in the stress response (Aston-Jones et al. 1991). Patients with PTSD have increased norepinephrine in blood and urine, increased norepinephrine response to traumatic reminders, and increased behavioral and biochemical response (Bremner et al. 1996a, 1996b; Southwick et al. 1993) as well as brain response (Bremner et al. 1997a) to yohimbine (which stimulates the norepinephrine system). Psychophysiology studies also are consistent with increased noradrenergic function. For example, PTSD is characterized by increased heart rate and blood pressure response to reminders of trauma, in addition to increased norepinephrine release (McFall et al. 1990); these physiological indicators are controlled by noradrenergic function, and they increase the risk of cardiac morbidity (Vaccarino and Bremner 2015).

TABLE 3–1. **Evidence for alterations in catecholaminergic function in anxiety disorders**

Finding	PTSD	Panic disorder
Increased resting heart rate and blood pressure	±	±
Increased heart rate and blood pressure response to traumatic reminders/panic attacks	+++	++
Increased resting urinary norepinephrine and epinephrine	+	++
Increased resting plasma norepinephrine or MHPG	–	–
Increased plasma norepinephrine with traumatic reminders/ panic attacks	+	±
Increased orthostatic heart rate response to exercise	+	+
Decreased binding to platelet α_2 receptors	+	±
Decrease in basal and stimulated activity of cAMP	±	+
Decrease in platelet monoamine oxidase activity	+	?
Increased symptoms, heart rate, and plasma MHPG with yohimbine noradrenergic challenge	+	+++
Differential brain metabolic response to yohimbine	+	+

Note. –=one or more studies did not support this finding (with no positive studies), or the majority of studies did not support this finding; ±=an equal number of studies supported and did not support this finding; +=at least one study supported this finding, with no studies not supporting the finding, or the majority of studies supported the finding; ++=two or more studies supported this finding, with no studies not supporting the finding; +++=three or more studies supported this finding, with no studies not supporting the finding; cAMP=cyclic adenosine monophosphate; MHPG=3-methoxy-4-hydroxyphenylglycol.

TABLE 3–2. **Evidence for alterations in CRF/HPA axis function in anxiety disorders**

Finding	PTSD	Panic disorder
Alterations in urinary cortisol	±*	±
Altered plasma cortisol with 24-hour sampling	++	+ (increased)
Supersuppression with DST	+++	–
Blunted ACTH response to CRF	±	±
Elevated CRF in cerebrospinal fluid	+++	+
Increased lymphocyte glucocorticoid receptors	++	NT

Note. –=one or more studies did not support this finding (with no positive studies), or the majority of studies did not support this finding; ±=an equal number of studies supported this finding and did not support this finding; +=at least one study supported this finding, with no studies not supporting the finding, or the majority of studies supported the finding; ++=two or more studies supported this finding, with no studies not supporting the finding; +++=three or more studies supported this finding, with no studies not supporting the finding; ACTH=adrenocorticotropic hormone; CRF=corticotropin-releasing factor; DST=dexamethasone suppression test; HPA=hypothalamic-pituitary-adrenal; NT=not tested (to our knowledge).
*Findings of decreased urinary cortisol levels in older male combat veterans and Holocaust survivors and increased cortisol levels in younger female abuse survivors may be explainable by differences in sex, age, trauma type, or developmental epoch at the time of the trauma.

TABLE 3–3.   **Evidence for alterations in other neurotransmitter systems in anxiety disorders**

Finding	PTSD	Panic disorder
Benzodiazepine		
Increased symptomatology with benzodiazepine antagonist	–	++
Opiate		
Naloxone-reversible analgesia	+	
Increased plasma β-endorphin response to exercise	+	
Increased endogenous opiates in CSF	+	
Serotonin		
Decreased serotonin reuptake site binding in platelets	++	
Decreased serotonin transmitter in platelets	–	
Blunted prolactin response to buspirone (5-HT$_{1A}$ probe)	–	
Altered serotonin effect on cAMP in platelets (5-HT$_{1A}$ probe)	–	
Thyroid		
Increased baseline thyroxine level	+	
Increased TSH response to TRH	+	
Somatostatin		
Increased somatostatin levels at baseline in CSF	+	
Cholecystokinin (CCK)		
Increased anxiety symptoms with CCK administration	NT	++

Note.   –=one or more studies did not support this finding (with no positive studies), or the majority of studies did not support this finding; +=at least one study supported this finding, with no studies not supporting the finding, or the majority of studies supported the finding; ++=two or more studies supported this finding, with no studies not supporting the finding; cAMP=cyclic adenosine monophosphate; CSF=cerebrospinal fluid; 5-HT$_{1A}$=serotonin type 1A; NT=not tested (to our knowledge); TRH=thyrotropin-releasing hormone; TSH=thyroid-stimulating hormone.

Neurohormonal Function in Panic Disorder

In patients with panic disorder, the responsiveness of the HPA system to a combined dexamethasone-CRF challenge test was higher than in psychiatrically healthy control subjects but lower than in patients with depression. The difference in responsiveness between patients with panic disorder and those with depression may be due to over-expression of vasopressin in major depression, which is known to synergize the effect of CRF at corticotropes. The results of the combined dexamethasone-CRF test indicate that a substantial portion of patients with panic disorder have disturbed HPA system regulation. If sensitization by repetitive panic attacks is indeed responsible for progressive HPA dysregulation, and if progressive HPA dysregulation is indeed of decisive importance for the pathogenesis of panic disorder, then therapeutic strategies capable of dampening the hyperactivity of the HPA–locus coeruleus "alarm system" are indicated. Patients with panic disorder also have been shown to have increased noradrenergic function as measured by increased responsiveness to yohimbine and other measures.

Release of glucocorticoids and catecholamines with stress may modulate the encoding of memories of the stressful event. Among the most characteristic features of anxiety disorders such as PTSD and panic disorder is that memories of the traumatic experience or original panic attack remain indelible for decades and are easily reawakened by various stimuli and stressors. The strength of traumatic memories relates, in part, to the degree to which certain neuromodulatory systems, particularly catecholamines and glucocorticoids, are activated by the traumatic experience. Evidence from experimental and clinical investigations suggests that memory processes remain susceptible to modulating influences after information has been acquired. Long-term alterations in these catecholaminergic and glucocorticoid systems also may be responsible for fragmentation of memories, hyperamnesia, amnesia, deficits in declarative memory, delayed recall of abuse, and other aspects of the wide range of memory distortions in PTSD.

Effects of Pharmacotherapy on Brain Circuits Mediating Anxiety

Pharmacotherapy for anxiety is associated with a modulation of neurohormonal systems mediating symptoms of anxiety. Administration of benzodiazepine medications acts directly on the GABA/benzodiazepine complex to promote release of the inhibitory neurotransmitter GABA. The SSRIs increase serotonin concentrations, which has secondary effects on glucocorticoid and noradrenergic systems. SSRIs have been shown to decrease cortisol response and autonomic response to stress in patients with PTSD (Vermetten et al. 2006). Antidepressants also promote nerve growth in the hippocampus, an effect that has been hypothesized to underlie the mechanism by which antidepressants are efficacious for anxiety and depression (Santarelli et al. 2003).

Working Model for the Neural Circuitry of Anxiety Disorders

Study findings reviewed in this chapter are consistent with dysfunction of an interrelated neurochemical and neuroanatomical system in human trauma-related and anxiety disorders. PTSD and panic disorder have several biological and phenomenological similarities that allow them to be considered in relation to each other. Investigation of phobic disorders and GAD is still in the early stages; although they have some phenomenological similarities to PTSD and panic disorder, it is premature to include these disorders in a model for human anxiety disorders. OCD is different in many ways from these other disorders and therefore has not been reviewed in this chapter. PTSD is related more to the deleterious effects of environmental stress, whereas panic disorder is not as clearly related to stress and may be related more to genetic variability in anxiety. Therefore, a model can be created that incorporates information from animal and clinical research relevant to these disorders, keeping in mind that working models are subject to modification with new information and that generalizations involving causality should be seen as merely speculative when derived from clinical studies that are, by their very nature, cross-sectional.

A biological model to explain pathological human anxiety should include both brain stem circuits and cortical and subcortical regions involved in memory and modulation of emotion. The evidence reviewed in this chapter is consistent with chronically increased function of neurochemical systems (CRF and norepinephrine) that mediate the stress response in trauma-related and anxiety disorders. Although activity at the central portion of the HPA axis is increased, responses at other portions of the HPA axis, including the pituitary and adrenal, and long-term effects on the hormonal final product, cortisol, do not show increased concentrations of the hormone. Instead, levels are normal or low. Increased norepinephrine and CRF released in the brain act on specific brain areas (including the hippocampus; medial prefrontal, temporal, and parietal cortices; and cingulate) that are dysfunctional in human anxiety disorders. Other neurochemical systems, including benzodiazepines, opiates, dopamine, cholecystokinin, and neuropeptide Y, also play a role.

Hippocampal dysfunction may play a role in the pathological symptoms of anxiety. In stress-related anxiety disorders (i.e., PTSD), symptoms and cognitive dysfunction associated with PTSD may be linked to hippocampal dysfunction. Several studies showed similar brain findings in trauma-related disorders (including patients with early trauma and a diagnosis of dissociative identity disorder or borderline personality disorder, neither of which is covered in this chapter) not seen in other anxiety disorders such as panic disorder or OCD. This led to the hypothesis of trauma spectrum disorders, which include PTSD (Bremner 2002). Subjective feelings of anxiety are common, however, in PTSD and the anxiety disorders and are likely related to elevated norepinephrine, autonomic function, CRF, and possibly neuropeptidal systems, although they differ in that a threat is more easily identified in the former.

The medial prefrontal cortex also plays a prominent role in fear and anxiety. Moving up in terms of species complexity, the most salient change in brain architecture is the massive increase in cortical gray matter, especially in the frontal cortex. It is therefore not surprising that the frontal lobe plays a role in the phenomenon uniquely associated with our species—that is, emotion. The medial portion of the prefrontal cortex has an important role in human emotion and anxiety, with inhibitory inputs that decrease amygdala responsiveness and mediate extinction of fear responses. This area also stimulates the peripheral cortisol and sympathetic response to stress. We have hypothesized that dysfunction in this area may mediate increased emotionality and failure of extinction to fear-inducing cues in trauma-related and anxiety disorders. Evidence to support this idea includes failure of normal activation in this area with yohimbine-induced provocation of anxiety in both PTSD and panic disorder as well as failure of activation and decreased blood flow with traumatic cue exposure in PTSD. Again, potentiated release of norepinephrine with stressors in PTSD and panic disorder is expected to be associated with a relative decrease in neuron function in this area. Findings in anxiety disorder research are consistently supportive of a role for the medial prefrontal cortex in emotionality, with a long history of literature, mostly from studies of lesions in human subjects.

Key Points

- Underlying the symptoms of trauma-related and anxiety disorders are alterations in the function and structure of brain areas involved in stress and memory.

- These alterations involve neurotransmitters and neural circuits that play a critical role in the stress response.

- Specific alterations include increased function of the neurochemical systems (i.e., corticotropin-releasing factor, cortisol, and norepinephrine) that mediate the stress response, as well as dysregulation of the hypothalamic-pituitary-adrenal axis.

- The affected neurotransmitters and neurohormones are released in specific brain areas (including the hippocampus; medial prefrontal, temporal, and parietal cortices; and cingulate) that are dysfunctional in human trauma-related and anxiety disorders.

- Other neurochemical systems, including benzodiazepines, opiates, dopamine, cholecystokinin, and neuropeptide Y, also play a role in the maintenance of anxiety symptoms.

- Studies performed to date are encouraging, in that many findings from animal studies have been successfully applied to human anxiety disorders.

- The past decade has seen an exciting expansion of research in human trauma-related and anxiety disorders. Future research must continue to apply findings from the revolution in neuroscience to increase understanding of human anxiety disorders.

References

Adamaszek M, D'Agata F, Ferrucci R, et al: Consensus paper: Cerebellum and emotion. Cerebellum 16(2):552–576, 2017 27485952

American Psychiatric Association: Diagnostic and Statistical Manual of Mental Disorders, 5th Edition. Arlington, VA, American Psychiatric Association, 2013

Aston-Jones G, Shipley MT, Chouvet G, et al: Afferent regulation of locus coeruleus neurons: anatomy, physiology and pharmacology. Prog Brain Res 88:47–75, 1991 1687622

Baker DG, Ekhator NN, Kasckow JW, et al: Higher levels of basal serial CSF cortisol in combat veterans with posttraumatic stress disorder. Am J Psychiatry 162(5):992–994, 2005 15863803

Bremner JD: Does Stress Damage the Brain? New York, WW Norton, 2002

Bremner JD: Functional neuroanatomical correlates of traumatic stress revisited 7 years later, this time with data. Psychopharmacol Bull 37(2):6–25, 2003 14566211

Bremner JD: Brain Imaging Handbook. New York, WW Norton, 2005

Bremner JD: Traumatic stress: effects on the brain. Dialogues Clin Neurosci 8(5):445–461, 2006 17290802

Bremner JD (ed): Posttraumatic Stress Disorder: From Neurobiology to Treatment. Hoboken, NJ, Wiley-Blackwell, 2016

Bremner JD, Charney DS: Neural circuits in fear and anxiety, in Textbook of Anxiety Disorders. Edited by Stein DJ, Hollander E, Rothbaum BO. Washington, DC, American Psychiatric Publishing, 2010, pp 55–71

Bremner JD, Pearce B: Neurotransmitter, neurohormonal, and neuropeptidal function in PTSD, in Posttraumatic Stress Disorder: From Neurobiology to Treatment. Edited by Bremner JD. Hoboken, NJ, Wiley-Blackwell, 2016, pp 181–232

Bremner JD, Vermetten E: The hippocampus and post-traumatic stress disorders, in The Clinical Neurobiology of the Hippocampus: An Integrative View. Edited by Bartsch T. New York, Oxford University Press, 2012, pp 262–272

Bremner JD, Randall P, Scott TM, et al: MRI-based measurement of hippocampal volume in patients with combat-related posttraumatic stress disorder. Am J Psychiatry 152(7):973–981, 1995 7793467

Bremner JD, Krystal JH, Southwick SM, et al: Noradrenergic mechanisms in stress and anxiety, I: preclinical studies. Synapse 23(1):28–38, 1996a 8723133

Bremner JD, Krystal JH, Southwick SM, et al: Noradrenergic mechanisms in stress and anxiety, II: clinical studies. Synapse 23(1):39–51, 1996b 8723134

Bremner JD, Innis RB, Ng CK, et al: Positron emission tomography measurement of cerebral metabolic correlates of yohimbine administration in combat-related posttraumatic stress disorder. Arch Gen Psychiatry 54(3):246–254, 1997a 9075465

Bremner JD, Licinio J, Darnell A, et al: Elevated CSF corticotropin-releasing factor concentrations in posttraumatic stress disorder. Am J Psychiatry 154(5):624–629, 1997b 9137116

Bremner JD, Southwick SM, Charney DS: The neurobiology of posttraumatic stress disorder: an integration of animal and human research, in Posttraumatic Stress Disorder: A Comprehensive Text. Edited by Saigh P, Bremner JD. New York, Allyn and Bacon, 1999a, pp 103–143

Bremner JD, Staib LH, Kaloupek D, et al: Neural correlates of exposure to traumatic pictures and sound in Vietnam combat veterans with and without posttraumatic stress disorder: a positron emission tomography study. Biol Psychiatry 45(7):806–816, 1999b 10202567

Bremner JD, Vermetten E, Schmahl C, et al: Positron emission tomographic imaging of neural correlates of a fear acquisition and extinction paradigm in women with childhood sexual-abuse-related post-traumatic stress disorder. Psychol Med 35(6):791–806, 2005 15997600

Bremner JD, Vermetten E, Kelley ME: Cortisol, dehydroepiandrosterone, and estradiol measured over 24 hours in women with childhood sexual abuse-related posttraumatic stress disorder. J Nerv Ment Dis 195(11):919–927, 2007 18000454

Campanella C, Bremner JD: Neuroimaging of PTSD, in Posttraumatic Stress Disorder: From Neurobiology to Treatment. Edited by Bremner JD. Hoboken, NJ, Wiley-Blackwell, 2016, pp 291–320

Cannon WB: The James-Lange theory of emotions: a critical examination and an alternative theory. By Walter B. Cannon, 1927. Am J Psychol 100(3–4):567–586, 1987 3322057

Chapman WP, Schroeder HR, Geyer G, et al: Physiological evidence concerning importance of the amygdaloid nuclear region in the integration of circulatory function and emotion in man. Science 120(3127):949–950, 1954 13216196

Charney DS, Bremner JD: The neurobiology of anxiety disorders, in Neurobiology of Mental Illness. Edited by Charney DS, Nestler EJ, Bunney SS. New York, Oxford University Press, 1999, pp 494–517

Charney DS, Sklar P, Buxbaum JD, et al (eds): Neurobiology of Mental Illness, 4th Edition. New York, Oxford University Press, 2014

Damasio H, Grabowski T, Frank R, et al: The return of Phineas Gage: clues about the brain from the skull of a famous patient. Science 264(5162):1102–1105, 1994 8178168

Davis M: The role of the amygdala in fear and anxiety. Annu Rev Neurosci 15:353–375, 1992 1575447

Devinsky O, Morrell MJ, Vogt BA: Contributions of anterior cingulate cortex to behaviour. Brain 118(pt 1):279–306, 1995 7895011

Diamond DM, Fleshner M, Ingersoll N, et al: Psychological stress impairs spatial working memory: relevance to electrophysiological studies of hippocampal function. Behav Neurosci 110(4):661–672, 1996 8864259

Duman RS, Malberg J, Nakagawa S: Regulation of adult neurogenesis by psychotropic drugs and stress. J Pharmacol Exp Ther 299(2):401–407, 2001 11602648

Elzinga BM, Schmahl CG, Vermetten E, et al: Higher cortisol levels following exposure to traumatic reminders in abuse-related PTSD. Neuropsychopharmacology 28(9):1656–1665, 2003 12838270

Gilbertson MW, Shenton ME, Ciszewski A, et al: Smaller hippocampal volume predicts pathologic vulnerability to psychological trauma. Nat Neurosci 5(11):1242–1247, 2002 12379862

Goldman-Rakic PS: Topography of cognition: parallel distributed networks in primate association cortex. Annu Rev Neurosci 11:137–156, 1988 3284439

Gray JA: The Neuropsychology of Anxiety. New York, Oxford University Press, 1982

Gunne LM, Reis DJ: Changes in brain catecholamines associated with electrical stimulation of amygdaloid nucleus. Life Sci (1962) 11:804–809, 1963 14078133

Hilton SM, Zbrozyna AW: Amygdaloid region for defence reactions and its efferent pathway to the brain stem. J Physiol 165:160–173, 1963 13954608

Iwata J, LeDoux JE, Meeley MP, et al: Intrinsic neurons in the amygdaloid field projected to by the medial geniculate body mediate emotional responses conditioned to acoustic stimuli. Brain Res 383(1–2):195–214, 1986 3768689

Kitayama N, Vaccarino V, Kutner M, et al: Magnetic resonance imaging (MRI) measurement of hippocampal volume in posttraumatic stress disorder: a meta-analysis. J Affect Disord 88(1):79–86, 2005 16033700

Kitayama N, Quinn S, Bremner JD: Smaller volume of anterior cingulate cortex in abuse-related posttraumatic stress disorder. J Affect Disord 90(2–3):171–174, 2006 16375974

LeDoux JE: Emotional memory systems in the brain. Behav Brain Res 58(1–2):69–79, 1993 8136051

LeDoux JE: The Emotional Brain: The Mysterious Underpinnings of Emotional Life. New York, Simon and Schuster, 1996

LeDoux JE, Cicchetti P, Xagoraris A, et al: The lateral amygdaloid nucleus: sensory interface of the amygdala in fear conditioning. J Neurosci 10(4):1062–1069, 1990 2329367

McDonald AJ: Organization of amygdaloid projections to the prefrontal cortex and associated striatum in the rat. Neuroscience 44(1):1–14, 1991a 1722886

McDonald AJ: Topographical organization of amygdaloid projections to the caudatoputamen, nucleus accumbens, and related striatal-like areas of the rat brain. Neuroscience 44(1):15–33, 1991b 1722890

McFall ME, Murburg MM, Ko GN, et al: Autonomic responses to stress in Vietnam combat veterans with posttraumatic stress disorder. Biol Psychiatry 27(10):1165–1175, 1990 2340325

Nibuya M, Morinobu S, Duman RS: Regulation of BDNF and trkB mRNA in rat brain by chronic electroconvulsive seizure and antidepressant drug treatments. J Neurosci 15(11):7539–7547, 1995 7472505

Papez JW: A proposed mechanism of emotion. AMA Arch Neurol Psychiatry 38:725–743, 1937

Phillips RG, LeDoux JE: Differential contribution of amygdala and hippocampus to cued and contextual fear conditioning. Behav Neurosci 106(2):274–285, 1992 1590953

Quirk GJ, Garcia R, González-Lima F: Prefrontal mechanisms in extinction of conditioned fear. Biol Psychiatry 60(4):337–343, 2006 16712801

Radley JJ, Sisti HM, Hao J, et al: Chronic behavioral stress induces apical dendritic reorganization in pyramidal neurons of the medial prefrontal cortex. Neuroscience 125(1):1–6, 2004 15051139

Rauch SL, Whalen PJ, Shin LM, et al: Exaggerated amygdala response to masked facial stimuli in posttraumatic stress disorder: a functional MRI study. Biol Psychiatry 47(9):769–776, 2000 10812035

Rauch SL, Shin LM, Segal E, et al: Selectively reduced regional cortical volumes in post-traumatic stress disorder. Neuroreport 14(7):913–916, 2003 12802174

Roth RH, Tam SY, Ida Y, et al: Stress and the mesocorticolimbic dopamine systems. Ann N Y Acad Sci 537:138–147, 1988 3059920

Santarelli L, Saxe M, Gross C, et al: Requirement of hippocampal neurogenesis for the behavioral effects of antidepressants. Science 301(5634):805–809, 2003 12907793

Sapolsky RM: Why stress is bad for your brain. Science 273(5276):749–750, 1996 8701325

Selemon LD, Goldman-Rakic PS: Common cortical and subcortical targets of the dorsolateral prefrontal and posterior parietal cortices in the rhesus monkey: evidence for a distributed neural network subserving spatially guided behavior. J Neurosci 8(11):4049–4068, 1988 2846794

Shin LM, Orr SP, Carson MA, et al: Regional cerebral blood flow in the amygdala and medial prefrontal cortex during traumatic imagery in male and female Vietnam veterans with PTSD. Arch Gen Psychiatry 61(2):168–176, 2004 14757593

Smith ME: Bilateral hippocampal volume reduction in adults with post-traumatic stress disorder: a meta-analysis of structural MRI studies. Hippocampus 15(6):798–807, 2005 15988763

Southwick SM, Krystal JH, Morgan CA, et al: Abnormal noradrenergic function in posttraumatic stress disorder. Arch Gen Psychiatry 50(4):266–274, 1993 8466387

Squire LR, Zola-Morgan S: The medial temporal lobe memory system. Science 253(5026):1380–1386, 1991 1896849

Stein MB, Goldin PR, Sareen J, et al: Increased amygdala activation to angry and contemptuous faces in generalized social phobia. Arch Gen Psychiatry 59(11):1027–1034, 2002 12418936

Vaccarino V, Bremner JD: Posttraumatic stress disorder and risk of cardiovascular disease, in Handbook of Psychocardiology. Edited by Alvarenga M, Byrne D. New York, Springer, 2015, pp 265–282

van Praag H, Kempermann G, Gage FH: Running increases cell proliferation and neurogenesis in the adult mouse dentate gyrus. Nat Neurosci 2(3):266–270, 1999 10195220

Vermetten E, Vythilingam M, Southwick SM, et al: Long-term treatment with paroxetine increases verbal declarative memory and hippocampal volume in posttraumatic stress disorder. Biol Psychiatry 54(7):693–702, 2003 14512209

Vermetten E, Vythilingam M, Schmahl C, et al: Alterations in stress reactivity after long-term treatment with paroxetine in women with posttraumatic stress disorder. Ann N Y Acad Sci 1071:184–202, 2006 16891570

Vogt BA, Finch DM, Olson CR: Functional heterogeneity in cingulate cortex: the anterior executive and posterior evaluative regions. Cereb Cortex 2(6):435–443, 1992 1477524

Woodward SH, Kaloupek DG, Streeter CC, et al: Decreased anterior cingulate volume in combat-related PTSD. Biol Psychiatry 59(7):582–587, 2006 16165099

Yehuda R: Advances in understanding neuroendocrine alterations in PTSD and their therapeutic implications. Ann NY Acad Sci 1071:137–166, 2006 16891568

Yehuda R, Southwick SM, Krystal JH, et al: Enhanced suppression of cortisol following dexamethasone administration in posttraumatic stress disorder. Am J Psychiatry 150(1):83–86, 1993 8417586

Yehuda R, Teicher MH, Levengood RA, et al: Circadian regulation of basal cortisol levels in posttraumatic stress disorder. Ann N Y Acad Sci 746(1):378–380, 1994 7825891

Yehuda R, Teicher MH, Trestman RL, et al: Cortisol regulation in posttraumatic stress disorder and major depression: a chronobiological analysis. Biol Psychiatry 40(2):79–88, 1996 8793040

Recommended Readings

Bremner JD: Does Stress Damage the Brain? Understanding Trauma-Related Disorders From a Mind-Body Perspective. New York, WW Norton, 2002

Bremner JD (ed): Posttraumatic Stress Disorder: From Neurobiology to Treatment. Hoboken, NJ, Wiley-Blackwell, 2016

Bremner JD, Elzinga B, Schmahl C, et al: Structural and functional plasticity of the human brain in posttraumatic stress disorder. Prog Brain Res 167:171–186, 2008

Charney DS: Psychobiological mechanisms of resilience and vulnerability: implications for successful adaptation to extreme stress. Am J Psychiatry 161:195–216, 2004

Charney DS, Bremner JD: The neurobiology of anxiety disorders, in Neurobiology of Mental Illness. Edited by Charney DS, Nestler EJ, Bunney SS. Oxford, UK, Oxford University Press, 1999, pp 494–517

Nemeroff CB, Bremner JD, Foa EB, et al: Posttraumatic stress disorder: a state-of-the-science review. J Psychiatr Res 40:1–21, 2006

Pitman RK: Investigating the pathogenesis of posttraumatic stress disorder with neuroimaging. J Clin Psychiatry 62:47–54, 2001

Rauch SL, Shin LM, Phelps EA: Neurocircuitry models of posttraumatic stress disorder and extinction: human neuroimaging research—past, present, and future. Biol Psychiatry 60:376–382, 2006

CHAPTER 4

Cultural and Social Aspects of Anxiety Disorders

Denise April Chavira, Ph.D.

Carolyn Ponting, M.A.

Roberto Lewis-Fernández, M.D.

In this chapter, we discuss cultural and social aspects of anxiety disorders. DSM-5 characterizes *culture* as "systems of knowledge, concepts, rules, and practices that are learned and transmitted across generations. Culture includes language, religion and spirituality, family structures, life-cycle stages, ceremonial rituals, and customs, as well as moral and legal systems" (American Psychiatric Association 2013, p. 749). As this broad definition suggests, our conception of culture in this chapter encompasses the entire process of meaning-making through which people make sense of their experience, including their health conditions. This process is "cultural" because it is constantly re-created by individuals based on their engagement with many traditions of meaning-making learned from their families, communities, and other social groups (e.g., professions, faith communities). All these traditions influence the person simultaneously and evolve constantly over time, patterning a rich and changing tapestry of cognitions, emotions, behaviors, values, and practices.

Experiences of anxiety and anxiety disorders also are influenced by individuals' social contexts and backgrounds, including their differential access to resources and power relations, class origins, levels of education, and group experiences such as migration and risk of adverse exposures (e.g., discrimination, crime). In addition, and just as important, individuals' experience is influenced by the social and cultural characteristics of their providers and the health care system. These include the professional traditions that underpin diagnostic classifications (e.g., mind-body dualism, tendency to obscure the social origin of embodied health conditions), personal forms of implicit bias, taken-for-granted ideologies that structure unequal access to health care, and policies regarding insurance coverage for specific treatments. We illustrate several of these aspects of the anxiety disorders, taking race/ethnicity as a key example given the focus of the literature in this area.

Prevalence

Anxiety disorders affect people worldwide, although estimates vary widely between and within countries (Table 4–1). According to a systematic review of 87 prevalence studies across 44 countries (Baxter et al. 2013), the worldwide lifetime prevalence of any anxiety disorder ranges from 4.8% to 10.9%. On average, African cultures report the lowest lifetime prevalence (5.4%) whereas Anglo/European cultures report the highest (10.4%). The last study to examine global prevalence of specific disorders found that generalized anxiety disorder (GAD; 6.2%) and specific phobias (4.9%) have the highest lifetime prevalence, and panic disorder has the lowest (1.2%) (Somers et al. 2006). Globally, specific phobias (4.9%) and GAD (6.2%) have the highest lifetime prevalence, and panic disorder has the lowest (1.2%). In the United States, non-Latino white individuals typically have a higher prevalence of anxiety disorders than do other racial/ethnic groups; however, the prevalence of agoraphobia and panic disorder has been comparable among Puerto Rican people, for example, indicating variability associated with sociocultural factors (Asnaani et al. 2010). Some studies find higher prevalence of anxiety disorders among Native Americans and of specific phobias and PTSD among African American persons, compared with non-Latino white individuals (Grant et al. 2005; Hofmann and Hinton 2014). Evidence also indicates that Asian American individuals tend to have the lowest prevalence of GAD and PTSD (Himle et al. 2009), tracking with the generally low prevalence of anxiety disorders in Asian countries (Lewis-Fernández et al. 2010b).

The similarities and differences in the prevalence of various disorders across sociocultural groups raise many questions, including whether differences are due to methodological issues (e.g., lack of measurement equivalence, variations in sample size, diverse caseness definitions), limited validity or precision inherent in the diagnostic criteria, or true differences in prevalence. Limited attention has been devoted to establishing cross-cultural measurement equivalence or ensuring representation of individuals from various sociocultural groups, and most cross-cultural research has been conducted in the United States and Europe. Social and contextual factors such as sex, age, nativity, economic status, and urbanicity also may account for significant variability in prevalence rates (Baxter et al. 2013).

In this chapter, we build on existing conceptual frameworks of sociocultural influences on mental health (Hwang et al. 2008) to understand how diverse cultural and social characteristics influence the phenomenology, etiology, and treatment of anxiety disorders. We use this model (Figure 4–1) to suggest that culture intersects with various social factors (e.g., socioeconomic status, gender, migration) to influence 1) the types of stressors one experiences; 2) conceptualizations of anxiety via traditional knowledge and culturally influenced attitudes, values, and norms; 3) perceptions of and behaviors to manage anxiety; 4) detection and diagnosis of anxiety disorders; and 5) availability, quality, and course of treatment, including as affected by 6) developments in health care policy. As an example, cultural processes, including attitudes

TABLE 4–1. **Prevalence and diagnostic rates of anxiety disorders in the United States and internationally**

Study	Study location	Findings related to prevalence/risk
United States		
Asnaani et al. 2010	United States	Lifetime prevalence: NLWs more likely to be diagnosed with SAD (12.6%), GAD (8.6%), and PD (5.1%) than African Americans (8.6%, 4.9%, 3.8%, respectively), Latinos (8.2%, 5.8%, 4.1%, respectively), and Asian Americans (5.3%, 2.4%, 2.1%, respectively)
		Lifetime prevalence: Asian Americans less likely to be diagnosed with GAD and PTSD than Latinos and NLWs
		Lifetime prevalence: African Americans more likely to be diagnosed with PTSD (8.6%) than Asian Americans (1.6%) and Latinos (5.6%)
Himle et al. 2009	United States	12-month prevalence: African Americans (3.8%) and Caribbean blacks (5.3%) more likely to meet criteria for PTSD than NLWs (3.5%)
		12-month prevalence: NLWs at elevated risk for GAD (2.7%), PD (2.6%), and SAD (7.1%) vs. African Americans (1.4%, 2.3%, 4.6%, respectively) and Caribbean blacks (1.4%, 2.7% [higher standard error], 4.7%, respectively)
International		
Baxter et al. 2013	Europe, Indo/Asia, Africa, Central/ Eastern Europe, North Africa, Middle East, Latin America	12-month prevalence: Euro/Anglo countries had the highest prevalence of anxiety disorders (10.4%); African countries had the lowest (5.3%)
		12-month prevalence: Populations exposed to conflict (e.g., exposure to war) had increased risk for PTSD vs. nonconflict areas (9.0% vs. 5.6%)
Hinton and Lewis-Fernández 2011	Africa, Europe, Asia, Middle East, North America, Australia	12-month prevalence: Rates of PTSD highest in United States (3.5%), followed by Australia (1.3%), Europe (0.9%), South Korea (0.7%), and Mexico and South Africa (both at 0.6%)
		12-month prevalence: Rates of PTSD lowest in Nigeria (0%), followed by China (0.2%) and Japan (0.4%)
Lewis-Fernández et al. 2010b	Africa, Europe, Asia, Middle East, North America, Australia	12-month prevalence: Rates of specific phobia considerably higher in United States (7.1%–8.7%) and Europe (6.4%) vs. non-European countries (e.g., China, 2.7%; Mexico, 4%; South Korea, 4.2%)

TABLE 4–1. **Prevalence and diagnostic rates of anxiety disorders in the United States and internationally** *(continued)*

Study	Study location	Findings related to prevalence/risk
Lewis-Fernández et al. 2010b *(continued)*		12-month prevalence: Rates of SAD in the United States (2.8%–6.8%) considerably higher vs. non-European countries (e.g., South Korea and China, 0.2%; Japan, 0.8%; Mexico, 1.7%)
		12-month prevalence: Rates of OCD highest in Turkey (3%), followed by United States (1%) and Australia (0.7%), and lowest in China (0%) and Nigeria (0.1%)
		12-month prevalence: Rates of GAD in United States (2.1%–2.9%) comparable to those in Australia (3.6%) and Europe (1.7%) and higher than those in Nigeria (0%) and Mexico (0.4%)
		12-month prevalence: Rates of agoraphobia highest in South Africa (4.8%) and lowest in metropolitan China (0%), with New Zealand (1.2%) and Europe (1.3%) falling in the middle
Lindert et al. 2009	Europe, Indo/Asia, Africa, Central/ Eastern Europe, North Africa, Middle East, Latin America, Australia	Combined lifetime prevalence across 35 studies ($N=24,051$) for any anxiety disorder was 21% among labor migrants and 40% among refugees

Note. GAD=generalized anxiety disorder; NLW=non-Latino white; PD=panic disorder; SAD=social anxiety disorder.

about stigma, holistic views of health and pathophysiology, and the importance of the family, may lead to the expression of anxiety primarily as somatic symptoms to communicate distress most effectively, adhere to social norms about symptom severity and gender roles, and preserve interpersonal harmony. In turn, this may affect whether one seeks help from informal or formal sources and whether a DSM-trained clinician is able to detect psychological distress. Such an integrative approach provides a model for the complex interplay of culture and social characteristics that influence anxiety disorders and their treatment.

Impact of Social and Cultural Characteristics on Stressors Related to Anxiety Disorders

The impact of social and cultural characteristics is present even in the risk of exposure to and quality of the stressors themselves that create vulnerability for anxiety disorders, such as experiences of migration and discrimination.

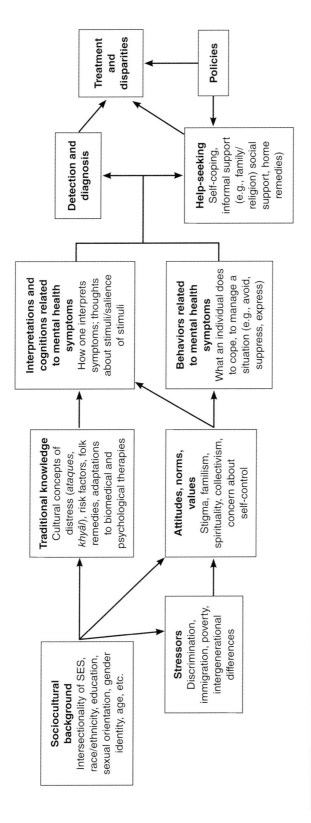

FIGURE 4–1. Sociocultural model of mental health.

SES=socioeconomic status.
Source. Adapted from Hwang et al. 2008.

Migration

Migration was initially thought to be associated with numerous challenges that would place immigrants at higher risk for mental health problems. However, this immigrant-risk hypothesis has received mixed empirical support (Alegría et al. 2008). Some studies that link immigrant status with a higher risk for anxiety disorders (Del Amo et al. 2011) have found that this relationship is connected to the level of stress in the host country and the migration process itself—often operationalized as acculturative stress—rather than the mere fact of being an immigrant. Furthermore, social determinants common among low-income groups, such as overcrowded housing and high unemployment, coupled with the risk of exclusion from social services and health care associated with migrant status, compound acculturative stress and increase risk for psychiatric disorders (Bas-Sarmiento et al. 2017). Evidence also exists for the opposite finding in the United States and other countries such as Australia, the United Kingdom, and Spain: foreign-born individuals have lower prevalence rates of anxiety, mood, and substance use disorders than do their non-foreign-born ("native") counterparts, a phenomenon labeled the *immigrant paradox*, given the paradoxical relationship between worse social conditions among migrants and better health indexes (Alegría et al. 2008; Polanco et al., in press). Diverse social, political, and historical contexts surrounding migration experiences likely account for some of this variability across groups.

Discrimination

Discrimination is another social factor that is a robust predictor of poor mental and physical health outcomes. In a meta-analysis of 293 studies largely from the United States (81%) and Europe (9%), racism/discrimination was associated with poorer mental health, including depression, anxiety, and stress-related symptoms. In the United States, perceived discrimination has been linked to anxiety, depression, suicidality, and substance use in Latino and Asian American community samples (Chou et al. 2012; Otiniano Verissimo et al. 2014). Among veterans, race-based discrimination and mistreatment in the military are possible mediators for higher rates of trauma-related stress (Ruef et al. 2000).

Traditional Knowledge and Conceptualizations of Distress and Anxiety

It is possible to speak of *anxiety*, at a high level of abstraction, as a common experience worldwide. At the same time, local variations may depend on specific culturally based attributions, behavioral responses, and patterns of interpersonal interaction so that they occur only when those modes of explanation and interaction are present. DSM-5 introduced the term *cultural concepts of distress* (replacing *culture-bound syndromes*) to indicate that these cultural conceptualizations represent not only syndromic presentations of symptoms that regularly "run together" but also a more diffuse set of complaints, symptoms, and predicaments that constitute *cultural idioms of distress*—general "languages" of suffering shaped by cultural understandings of what are meaningful ways of denoting affliction, such as concepts of "nerves" or "thinking too much"—and *causal explanations*—often referencing local ethnophysiological ideas about etiology, such as frightening experiences (e.g., *susto*) and stress (Lewis-Fernández et al. 2017b).

Many cultural concepts of distress involve anxiety symptoms. For example, *khyâl* attacks are panic attack–like episodes prevalent among Cambodians that are attributed to the internal dysregulation of *khyâl*, a wind-like substance integral to local ethnophysiology (Hinton et al. 2005); related wind-like concepts are common among Tibetans, Vietnamese, Chinese, and Mongolians (Hinton et al. 2004, 2005). These ethnophysiological explanations pattern the symptoms and treatment expectations of those experiencing *khyâl* attacks. For example, panic symptoms are accompanied by signs of autonomic arousal (e.g., tinnitus), associated symptoms (e.g., "neckache"), and catastrophic cognitions ("my neck vessels will explode") that are attributed to the dysregulated flow of *khyâl*. Traditional treatment often includes *coining*, in which healers raise welts on the skin in specific shapes by rubbing with coins and liniment to rebalance the flow of *khyâl*.

Cultural concepts of distress can also pattern the ways in which people react to adversity. For example, *ataque de nervios* (attack of nerves) is a cultural syndrome with a lifetime prevalence of 5%–11% among U.S. Latino persons (depending on subgroup) that is characterized by trembling, crying, screaming uncontrollably, and sudden verbal and physical aggression, usually in response to a stressful life event or significant loss. Additional symptoms may include dizziness or fainting, dissociation, and suicidal gestures. Although overlapping phenomenologically with panic attacks and disorder, only 17%–33% of *ataques* met criteria for panic disorder in one study (Lewis-Fernández et al. 2002). In clinical samples, anxiety sensitivity and dissociative capacity are significant risk factors for the onset and severity of *ataque* in response to adversity (Lewis-Fernández et al. 2010a). Certain cultural views—such as a self-construal that prioritizes equanimity/tranquility (*tranquilidad*) and always being "in control" as well as fear that strong "negative" emotions, such as anger, may lead to personal and social catastrophe—also may constitute risk factors (Lewis-Fernández and Aggarwal 2015). *Ataque* conveys useful information as a clinical marker beyond psychiatric diagnosis: its presence is associated with higher risk of suicidal ideation, disability due to mental health problems, and mental health service use, after adjusting for psychiatric disorders, trauma exposure, and other clinical and demographic variables (Lewis-Fernández et al. 2009).

Taijin kyofusho ("interpersonal fear disorder" in Japanese) is a cultural syndrome common in Japan and Korea (as *taein kong po*) that combines elements of social anxiety and body dysmorphic disorder, including in some cases delusional features, in novel ways that can help identify common etiologies and treatments for these conditions (Kirmayer and Young 1998). *Taijin kyofusho* embodies the cultural priority given to other-focused (*allocentric*) concerns in addition to self-focused embarrassment fears: the person worries that he or she will do something or appear offensive to others, such as displaying physical flaws and socially inappropriate behaviors (e.g., staring at others' bodies). Research on this aspect of social anxiety has since found that it is also salient among non-Asian populations, such as in the United States (Choy et al. 2008). Given their international salience, *allocentric fears* have been included in the definition of social anxiety disorder, facilitating its identification across cultures (Lewis-Fernández et al. 2010b).

Culturally Influenced Attitudes, Norms, and Values

Cultural and social characteristics of families and communities help pattern the attitudes, norms, and values that influence a person's development. These group characteristics can act as risk factors (e.g., by heightening stigma) or as protective factors (e.g., by promoting family support) for anxiety disorders.

Collectivism is a cultural orientation that emphasizes connectedness with others and places a high value on harmonious interpersonal relationships. Collectivism may protect against depressive symptoms via its greater relational and community emphases, which are associated with social support and subjective well-being (Triandis 2000). However, individuals with high collectivism tend to attribute great significance to social context and may be more likely to experience social anxiety than individuals with low collectivism (Okazaki 1997). Data from a growing cultural neuroscience literature are congruent with this hypothesis; electroencephalogram activity was heightened in response to social cues and feedback in Asian versus non-Asian participants (Park and Kitayama 2014).

Mental health–related *stigma* is a socially constructed orientation associated with attitudes, values, and norms that affect the conceptualization of mental illness and help-seeking behavior (Clement et al. 2015). Sociocultural groups vary in their attributions of stigma to mental illness, even within the same society. One theory holds that high stigma is associated with an embodied emphasis on somatic symptoms as signs of emotional distress to distance the patient from more severe and stigmatized forms of mental illness (Ryder et al. 2002). Somatization may be a culturally appropriate way of expressing emotional or social distress in an individual's cultural context, whereas other symptoms, including cognitive symptoms of anxiety, represent stigmatized mental health dysfunction (Kirmayer and Young 1998).

Interpretations, Cognitions, and Behaviors Related to Mental Health Symptoms

Exposed to traditional knowledge about illness and care and to group attitudes, norms, and values in their communities, individuals reinterpret these learned orientations in their own ways, influenced by their particular hybridity or intersectionality of background and by the social conditions in which they live. These interpretations are not only cognitive but also embodied as taken-for-granted emotions and behaviors, all of which influence the experience of anxiety disorders and associated help-seeking activities. For example, individuals' cultural backgrounds can influence whether they view biological causation of anxiety disorders as obvious or surprising and therefore view pharmacotherapy as helpful or reductive and even dangerous (e.g., putting them at risk for addiction; Vargas et al. 2015). Some individuals and groups prioritize a spiritual or religious orientation. In a large study of ethnically diverse British individuals with anxiety and depression, those of Bangladeshi ethnicity were the most likely to interpret their symptoms as spiritual in origin and to prefer spiritual treatments (Bhui et al. 2006). Perhaps most individuals endorse a combined explanation for common mental disorders such as anxiety, integrating in more-or-less seamless ways biological (e.g., genetic), social (e.g., work-related), psychological (e.g., temperament), and spiritual or supernatural (e.g., fate) causes into their explanatory models (Kendler 2008).

Many anxiety symptoms, such as phobias, worries, and obsessions, are universal phenomena that may be shaped by specific life contexts with unique experiences and interpretations of surrounding stimuli. In an international review of OCD, Fontenelle et al. (2004) found that aggressive and religious obsessions were predominant in Brazilian and Middle Eastern samples, respectively, whereas in other countries, themes of contamination were predominant. This may be related to the effect of extrinsic factors such as religion, geographical location, and socioeconomic status on the content of obsessions and compulsions. For example, Brazilian patients with OCD may be influenced by increased levels of violence in Brazil over recent decades, leading to salient obsessions about aggression. Okasha et al. (1994) argued that Egyptian patients with OCD commonly present with religious obsessions and repeating compulsions, even when not religiously observant, because of the regional, national, and cultural emphasis on religious rituals and the practice of warding off blasphemous thoughts by repeating religious phrases.

External Help-Seeking

The World Health Organization has noted marked unmet mental health need and severe shortages of psychiatrists and mental health providers in both low- and middle-income countries (Bruckner et al. 2011). In these settings, many individuals rely on traditional healers or religious leaders to help manage mental health concerns. Gureje et al. (2015) reported that even among participants who ultimately accessed formal mental health care services, a substantial proportion of the inhabitants of Nigeria (32.0%), India (43.5%), the United Arab Emirates (44.4%), Zimbabwe (44.5%), and Malaysia (69.0%) first sought help for anxiety and depressive disorders from traditional or faith-based healers.

In the United States, racial/ethnic minority individuals with mental health needs are more likely than their non-Latino counterparts to delay formal mental health care (Chen and Dagher 2016) and show less adherence to treatments (Aggarwal et al. 2016), often ending care prematurely (Delphin-Rittmon et al. 2015). This pattern is also found in primary care settings, where racial/ethnic minorities are less likely to receive adequate levels of psychotherapy or pharmacotherapy for anxiety disorders (Weisberg et al. 2014). Health insurance coverage is a key determinant of differential use of mental health services, yet disparities often remain even when social factors such as insurance are addressed (Chow et al. 2003).

Although they are less likely to use formal mental health services, underserved racial/ethnic groups are more likely to engage informal supports such as religious advisors and healers than are non-Latino white individuals (Abe-Kim et al. 2004); for example, African American people often report receiving more social support in their churches than do Latino or non-Latino white individuals (Krause 2016). Perhaps because of concerns about stigma and disrupting community harmony, Americans of Chinese, Japanese, Korean, and Vietnamese descent tend to use fewer social supports to cope with mental illness compared with non-Latino white individuals (Kim et al. 2008). Finally, cultural background and formal health care use can intersect in complex ways; for example, among Latino persons, high levels of family support can deter use of specialty or medical services (Villatoro et al. 2014).

Detection and Diagnosis

Underdetection and misdiagnosis may occur when clinicians apply measures and diagnostic criteria for anxiety disorders without proven validity across cultural groups. Similarly, DSM primarily assesses psychological symptoms, biasing the diagnosis of anxiety disorders toward individuals who attend to psychological over physical symptoms (Marques et al. 2011), whereas somatization tends to be reported more frequently by individuals from non-Western cultures (Ryder et al. 2002). In specific contexts, provider- and system-level factors, such as limited time, linguistic barriers, and lack of cultural competency training, also can deter detection of anxiety disorders across cultural groups (Stockdale et al. 2008). These effects are compounded by the effects of socioeconomic disadvantage, which limit access to and quality of care.

Treatment

Evidence-based practices such as cognitive-behavioral therapy have shown efficacy for patients from underserved racial/ethnic groups with anxiety disorders, including PTSD, GAD, and panic disorder (Horrell 2008). Several large randomized clinical trials have reported that Latino, African American, and Asian American patients respond as well to evidence-based psychotherapy and pharmacological interventions as non-Latino white patients (e.g., Chavira et al. 2014). Nevertheless, meta-analyses show that even better efficacy is possible when psychotherapies are culturally adapted (Hall et al. 2016).

A practical question remains about how to disseminate culturally adapted treatments. The implementation of psychotherapies and other treatments in low- and middle-income countries has been the focus of the emerging discipline of global mental health. A good deal of evidence indicates that treatments can be adapted for use in contextually relevant ways in a range of settings around the world, including their effective delivery by nonspecialists.

Underserved racial/ethnic groups are less likely to receive pharmacotherapy for anxiety-related disorders (Moitra et al. 2014). This is partly because of the lower acceptability of psychopharmacological treatments in these groups, including when compared with psychological interventions (Williams et al. 2012). Yet given the overall environment of lower quality of mental health care for racial/ethnic minorities—encompassing lower detection rates, misdiagnosis, lower likelihood of guideline-concordant treatment, less participatory engagement, and use of earlier-generation medications—some form of systemic or individual implicit bias is also likely at work (Lewis-Fernández et al. 2017a).

Researchers also have studied culturally adapted interventions (Table 4–2). Most of these treatments for anxiety disorders have been conducted in a group format and include psychoeducation to address the cultural explanatory models of the target population (van Loon et al. 2013). The work of Hinton et al. (2004, 2005, 2011) with

TABLE 4–2.   Characteristics of research on cultural adaptations of interventions to treat anxiety in adults

Study	Sample size; race/ethnicity	Diagnosis	Culturally adapted treatment	Incorporation of cultural values, beliefs, and symptoms
Carter et al. 2003	25; African American	Panic symptoms	Group panic control therapy	In group discussions
Hinton et al. 2004	12; Vietnamese	PTSD	Group CBT	Psychoeducation about relation between headache, orthostatic panic, trauma, and panic response and visualizations
Hinton et al. 2005	40; Cambodian	PTSD	CBT	Psychoeducation, presentation of symptoms, and in visualizations
Gone 2009[a]	16; Native American	PTSD	Trauma narrative	Use of narration of historical trauma to reclaim indigenous heritage, identity, and spirituality
Hinton et al. 2011	24; Latino American	PTSD	Group CBT	Focus on culturally specific syndromes, use of culturally consonant imagery
Neal-Barnett et al. 2011[a]	37; African American (women)	Generalized anxiety and panic attacks	Group CBT	Use of racially homogeneous group, minimization of homework, use of culturally relevant metaphors
Pan et al. 2011	30; Asian American	Specific phobia	Exposure therapy	Evaluating the explanatory model of the patient and extensive psychoeducation
Wagner et al. 2012	15; Iraqi	PTSD	CBT	Focus on war-related trauma experiences
Hovey et al. 2014	6; Mexican (women in United States)	Any anxiety	Group CBT	Use of *promotoras*,[b] use of relevant life experiences (e.g., discrimination)

Note.   CBT = cognitive-behavioral therapy.
[a]Studies focused on stakeholder acceptability of interventions but did not test their effect on reducing anxiety symptoms.
[b]*Promotoras* are trusted community members who serve as health educators and often link the community with health services, delivering culturally nuanced care. Promotoras are particularly utilized in Latino communities.
Source.   Adapted from van Loon et al. 2013.

Cambodian and Vietnamese patients and of Gone (2009) with Native American patients with PTSD included case conceptualizations and treatment strategies that are consistent with cultural understandings. Several small-scale studies have examined cultural adaptations for phobias and anxiety disorders more broadly. Noticeably absent from this literature are randomized controlled trials with indigenous groups and interventions with undocumented immigrants and non–English speakers.

Policy Implications

Systemic change beyond mental health can also serve to reduce disparities related to anxiety disorders in underserved populations. A landmark experiment conducted in the 1990s evaluated the outcomes of 4,248 mostly racial/ethnic minority individuals randomly assigned to receive Section 8 subsidized housing vouchers allowing them to move to neighborhoods where less than 10% of the residents lived in poverty (Feins and Shroder 2005). Adults receiving the vouchers reported fewer anxiety symptoms than did control adults (Katz et al. 2001). In addition to policies to prevent the onset of anxiety symptoms, policies that encourage language inclusivity are warranted. The recruitment and training of bilingual health professionals is part of the solution, and financial incentives for bilingual students may increase the feasibility of attending graduate school for those interested in addressing these gaps.

Conclusion

In this chapter, we provided an integrative conceptual model to explain how aspects of culture converge to affect the experience and expression of anxiety disorders across ethnic groups. In doing so, we moved beyond a discussion of between-group ethnic differences, which can be vulnerable to overgeneralizing and stereotypes. Continued research examining social and cultural processes that influence anxiety, inclusive of contextual stressors and cultural values, knowledge, and attitudes, is critical to improving our understanding of mechanisms that may account for differential rates of as well as risk for anxiety disorders across ethnic groups. Such research is fundamental to improving diagnosis, detection, and treatment of anxiety disorders in diverse social and cultural groups.

Key Points

- Anxiety symptoms, such as phobias, worries, and obsessions, are likely universal phenomena that are also shaped by specific life contexts.

- Cultural and social contexts have the potential to influence stressors, traditional knowledge, and attitudes, values, and norms and to impact the phenomenology, etiology, and treatment of anxiety disorders.

- Culturally informed assessment incorporates information on cultural and social contexts and facilitates accurate detection, diagnosis, and treatment.

- Evidence-based practices are effective for ethnic minorities with anxiety disorders, yet emerging data suggest potentially larger effects when interventions are culturally adapted.

References

Abe-Kim J, Gong F, Takeuchi D: Religiosity, spirituality, and help-seeking among Filipino Americans: religious clergy or mental health professionals? J Community Psychol 32(6):675–689, 2004

Aggarwal NK, Pieh MC, Dixon L, et al: Clinician descriptions of communication strategies to improve treatment engagement by racial/ethnic minorities in mental health services: a systematic review. Patient Educ Couns 99(2):198–209, 2016 26365436

Alegría M, Canino G, Shrout PE, et al: Prevalence of mental illness in immigrant and non-immigrant U.S. Latino groups. Am J Psychiatry 165(3):359–369, 2008 18245178

American Psychiatric Association: Diagnostic and Statistical Manual of Mental Disorders, 5th Edition. Arlington, VA, American Psychiatric Association, 2013

Asnaani A, Richey JA, Dimaite R, et al: A cross-ethnic comparison of lifetime prevalence rates of anxiety disorders. J Nerv Ment Dis 198(8):551–555, 2010 20699719

Bas-Sarmiento P, Saucedo-Moreno MJ, Fernández-Gutiérrez M, et al: Mental health in immigrants versus native population: a systematic review of the literature. Arch Psychiatr Nurs 31(1):111–121, 2017 28104048

Baxter AJ, Scott KM, Vos T, et al: Global prevalence of anxiety disorders: a systematic review and meta-regression. Psychol Med 43(5):897–910, 2013 22781489

Bhui K, Rüdell K, Priebe S: Assessing explanatory models for common mental disorders. J Clin Psychiatry 67(6):964–971, 2006 16848657

Bruckner TA, Scheffler RM, Shen G, et al: The mental health workforce gap in low- and middle-income countries: a needs-based approach. Bull World Health Organ 89(3):184–194, 2011 21379414

Carter MM, Sbrocco T, Gore KL, et al: Cognitive-behavioral group therapy versus a wait-list control in the treatment of African American women with panic disorder. Cognit Ther Res 27(5):505–518, 2003

Chavira DA, Golinelli D, Sherbourne C, et al: Treatment engagement and response to CBT among Latinos with anxiety disorders in primary care. J Consult Clin Psychol 82(3):392–403, 2014 24660674

Chen J, Dagher R: Gender and race/ethnicity differences in mental health care for use before and during the great recession. J Behav Health Ser R 43(2):187–199, 2016

Chou T, Asnaani A, Hofmann SG: Perception of racial discrimination and psychopathology across three U.S. ethnic minority groups. Cultur Divers Ethnic Minor Psychol 18(1):74–81, 2012 21967527

Chow JCC, Jaffee K, Snowden L: Racial/ethnic disparities in the use of mental health services in poverty areas. Am J Public Health 93(5):792–797, 2003 12721146

Choy Y, Schneier FR, Heimberg RG, et al: Features of the offensive subtype of Taijin-Kyofu-Sho in US and Korean patients with DSM-IV social anxiety disorder. Depress Anxiety 25(3):230–240, 2008 17340609

Clement S, Schauman O, Graham T, et al: What is the impact of mental health-related stigma on help-seeking? A systematic review of quantitative and qualitative studies. Psychol Med 45(1):11–27, 2015 24569086

Del Amo J, Jarrín I, García-Fulgueiras A, et al: Mental health in Ecuadorian migrants from a population-based survey: the importance of social determinants and gender roles. Soc Psychiatry Psychiatr Epidemiol 46(11):1143–1152, 2011 20878144

Delphin-Rittmon ME, Flanagan EH, Andres-Hyman R, et al: Racial-ethnic differences in access, diagnosis and outcomes in public-sector inpatient mental health treatment. Psych Serv 12(2):158, 2015

Feins JD, Shroder MD: Moving to opportunity: the demonstration's design and its effects on mobility. Urban Stud 42(8):1275–1299, 2005

Fontenelle LF, Mendlowicz MV, Marques C, et al: Trans-cultural aspects of obsessive-compulsive disorder: a description of a Brazilian sample and a systematic review of international clinical studies. J Psychiatr Res 38(4):403–411, 2004 15203292

Gone JP: A community-based treatment for Native American historical trauma: prospects for evidence-based practice. J Consult Clin Psychol 77(4):751–762, 2009 19634967

Grant BF, Stinson FS, Hasin DS, et al: Prevalence, correlates, and comorbidity of bipolar I disorder and Axis I and II disorders: results from the National Epidemiologic Survey on Alcohol and Related Conditions. J Clin Psychiatry 66(10):1205–1215, 2005 16259532

Gureje O, Nortje G, Makanjuola V, et al: The role of global traditional and complementary systems of medicine in the treatment of mental health disorders. Lancet Psychiatry 2(2):168–177, 2015 26359753

Hall GC, Ibaraki AY, Huang ER, et al: A meta-analysis of cultural adaptations of psychological interventions. Behav Ther 47(6):993–1014, 2016 27993346

Himle JA, Baser RE, Taylor RJ, et al: Anxiety disorders among African Americans, blacks of Caribbean descent, and non-Hispanic whites in the United States. J Anxiety Disord 23(5):578–590, 2009 19231131

Hinton DE, Lewis-Fernández R: The cross-cultural validity of postraumatic stress disorder: implications for DSM-5. Depress Anxiety 28(9):783–801, 2011

Hinton DE, Pham T, Tran M, et al: CBT for Vietnamese refugees with treatment-resistant PTSD and panic attacks: a pilot study. J Trauma Stress 17(5):429–433, 2004 15633922

Hinton DE, Chhean D, Pich V, et al: A randomized controlled trial of cognitive-behavior therapy for Cambodian refugees with treatment-resistant PTSD and panic attacks: a cross-over design. J Trauma Stress 18(6):617–629, 2005 16382423

Hinton DE, Hofmann SG, Rivera E, et al: Culturally adapted CBT (CA-CBT) for Latino women with treatment-resistant PTSD: a pilot study comparing CA-CBT to applied muscle relaxation. Behav Res Ther 49(4):275–280, 2011 21333272

Hofmann SG, Hinton DE: Cross-cultural aspects of anxiety disorders. Curr Psychiatry Rep 16(6):450, 2014

Horrell SCV: Effectiveness of cognitive-behavioral therapy with adult ethnic minority clients: a review. Prof Psychol Res Pr 39(2):60–168, 2008

Hovey JD, Hurtado G, Seligman LD: Findings for a CBT support group for Latina migrant farmworkers in Western Colorado. Curr Psychol 33:271–281, 2014

Hwang WC, Myers HF, Abe-Kim J, et al: A conceptual paradigm for understanding culture's impact on mental health: the cultural influences on mental health (CIMH) model. Clin Psychol Rev 28(2):211–227, 2008 17587473

Katz LF, Kling JR, Liebman JB: Moving to opportunity in Boston: early results of a randomized mobility experiment. Q J Econ 116(2):607–654, 2001

Kendler KS: Explanatory models for psychiatric illness. Am J Psychiatry 165(6):695–702, 2008 18483135

Kim HS, Sherman DK, Taylor SE: Culture and social support. Am Psychol 63(6):518–526, 2008 18793039

Kirmayer LJ, Young A: Culture and somatization: clinical, epidemiological, and ethnographic perspectives. Psychosom Med 60(4):420–430, 1998 9710287

Krause N: Assessing supportive social exchanges inside and outside religious institutions: exploring variations among whites, Hispanics, and blacks. Soc Indic Res 128(1):131–146, 2016

Lewis-Fernández R, Aggarwal NK: Psychiatric classification beyond the DSM: an interdisciplinary approach, in Revisioning Psychiatry: Cultural Phenomenology, Critical Neuroscience, and Global Mental Health. Edited by Kirmayer LJ, Lemelson RB, Cummings CA. New York, Cambridge University Press, 2015, pp 434–468

Lewis-Fernández R, Guarnaccia PJ, Martínez IE, et al: Comparative phenomenology of ataques de nervios, panic attacks, and panic disorder. Cult Med Psychiatry 26(2):199–223, 2002 12211325

Lewis-Fernández R, Horvitz-Lennon M, Blanco C, et al: Significance of endorsement of psychotic symptoms by US Latinos. J Nerv Ment Dis 197(5):337–347, 2009 19440107

Lewis-Fernández R, Gorritz M, Raggio GA, et al: Association of trauma-related disorders and dissociation with four idioms of distress among Latino psychiatric outpatients. Cult Med Psychiatry 34(2):219–243, 2010a 20414799

Lewis-Fernández R, Hinton DE, Laria AJ, et al: Culture and the anxiety disorders: recommendations for DSM-V. Depress Anxiety 27(2):212–229, 2010b 20037918

Lewis-Fernández R, Aggarwal NK, Lam PC, et al: Feasibility, acceptability and clinical utility of the Cultural Formulation Interview: mixed-methods results from the DSM-5 international field trial. Br J Psychiatry 210(4):290–297, 2017a 28104738

Lewis-Fernández R, Kirmayer LJ, Guarnaccia PJ, et al: Cultural concepts of distress, in Kaplan and Sadock's Comprehensive Textbook of Psychiatry, Vol II. Edited by Sadock BJ, Sadock VA, Ruiz R. New York, Lippincott, Williams & Wilkins, 2017b, pp 2443–2460

Lindert J, Ehrenstein OS, Priebe S, et al: Depression and anxiety in labor migrants and refugees—a systematic review and meta-analysis. Soc Sci Med 69(2):246–257, 2009 19539414

Marques L, Robinaugh DJ, LeBlanc NJ, et al: Cross-cultural variations in the prevalence and presentation of anxiety disorders. Expert Rev Neurother 11(2):313–322, 2011 21306217

Moitra E, Lewis-Fernández R, Stout RL, et al: Disparities in psychosocial functioning in a diverse sample of adults with anxiety disorders. J Anxiety Disord 28(3):335–343, 2014 24685821

Neal-Barnett A, Stadulis R, Murray M, et al: Sister circles as a culturally relevant intervention for anxious African American women. Clin Psychol (New York) 18(3):266–273, 2011 22081747

Okasha A, Saad A, Khalil AH, et al: Phenomenology of obsessive-compulsive disorder: a transcultural study. Compr Psychiatry 35(3):191–197, 1994 8045109

Okazaki S: Sources of ethnic differences between Asian American and white American college students on measures of depression and social anxiety. J Abnorm Psychol 106(1):52–60, 1997 9103717

Otiniano Verissimo AD, Gee GC, Ford CL, et al: Racial discrimination, gender discrimination, and substance abuse among Latina/os nationwide. Cultur Divers Ethnic Minor Psychol 20(1):43–51, 2014 24491127

Pan D, Huey SJ, Hernandez D: Culturally adapted versus standard exposure treatment for phobic Asian Americans: treatment efficacy, moderators and predictors. Cultur Divers Ethnic Minor Psychol 17(1):11, 2011

Park J, Kitayama S: Interdependent selves show face-induced facilitation of error processing: cultural neuroscience of self-threat. Soc Cogn Affect Neurosci 9(2):201–208, 2014 23160814

Polanco L, Duarte C, Lewis-Fernández R: Acculturation and suicide-related risk among Latin American migrants, in Oxford Textbook of Migrant Psychiatry. Edited by Bhugra D. New York, Oxford University Press, in press

Ruef AM, Litz BT, Schlenger WE: Hispanic ethnicity and risk for combat-related posttraumatic stress disorder. Cultur Divers Ethnic Minor Psychol 6(3):235–251, 2000 10938633

Ryder AG, Yang H, Heine SJ: Somatization vs. psychologization of emotional distress: a paradigmatic example for cultural psychopathology. Online Readings in Psychology and Culture 10(2):3–22, 2002

Somers JM, Goldner EM, Waraich P, et al: Prevalence and incidence studies of anxiety disorders: a systematic review of the literature. Can J Psychiatry 51:100–113, 2006

Stockdale SE, Lagomasino IT, Siddique J, et al: Racial and ethnic disparities in detection and treatment of depression and anxiety among psychiatric and primary health care visits, 1995–2005. Med Care 46(7):668–677, 2008 18580385

Triandis HC: Cultural syndromes and subjective well-being, in Culture and Subjective Well-Being. Edited by Diener E, Suh EM. Cambridge, MA, MIT Press, 2000, pp 13–36

van Loon A, van Schaik A, Dekker J, et al: Bridging the gap for ethnic minority adult outpatients with depression and anxiety disorders by culturally adapted treatments. J Affect Disord 147(1–3):9–16, 2013 23351566

Vargas SM, Cabassa LJ, Nicasio A, et al: Toward a cultural adaptation of pharmacotherapy: Latino views of depression and antidepressant therapy. Transcult Psychiatry 52(2):244–273, 2015 25736422

Villatoro AP, Morales ES, Mays VM: Family culture in mental health help-seeking and utilization in a nationally representative sample of Latinos in the United States: the NLAAS. Am J Orthopsychiatry 84(4):353–363, 2014 24999521

Wagner B, Schulz W, Knaevelsrud C: Efficacy of an Internet-based intervention for posttraumatic stress disorder in Iraq: a pilot study. Psychiatry Res 195(1–2):85–88, 2012 21813187

Weisberg RB, Beard C, Moitra E, et al: Adequacy of treatment received by primary care patients with anxiety disorders. Depress Anxiety 31(5):443–450, 2014 24190762

Williams MT, Domanico J, Marques L, et al: Barriers to treatment among African Americans with obsessive-compulsive disorder. J Anxiety Disord 26(4):555–563, 2012 22410094

Recommended Readings

Asnaani A, Richey JA, Dimaite R, et al: A cross-ethnic comparison of lifetime prevalence rates of anxiety disorders. J Nerv Ment Dis 198:551–555, 2010

Hinton DE: Multicultural challenges in the delivery of anxiety treatment. Depress Anxiety 29:1–3, 2012

Hinton DE, Lewis-Fernández R: The cross-cultural validity of posttraumatic stress disorder: implications for DSM-5. Depress Anxiety 28:783–801, 2011

Kohrt BA, Rasmussen A, Kaiser BN, et al: Cultural concepts of distress and psychiatric disorders: literature review and research recommendations for global mental health epidemiology. Int J Epidemiol 43(2):365–406, 2014

Lewis-Fernandez R, Hinton DE, Laria AJ, et al: Culture and the anxiety disorders: recommendations for DSM-V. Depress Anxiety 27:212–229, 2010

Wheaton MG, Berman NC, Fabricant LE, et al: Differences in obsessive-compulsive symptoms and obsessive beliefs: a comparison between African Americans, Asian Americans, Latino Americans, and European Americans. Cogn Behav Ther 42(1):9–20, 2013 23134374

CHAPTER 5

Economic and Social Burden of Anxiety, Trauma-Related, and Obsessive-Compulsive and Related Disorders

David F. Tolin, Ph.D.

In 2015, the United States spent $3.2 trillion on health care, or 17.8% of the gross domestic product (Centers for Disease Control and Prevention 2017). Chronic diseases cost more than $1 trillion, with mental disorders accounting for 16% of this cost (DeVol and Bedroussian 2007). Globally, mental disorders account for 5 of the top 10 causes of years lived with disability (Murray and Lopez 1996). The aim of this chapter is to describe the burden of anxiety, trauma-related, and obsessive-compulsive and related disorders from an economic and quality-of-life perspective. After reviewing research on the prevalence of anxiety-related disorders, I describe the financial burden of anxiety in terms of its direct and indirect costs, including analyses showing the effect of anxiety-related disorders on work impairment and income. I also discuss the effect of anxiety on quality of life at the individual and family level.

Estimating the Economic Burden of Anxiety, Trauma, and OCD-Related Disorders

Psychiatric Work Impairment

One way to measure the economic burden of anxiety disorders is to examine the extent of work or role impairment. In the National Comorbidity Survey (NCS), participants were asked about *psychiatric work loss days* (number of days that the respondent was unable to work or carry out usual activities because of mental health issues) and *psychiatric work cutback days* (number of days that the respondent was less effective at work or in activities because of mental health issues) in the past 30 days (Kessler and Frank 1997). *Psychiatric work impairment days* are then calculated from the combination of both. Previous research with the NCS (Kessler and Frank 1997) and the Australian National Survey of Mental Health and Well-Being (Lim et al. 2000) indicated that all of the anxiety disorders assessed in those surveys were associated with a significantly increased number of psychiatric work impairment days, with particularly high rates of work impairment days seen in respondents meeting criteria for panic disorder, generalized anxiety disorder (GAD), PTSD, and agoraphobia.

In this chapter, I examine psychiatric work impairment in the Collaborative Psychiatric Epidemiology Surveys (CPES; Alegria et al. 2008), a compilation of three nationally representative surveys (N=20,013) conducted by the Institute for Social Research at the University of Michigan. The core CPES questionnaire was based largely on the World Mental Health Composite International Diagnostic Interview, a standardized psychiatric diagnostic interview developed for administration by lay interviewers. The CPES include the following three surveys:

NCS-Replication (NCS-R; Kessler and Merikangas 2004): The NCS-R was administered in two parts. Part one included a core diagnostic assessment of all 9,282 respondents. Part two included questions about risk factors, consequences, other correlates, and additional disorders. Part two was administered to only 5,692 of the 9,282 part-one respondents.

National Survey of American Life (Jackson et al. 2004): The National Survey of American Life was designed to explore racial/ethnic differences in mental disorders and service use in African American (n=3,570) and Afro-Caribbean (n=1,621) populations of the United States as compared with non-Hispanic white respondents (n=891) living in the same communities.

National Latino and Asian American Study (NLAAS; Alegria et al. 2004): The NLAAS examined the prevalence of mental disorders and service use by Latino and Asian American adults in the United States. The NLAAS survey was administered to Latino (n=2,554) and Asian American (n=2,095) adults as well as a small sample of non-Latino white adults (n=215).

All of these surveys consisted of home-based interviews of noninstitutionalized adults aged 18 years and older living in the United States. The NCS-R and National Survey of American Life were conducted from 2001 to 2003; the NLAAS was conducted from 2002 to 2003.

As was done with previous research (Kessler et al. 2001), the current analyses calculated the number of psychiatric work impairment days as the number of psychiatric work loss days plus 50% of the number of psychiatric work cutback days. Although studies have differed in how psychiatric work impairment was calculated, this method is now preferred (R.C. Kessler, personal communication, February 10, 2007).

Information about psychiatric work loss and work cutback days was available from 14,162 CPES respondents, allowing for the calculation of psychiatric work impairment days over the previous 30-day period. Table 5–1 shows the average number of psychiatric work impairment days for respondents meeting DSM-IV (American Psychiatric Association 1994) criteria for anxiety disorders within the past 30 days.

TABLE 5–1.   **Psychiatric work impairment days in the past 30 days, according to 30-day anxiety disorder diagnoses, from the Collaborative Psychiatric Epidemiology Surveys (N=20,013)**

DSM-IV diagnosis	N	Mean impairment days, N (SD)	t vs. those without disorder[a]	d vs. those without disorder
Adult separation anxiety disorder	72	4.74 (8.14)	12.49	0.68
Agoraphobia without panic disorder	99	5.57 (8.70)	19.81	0.80
Generalized anxiety disorder	105	1.52 (4.24)	4.01	0.29
OCD[b]	92	3.23 (6.01)	9.92	0.60
Panic disorder	146	3.50 (6.03)	14.13	0.65
PTSD	131	3.90 (7.16)	13.84	0.62
Social phobia	432	2.59 (5.82)	17.12	0.48
Specific phobia	492	1.97 (5.20)	11.27	0.37
Any anxiety disorder	1,245	2.23 (5.40)	19.08	0.47

Note. t=Student t test; d=Cohen's d (effect size).
[a]$P=0.001$.
[b]Calculated according to the presence of obsessions or compulsions plus interference attributed to obsessions or compulsions or presence of symptoms for more than 60 minutes/day.

For each anxiety disorder, those with and without the condition (even if other mental disorders were present) were compared with independent-sample t tests as well as the effect size estimate d, for which values of 0.2, 0.5, and 0.8 are interpreted conventionally to mean small, medium, and large effects, respectively (Cohen 1988). As shown in Table 5–1, anxiety disorders overall were associated with a mean 2.2 psychiatric work impairment days per month, with the greatest number of impairment days seen in respondents meeting criteria for agoraphobia, adult separation anxiety disorder, PTSD, panic disorder, and OCD. All anxiety disorders were associated with a significantly higher rate of work impairment than found for those without these disorders.

Next, I compared respondents with current anxiety disorders (n=1,433), those with remitted anxiety disorders (n=1,491), and those with no history of anxiety disorders (n=2,644). The three groups differed in psychiatric work impairment days ($F_{2, 5,565}$= 196.84; $P<0.001$). Tukey honestly significant difference post hoc tests indicated significant differences among all three groups ($P<0.05$; Figure 5–1). Thus, even individuals with remitted anxiety disorders show residual work impairment.

Income

I identified the proportion of respondents in each group whose household income was below the federal poverty line for a family of that size. Chi-square analysis indicated that the three groups differed: $\chi^2(2)=125.971$; $P=0.001$. Respondents with current anxiety disorders were more likely to live below the federal poverty threshold (22.4%) than were those with remitted (10.2%) or no anxiety disorders (11.5%). As shown in Figure 5–2, the highest poverty rates were seen among respondents with OCD. More than one-third of the respondents with OCD or agoraphobia lived below

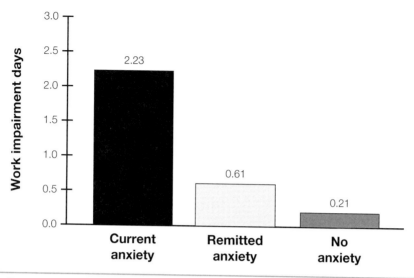

FIGURE 5–1.   Psychiatric work impairment in respondents with current, remitted, or no anxiety disorders.

Mean (standard error) psychiatric work impairment days in the past month for respondents with current anxiety disorders, those with remitted (lifetime but not in the past 30 days) anxiety disorders, and those with no history of anxiety disorders.

the federal poverty line; more than one-quarter of those with panic disorder, separation anxiety disorder, and social phobia lived below the poverty line.

Overall Cost to Society

Psychiatric work impairment is only one of several possible contributors to the economic burden of anxiety. Historically, economic burden of illness has been defined as including *direct costs* and *indirect costs*. Direct costs include psychiatric service costs (e.g., counseling and hospitalizations), nonpsychiatric medical costs (e.g., emergency department treatment), and the costs of medications. Indirect costs include lost productivity resulting from suicide (mortality), excessive absenteeism, or reduced work capacity.

In the first major examination of the overall financial costs of anxiety disorders, DuPont et al. (1996) reanalyzed data from survey respondents with panic disorder with and without agoraphobia, social phobia, simple phobia, OCD, and GAD (importantly, however, PTSD was not assessed). Similarly, Greenberg et al. (1999) reanalyzed data from the NCS, supplemented by cost data from a health maintenance organization and the U.S. Census Bureau, costs from professional associations and news periodicals, suicide data from the National Center for Health Statistics, and industry sources regarding prescription drugs. Anxiety disorders included in this review were panic disorder, agoraphobia, PTSD, social anxiety disorder, specific phobia, and GAD (however, OCD and related disorders were not assessed).

Overall, these two studies found relatively similar costs of anxiety disorders: DuPont et al. (1996) estimated the total cost to be $46.6 billion in 1990 (approximately $73.9 billion in 2007 dollars), or 31.5% of the total economic burden of mental illness. Greenberg et al. (1999) estimated this cost to be $42.3 billion in 1990 (approximately

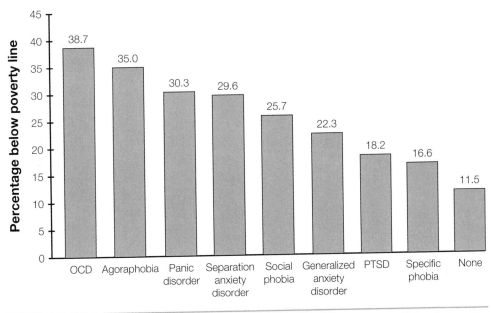

Figure 5-2. Proportion of respondents with current anxiety disorders living below the federal poverty line.

$67.1 billion in 2007 dollars). However, as shown in Figure 5–3, the distribution of costs was quite different between the two studies. DuPont and colleagues reported that approximately three-quarters of the total cost of anxiety disorders stemmed from indirect costs, particularly income loss from work ($34.2 billion, or $54.2 billion in 2007 dollars). Mortality costs added $1.3 billion ($2.1 billion in 2007 dollars) to the indirect costs. Direct costs accounted for less than one-quarter of the total cost, $10.7 billion ($17.0 billion in 2007 dollars). Of the direct costs, nursing home costs accounted for the largest percentage ($5.5 billion, or $8.7 billion in 2007 dollars), followed by prescription drug costs ($1.2 billion, or $1.9 billion in 2007 dollars), nonphysician mental health visits ($645 million, or $1.0 billion in 2007 dollars), short-stay hospital care ($388 million, or $615 million in 2007 dollars), and office-based physician visits ($356 million, or $564 million in 2007 dollars).

Conversely, Greenberg et al. (1999) reported that 85% of the total costs were due to direct costs, particularly nonpsychiatric medical treatment ($23.0 billion, or $36.5 billion in 2007 dollars). Psychiatric treatment costs accounted for $13.3 billion ($21.1 billion in 2007 dollars), and pharmaceutical costs accounted for $759 million ($1.2 billion in 2007 dollars). Indirect costs, on the other hand, represented a much smaller proportion of the total costs. Total workplace costs accounted for $4.1 billion ($6.5 billion in 2007 dollars), followed by mortality costs ($1.2 billion, or $1.9 billion in 2007 dollars).

Why was the cost distribution so different, with DuPont et al. (1996) showing mostly indirect costs and Greenberg et al. (1999) showing mostly direct costs? One possible contributor is the difference in patient groups between the two studies. DuPont's group did not examine individuals with PTSD. In the Greenberg et al. study, individuals with PTSD were among the highest users of health care services and were significantly more likely than those without PTSD to use virtually all levels of mental

Dupont et al. 1996

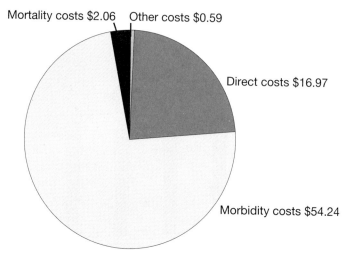

Greenberg et al. 1996

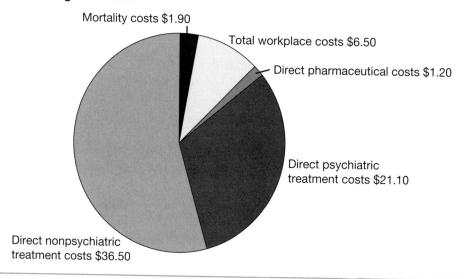

FIGURE 5–3. Economic costs of anxiety disorders.

Adjusted to 2007 dollars, in billions of dollars.

Source.   *Top:* DuPont et al. 1996; *Bottom:* Greenberg et al. 1999.

health treatment, including psychiatric hospitalization. Among veterans seen in a Veterans Affairs medical center, those with PTSD had a greater number of medical conditions and complaints than did those without PTSD (Deykin et al. 2001) and were more likely to have received recent inpatient or outpatient medical treatment (Schnurr et al. 2000). PTSD is associated with substantially higher health care costs than are other anxiety disorders (Marciniak et al. 2005). Therefore, the inclusion of individuals with PTSD (as well as attention to the nonpsychiatric medical treatment in such individuals) might well have increased the direct cost estimates in that study. Greenberg et al. (1999; using NCS data) did not examine individuals with OCD. Given the high rates of unemployment and reduced work capacity among individuals with OCD (Murray and Lopez 1996), the inclusion of this population might have increased the indirect cost estimate. Another likely contributor to the difference is the expanded inclusion of direct nonpsychiatric medical costs in the Greenberg study. In the DuPont et al. (1996) study, medical treatment visits were included only if they were associated with a primary or secondary diagnosis of an anxiety disorder.

Thus, in addition to being the most common forms of mental disorder, anxiety disorders are among the most costly. All of the anxiety disorders are associated with significant impairment in work and role functioning, and even individuals whose anxiety disorders have remitted continue to report residual functional impairment. Individuals with anxiety disorders are significantly more likely than those without anxiety disorders to live below the poverty threshold, with poverty particularly common in individuals with OCD and agoraphobia. The relationship between anxiety and income might well be bidirectional: low socioeconomic status may increase the risk of developing anxiety disorders, and the presence of anxiety-related symptoms can add to work impairment and subsequently reduce income from work. The overall economic burden of anxiety disorders was estimated at $67–$74 billion in 2007 dollars (or $83–$92 billion in today's dollars). The breakdown of expenditures (e.g., direct vs. indirect costs) is not clear, although direct costs of psychiatric treatment clearly do not account for most of the cost. Rather, the direct costs of nonpsychiatric medical treatment (e.g., emergency department visits, general practitioner visits) and lost revenue from work appear to be stronger contributors. The financial burden of the obsessive-compulsive and related disorders is not detailed here; however, the relation between these disorders and health-related quality of life is addressed later in this chapter in the "Quality of Life" subsection.

Estimating the Social Burden of Anxiety, Trauma, and OCD-Related Disorders

Family Burden

Although considerable research has been conducted on the effect of mental illness (e.g., schizophrenia) on the family, anxiety disorders have received considerably less attention in this regard; most of the existing studies have examined family burden in relation to OCD and (typically combat-related) PTSD. Overall, family members of patients with OCD and PTSD generally report levels of distress, impairment, and burden comparable with those of family members of patients with severe mental illness, such as schizophrenia (Kalra et al. 2008; Veltro et al. 1994).

Anxiety disorders such as OCD and PTSD appear to have a negative impact on partner relationships, with patients and their partners in both groups reporting high levels of relationship distress (Cooper 1996; Jordan et al. 1992; Riggs et al. 1998). Among veterans with PTSD, emotional numbing has been identified as a specific symptom associated with greater relationship distress (Riggs et al. 1998). Furthermore, the presence of combat-related PTSD appears to increase the risk for interpersonal physical and verbal aggression, including domestic violence (Taft et al. 2007).

In addition to partner relationship problems and distress, some evidence suggests that anxiety disorders may negatively affect other aspects of family functioning. Individuals with OCD and veterans with PTSD both report problems with family functioning (Davidson and Mellor 2001; Hollander et al. 1996). Family members also report general family dysfunction (Davidson and Mellor 2001; Van Noppen and Steketee 2003) as well as specific burden in areas such as financial strain, disruption of family activities, and impaired family interactions (Black et al. 1998; Calvocoressi et al. 1995; Van Noppen and Steketee 2003; Verbosky and Ryan 1988). Similar to research findings on the potential impact of PTSD on partner relationships among veterans, emotional numbing appears to be particularly related to impairment in the relationship between the child and the veteran parent with PTSD (Ruscio et al. 2002).

Finally, an anxiety disorder in a family member has been associated with psychological distress, poor psychosocial functioning, and reduced quality of life among other members of the family. In some studies, family members of individuals with PTSD or OCD reported impairment in their social and leisure functioning as a result of their family member's illness (Black et al. 1998; Cooper 1996; Stengler-Wenzke et al. 2006). In comparison with the general population, family members also reported lower levels of physical and psychological well-being (Stengler-Wenzke et al. 2006) and life satisfaction (Jordan et al. 1992). Among family members of relatives with OCD, severity of family members' depressive and anxious symptoms was found to be related to degree of modifications made in routine activities because of OCD and the patient's reactions when the family member refused to assist in rituals (Amir et al. 2000). Some evidence indicates that children of veterans with PTSD have greater behavioral, academic, and psychiatric problems than do children of veterans without PTSD or children of civilians (Davidson et al. 1989; Harkness 1991; Jordan et al. 1992).

Quality of Life

Quality of life is a multidimensional construct that extends beyond anxiety symptoms to include subjective well-being and life satisfaction. Documented quality-of-life problems in the anxiety disorders have included marital and financial problems in panic disorder (Weissman 1991), impaired relationships in social anxiety disorder (Eng et al. 2005; Stein and Kean 2000), high rates of public financial assistance and diminished subjective well-being in PTSD (Zatzick et al. 1997), role limitations in OCD (Hollander et al. 1996; Koran et al. 1996), and high rates of disability in GAD (Wittchen 2002).

Olatunji et al. (2007) conducted a quantitative review of 32 patient samples from 23 separate studies ($N=2,892$). Effect size estimates were calculated between anxiety and control samples. Overall, a large effect size was found ($d=1.31$), indicating poorer quality of life among patients with anxiety than among control subjects, with no significant difference seen between studies that used epidemiological samples and studies that used treatment-seeking clinical samples. No diagnosis was associated with significantly poorer overall quality of life (compared with control samples) than was any other diagnosis. Across anxiety disorders, mental health and social functioning were rated as more impaired than was physical health.

Figure 5–4 shows, for each anxiety disorder, mean effect size estimates for specific quality-of-life domains (physical health, mental health, work, social, home and family). With few exceptions, each anxiety disorder was associated with large and significant effect sizes compared with control samples. For physical health, all disorders

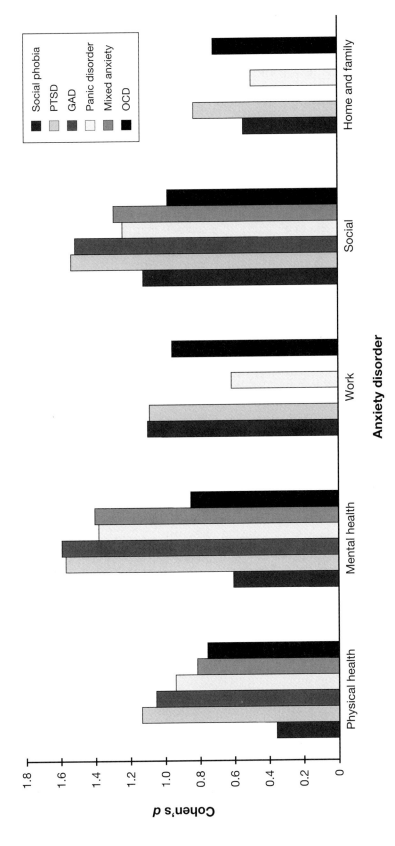

FIGURE 5–4. Effect size estimates for specific domains of quality of life in subjects with specific anxiety disorders compared with control samples.

GAD=generalized anxiety disorder.
Source. Adapted from Olatunji et al. 2007.

except social phobia were associated with significant impairment. For mental health, the effect sizes for PTSD, GAD, panic disorder, and mixed anxiety were significantly higher than that for social phobia. For work, PTSD was associated with a significantly larger effect size estimate than was panic disorder. For social and home and family, no significant differences were found among the anxiety disorders.

Significant deficits in health-related quality of life also have been identified in the obsessive-compulsive and related disorders. Hoarding disorder is associated with high levels of functional impairment (Lochner et al. 2005), as well as substantial safety risk (Frost et al. 2000); as an example, an analysis of house fires in Melbourne, Australia, over a 10-year period found that hoarding was determined to be a factor in 24% of all preventable fire fatalities (Lucini et al. 2009). Patients with hoarding disorder reported significantly lower quality of life across multiple domains than did nonhoarding patients with OCD (Saxena et al. 2011). In a self-selected sample, people with hoarding disorder reported a level of psychiatric work impairment that equaled or exceeded that of most individuals with anxiety and depressive disorders and was comparable with that reported by those with bipolar disorder (Tolin et al. 2008). These participants also reported high rates of threats of eviction and removal of children or elderly from the home by government agencies (Tolin et al. 2008). Involvement of government agencies, including the public health department, is not uncommon in hoarding disorder cases: approximately 64% of surveyed health officials reported receiving at least one complaint of hoarding during a 5-year period (Frost et al. 2000).

Body dysmorphic disorder is associated with substantial functional impairments and reduced quality of life. In epidemiological research, 21% of individuals with body dysmorphic disorder report substantial social impairment resulting from appearance preoccupations, and 9% report work or school impairment because of these concerns (Koran et al. 2008). In one study of treatment-seeking patients, fewer than half were working full-time, and 23% were receiving disability payments. Thirty-nine percent of the sample reported not working in the past month because of psychiatric illness, and of those who were working, 80% reported impairment in work functioning because of psychiatric illness (Didie et al. 2008). Many avoid social interactions because they fear that others will see their perceived physical defects (Kelly et al. 2010), and between one-quarter and one-third report having been completely housebound at some point (Phillips et al. 2005). The majority (77%) report a history of suicidal ideation, and 24% report a history of suicide attempts (Phillips et al. 2006).

Individuals with trichotillomania show elevated levels of depression and anxiety, as well as lower self-esteem, compared to those without trichotillomania (Duke et al. 2009). Among treatment-seeking and other selected samples, patients with trichotillomania often report significant impairments in social functioning, such as problems with peer relationships, teasing, and feeling isolated (Marcks et al. 2005). Most adults with trichotillomania report behaviors to conceal hair loss; physical pain or skin irritation; being secretive about hair pulling; avoiding certain recreational activities so that hair loss will not be detected; problems with concentration; and feeling alone, guilty, or unattractive (Diefenbach et al. 2005). Impairment in academic and occupational functioning is common (Woods et al. 2006). In severe cases of hair ingestion, trichobezoars (masses of hair in the digestive tract) can lead to intestinal obstructions and associated medical complications.

Studies of selected skin-picking disorder samples indicate that the disorder can be time consuming, with some patients reporting spending 6–8 hours per day picking skin (Odlaug and Grant 2008). Approximately half experience "deep craters" and infections caused by skin picking (Wilhelm et al. 1999). Many report avoiding social or entertainment events, or going out into public, because of the effects of skin picking, and more than one-third report daily interference with work duties (Flessner and Woods 2006).

Key Points

- Anxiety-related disorders were associated with an average of 2 psychiatric work impairment days per month, with the greatest number of impairment days seen in individuals with agoraphobia, adult separation anxiety disorder, PTSD, panic disorder, and OCD. Even individuals with remitted anxiety-related disorders report residual work impairment.

- Individuals with anxiety-related disorders are more likely to live below the federal poverty threshold than are those without anxiety disorders, with more than one-third of respondents with OCD or agoraphobia living below the federal poverty line.

- The overall cost of anxiety-related disorders was estimated to be $67–$74 billion in 2007 dollars (or $83–$92 billion in today's dollars). Direct costs of nonpsychiatric medical treatment and lost revenue from work appear to be major contributors to the overall cost.

- Family members of individuals with anxiety-related disorders report high levels of distress, impairment, and caregiver burden.

- Anxiety-related disorders are associated with reduced quality of life, with no clear difference across diagnoses.

References

Alegria M, Takeuchi D, Canino G, et al: Considering context, place and culture: the National Latino and Asian American Study. Int J Methods Psychiatr Res 13(4):208–220, 2004 15719529

Alegria M, Jackson JS, Kessler RC, et al: Collaborative Psychiatric Epidemiology Surveys. Ann Arbor, MI, Inter-University Consortium for Political and Social Research, Institute for Social Research, Survey Research Center, University of Michigan, 2008

American Psychiatric Association: Diagnostic and Statistical Manual of Mental Disorders, 4th Edition. Washington, DC, American Psychiatric Association, 1994

Amir N, Freshman M, Foa EB: Family distress and involvement in relatives of obsessive-compulsive disorder patients. J Anxiety Disord 14(3):209–217, 2000 10868980

Black DW, Gaffney G, Schlosser S, et al: The impact of obsessive-compulsive disorder on the family: preliminary findings. J Nerv Ment Dis 186(7):440–442, 1998 9680047

Calvocoressi L, Lewis B, Harris M, et al: Family accommodation in obsessive-compulsive disorder. Am J Psychiatry 152(3):441–443, 1995 7864273

Centers for Disease Control and Prevention: Health Expenditures. May 3, 2017. Available at: https://www.cdc.gov/nchs/fastats/health-expenditures.htm. Accessed June 11, 2019.

Cohen J: Statistical Power Analysis for the Behavioral Sciences, 2nd Edition. Hillsdale, NJ, Erlbaum, 1988

Cooper M: Obsessive-compulsive disorder: effects on family members. Am J Orthopsychiatry 66(2):296–304, 1996 8860758

Davidson AC, Mellor DJ: The adjustment of children of Australian Vietnam veterans: is there evidence for the transgenerational transmission of the effects of war-related trauma? Aust N Z J Psychiatry 35(3):345–351, 2001 11437808

Davidson J, Smith R, Kudler H: Familial psychiatric illness in chronic posttraumatic stress disorder. Compr Psychiatry 30(4):339–345, 1989 2758806

DeVol R, Bedroussian A: An Unhealthy America: The Economic Burden of Chronic Disease. Santa Monica, CA, Milken Institute, 2007

Deykin EY, Keane TM, Kaloupek D, et al: Posttraumatic stress disorder and the use of health services. Psychosom Med 63(5):835–841, 2001 11573033

Didie ER, Menard W, Stern AP, et al: Occupational functioning and impairment in adults with body dysmorphic disorder. Compr Psychiatry 49(6):561–569, 2008 18970904

Diefenbach GJ, Tolin DF, Hannan S, et al: Trichotillomania: impact on psychosocial functioning and quality of life. Behav Res Ther 43(7):869–884, 2005 15896284

Duke DC, Bodzin DK, Tavares P, et al: The phenomenology of hairpulling in a community sample. J Anxiety Disord 23(8):1118–1125, 2009 19651487

DuPont RL, Rice DP, Miller LS, et al: Economic costs of anxiety disorders. Anxiety 2(4):167–172, 1996 9160618

Eng W, Coles ME, Heimberg RG, et al: Domains of life satisfaction in social anxiety disorder: relation to symptoms and response to cognitive-behavioral therapy. J Anxiety Disord 19(2):143–156, 2005 15533701

Flessner CA, Woods DW: Phenomenological characteristics, social problems, and the economic impact associated with chronic skin picking. Behav Modif 30(6):944–963, 2006 17050772

Frost RO, Steketee G, Williams L: Hoarding: a community health problem. Health Soc Care Community 8(4):229–234, 2000 11560692

Greenberg PE, Sisitsky T, Kessler RC, et al: The economic burden of anxiety disorders in the 1990s. J Clin Psychiatry 60(7):427–435, 1999 10453795

Harkness LL: The effect of combat-related PTSD on children. National Center for PTSD Clinical Newsletter 2(1):12–13, 1991

Hollander E, Kwon JH, Stein DJ, et al: Obsessive-compulsive and spectrum disorders: overview and quality of life issues. J Clin Psychiatry 57(suppl 8):3–6, 1996 8698678

Jackson JS, Torres M, Caldwell CH, et al: The National Survey of American Life: a study of racial, ethnic and cultural influences on mental disorders and mental health. Int J Methods Psychiatr Res 13(4):196–207, 2004 15719528

Jordan BK, Marmar CR, Fairbank JA, et al: Problems in families of male Vietnam veterans with posttraumatic stress disorder. J Consult Clin Psychol 60(6):916–926, 1992 1460153

Kalra H, Kamath P, Trivedi JK, et al: Caregiver burden in anxiety disorders. Curr Opin Psychiatry 21(1):70–73, 2008 18281843

Kelly MM, Walters C, Phillips KA: Social anxiety and its relationship to functional impairment in body dysmorphic disorder. Behav Ther 41(2):143–153, 2010 20412881

Kessler RC, Frank RG: The impact of psychiatric disorders on work loss days. Psychol Med 27(4):861–873, 1997 9234464

Kessler RC, Merikangas KR: The National Comorbidity Survey Replication (NCS-R): background and aims. Int J Methods Psychiatr Res 13(2):60–68, 2004 15297904

Kessler RC, Mickelson KD, Barber CB, et al: The effects of chronic medical conditions on work impairment, in Caring and Doing for Others: Social Responsibility in the Domains of the Family, Work, and Community. Edited by Rossi AS. Chicago, IL, University of Chicago Press, 2001, pp 403–426

Koran LM, Thienemann ML, Davenport R: Quality of life for patients with obsessive-compulsive disorder. Am J Psychiatry 153(6):783–788, 1996 8633690

Koran LM, Abujaoude E, Large MD, et al: The prevalence of body dysmorphic disorder in the United States adult population. CNS Spectr 13(4):316–322, 2008 18408651

Lim D, Sanderson K, Andrews G: Lost productivity among full-time workers with mental disorders. J Ment Health Policy Econ 3(3):139–146, 2000 11967449

Lochner C, Kinnear CJ, Hemmings SM, et al: Hoarding in obsessive-compulsive disorder: clinical and genetic correlates. J Clin Psychiatry 66(9):1155–1160, 2005 16187774

Lucini G, Monk I, Szlatenyi C: An Analysis of Fire Incidents Involving Hoarding Households. Worcester, MA, Worcester Polytechnic Institute, 2009

Marciniak MD, Lage MJ, Dunayevich E, et al: The cost of treating anxiety: the medical and demographic correlates that impact total medical costs. Depress Anxiety 21(4):178–184, 2005 16075454

Marcks BA, Woods DW, Ridosko JL: The effects of trichotillomania disclosure on peer perceptions and social acceptability. Body Image 2(3):299–306, 2005 18089196

Murray CJ, Lopez AD (eds): The Global Burden of Disease: A Comprehensive Assessment of Mortality and Disability From Diseases, Injuries, and Risk Factors in 1990 and Projected to 2020. Cambridge, MA, Harvard University Press, 1996

Odlaug BL, Grant JE: Clinical characteristics and medical complications of pathologic skin picking. Gen Hosp Psychiatry 30(1):61–66, 2008 18164942

Olatunji BO, Cisler JM, Tolin DF: Quality of life in the anxiety disorders: a meta-analytic review. Clin Psychol Rev 27(5):572–581, 2007 17343963

Phillips KA, Menard W, Fay C, et al: Demographic characteristics, phenomenology, comorbidity, and family history in 200 individuals with body dysmorphic disorder. Psychosomatics 46(4):317–325, 2005 16000674

Phillips KA, Didie ER, Menard W, et al: Clinical features of body dysmorphic disorder in adolescents and adults. Psychiatry Res 141(3):305–314, 2006 16499973

Riggs DS, Byrne CA, Weathers FW, et al: The quality of the intimate relationships of male Vietnam veterans: problems associated with posttraumatic stress disorder. J Trauma Stress 11(1):87–101, 1998 9479678

Ruscio AM, Weathers FW, King LA, et al: Male war-zone veterans' perceived relationships with their children: the importance of emotional numbing. J Trauma Stress 15(5):351–357, 2002 12392222

Saxena S, Ayers CR, Maidment KM, et al: Quality of life and functional impairment in compulsive hoarding. J Psychiatr Res 45(4):475–480, 2011 20822778

Schnurr PP, Friedman MJ, Sengupta A, et al: PTSD and utilization of medical treatment services among male Vietnam veterans. J Nerv Ment Dis 188(8):496–504, 2000 10972568

Stein MB, Kean YM: Disability and quality of life in social phobia: epidemiologic findings. Am J Psychiatry 157(10):1606–1613, 2000 11007714

Stengler-Wenzke K, Kroll M, Matschinger H, et al: Quality of life of relatives of patients with obsessive-compulsive disorder. Compr Psychiatry 47(6):523–527, 2006 17067878

Taft CT, Street AE, Marshall AD, et al: Posttraumatic stress disorder, anger, and partner abuse among Vietnam combat veterans. J Fam Psychol 21(2):270–277, 2007 17605549

Tolin DF, Frost RO, Steketee G, et al: The economic and social burden of compulsive hoarding. Psychiatry Res 160(2):200–211, 2008 18597855

Van Noppen BL, Steketee G: Family responses and multifamily behavioral treatment for obsessive-compulsive disorder. Brief Treat Crisis Interv 3(2):231–247, 2003

Veltro F, Magliano L, Lobrace S, et al: Burden on key relatives of patients with schizophrenia vs neurotic disorders: a pilot study. Soc Psychiatry Psychiatr Epidemiol 29(2):66–70, 1994 8009321

Verbosky SJ, Ryan DA: Female partners of Vietnam veterans: stress by proximity. Issues Ment Health Nurs 9(1):95–104, 1988 3356550

Weissman MM: Panic disorder: impact on quality of life. J Clin Psychiatry 52(suppl):6–8, discussion 9, 1991 1995601

Wilhelm S, Keuthen NJ, Deckersbach T, et al: Self-injurious skin picking: clinical characteristics and comorbidity. J Clin Psychiatry 60(7):454–459, 1999 10453800

Wittchen HU: Generalized anxiety disorder: prevalence, burden, and cost to society. Depress Anxiety 16(4):162–171, 2002

Woods DW, Flessner CA, Franklin ME, et al: The Trichotillomania Impact Project (TIP): exploring phenomenology, functional impairment, and treatment utilization. J Clin Psychiatry 67(12):1877–1888, 2006 17194265

Zatzick DF, Marmar CR, Weiss DS, et al: Posttraumatic stress disorder and functioning and quality of life outcomes in a nationally representative sample of male Vietnam veterans. Am J Psychiatry 154(12):1690–1695, 1997 9396947

Recommended Readings

DuPont RL, Rice DP, Shiraki S, et al: Economic costs of obsessive-compulsive disorder. Med Interface 8:102–109, 1996

Greenberg PE, Sisitsky T, Kessler RC, et al: The economic burden of anxiety disorders in the 1990s. J Clin Psychiatry 60:427–435, 1999

Kessler RC, Frank RG: The impact of psychiatric disorders on work loss days. Psychol Med 27:861–873, 1997

Murray CJ, Lopez AD (eds): The Global Burden of Disease: A Comprehensive Assessment of Mortality and Disability From Diseases, Injuries, and Risk Factors in 1990 and Projected to 2020. Cambridge, MA, Harvard University Press, 1996

Olatunji BO, Cisler JM, Tolin DF: Quality of life in the anxiety disorders: a meta-analytic review. Clin Psychol Rev 27:572–581, 2007

PART II

Core Principles for Treating
Anxiety Disorders

CHAPTER 6

Cognitive-Behavioral Concepts of Anxiety

Alexandra S. Tanner, M.A.

Michelle G. Craske, Ph.D.

Fear and anxiety are adaptive for human survival in the presence of actual threat. The human autonomic nervous system is designed to prepare us to respond effectively to threat in our environment. This process, commonly referred to as the fight-or-flight response (Cannon 1915), is initiated in the presence of both real and perceived threats. Pathological anxiety is characterized by a hypervigilance to threat, a tendency to perceive neutral or ambiguous stimuli as threatening, catastrophic interpretations of perceived threat, physiological hyperarousal in response to neutral or ambiguous stimuli, distorted beliefs regarding one's ability to tolerate or cope with threat, and reliance on escape and safety behaviors.

Cognitive-behavioral therapies (CBTs) are rooted in the science and theories of associative learning (i.e., classical and operant conditioning), social learning, and cognitive appraisal. CBT assumes that maladaptive thoughts, behaviors, and emotions have been acquired, at least in part, through learning and experience and therefore are amenable to change through new learning and experiences. In this chapter we provide overviews of these three theories of anxiety and their corresponding therapeutic principles.

Associative Learning Theory

Associative learning theory suggests that anxiety can be conditioned through direct experience of, vicarious observation of, and consumption of information about negative events (Mineka and Zinbarg 2006). Additionally, anxiety is maintained through negative reinforcement of avoidance behaviors, which provide temporary alleviation of anxiety symptoms. Thus, corresponding treatments include exposure therapy, which encourages approach behaviors and aims to extinguish conditioned fears by disrupting the association between the conditioned stimulus (i.e., neutral stimulus evoking fear) and unconditioned stimulus (i.e., aversive outcome).

Social Learning Theory

Social learning theory identified the importance of self-efficacy as a cognitive mediator of learning. *Self-efficacy* is defined as "the conviction that one can successfully execute the behavior required to produce an outcome" (Bandura 1977). With regard to anxiety, poor self-efficacy is likely to contribute to beliefs about one's inability to cope with threat, anxiety, and distress; these beliefs, in turn, facilitate escape and safety behaviors. Thus, corresponding interventions include behavioral experiments and exposure-based therapies encouraging accomplishment and mastery and cognitive restructuring interventions highlighting adaptive self-coping experiences (i.e., positivity reorientation; Clark 2014).

Cognitive Appraisal Theory

Cognitive appraisal theory assumes that distorted and dysfunctional thinking is present in all psychological disorders and mediates the impact of situational factors on mood and behaviors. Albert Ellis's (1962) theory of rational-emotive behavior therapy suggests that 1) thoughts can be confirmed or disproved by the environment and 2) emotional responses are mediated by thoughts; thus, maladaptive responses or reactions reflect inaccurate cognitions about the situation. In the context of anxiety, an individual's fearful response to a neutral situation reflects inappropriate thoughts about the danger or threat of that situation (e.g., an individual with social anxiety experiencing anxiety at a party). Thus, corresponding interventions include challenging and disproving the inaccurate thoughts to promote more adaptive responding.

Aaron Beck's (1976) theory of cognitive therapy similarly identifies rigid and inaccurate cognitions as a primary precipitant of maladaptive behaviors and emotional distress. More specifically, Beck (2005) suggested that underlying negative schemas about the self and world (hypothesized to originate from genetic predisposition and direct or observed life events) are activated by external events and subsequently bias information processing, which in turn results in distorted beliefs about experiences and cognitive errors. Among the anxiety disorders, underlying core beliefs/schemas often involve expectations of threat or danger and beliefs about one's inability to cope with threat or danger. Common cognitive errors include catastrophic interpretations of stimuli or events and biased expectations of negative outcomes. Cognitive errors are thought to mediate effects of schemas on automatic thoughts and typically result in actions that reinforce underlying schemas. Corresponding interventions thus include verbal cognitive restructuring interventions, such as schema-related evidence gathering; consequential analysis; cognitive bias identification; generating alternative representations of the self; normalization; decatastrophizing; problem solving; imaginal exposure to unwanted thoughts, images, and emotions; distancing; reframing or perspective taking; reattribution; and positivity reorientation (Clark 2014). Additionally, behavioral interventions include empirical hypothesis testing to gather new evidence for the formation of more accurate and balanced thinking (Clark 2014).

Cognitive-Behavioral Theory

Cognitive-behavioral theory represents a melding of learning theory and cognitive theory. CBTs emphasize the reciprocal interaction of thoughts, behaviors, and emotions with both the maintenance of psychopathology and its improvement (i.e., maladaptive reciprocal interactions vs. adaptive reciprocal interactions). More recently, "third-wave" cognitive-behavioral interventions such as mindfulness and acceptance-based therapies emphasize function rather than content of cognitions.

In this chapter, we outline the therapeutic interventions and summarize the literature for empirically supported CBTs for anxiety disorders. Additionally, we discuss emerging interventions and augmentation strategies that show promise for the treatment of anxiety. Last, we address concerns about the effect of comorbidity on the success of anxiety treatment as well as other practical considerations.

Empirically Based Treatments

CBT is a short-term, skills-based, goal-oriented treatment that, as discussed earlier, uses various strategies to target cognitive (e.g., maladaptive threat biases), behavioral (e.g., avoidant and safety-seeking behaviors), and physical (e.g., excessive autonomic arousal) anxiety symptoms. Interventions include psychoeducation and the self-monitoring of thoughts, behaviors, and feelings to increase awareness of the links between thoughts, behaviors, and feelings and the impact of these on mood; cognitive restructuring (i.e., identifying, challenging, and replacing) of catastrophic and inaccurate thinking patterns to encourage cognitive flexibility and more accurate thinking; in-vivo (i.e., real life), interoceptive, or imaginal exposure to feared stimuli to encourage approach and coping behaviors; and relaxation techniques and breathing retraining to downregulate autonomic arousal (Craske et al. 2017).

CBT is the most empirically supported treatment for anxiety disorders (Craske et al. 2017). Meta-analyses comparing CBT with waitlist control or treatment-as-usual conditions suggest that CBT is effective in reducing symptoms of generalized anxiety disorder (GAD; Cuijpers et al. 2014), social anxiety disorder (Mayo-Wilson et al. 2014), panic disorder (Pompoli et al. 2016), OCD (Öst et al. 2015), PTSD (Bisson et al. 2013), and mixed anxiety disorder samples (Bandelow et al. 2015; Cuijpers et al. 2016; Watts et al. 2015). A recent meta-analysis by Carpenter et al. (2018) examining 41 randomized placebo-controlled trials found moderate effects of CBT on target disorder symptoms, with large effect sizes for OCD, GAD, and acute stress disorder and small to moderate effect sizes for PTSD, social anxiety disorder, and panic disorder. When compared with pharmacotherapy, meta-analyses suggest CBT is equally efficacious for reducing anxiety (Cuijpers et al. 2013). CBT has also shown moderate improvements in patients' quality of life across anxiety disorders compared with that of patients receiving placebo, receiving an active comparator treatment, or on the waitlist (Hofmann et al. 2014).

Albeit with a smaller body of literature, empirical support exists for mindfulness- and acceptance-based therapies, such as acceptance and commitment therapy (ACT), in the treatment of anxiety disorders. Rooted in relational frame theory, ACT aims to increase psychological flexibility using acceptance and mindfulness strategies, combined with commitment and behavior-change strategies to alleviate suffering (Hayes and Pierson 2005). ACT focuses on acceptance of negative experiences and helps clients see how their continued distress stems from failed attempts to control or change anxious thoughts and feelings. Clients also are encouraged to engage in values-driven behavior with a willingness to experience anxiety in the pursuit of their goals. ACT uses six core principles to guide therapeutic interventions and achieve psychological flexibility: 1) challenging the control agenda, 2) cognitive defusion, 3) willingness/acceptance, 4) being present/the self as context, 5) values, and 6) commitment (Hayes and Pierson 2005).

Reviews of the literature suggest that ACT is an effective and promising intervention for anxiety disorders. A 2014 meta-analysis examining nine randomized controlled trials (RCTs) of ACT versus waitlist control or active control conditions for anxiety and OCD spectrum disorders found no significant difference in effect sizes between treatments (Bluett et al. 2014). A 2015 review examining four RCTs comparing ACT with alternative established treatments for GAD, social anxiety disorder, and mixed anxiety samples showed that ACT was a viable alternative to comparator treatments in reducing anxiety symptoms and improving quality of life and psychological flexibility (Landy et al. 2015). Additionally, mediation analyses suggested substantial overlap in treatment mechanisms of ACT and traditional CBT, indicating that both interventions may be targeting similar underlying processes. A 2012 review examining open trials of ACT for PTSD suggested that ACT may be beneficial for treatment of PTSD (Bomyea and Lang 2012); however, a recent RCT comparing ACT with present-centered therapy for PTSD in veterans found modest and similar effects for both treatments (Lang et al. 2017). Overall, preliminary research suggests ACT is a comparable intervention to traditional CBT for the treatment of OCD and anxiety disorders, but additional research is necessary to elucidate the effect of ACT on PTSD.

Novel or Emerging Treatments

Numerous novel cognitive-behavioral interventions show promise for the treatment of anxiety disorders. This section discusses the existing evidence for 1) an inhibitory model of exposure therapy, 2) D-cycloserine (DCS)-augmented exposure therapy, and 3) digital health interventions.

Inhibitory Learning Model

Craske et al. (2008, 2014) proposed a new theoretical framework for exposure therapy, known as the *inhibitory learning model*, which is grounded in basic science principles of associative extinction learning. The inhibitory learning model posits that new non-threat associations are learned during exposure and compete with the original threat association (Bouton 2000; Rescorla 2001). As demonstrated by the animal extinction literature, because original threat associations remain intact after extinction training, fear can return over time (i.e., spontaneous recovery), in novel contexts (i.e., context-renewal), and following unexpected exposure to an actual threat (i.e., reinstatement) (Bouton 2002). Consistent with this hypothesis, a substantial number of individuals with anxiety do not experience clinically significant reductions in symptoms following exposure-based therapies (Arch and Craske 2009) or relapse after treatment (Craske and Mystkowski 2006). Furthermore, individuals with anxiety demonstrate deficits in inhibitory learning and inhibitory neural regulation during extinction (Craske et al. 2012). Therefore, Craske et al. (2014) proposed strategies to optimize inhibitory learning and retrieval during exposure therapy to enhance treatment outcomes and compensate for inhibitory learning deficits among anxious individuals. Optimization strategies include 1) expectancy violation, 2) deepened extinction, 3) occasional reinforced extinction, 4) removal of safety signals, 5) variability, 6) retrieval cues, 7) multiple contexts, and 8) affect labeling (Craske et al. 2014).

A 2018 review of studies examining inhibitory learning optimization strategies in both human and animals suggested that some of the proposed strategies show promise for enhancing exposure therapy, particularly removal of safety signals and enhancing expectancy violations (Weisman and Rodebaugh 2018). Enhancing expectancy violations involves designing exposures that maximally violate the expectancy of the negative outcome (Craske et al. 2014) and has been shown to enhance exposure learning in acrophobia and interoceptive exposure compared with traditional exposure (Baker et al. 2010; Deacon et al. 2013). However, because of the limited number of studies and methodological limitations of the present literature, Weisman and Rodebaugh (2018) suggested areas of continued investigation. Given the strength of the theoretical basis for the inhibitory learning model, additional research on strategies to optimize inhibitory learning during exposure is warranted.

D-Cycloserine-Augmented Exposure Therapy

DCS is an NMDA partial agonist that has been studied in animal models and found to facilitate fear extinction when given before or shortly after extinction training (Davis et al. 2006). Over the past decade or so, DCS has gained popularity as a potential augmentation strategy of exposure-based therapy for anxiety disorders. Reviews and meta-analyses of the literature have indicated mixed results on the benefits of DCS augmentation on extinction learning (Bürkner et al. 2017; Hofmann et al. 2015; Mataix-Cols et al. 2017; McGuire et al. 2017; Ori et al. 2015). Whereas some studies found that DCS enhances extinction learning, others suggested DCS accelerates extinction learning (Hofmann et al. 2015); further studies have indicated null or adverse effects (Bürkner et al. 2017; McGuire et al. 2017; Hofmann et al. 2015). Inconsistent results across clinical trials hamper conclusions but likely reflect the presence of treatment-moderating variables. For example, DCS dose and timing of administration may contribute to varying results (Hofmann et al. 2015). Additionally, among individuals reporting high levels of fear after exposure, DCS appears to augment reconsolidation of fear memories rather than exposure learning (Hofmann et al. 2015).

In 2017, three meta-analyses were published by three independent research groups. Results of one meta-analysis examining 21 double-blind RCTs of DCS-augmented exposure therapy for OCD, PTSD, and anxiety disorders demonstrated small effects of augmentation on exposure therapy from pre- to posttreatment (Mataix-Cols et al. 2017). Moreover, results determined that DCS is not moderated by concurrent antidepressant use. The second meta-analysis examined 20 RCTs of DCS augmentation versus placebo augmentation for anxiety disorders, OCD, and PTSD (McGuire et al. 2017). Overall, results found nonsignificant differences between DCS and placebo augmentation across diagnoses on acute efficacy, treatment response, and treatment remission as well as follow-up efficacy, treatment response, and diagnostic remission. When examining diagnostic groups separately, however, DCS augmentation had a moderately significant effect on acute efficacy for anxiety disorders. Additionally, results elucidated numerous moderators of DCS augmentation, such as concurrent selective serotonin reuptake inhibitor use, age, study quality, and year of publication. The third meta-analysis examined 23 studies of DCS-augmented exposure therapy for OCD and anxiety disorders (Bürkner et al. 2017). Results revealed small effects of DCS at posttreatment and 1-month follow-up across diagnoses. Additionally, study quality and year of publication were significant moderators of DCS effects, with higher-quality and more-recent studies reporting smaller DCS effects. The most recent meta-analyses are limited by small sample sizes, particularly when diagnostic groups are examined separately, which reduces the power to find reliable moderators. Thus, conclusions should be interpreted with caution but may suggest a small benefit of DCS for enhancing exposure learning. Additional research is needed to identify better treatment and patient moderators of DCS to optimize augmentation effects on exposure-based therapies.

Digital Health Interventions

Treatment cost and accessibility remain barriers to therapy for many anxious individuals. Computer-based psychotherapy (CP) represents a promising solution to this problem. A 2009 meta-analysis examining 23 RCTs of CP (administered via standalone or internet-linked computers, palmtop computers, phone-interactive voice response, DVDs, and cell phones) versus non-CP for phobias, panic with and without agoraphobia, PTSD, and OCD found that CP and non-CP were equally effective (Cuijpers et al. 2009). Additionally, CP effects were not moderated by type of anxiety disorder or form of delivery. A 2010 meta-analysis examining 22 studies comparing CP with a waitlist or active treatment control condition for individuals with major depression, panic disorder, social anxiety disorder, or GAD found CP superior to control conditions in reducing depression and anxiety symptoms (Andrews et al. 2010). Furthermore, benefits of CP were maintained at a median of 26-week follow-up. The majority of comparator conditions were waitlist control. Among a subset of five studies comparing CP to face-to-face CBT, both treatments were equally beneficial.

With rapidly evolving smartphone technology, capabilities, and accessibility, interest has expanded to smartphone-administered interventions. A 2017 systematic review and meta-analysis indicated nine RCTs comparing smartphone interventions with control conditions for anxiety symptoms (subclinical and clinical samples; Firth et al. 2017). Smartphone interventions yielded significantly greater reductions in anxiety scores. The differences in effect sizes between smartphone interventions and control conditions were significantly greater for waitlist/inactive controls than for active controls. Because of the limited number of studies, varying study quality, and heterogeneity across treatments, conclusions should be interpreted with caution. Nevertheless, preliminary evidence suggests computer- and smartphone-administered interventions can reduce anxiety, which could have significant implications for our ability to meet the ever-growing demand for treatment.

Comorbidity and Practical Considerations

Comorbidity among anxiety disorders and mood disorders occurs frequently (Brown et al. 2001; Fava et al. 2000; Kessler et al. 2005). Studies indicate that the presence of comorbid depression does not minimize the effects of CBT for anxiety (Emmrich et al. 2012). Additionally, evidence suggests transdiagnostic CBT reduces anxiety among individuals with and without comorbid diagnoses (Norton et al. 2013) and is equally as effective as diagnosis-specific CBT for panic disorder, social anxiety disorder, and GAD (Norton and Barrera 2012). The benefits of transdiagnostic CBT likely reflect the underlying theoretical basis of CBT; more specifically, although the content of threat may vary across anxiety disorders, nonspecific CBT treatments can still be effective by targeting constructs such as threat biases and associative fear learning, which are common to all anxiety disorders.

Between-session practice, commonly referred to as "homework," is an integral component of CBTs. Homework compliance is considered a measure of treatment engagement (Lebeau et al. 2013), and meta-analyses suggest that compliance (i.e., quantity of homework completed) significantly predicts better treatment outcomes with small to moderate effect sizes (Kazantzis et al. 2010; Mausbach et al. 2010). In addition, homework completion quality—that is, how well the homework was completed—also significantly predicts better treatment response (Kazantzis et al. 2016). These findings highlight the importance of using homework during treatment and addressing issues of homework compliance during the course of therapy to increase treatment benefits.

Conclusion

Robust evidence exists for the benefits of CBT in reducing symptoms across anxiety, OCD, and stress disorders. Emerging treatments grounded in empirical science are building on existing interventions to increase efficacy and reduce the number of individuals who either do not respond to therapy or relapse following its termination. This chapter highlighted the importance of developing sound theoretical models of disorders and interventions to yield positive results. Mechanistic, translational, and clinical research is ongoing to enhance treatment techniques and identify individuals most likely to respond favorably.

Key Points

- Cognitive-behavioral therapies (CBTs) are grounded in associative learning, social learning, and cognitive appraisal theory.

- CBT is the most empirically supported treatment for anxiety disorders.

- Support for "third-wave" cognitive-behavioral interventions, such as acceptance and commitment therapy, for the treatment of anxiety is growing and suggests benefits comparable with those of traditional CBT.

- Novel interventions focused on enhancing consolidation and retrieval of new learning during therapy, such as the inhibitory learning model of exposure and D-cycloserine-augmented exposure therapy, show promise for enhancing treatment response and retention.

- Digitally administered CBT significantly reduces anxiety and may help address issues of treatment accessibility.

- Comorbidity among anxiety disorders and mood disorders is common, and transdiagnostic CBT is effective in reducing anxiety with and without comorbid diagnoses.

- Quantity and quality of homework compliance are significant predictors of treatment outcome and should be monitored and addressed throughout treatment.

References

Andrews G, Cuijpers P, Craske MG, et al: Computer therapy for the anxiety and depressive disorders is effective, acceptable and practical health care: a meta-analysis. PLoS ONE 5(10):e13196, 2010 20967242

Arch JJ, Craske MG: First-line treatment: a critical appraisal of cognitive behavioral therapy developments and alternatives. Psychiatr Clin North Am 32(3):191–215, 2009 19716989

Bandelow B, Reitt M, Röver C, et al: Efficacy of treatments for anxiety disorders: a meta-analysis. Int Clin Psychopharmacol 30(4):183–192, 2015 25932596

Bandura A: Self-efficacy: toward a unifying theory of behavioral change. Psychol Rev 84(2):191–215, 1977 847061

Baker A, Mystkowski J, Culver N, et al: Does habituation matter? Emotional processing theory and exposure therapy for acrophobia. Behav Res Ther 84(2):191–215, 2010 20723886

Beck AT: Cognitive Therapy and the Emotional Disorders. New York, International Universities Press, 1976

Beck AT: The current state of cognitive therapy: a 40-year retrospective. Arch Gen Psychiatry 62(9):953–959, 2005 16143727

Bisson JI, Roberts NP, Andrew M, et al: Psychological therapies for chronic post-traumatic stress disorder (PTSD) in adults. Cochrane Database Syst Rev 12(12):CD003388, 2013 24338345

Bluett EJ, Homan KJ, Morrison KL, et al: Acceptance and commitment therapy for anxiety and OCD spectrum disorders: an empirical review. J Anxiety Disord 28(6):612–624, 2014 25041735

Bomyea J, Lang AJ: Emerging interventions for PTSD: future directions for clinical care and research. Neuropharmacology 62(2):607–616, 2012 21664365

Bouton ME: A learning theory perspective on lapse, relapse, and the maintenance of behavior change. Health Psychol 19(1S):57–63, 2000 10709948

Bouton ME: Context, ambiguity, and unlearning: sources of relapse after behavioral extinction. Biol Psychiatry 52(10):976–986, 2002 12437938

Brown TA, Campbell LA, Lehman CL, et al: Current and lifetime comorbidity of the DSM-IV anxiety and mood disorders in a large clinical sample. J Abnorm Psychol 110(4):585–599, 2001 11727948

Bürkner PC, Bittner N, Holling H, et al: D-cycloserine augmentation of behavior therapy for anxiety and obsessive-compulsive disorders: a meta-analysis. PLoS ONE 12(3):e173660, 2017 28282427

Cannon WB: Bodily Changes in Pain, Hunger, Fear, and Rage. New York, Appleton-Century-Crofts, 1915

Carpenter JK, Andrews LA, Witcraft SM, et al: Cognitive behavioral therapy for anxiety and related disorders: a meta-analysis of randomized placebo-controlled trials. Depress Anxiety 35(6):502–514, 2018 29451967

Clark DA: Cognitive restructuring, in The Wiley Handbook of Cognitive Behavioral Therapy, Vol 1. Edited by Hofmann SG (Series Editor), Dozois DJA (Volume Editor). Hoboken, NJ, Wiley, 2014, pp 23–44

Craske MG, Mystkowski J: Exposure therapy and extinction: clinical studies, in Fear and Learning: From Basic Processes to Clinical Implications. Edited by Craske MG, Hermans D, Vansteenwegen D. Washington, DC, American Psychological Association, 2006, pp 217–233

Craske MG, Kircanski K, Zelikowsky M, et al: Optimizing inhibitory learning during exposure therapy. Behav Res Ther 46(1):5–27, 2008 18005936

Craske MG, Liao B, Brown L, et al: Role of inhibition in exposure therapy. J Exp Psychopathol 3:322–345, 2012

Craske MG, Treanor M, Conway CC, et al: Maximizing exposure therapy: an inhibitory learning approach. Behav Res Ther 58:10–23, 2014 24864005

Craske MG, Stein MB, Eley TC, et al: Anxiety disorders. Nat Rev Dis Primers 3:17024, 2017 28470168

Cuijpers P, Marks IM, van Straten A, et al: Computer-aided psychotherapy for anxiety disorders: a meta-analytic review. Cogn Behav Ther 38(2):66–82, 2009 20183688

Cuijpers P, Sijbrandij M, Koole SL, et al: The efficacy of psychotherapy and pharmacotherapy in treating depressive and anxiety disorders: a meta-analysis of direct comparisons. World Psychiatry 12(2):137–148, 2013 23737423

Cuijpers P, Sijbrandij M, Koole S, et al: Psychological treatment of generalized anxiety disorder: a meta-analysis. Clin Psychol Rev 34(2):130–140, 2014 24487344

Cuijpers P, Cristea IA, Weitz E, et al: The effects of cognitive and behavioural therapies for anxiety disorders on depression: a meta-analysis. Psychol Med 46(16):3451–3462, 2016 27659840

Davis M, Ressler K, Rothbaum BO, et al: Effects of D-cycloserine on extinction: translation from preclinical to clinical work. Biol Psychiatry 60(4):369–375, 2006 16919524

Deacon B, Kemp JJ, Dixon LJ, et al: Maximizing the efficacy of interoceptive exposure by optimizing inhibitory learning: a randomized controlled trial. Behav Res Ther 51(9):588–596, 2013 16919524

Ellis A: Reason and Emotion in Psychotherapy. New York, Stuart, 1962

Emmrich A, Beesdo-Baum K, Gloster AT, et al: Depression does not affect the treatment outcome of CBT for panic and agoraphobia: results from a multicenter randomized trial. Psychother Psychosom 81(3):161–172, 2012 22399019

Fava M, Rankin MA, Wright EC, et al: Anxiety disorders in major depression. Compr Psychiatry 41(2):97–102, 2000 10741886

Firth J, Torous J, Nicholas J, et al: The efficacy of smartphone-based mental health interventions for depressive symptoms: a meta-analysis of randomized controlled trials. World Psychiatry 16(3):287–298, 2017 28941113

Hayes SC, Pierson H: Acceptance and commitment therapy, in Encyclopedia of Cognitive Behavior Therapy. Edited by Freeman A, Felgoise SH, Nezu CM, et al. New York, Springer Science + Business Media, 2005, pp 1–4

Hofmann SG, Wu JQ, Boettcher H: Effect of cognitive-behavioral therapy for anxiety disorders on quality of life: a meta-analysis. J Consult Clin Psychol 82(3):375–391, 2014 24447006

Hofmann SG, Otto MW, Pollack MH, et al: D-cycloserine augmentation of cognitive behavioral therapy for anxiety disorders: an update. Curr Psychiatry Rep 17(1):532, 2015 25413638

Kazantzis N, Whittington C, Dattilio F: Meta-analysis of homework effects in cognitive and behavioral therapy: a replication and extension. Clin Psychol Sci Pract 17(2):144–156, 2010

Kazantzis N, Whittington C, Zelencich L, et al: Quantity and quality of homework compliance: a meta-analysis of relations with outcome in cognitive behavior therapy. Behav Ther 47(5):755–772, 2016 27816086

Kessler RC, Berglund P, Demler O, et al: Lifetime prevalence and age-of-onset distributions of DSM-IV disorders in the National Comorbidity Survey Replication. Arch Gen Psychiatry 62(6):593–602, 2005 15939837

Landy LN, Schneider RL, Arch JJ: Acceptance and commitment therapy for the treatment of anxiety disorders: a concise review. Curr Opin Psychol 2:70–74, 2015

Lang AJ, Schnurr PP, Jain S, et al: Randomized controlled trial of acceptance and commitment therapy for distress and impairment in OEF/OIF/OND veterans. Psychol Trauma 9(suppl 1):74–84, 2017 27322609

Lebeau RT, Davies CD, Culver NC, et al: Homework compliance counts in cognitive-behavioral therapy. Cogn Behav Ther 42(3):171–179, 2013 23419077

Mataix-Cols D, Fernández de La Cruz L, Monzani B, et al: D-cycloserine augmentation of exposure-based cognitive behavior therapy for anxiety, obsessive-compulsive, and post-traumatic stress disorders: a systematic review and meta-analysis of individual participant data. JAMA Psychiatry 74(5):501–510, 2017 28122091

Mausbach BT, Moore R, Roesch S, et al: The relationship between homework compliance and therapy outcomes: an updated meta-analysis. Cognit Ther Res 34(5):429–438, 2010 20930925

Mayo-Wilson E, Dias S, Mavranezouli I, et al: Psychological and pharmacological interventions for social anxiety disorder in adults: a systematic review and network meta-analysis. Lancet Psychiatry 1(5):368–376, 2014 26361000

McGuire JF, Wu MS, Piacentini J, et al: A meta-analysis of d-cycloserine in exposure-based treatment: moderators of treatment efficacy, response, and diagnostic remission. J Clin Psychiatry 78(2):196–206, 2017 27314661

Mineka S, Zinbarg R: A contemporary learning theory perspective on the etiology of anxiety disorders: it's not what you thought it was. Am Psychol 61(1):10–26, 2006 16435973

Norton PJ, Barrera TL: Transdiagnostic versus diagnosis-specific CBT for anxiety disorders: a preliminary randomized controlled noninferiority trial. Depress Anxiety 29(10):874–882, 2012 22767410

Norton PJ, Barrera TL, Mathew AR, et al: Effect of transdiagnostic cbt for anxiety disorders on comorbid diagnoses. Depress Anxiety 30(2):168–173, 2013 23212696

Ori R, Amos T, Bergman H, et al: Augmentation of cognitive and behavioural therapies (CBT) with d-cycloserine for anxiety and related disorders. Cochrane Database Syst Rev 10(5):CD007803, 2015 25957940

Öst LG, Havnen A, Hansen B, et al: Cognitive behavioral treatments of obsessive-compulsive disorder. A systematic review and meta-analysis of studies published 1993–2014. Clin Psychol Rev 40:156–169, 2015 26117062

Pompoli A, Furukawa TA, Imai H, et al: Psychological therapies for panic disorder with or without agoraphobia in adults: a network meta-analysis. Cochrane Database Syst Rev 4:CD011004, 2016 27071857

Rescorla RA: Experimental extinction, in Handbook of Contemporary Learning Theories. Edited by Mowrer R, Klein S. Mahwah, NJ, Erlbaum, 2001, pp 119–154

Watts SE, Turnell A, Kladnitski N, et al: Treatment-as-usual (TAU) is anything but usual: a meta-analysis of CBT versus TAU for anxiety and depression. J Affect Disord 175:152–167, 2015 25618002

Weisman JS, Rodebaugh TL: Exposure therapy augmentation: a review and extension of techniques informed by an inhibitory learning approach. Clin Psychol Rev 59:41–51, 2018 29128146

Recommended Readings

Carpenter JK, Andrews LA, Witcraft SM, et al: Cognitive behavioral therapy for anxiety and related disorders: a meta-analysis of randomized placebo-controlled trials. Depress Anxiety 35(6):502–514, 2018

Craske MG, Treanor M, Conway CC, et al: Maximizing exposure therapy: an inhibitory learning approach. Behav Res Ther 58:10–23, 2014

Craske MG, Stein MB, Eley TC, et al: Anxiety disorders. Nat Rev Dis Prim 3:17024, 2017

CHAPTER 7

Psychodynamic Concepts and Treatment of Anxiety

Fredric N. Busch, M.D.

Barbara L. Milrod, M.D.

Psychoanalytic concepts and techniques are of immense clinical value for patients with anxiety disorders. Since the 1980s, clinicians and researchers developing approaches to anxiety disorders have employed psychodynamic psychotherapy, a less intensive form of psychotherapy that is derived from psychoanalysis and shares many of its theoretical and clinical constructs. Since the 1990s, psychodynamic researchers have been systematically testing manualized, symptom-focused psychodynamic treatments for DSM anxiety disorders. Some of these treatments are efficacious. Efforts are being made to measure and assess potential mediators of psychodynamic treatment effects. The purpose of this chapter is to give an overview of psychoanalytic theory, psychodynamic treatment approaches, and research in anxiety disorders (Table 7–1).

Basic Psychoanalytic Concepts Relating to Mental Life and Anxiety

The Unconscious

From a psychoanalytic perspective, mental life exists on two levels: 1) within consciousness and 2) in a more inaccessible realm called the *unconscious* (Freud 1893–1895/1955). *Psychic or emotional symptoms arise from aspects of mental life that are, at least in part, unconscious.* This includes unacceptable fantasies (Shapiro 1992), affects, and wishes. Clinical observations and studies have indicated that patients with panic disorder often are unaware of angry feelings and vengeful fantasies that are perceived as a threat to important attachment figures (Busch et al. 1991; Shear et al. 1993). Psy-

TABLE 7–1.   **Core psychoanalytic constructs**

Concept	Description
The unconscious	Mental life exists on two levels: consciousness and unconscious. Anxiety and panic symptoms arise from aspects of mental life that are in part unconscious.
Defense mechanisms	Unconscious psychological processes that screen unacceptable feelings and fantasies from consciousness. Identification aids in gaining access to unconscious material.
Compromise formation	Aspects of mental life, including symptoms, that symbolically represent a compromise between a wish and a defense.
Representation of self and others	Internalized representations of self and others that affect relationships and the development of symptoms.
Transference	Models of developmentally formative relationships emerge in the relationship with the therapist and help to identify contributors to symptoms.
Ambivalence	Anxiety and phobic symptoms can arise from conflicts about angry feelings and fantasies and their potential impact on close attachment relationships.
Attachment style	Patients with anxiety disorders often have an insecure attachment style, feeling that important attachment figures will not be responsive to their needs. This style interferes with mentalization, the capacity to understand the minds of oneself and others.

chodynamic treatments help patients become aware of these affects and fantasies, articulate them, and render them less threatening once they are better understood. This process leads to symptomatic change.

Defense Mechanisms

People unconsciously avoid "unpleasure," and ideas and feelings that produce "unpleasure" are screened from consciousness by unconscious psychological processes called *defense mechanisms* (Freud 1911/1958). Defenses frequently employed by patients with panic disorder include *reaction formation, undoing,* and *denial* (Busch et al. 1995, 2012). Reaction formation and undoing involve management of attachment fears in these patients. By unconsciously attempting to convert anger to more affiliative affects, patients reduce the threat they perceive because of their rage at an attachment figure. Somatization represents an important defense in many anxiety disorders. It allows avoidance of fantasies and feelings through focus on the body. In a psychodynamic treatment, the therapist focuses on meanings of defenses to identify emotions and fantasies that trigger symptoms.

Compromise Formation

Many aspects of mental life, including symptoms (e.g., anxiety), dreams, fantasies, and aspects of character, result from *compromise formations* (Freud 1893–1895/1955). A compromise formation symbolically represents a compromise between a forbidden wish and the defense against the wish. Panic attacks can represent a compromise between aggressive fantasies, which are viewed as dangerous, and self-punishment for the fantasies, which is experienced by the patient as terror and disability. The vulnerability triggered by panic attacks also can reduce the perceived threat from aggressive fantasies. Although usually unconscious, aggressive impulses can be expressed by coercive efforts to control ambivalently held others. The following case illustrates panic disorder symptoms that represent a compromise formation:

> Ms. C was driving from one city to another to attend her eighteenth birthday party when she experienced her first panic attack. The attack was so severe that she had to pull off the road and call her mother in the destination city and ask her to pick her up on the highway. It took her mother several hours to find another person to drive with her who could also drive the car back, and meanwhile, Ms. C's party had to be canceled.
>
> At the moment she experienced the attack, Ms. C found herself thinking that her eighteenth birthday was very important: it symbolized her "total independence" from her family and a new ability "to get rid of them." In unraveling the onset of her illness in psychotherapy, it became clear that in her fantasy, turning 18 and being "independent" represented the emotional equivalent of killing her parents and siblings, all of whom enraged her. The fantasy had been so appealing yet terrifying for her that she had her first panic attack. The panic attack represented both the *wish* to be rid of her family (suddenly, Ms. C in fantasy found herself feeling entirely alone and unable to function) and the *defense* against this wish—a sudden-onset, severe illness that made "independence" from her family (and the existence of her birthday celebration) impossible and effectively immobilized her in her escape/fantasy plan. The panic also represented a real way in which she punished herself for her unacceptable fantasies—now she could never be free of her family—and also punished her mother, who spent hours canceling everything she had planned in order to take care of Ms. C.

Representation of Self and Others/Transference

During development, individuals form internalized representations of themselves and others, including significant attachment relationships (Freud 1905/1953). From a psychoanalytic perspective, these representations affect the development of psychic symptoms such as anxiety. Current relationships with others are affected by perceptions of developmentally formative relationships that continue to exert compelling unconscious influence. Patients with panic often view themselves as unsafe, requiring others for protection, but often also perceive others as temperamental, frightening, controlling, or rejecting, which aggravates their sense of insecurity (Busch et al. 2012). Their perceptions add to a sense of fearful dependency on significant others. Identification of these self and object representations aids in developing a psychodynamic formulation to understand and address the emotional/attachment sources of anxiety and panic.

Patterns of perceptions of significant others typically emerge in the relationship with the therapist; this universal psychological phenomenon, *transference* (Freud 1905/1953), is a cornerstone of psychoanalytic theory and practice. In any clinical practice, focus on the transference can help patients recognize underlying, organizing fantasies that surround the therapeutic relationship, regardless of the type of treatment in which they are engaged or the therapeutic orientation of the therapist. Patients with anxiety disorders commonly experience tremendous distress at times of separation from the significant people in their lives (Milrod et al. 2014), including their therapists. Anxiety symptoms can worsen when ongoing treatment, regardless of modality, is temporarily or permanently discontinued. These separations or terminations can provide important opportunities for patients to better articulate, understand, and manage their mixed feelings about autonomy in the context of the transference.

Ambivalent Feelings

Unconscious angry and ambivalent aspects of intense love attachments can result in agoraphobia and the need for a phobic companion (Deutsch 1929). Partly in an unconscious attempt to prevent destruction of their love objects by hostile, compelling, destructive fantasies, patients must have their phobic companion present at all times to prove to themselves that their fantasies have not come true. Need for a phobic companion also commonly emerges from an unconscious passive wish to control this person. The conflict between anger and its associated threats to attachment is a core dynamic contributor to anxiety and panic (Busch et al. 2012).

Attachment Style

Patients with anxiety disorders tend to have an insecure attachment style, in which they feel that others cannot be depended on to be emotionally responsive (Bowlby 1973; Main and Goldwyn 1994; Milrod et al. 2014). This can interfere with the development of *mentalization*, the capacity to understand the minds of oneself and others (Fonagy and Target 1997). Limitations in one's ability to mentalize can interfere with identifying internal factors that contribute to anxiety and can also interfere with understanding relationships with others, adding to perceived threats of abandonment and intrusion.

Clinical Psychodynamic Approach to Patients With Anxiety

The initial focus in a psychodynamically informed treatment of any anxiety disorder is to gain adequate information necessary to delineate the specific fantasies, conflicts, and feelings underlying the symptoms. When evaluating an anxious patient, the psychodynamically informed clinician must obtain a very detailed psychological history, focusing on the circumstances, meanings, and feelings associated with episodes of intense anxiety or panic. A goal of treatment is for patients to become consciously aware of underlying emotional conflicts and, with this awareness, begin to handle them differently, in ways that are verbally rather than somatically mediated. The following case example illustrates the underlying meaning of panic symptoms in a recently married woman:

> Ms. E, a 25-year-old newly married woman, presented in a constant state of severe panic and agoraphobia. It was impossible for her to leave her apartment unaccompanied. She was unable to eat, lost 15 pounds, and slept only a few hours each night. She did not respond to several medication trials, including benzodiazepines, tricyclic antidepressants, selective serotonin reuptake inhibitors, and, finally, chlorpromazine.
>
> Ms. E reported being well until 3 months before her marriage, the day she first tried on her wedding dress. Her most prominent symptoms during panic attacks were se-

vere nausea (she never vomited) and dizziness, symptoms she described as "being like the first trimester of pregnancy." She had been given pregnancy tests on numerous visits to medical emergency departments, the results of which were negative.

Ms. E's panic and agoraphobia ultimately remitted after 3 months of thrice-weekly psychodynamic psychotherapy. Yet from the information presented, which was obtained during the first 10 minutes of her first contact, the following important dynamic information became clear, simply as a result of careful focus on the time and place of her initial symptoms and a brief discussion of her fantasies about the meanings of her symptoms: 1) Ms. E had mixed feelings, of which she was not aware, about getting married, and 2) Ms. E thought of her panic attacks as, somehow, oddly like the first part of a pregnancy. Given that these ideas co-occurred with her illness onset, it seemed highly likely that one of the elements of her strong unconscious mixed feelings about getting married concerned her newly awakened ambivalence about becoming pregnant once she was married. These dynamisms proved to be of central importance later in her treatment and in the resolution of her symptoms and formed a starting place for the therapist to approach the patient.

In working psychodynamically with patients who have severe symptoms such as those described for Ms. E, clinicians must refrain from joining in patients' severe anxiety and must impart the idea that symptoms are understandable psychological phenomena. The goal of psychodynamic psychotherapy for anxiety disorders is to determine how the symptoms make sense as psychological phenomena and thus help patients recognize their own feelings and thoughts in a more coherent way.

A Psychodynamic Formulation for Panic Disorder

Our psychodynamic formulation for panic disorder with and without agoraphobia was developed from psychoanalytic precepts about anxiety and from psychological studies and clinical observations of panic patients (Busch et al. 1991; Shear et al. 1993). Personality traits, including dependency and difficulty in being assertive, appear to predispose to the onset of panic disorder, which is then triggered by particular life stressors (Busch et al. 2012). Many studies suggest that acute stressors, described in the literature as "life events," frequently occur just prior to panic onset (Busch et al. 2012; Faravelli 1985; Klass et al. 2009; Milrod et al. 2004; Roy-Byrne et al. 1986). Despite the DSM-5 description of panic attacks as coming "out of the blue" (American Psychiatric Association 2013, p. 209), from a psychodynamic perspective, the meaning of these events to the individual (including the unconscious significance they carry) and the affects triggered in response to these events play a central role in the development of panic attacks. Fantasies surrounding separation and autonomy are common areas of conflict for panic patients. Several lines of evidence provide support for this finding (Kossowsky et al. 2013; Milrod et al. 2014; Silove et al. 2015). Patients with panic disorder have difficulty tolerating (and sometimes modulating) angry feelings and fantasies (Busch et al. 1991, 2012; Shear et al. 1993). Panic attacks can be self-punitive; patients may unconsciously atone for fantasies and feelings that trigger guilt with panic.

Clinical Psychodynamic Approaches to Panic Disorder

Milrod et al. (1997) and Busch et al. (2012) developed a manualized treatment, panic-focused psychodynamic psychotherapy (PFPP), based on the psychodynamic formulation described earlier, which has been modified and extended to treatment of other anxiety disorders. The treatment targets the core dynamics of panic disorder, including separation anxiety, abandonment fears, and difficulties in managing ambivalence, conflicted rage, and guilt. Psychodynamic techniques of clarification, confrontation, interpretation, and focus on the transference are employed, but PFPP differs from traditional psychodynamic psychotherapy in its pursuit of the unconscious significance of anxiety symptoms.

Psychodynamic Perspectives on Non-Panic Anxiety Disorders

Many aspects of the psychodynamic understanding of panic disorder are applicable to a psychodynamic approach to other anxiety disorders. Psychodynamic constellations have been suggested for specific anxiety disorders (Busch et al. 2012), and a large psychoanalytic and psychodynamic literature about PTSD is available (Busch and Milrod 2018; Freud 1920/1955; Horowitz 1999; Kanas et al. 1994). Psychodynamic researchers have been developing treatment approaches to specific anxiety disorders and systematically assessing treatment outcomes. Several of these studies (Leichsenring et al. 2009, 2013) use a less symptom-focused form of psychodynamic psychotherapy, supportive expressive therapy (SET) (Luborsky 1984).

SET identifies and addresses the "core conflictual relationship theme" that formulates core dynamics in terms of the patient's wish, the response of the other, and the response of the self. SET operationally captures many core domains of psychodynamic psychotherapy but has limited inclusion of other domains, such as focus on attachment and reflection (Fonagy and Target 1997) and the centrality of unconscious symbolic fantasy and development (Busch et al. 2012). SET's more narrow range compared with subsequent broader manualized psychodynamic psychotherapies may have curtailed the degree of improvement with this approach in the treatment of anxiety disorders (Milrod 2013).

Combining Psychodynamic Treatments With Medication

Although some anxious patients wish to start medication quickly to diminish discomfort, many highly anxious patients are too frightened of medication to consider taking it (Cross-National Collaborative Panic Study 1992; Hofmann et al. 1998). Medication should be considered and discussed as an efficacious treatment option alongside effective psychotherapies.

Limited systematic evidence evaluating medication added to psychodynamic treatment of anxiety disorders is available (Wiborg and Dahl 1996). Psychodynamic treatments can be combined effectively with antianxiety medication (Busch and Sandberg 2007; Milrod and Busch 1998). In more severe cases, medication can aid psychotherapy by relieving severe anxiety, thus permitting patients to explore more productively the underlying significance of symptoms. In psychodynamic treatments, therapist and patient examine the emotional meanings of taking medication (Busch and Sandberg 2007; Milrod and Busch 1998).

Review of Psychodynamic Research on Anxiety Disorders

Randomized controlled trial (RCT) evidence of efficacy for psychodynamic psycho-therapies now exists for panic disorder with or without agoraphobia, social anxiety disorder in adults and adolescents, and generalized anxiety disorder (GAD), and two groups of psychodynamic researchers are now starting RCTs of psychodynamic inter-ventions for PTSD (Leichsenring et al. 2018; Milrod and Chen 2018). Increasing num-bers and better quality of systematic studies of psychodynamic psychotherapy as well as cognitive-behavioral therapy (CBT) have been performed over the past de-cade (Thoma et al. 2012), and recent, relatively well-controlled meta-analyses suggest that psychodynamic psychotherapies are often equivalently efficacious in compari-son with other treatments (Milrod 2017; Steinert et al. 2017).

Panic Disorder

Milrod et al. (2007) conducted an RCT of 49 patients with primary DSM-IV panic dis-order with and without agoraphobia (American Psychiatric Association 1994), com-paring PFPP with a less active psychotherapy for panic disorder, applied relaxation therapy (ART; Cerny et al. 1984). PFPP had a significantly better response rate than ART (73% vs. 39%; $P=0.016$), using the standard definition of "response": a 40% de-crease in total Panic Disorder Severity Scale (PDSS) score from baseline (Barlow et al. 2000). Subjects in the PFPP condition experienced significantly greater improvement in panic disorder symptoms as measured by the PDSS ($P=0.002$) and psychosocial function as measured by the Sheehan Disability Scale (Sheehan 1983; $P=0.014$). A study of *reflective function* (Rudden et al. 2006) conducted in conjunction with this first PFPP RCT indicated that a measure of awareness of the link between emotional expe-rience and symptoms—symptom-specific reflective functioning—improved signifi-cantly from baseline to posttreatment in patients treated with PFPP but not in those treated with ART. The efficacy of PFPP was replicated in a study by Beutel et al. (2013).

Milrod et al. (2016) conducted a two-site RCT of 201 patients with primary DSM-IV panic disorder with and without agoraphobia, comparing PFPP, CBT, and ART. Attri-tion was significantly higher in the ART condition, and patients who were most symptomatic dropped out of ART significantly more (69% in ART, 26% in PFPP, 24% in CBT; $P=0.013$), indicating that ART is less tolerable for the sickest panic patients. The authors found significant site-by-treatment differences in outcome: patients at one site (Weill Cornell Medical College [Cornell]) improved at the same rate in all three treatments, whereas patients at the other (University of Pennsylvania [Penn]) improved faster in ART and CBT than PFPP. At termination, Cornell patients re-sponded better to PFPP and CBT compared with ART, whereas Penn patients did not show a significant differential response across treatments. Overall response rates on the PDSS across both sites were ART 46%, CBT 63%, and PFPP 59%. A process and outcome study (Keefe et al. 2018b) involving the two-site study found that the degree to which panic-focused interpretations were used in PFPP in midtreatment uniquely correlated with the level of subsequent improvement in panic symptoms. Patients with more severe personality disorders, particularly Cluster B, experienced more improvement in their personality disorder cluster symptoms in PFPP than in CBT (Keefe et al. 2018a).

Posttraumatic Stress Disorder

Brom et al. (1989) compared 112 patients with PTSD, diagnosed according to DSM-III criteria (American Psychiatric Association 1980), who were randomly assigned to receive either psychodynamic psychotherapy ($n=29$), hypnotherapy ($n=29$), or trauma desensitization ($n=31$) or were designated to a waitlist control group ($n=23$). Posttraumatic symptoms were assessed with the Symptom Checklist–90 (Arrindell and Ettema 1981) and the Impact of Event Scale (Horowitz et al. 1979). All three treatment groups showed significant improvement in trauma-related symptoms from baseline and compared with the control group, although this study was conducted before the development of the Clinician Administered PTSD Scale (Weathers et al. 2018), making comparisons to more recent studies of PTSD outcome difficult. Busch and Milrod (2018) developed a manualized treatment for PTSD for veterans treated at Veterans Health Administration medical centers that is currently undergoing RCT evaluation. Leichsenring et al. (2018) are starting an eight-site study of a trauma-focused psychodynamic treatment for PTSD (Wöller et al. 2012).

Social Anxiety Disorder

Leichsenring et al. (2013) studied 495 patients with social anxiety disorder treated with either manualized CBT ($n=209$) or SET ($n=207$) or assigned to a waitlist. Response and remission were significantly superior for CBT and dynamic therapy compared with the waitlist condition (response: CBT 60%, psychodynamic therapy 52%, and waitlist 15%; remission: 36%, 26%, 9%, respectively) on the Liebowitz Social Anxiety Scale (Liebowitz 1987). CBT was significantly superior to psychodynamic therapy in remission but not response rates. At 24-month follow-up (Leichsenring et al. 2014), remission rates for the two treatments were nearly identical (40%). Bögels et al. (2014) studied patients with primary social anxiety disorder ($n=47$) randomly assigned to psychodynamic psychotherapy ($n=22$) or CBT ($n=27$). Treatments were highly efficacious, with large within-subject effect sizes for social anxiety but no differences between groups on general or treatment-specific measures. Remission rates were more than 50% and similar for psychodynamic psychotherapy and CBT.

Generalized Anxiety Disorder

Leichsenring et al. (2009) studied patients with DSM-IV GAD treated with CBT ($n=29$) or SET ($n=28$). Patients in each group showed large and significant gains, and no difference in outcome was found between the treatments on the primary outcome measure, the Hamilton Anxiety Rating Scale (Hamilton 1959). CBT was superior, however, on measures of trait anxiety, worry, and depression.

Psychodynamic Research on Pediatric Anxiety

Salzer et al. (2018) examined the efficacy of CBT and SET compared with a waiting list condition in adolescents ages 14–20 who met criteria for social anxiety disorder. In a multicenter RCT, 107 patients were randomized to CBT ($n=34$), SET ($n=34$), or a waitlist ($n=39$). Response rates were 66%, 54%, and 20%, respectively. Corresponding remission rates were 47%, 34%, and 6%, respectively. CBT and SET were significantly superior to the waitlist condition in response and remission; results were stable at 6- and 12-month follow-up.

Conclusion

In addition to a wealth of theoretical conceptualizations concerning anxiety, psychoanalysis and psychodynamic therapy have important contributions to make to anxiety treatment. Dynamic researchers have been performing efficacy studies of manualized psychodynamic interventions for anxiety disorders, providing a clear picture of the efficacy and utility of psychodynamic psychotherapy. Although the number of studies is limited, and those involving DSM-5 have yet to be completed, studies thus far for a variety of anxiety disorders generally demonstrate efficacy and an equivalence to CBT. Process and outcome studies are identifying mechanisms that contribute to the efficacy of psychodynamic treatments. Further studies should identify which patients benefit most from specific interventions. Understanding for whom treatments work and the mechanisms of action can lead to the development of more specific interventions for individual patients.

Key Points

- Psychodynamic models conceptualize anxiety disorders as developing from wishes, feelings, and fantasies, often unconscious, that are experienced as frightening or intolerable.

- In psychodynamic psychotherapy, therapist and patient work to identify and reappraise emotional conflicts, rendering them less threatening.

- A manualized psychodynamic approach to panic disorder has demonstrated efficacy when compared with a less active treatment and did not significantly differ in outcome when compared with cognitive-behavioral therapy.

- A manualized psychodynamic psychotherapy for social anxiety disorder in adults and children has been shown to be efficacious.

- Further studies will help to determine the role of psychodynamic psychotherapy among the available treatments for anxiety disorders.

References

American Psychiatric Association: Diagnostic and Statistical Manual of Mental Disorders, 3rd Edition. Washington, DC, American Psychiatric Association, 1980

American Psychiatric Association: Diagnostic and Statistical Manual of Mental Disorders, 4th Edition. Washington, DC, American Psychiatric Association, 1994

American Psychiatric Association: Diagnostic and Statistical Manual of Mental Disorders, 5th Edition. Arlington, VA, American Psychiatric Association, 2013

Arrindell W, Ettema H: Dimensional structure, reliability, and validity of the Dutch version of the Symptom Checklist (SCL-90): data based on a phobic and "normal" population [in Dutch]. Ned Tijdschr Psychol 36:77–108, 1981

Barlow DH, Gorman JM, Shear MK, et al: Cognitive-behavioral therapy, imipramine, or their combination for panic disorder: a randomized controlled trial. JAMA 283(19):2529–2536, 2000 10815116

Beutel ME, Scheurich V, Knebel A, et al: Implementing panic-focused psychodynamic psychotherapy into clinical practice. Can J Psychiatry 58(6):326–334, 2013 23768260

Bögels SM, Wijts P, Oort FJ, et al: Psychodynamic psychotherapy versus cognitive behavior therapy for social anxiety disorder: an efficacy and partial effectiveness trial. Depress Anxiety 31(5):363–373, 2014 24577880

Bowlby J: Attachment and Loss, Vol II: Separation, Anxiety, and Anger. New York, Basic Books, 1973

Brom D, Kleber RJ, Defares PB: Brief psychotherapy for posttraumatic stress disorders. J Consult Clin Psychol 57(5):607–612, 1989 2571625

Busch FN, Milrod BL: Trauma-focused psychodynamic psychotherapy. Psychiatr Clin North Am 41(2):277–287, 2018 29739526

Busch FN, Sandberg L: Psychotherapy and Medication: The Challenge of Integration. Hillsdale, NJ, Analytic Press, 2007

Busch F, Cooper AM, Klerman GL, et al: Neurophysiological, cognitive-behavioral, and psychoanalytic approaches to panic disorder: toward an integration. Psychoanal Inq 11:316–332, 1991

Busch FN, Shear MK, Cooper AM, et al: An empirical study of defense mechanisms in panic disorder. J Nerv Ment Dis 183(5):299–303, 1995 7745383

Busch FN, Milrod BL, Singer MB, et al: Manual of Panic Focused Psychodynamic Psychotherapy, eXtended Range. New York, Routledge, 2012

Cerny JA, Vermilyea BB, Barlow DH, et al: Anxiety Treatment Project Relaxation Treatment Manual. Unpublished manual, 1984

Cross-National Collaborative Panic Study: Drug treatment of panic disorder: comparative efficacy of alprazolam, imipramine, and placebo. Cross-National Collaborative Panic Study, Second Phase Investigators. Br J Psychiatry 160:191–202, 1992 1540759

Deutsch H: The genesis of agoraphobia. Int J Psychoanal 10:51–69, 1929

Faravelli C: Life events preceding the onset of panic disorder. J Affect Disord 9(1):103–105, 1985 3160742

Fonagy P, Target M: Attachment and reflective function: their role in self-organization. Dev Psychopathol 9(4):679–700, 1997 9449001

Freud S: Fragment of an analysis of a case of hysteria (1905), in Standard Edition of the Complete Psychological Works of Sigmund Freud, Vol 7. Translated and edited by Strachey J. London, Hogarth, 1953, pp 3–122

Freud S: Studies on hysteria (1893–1895), in Standard Edition of the Complete Psychological Works of Sigmund Freud, Vol 2. Translated and edited by Strachey J. London, Hogarth, 1955, pp 1–181

Freud S: Beyond the pleasure principle (1920), in Standard Edition of the Complete Psychological Works of Sigmund Freud, Vol 18. Translated and edited by Strachey J. London, Hogarth, 1955, pp 3–64

Freud S: Formulations on the two principles of mental functioning (1911), in Standard Edition of the Complete Psychological Works of Sigmund Freud, Vol 12. Translated and edited by Strachey J. London, Hogarth, 1958, pp 213–226

Hamilton M: The assessment of anxiety states by rating. Br J Med Psychol 32(1):50–55, 1959 13638508

Hofmann SG, Barlow DH, Papp LA, et al: Pretreatment attrition in a comparative treatment outcome study on panic disorder. Am J Psychiatry 155(1):43–47, 1998 9433337

Horowitz MJ: Essential Papers on Posttraumatic Stress Disorder. New York, New York University Press, 1999

Horowitz M, Wilner N, Alvarez W: Impact of Event Scale: a measure of subjective stress. Psychosom Med 41(3):209–218, 1979 472086

Kanas N, Schoenfeld F, Marmar C, et al: Process and content in a long-term PTSD therapy group for Vietnam veterans. Group 18(3):78–88, 1994

Keefe JR, Milrod BL, Gallop R, et al: What is the effect on comorbid personality disorder of brief panic-focused psychotherapy in patients with panic disorder? Depress Anxiety 35(3):239–247, 2018a 29212135

Keefe JR, Solomonov N, Derubeis RJ, et al: Focus is key: panic-focused interpretations are associated with symptomatic improvement in panic-focused psychodynamic psychotherapy. Psychother Res 18:1–12, 2018b 29667870

Klass ET, Milrod BL, Leon AC, et al: Does interpersonal loss preceding panic disorder onset moderate response to psychotherapy? An exploratory study. J Clin Psychiatry 70(3):406–411, 2009 19026262

Kossowsky J, Pfaltz MC, Schneider S, et al: The separation anxiety hypothesis of panic disorder revisited: a meta-analysis. Am J Psychiatry 170(7):768–781, 2013 23680783

Leichsenring F, Salzer S, Jaeger U, et al: Short-term psychodynamic psychotherapy and cognitive-behavioral therapy in generalized anxiety disorder: a randomized, controlled trial. Am J Psychiatry 166(8):875–881, 2009 19570931

Leichsenring F, Salzer S, Beutel ME, et al: Psychodynamic therapy and cognitive-behavioral therapy in social anxiety disorder: a multicenter randomized controlled trial. Am J Psychiatry 170(7):759–767, 2013 23680854

Leichsenring F, Salzer S, Beutel ME, et al: Long-term outcome of psychodynamic therapy and cognitive-behavioral therapy in social anxiety disorder. Am J Psychiatry 171(10):1074–1082, 2014 25016974

Leichsenring F, Bennecke C, Beutel M, et al: Trauma-Focused Psychodynamic Therapy and STAIR Narrative Therapy in PTSD Related to Childhood Maltreatment: A Multi-Center Randomized Controlled Trail. Bonn, Germany, German Ministry of Research and Education, 2018

Liebowitz MR: Social phobia. Mod Probl Pharmacopsychiatry 22:141–173, 1987 2885745

Luborsky L: Principles of Psychoanalytic Psychotherapy: A Manual for Supportive-Expressive Treatment. New York, Basic Books, 1984

Main M, Goldwyn R: Adult Attachment Rating and Classification System: Manual Draft, Version 6.0. Unpublished manuscript, University of California at Berkeley, 1994

Milrod B: The Gordian knot of clinical research in anxiety disorders: some answers, more questions. Am J Psychiatry 170(7):703–706, 2013 23680919

Milrod B: The evolution of meta-analysis in psychotherapy research. Am J Psychiatry 174(10):913–914, 2017 28965459

Milrod B, Busch F: Integrating the use of medication with psychodynamic psychotherapy in the treatment of panic disorder. Psychoanal Inq 18:702–715, 1998

Milrod B, Chen C: A Pilot Randomized Controlled Trial of PTSD-Specific Psychodynamic Psychotherapy [PTSD-FPP] at the VA in Veterans With PTSD. Clinical Translational Sciences Center Pilot Award, UL1-TR-002348935. New York, Weill Cornell Medical College, 2018

Milrod B, Busch F, Cooper A, et al: Manual of Panic-Focused Psychodynamic Psychotherapy. Washington, DC, American Psychiatric Press, 1997

Milrod B, Leon AC, Shear MK: Can interpersonal loss precipitate panic disorder? Am J Psychiatry 161(4):758–759, 2004 15056531

Milrod B, Leon AC, Busch F, et al: A randomized controlled clinical trial of psychoanalytic psychotherapy for panic disorder. Am J Psychiatry 164(2):265–272, 2007 17267789

Milrod B, Markowitz JC, Gerber AJ, et al: Childhood separation anxiety and the pathogenesis and treatment of adult anxiety. Am J Psychiatry 171(1):34–43, 2014 24129927

Milrod B, Chambless DL, Gallop R, et al: Psychotherapies for panic disorder: a tale of two sites. J Clin Psychiatry 77(7):927–935, 2016 27464313

Roy-Byrne PP, Geraci M, Uhde TW: Life events and the onset of panic disorder. Am J Psychiatry 143(11):1424–1427, 1986 3777233

Rudden M, Milrod B, Target M, et al: Reflective functioning in panic disorder patients: a pilot study. J Am Psychoanal Assoc 54(4):1339–1343, 2006 17354509

Salzer S, Stefini A, Kronmüller KT, et al: Cognitive-behavioral and psychodynamic therapy in adolescents with social anxiety disorder: a multicenter randomized controlled trial. Psychother Psychosom 87(4):223–233, 2018 29895001

Shapiro T: The concept of unconscious fantasy. Journal of Clinical Psychoanalysis 1(4):517–524, 1992

Shear MK, Cooper AM, Klerman GL, et al: A psychodynamic model of panic disorder. Am J Psychiatry 150(6):859–866, 1993 8192722

Sheehan DV: The Sheehan disability scales, in The Anxiety Disease. New York, Charles Scribner and Sons, 1983, p 151

Silove D, Alonso J, Bromet E, et al: Pediatric-onset and adult-onset separation anxiety disorder across countries in the world mental health survey. Am J Psychiatry 172(7):647–656, 2015 26046337

Steinert C, Munder T, Rabung S, et al: Psychodynamic therapy: as efficacious as other empirically supported treatments? A meta-analysis testing equivalence of outcomes. Am J Psychiatry 174(10):943–953, 2017 28541091

Thoma NC, McKay D, Gerber AJ, et al: A quality-based review of randomized controlled trials of cognitive-behavioral therapy for depression: an assessment and metaregression. Am J Psychiatry 169(1):22–30, 2012 22193528

Weathers FW, Blake DD, Schnurr PP, et al: The Clinician-Administered PTSD Scale for DSM-5. April 16, 2018. Available at: https://www.ptsd.va.gov/professional/assessment/documents/CAPS_5_Past_Week.pdf. Accessed June 12, 2019.

Wiborg IM, Dahl AA: Does brief dynamic psychotherapy reduce the relapse rate of panic disorder? Arch Gen Psychiatry 53(8):689–694, 1996 8694682

Wöller W, Leichsenring F, Leweke F, et al: Psychodynamic psychotherapy for posttraumatic stress disorder related to childhood abuse—principles for a treatment manual. Bull Menninger Clin 76(1):69–93, 2012 22409207

Recommended Readings

Busch FN, Milrod BL, Singer MB, et al: Manual of Panic Focused Psychodynamic Psychotherapy, eXtended Range. New York, Routledge, 2012

Freud S: Inhibitions, symptoms and anxiety (1926), in Standard Edition of the Complete Psychological Works of Sigmund Freud, Vol 20. Translated and edited by Strachey J. London, Hogarth, 1959, pp 77–175

CHAPTER 8

Unified Protocol

A Transdiagnostic Cognitive-Behavioral Therapy Approach

Todd J. Farchione, Ph.D.

Stephanie Jarvi Steele, Ph.D.

Brittany K. Woods, M.A.

Andrew J. Curreri, M.A.

Mengxing Wang, M.A.

David H. Barlow, Ph.D., ABPP

Over the past several decades, many advances have been made in the psychological treatment of anxiety, depressive, and related disorders. One of the most notable was the development of individual manualized treatment protocols that focus on addressing discrete symptoms associated with specific disorders (e.g., *Mastery of Your Anxiety and Panic* for panic disorder [Craske and Barlow 2007], *Managing Social Anxiety* for social anxiety disorder [Hope et al. 2006]). Many of these treatments have gained strong empirical support (Barlow et al. 2014). However, in recent years, several different lines of research have come together to provide a strong rationale for a more unified transdiagnostic approach to treating these common disorders. First, research suggests that a substantial phenotypic overlap in symptoms exists across these common conditions, with correspondingly high rates of diagnostic comorbidity (Allen et al. 2010; Brown et al. 2001; Kessler et al. 1996; Roy-Byrne et al. 2006; Tsao et al. 2002, 2005). For example, in a study of 1,127 patients presenting with a principal anxiety disorder at the Center for Anxiety and Related Disorders at Boston University, 55% of patients had at least one additional anxiety or depressive disorder at the time of assessment, and this number increased to 76% when including lifetime diagnoses (Brown et al. 2001). Second, psychological treatments that target a single disorder often result in improvements in comorbid conditions that were not specifically addressed in treatment, suggesting a broad treatment response (Allen et al. 2010; Borkovec et al. 1995; Steele et al. 2018; Tsao et al. 1998, 2002). Third, research from affective neuroscience supports shared biological mechanisms across disorders of emotion. For example, increased negative emotionality has been associated with hyperexcitability of limbic structures and limited inhibitory control by cortical structures (Etkin and Wager 2007; Porto et al. 2009; Shin and Liberzon 2010). Furthermore, dysregulated cortical inhibition of amygdala responses has been found in studies of various anxiety and related disorders (Etkin et al. 2010; Holmes et al. 2012; Phan et al. 2006).

Additional findings support the existence of a higher-order temperament, neuroticism, that appears to be shared among all anxiety and depressive disorders. *Neuroticism* has been characterized as the frequent experience of intense negative affect accompanied by a sense of loss of control and inability to cope with the negative emotional experience (Barlow et al. 2014). Indeed, individuals with anxiety and depressive disorders tend to have higher baseline levels of negative affect/neuroticism (Brown and Barlow 2009) and express negative emotions more frequently than healthy counterparts (Campbell-Sills et al. 2006; Mennin et al. 2005), findings that have been supported statistically in a hierarchical structure of emotional disorders generated by Brown et al. (1998). Furthermore, these individuals tend to react more negatively to their emotional experiences (Barlow 1991; Barlow et al. 2011a; Brown and Barlow 2009; Campbell-Sills et al. 2006). Unfortunately, this can lead to a cycle of responding in which attempts to avoid or downregulate negative emotional experiences inadvertently result in an increase in the frequency and intensity of negative emotion and related distress, which contributes to the persistence of symptoms (Sauer-Zavala et al. 2017). Based on this model, avoidance and suppression of negative emotional experiences is viewed as a core underlying mechanism, important to the development and maintenance of anxiety and depressive disorders, that reflects the expression of neuroticism. Given the role of these dysfunctional emotion regulation processes in the development and maintenance of these conditions, we refer to them as "emotional disorders" to emphasize this common feature. For more information on the nature of emotional disorders, see Barlow et al. (2014) and Bullis et al. (2019).

Description of the Unified Protocol

Based on these advances, the Unified Protocol for Transdiagnostic Treatment of Emotional Disorders (UP; Barlow et al. 2011b, 2017b) was developed to target temperamental characteristics, particularly neuroticism, and including emotional lability, overreactivity to emotion, and resulting emotion dysregulation (Barlow et al. 2014). Specifically, the UP targets aversive, avoidant reactions to emotions. Its overarching goal is to decrease the frequency of negative emotions by helping patients learn new, more adaptive ways of responding to intense emotional experiences, thereby facilitating extinction of anxiety and distress triggered by emotional experience. The UP is a modular treatment designed to be administered in 12–16 sessions, not including an initial session dedicated to assessment and case formulation within a transdiagnostic framework. The UP consists of eight different treatment modules (Table 8–1), five of

TABLE 8–1.	Uniform Protocol modules and recommended session lengths

Module 1: Setting goals and maintaining motivation (1 session)

Module 2: Understanding emotions (1–2 sessions)

Module 3: Mindful emotion awareness (1–2 sessions)

Module 4: Cognitive flexibility (1–2 sessions)

Module 5: Countering emotional behaviors (1–2 sessions)

Module 6: Understanding and confronting physical sensations (1 session)

Module 7: Emotion exposures (4–6 sessions)

Module 8: Recognizing accomplishments and looking to the future (1 session)

Note. Core modules are in **bold**.

which are considered "core": 1) present-focused emotional awareness, 2) cognitive flexibility, 3) changing emotional behaviors, 4) awareness and tolerance of physical sensations, and 5) emotion exposures. In addition, these five core modules are preceded by a module designed to help increase motivation and readiness for change as well as an introductory module that provides psychoeducation and a framework for tracking emotional experiences. After the five core modules are completed, a final module on relapse prevention is provided. Flexibility is built into the treatment administration to allow for more or fewer sessions to be spent on specific modules, determined on a case-by-case basis. Session length is typically between 50 and 60 minutes. The general structure of sessions is as follows: tracking of general levels of anxiety and depressive symptoms, homework review (troubleshooting noncompliance, if necessary), introduction of a new skill or continued practice with a previously presented concept, and assignment of homework. In the following sections, we briefly review each module.

Module 1: Setting Goals and Maintaining Motivation

The first module of the UP focuses on increasing patients' readiness and motivation for change. The importance of goal setting is directly addressed, and time is spent establishing concrete treatment goals and identifying specific steps to achieve them. A goal-setting worksheet helps facilitate this discussion; at times, completion of this worksheet is assigned as homework, because patients often put considerable time and effort into detailing their plans for change. A second component of this module is a "decisional balance" exercise designed to help patients build and maintain motivation for change during treatment. This exercise offers patients an opportunity to weigh the benefits and costs of change against those of staying the same. This helps patients establish the necessary motivation to work hard in treatment while simultaneously acknowledging how motivation may wax and wane and shows that ambivalence is a natural and expected part of the change process. We often return to patients' previous responses to these exercises during treatment as a reminder of the specific reasons they originally set out to change, particularly when motivation is low and stress/distress is high. Specific goals also are revisited throughout treatment to ensure that they are being adequately addressed and that progress is being made toward meeting them.

Module 2: Understanding Emotions

In the second module, patients receive psychoeducation on the nature and function of emotions. For example, the therapist and patient discuss how anxiety alerts us to pay attention and may motivate us to prepare or take proactive steps toward a particular goal. Patients are taught to process an "emotional experience" in accordance with a three-component model; specifically, emotional experiences are broken down into cognitions (e.g., "If I go to the party, I won't have anyone to talk to"), physical sensations (e.g., racing heart, shortness of breath), and behaviors (e.g., staying home). The therapist may assign observation and tracking homework to enhance patients' understanding of emotional experiences as they unfold in daily life.

This module includes discussion of antecedents to emotional experiences as well as short- and long-term consequences of reactions to emotions. The focus here is on strong emotions that patients have difficulty experiencing fully or to which they react with problematic, avoidant behaviors. We refer to these reactions to strong (often painful, distressing) emotions as "emotional behaviors," meaning the behavior is related to and consistent with the feeling state (e.g., avoiding a party when feeling anxious). Observation and tracking of short- and long-term consequences (i.e., outcomes) of behavior begins to lay important groundwork for upcoming modules that promote behavior change through reduction of emotional behaviors.

Module 3: Mindful Emotion Awareness

The first core module, Module 3, builds on the previous module by teaching patients not only to notice their emotional experiences but also to cultivate a nonjudgmental, present-focused attitude toward them. Patients are asked to refrain from judging emotions when they come up and to ground themselves in the present moment so that they can be more aware of their emotional experiences as they unfold. The rationale for this module is based on mindfulness research showing that emotional acceptance facilitates more adaptive emotion regulation (Hayes and Feldman 2004). The module is meant to foster an approach-oriented relationship with emotions that is consistent with the overarching goal of the UP.

Patients are asked to participate in a guided meditation exercise in a session designed to help them practice becoming more aware of present (emotional) experiences in a nonjudgmental way. They learn to apply this new level of awareness to emotions induced in session through music or video clips. For example, a patient might be asked to identify a personally relevant and emotionally provoking song clip that is then played during the session. The patient then tries to attend mindfully to the primary components of his or her emotional response. Patients are taught how to use a deep breath as a behavioral cue to help "anchor in the present" and to practice mindful awareness of emotions coming up in daily life.

Module 4: Cognitive Flexibility

The next three modules focus on each of the three components introduced in Module 2: thoughts, behaviors, and physical sensations. Based on principles of cognitive therapy, Module 4 teaches patients to identify cognitive distortions, or "thinking traps," that contribute to emotions. Patients are taught to acknowledge that their thoughts are not always true and to consider alternatives. This kind of flexibility in thinking helps patients be more objective in their appraisals of situations, which may ease some of the distress associated with emotional experiences.

Module 5: Countering Emotional Behaviors

In Module 5, patients learn about the relationship between emotions and behaviors and how to identify (maladaptive) emotional behaviors such as engaging in compulsions, seeking reassurance, or avoiding feared situations. Emotional behaviors are evaluated in terms of their short- and long-term consequences; usually, these behaviors provide short-term relief from strong emotions but lead to unhelpful long-term consequences. Another objective of this module is to help patients develop alternative actions for their emotional behaviors, to correct the behavioral patterns for responding to strong emotions that have been contributing to their continued distress. For avoidant behaviors, for example, the alternative action is usually to face the avoided situations. This change in behavior is facilitated more directly through exposure exercises introduced in Module 7.

Module 6: Confronting Physical Sensations

Module 6 targets the third component of the three-component model—physical sensations. It contains interoceptive exposures (exposure to physical sensations) that traditionally have been used in panic protocols, but research supports the association of anxiety sensitivity—a trait-like fear of physical sensations—in other emotional disorders as well (Boswell et al. 2013). Various physical sensations are associated with a range of emotional experiences. For example, warm cheeks (blushing) or sweaty palms may be associated with social anxiety or muscle fatigue and heaviness with depression. Sometimes these sensations are at the forefront of a strong emotional experience for a patient, while at other times they interact with other components of the emotional response to make it more intense or overwhelming. For this reason, we suggest administering interoceptive exposures to all patients.

In this module, patients are asked repeatedly to elicit physical sensations that often accompany an emotional response to help them become more comfortable with these sensations and to learn that feared outcomes related to the sensations do not occur. It begins by presenting this rationale to patients and follows with a series of activities designed to elicit various physical sensations. The goal is to identify the activities that are most similar to "real-life" emotional experiences and cause at least moderate distress. Specific activities such as breathing through a thin straw, hyperventilating, and spinning in a chair are practiced repeatedly in session, back-to-back, with little break in between. Patients are asked to refrain from avoidance behaviors and are often pushed beyond their standard level of comfort to maximize learning.

Module 7: Emotional Exposures

In this module, patients work to apply all of the skills acquired during the course of treatment to situations that elicit strong emotions and are often avoided as a result. Exposures are a common component of most cognitive-behavioral treatments for anxiety and related disorders. In the UP, exposure focuses more directly on the experience of emotion than on the situation, image, or activity that elicits that emotion, thus the name "emotion exposures." These exposures, in addition to interoceptive exposures, can be situational (in vivo) or imaginal. The therapist helps patients create a hierarchy of situations that tend to trigger strong emotions or have historically been avoided, rating them according to distress. Prior to each exposure, therapist and patient discuss anticipated reactions during the exposure and predicted outcomes. The therapist helps during the exposure by discouraging avoidance when necessary. Afterward, the therapist guides patients in processing the exposure, which includes identifying the components of the emotional experience, what skills were used and how well, and what was learned from the exposure. The emotion exposure provides patients an opportunity to apply the emotion regulation skills learned during treatment. Over time, patients are expected to show increased tolerance of emotions, including confidence that they are able to handle emotional experiences and changes in patterns of responding. For this learning to generalize to "real-world" situations, patients are encouraged to continue to practice these skills between sessions in emotion-provoking situations.

Module 8: Relapse Prevention

Module 8 begins with a review of treatment skills, often presenting patients with examples relevant to their lives and how they would react to such a scenario. Patient and therapist review the patient's progress over the course of treatment, including how skills were implemented and the resulting changes in symptomatology. Throughout the course of treatment, patients are encouraged to track their progress with measures of anxiety, depression, and positive and negative affect, and the trajectories of these measures are discussed in relation to timing within treatment and skill acquisition. To maintain gains or continue improving in areas of difficulty, patients work with the therapist to create a detailed practice plan to follow after therapy ends. Patients produce long-term goals to work toward and anticipate future roadblocks to achieving these goals and how to troubleshoot them when they arise.

Efficacy and Effectiveness

The UP has been shown to reduce anxiety and depressive symptoms in samples of individuals with anxiety and depressive disorders (Ellard et al. 2010; Farchione et al. 2012), and these reductions in symptoms were maintained 18 months posttreatment (Bullis et al. 2014). Additionally, in a preliminary exploration of group delivery of the UP, results evidenced decreases in anxiety and depression and related functional impairment and improvements in quality of life and emotion regulation (Bullis et al. 2015). Recently, in a large clinical trial, the UP was compared with existing single-disorder protocols for principal diagnoses of generalized anxiety disorder, social anxiety disorder, OCD, or panic disorder and a waitlist control group. Equivalent reductions in symptoms were observed in patients' principal diagnosis at posttreatment and at 6-month follow-up for the UP and single-disorder protocol conditions. Both treatment conditions were clearly superior to waitlist. In this study, 62% of patients treated with the UP no longer met diagnostic criteria for an emotional disorder following treatment, and these improvements were largely maintained 6 months later (Barlow et al. 2017a). In addition to these clinical trials focusing primarily on treatment of anxiety disorders, the UP has been shown to reduce symptoms associated with clinically significant comorbid disorders not directly targeted in treatment (Steele et al. 2018) and has been successfully applied across various clinical presentations (Barlow and Farchione 2017), including substance abuse disorders (Ciraulo et al. 2013).

Addressing Comorbidity/Practical Considerations

High rates of current and lifetime comorbidity among the emotional disorders pose a potential challenge to the application of cognitive-behavioral treatments focused on single disorders (Brown et al. 2001; Kessler et al. 2005; Merikangas et al. 2003). Although the effects of comorbidity on treatment outcome are somewhat mixed, with some studies finding that patients tend to improve on the principal targeted diagnosis regardless of the presence of additional diagnoses (Allen et al. 2010; Brown et al. 1995; Tsao et al. 2002, 2005), comorbidity has the potential to interfere with treatment. For example, if a co-occurring disorder necessitates prioritization for immediate treatment or requires simultaneous treatment, it might shift the course of treatment or prevent the therapist from applying treatment procedures as initially intended. The presence of comorbidity does not present as much of a potential challenge clinically with the UP because it was designed to handle comorbidity without requiring significant modifications to the protocol, such as adding or prioritizing treatment components or determining the sequencing of treatment.

Conclusion

In this chapter, we provided a brief overview of the UP, a transdiagnostic cognitive-behavioral treatment designed to target underlying mechanisms related to the development and maintenance of anxiety, depressive, and related disorders. Support for the efficacy of the UP has now been established, and modification of the protocol for potential group and other treatment applications, including cultural adaptations, is being evaluated. We believe that this approach offers specific advantages for training and dissemination because therapists only need to become proficient in the delivery of a single protocol for a range of disorders, rather than completing costly and time-intensive training for multiple interventions (McHugh et al. 2009). This more efficient approach to training could, in turn, facilitate dissemination efforts and increase the availability of evidence-based treatments to meet a significant public health need (McHugh and Barlow 2010; Stewart et al. 2012).

Key Points

- Transdiagnostic treatment protocols have shown efficacy for the treatment of common emotional disorders seen in routine clinical practice (e.g., anxiety, depression).

- The Unified Protocol for Transdiagnostic Treatment of Emotional Disorders (UP) is a transdiagnostic treatment with empirical support for reduction of both symptoms and higher-order temperamental changes, such as changes in neuroticism, an underlying mechanism associated with onset and maintenance of emotional disorders.

- The UP has shown efficacy in treating comorbid psychopathology in addition to single-disorder patient presentations.

- The UP is associated with less attrition than single-disorder protocols.

- The UP offers opportunities for cost-effective streamlined training, with the potential to improve dissemination of science-based treatments to more patients in need of services compared with training clinicians to treat multiple individual diagnoses.

References

Allen LB, White KS, Barlow DH, et al: Cognitive-behavior therapy (CBT) for panic disorder: relationship of anxiety and depression comorbidity with treatment outcome. J Psychopathol Behav Assess 32(2):185–192, 2010 20421906

Barlow DH: Disorders of emotion. Psychol Inq 2(1):58–71, 1991

Barlow DH, Farchione TJ: Applications of the Unified Protocol for Transdiagnostic Treatment of Emotional Disorders. New York, Oxford University Press, 2017

Barlow DH, Farchione TJ, Boisseau CL, et al: Unified Protocol for Transdiagnostic Treatment of Emotional Disorders: Clinical Demonstrations. Boston, MA, Boston University Productions, 2011a

Barlow DH, Farchione TJ, Fairholme CP, et al: Unified Protocol for Transdiagnostic Treatment of Emotional Disorders: Therapist Guide. New York, Oxford University Press, 2011b

Barlow DH, Sauer-Zavala S, Carl JR, et al: The nature, diagnosis, and treatment of neuroticism: back to the future. Clin Psychol Sci 2:344–365, 2014

Barlow DH, Farchione TJ, Bullis JR, et al: The Unified Protocol for Transdiagnostic Treatment of Emotional Disorders compared with diagnosis-specific protocols for anxiety disorders: a randomized clinical trial. JAMA Psychiatry 74(9):875–884, 2017a 28768327

Barlow DH, Farchione TJ, Sauer-Zavala S, et al: Unified Protocol for Transdiagnostic Treatment of Emotional Disorders: Therapist Guide. New York, Oxford University Press, 2017b

Borkovec TD, Abel JL, Newman H: Effects of psychotherapy on comorbid conditions in generalized anxiety disorder. J Consult Clin Psychol 63(3):479–483, 1995 7608362

Boswell JF, Farchione TJ, Sauer-Zavala S, et al: Anxiety sensitivity and interoceptive exposure: a transdiagnostic construct and change strategy. Behav Ther 44(3):417–431, 2013 23768669

Brown TA, Barlow DH: A proposal for a dimensional classification system based on the shared features of the DSM-IV anxiety and mood disorders: implications for assessment and treatment. Psychol Assess 21(3):256–271, 2009 19719339

Brown TA, Antony MM, Barlow DH: Diagnostic comorbidity in panic disorder: effect on treatment outcome and course of comorbid diagnoses following treatment. J Consult Clin Psychol 63(3):408–418, 1995 7608353

Brown TA, Chorpita BF, Barlow DH: Structural relationships among dimensions of the DSM-IV anxiety and mood disorders and dimensions of negative affect, positive affect, and autonomic arousal. J Abnorm Psychol 107(2):179–192, 1998 9604548

Brown TA, Campbell LA, Lehman CL, et al: Current and lifetime comorbidity of the DSM-IV anxiety and mood disorders in a large clinical sample. J Abnorm Psychol 110(4):585–599, 2001 11727948

Bullis JR, Fortune MR, Farchione TJ, et al: A preliminary investigation of the long-term outcome of the Unified Protocol for Transdiagnostic Treatment of Emotional Disorders. Compr Psychiatry 55(8):1920–1927, 2014 25113056

Bullis JR, Sauer-Zavala S, Bentley KH, et al: The Unified Protocol for Transdiagnostic Treatment of Emotional Disorders: preliminary exploration of effectiveness for group delivery. Behav Modif 39(2):295–321, 2015 25316034

Bullis JR, Boettcher H, Sauer-Zavala S, et al: What is an emotional disorder? A transdiagnostic mechanistic definition with implications for assessment, treatment, and prevention. Clin Psychol Sci Pract 26(2):e12278, 2019

Campbell-Sills L, Barlow DH, Brown TA, et al: Effects of suppression and acceptance on emotional responses of individuals with anxiety and mood disorders. Behav Res Ther 44(9):1251–1263, 2006 16300723

Ciraulo DA, Barlow DH, Gulliver SB, et al: The effects of venlafaxine and cognitive behavioral therapy alone and combined in the treatment of co-morbid alcohol use-anxiety disorders. Behav Res Ther 51(11):729–735, 2013 24055681

Craske MG, Barlow DH: Mastery of Your Anxiety and Panic: Therapist Guide. New York, Oxford University Press, 2007

Ellard KK, Fairholme CP, Boisseau CL, et al: Unified protocol for the transdiagnostic treatment of emotional disorders: protocol development and initial outcome data. Cognit Behav Pract 17(11):88–101, 2010 23997572

Etkin A, Wager TD: Functional neuroimaging of anxiety: a meta-analysis of emotional processing in PTSD, social anxiety disorder, and specific phobia. Am J Psychiatry 164(10):1476–1488, 2007 17898336

Etkin A, Prater KE, Hoeft F, et al: Failure of anterior cingulate activation and connectivity with the amygdala during implicit regulation of emotional processing in generalized anxiety disorder. Am J Psychiatry 167(5):545–554, 2010 20123913

Farchione TJ, Fairholme CP, Ellard KK, et al: Unified protocol for transdiagnostic treatment of emotional disorders: a randomized controlled trial. Behav Ther 43(3):666–678, 2012 22697453

Hayes AM, Feldman G: Clarifying the construct of mindfulness in the context of emotion regulation and the process of change in therapy. Clin Psychol Sci Pract 11(3):255–262, 2004

Holmes AJ, Lee PH, Hollinshead MO, et al: Individual differences in amygdala-medial prefrontal anatomy link negative affect, impaired social functioning, and polygenic depression risk. J Neurosci 32(50):18087–18100, 2012 23238724

Hope DA, Heimberg RG, Turk C: Managing Social Anxiety. New York, Oxford University Press, 2006

Kessler RC, Nelson CB, McGonagle KA, et al: Comorbidity of DSM-III-R major depressive disorder in the general population: results from the US National Comorbidity Survey. Br J Psychiatry Suppl 168(30):17–30, 1996 8864145

Kessler RC, Berglund P, Demler O, et al: Lifetime prevalence and age-of-onset distributions of DSM-IV disorders in the National Comorbidity Survey Replication. Arch Gen Psychiatry 62(6):593–602, 2005 15939837

McHugh RK, Barlow DH: The dissemination and implementation of evidence-based psychological treatments. A review of current efforts. Am Psychol 65(2):73–84, 2010 20141263

McHugh RK, Murray HW, Barlow DH: Balancing fidelity and adaptation in the dissemination of empirically supported treatments: the promise of transdiagnostic interventions. Behav Res Ther 47(11):946–953, 2009 19643395

Mennin DS, Heimberg RG, Turk CL, et al: Preliminary evidence for an emotion dysregulation model of generalized anxiety disorder. Behav Res Ther 43(10):1281–1310, 2005 16086981

Merikangas KR, Zhang H, Avenevoli S, et al: Longitudinal trajectories of depression and anxiety in a prospective community study: the Zurich Cohort Study. Arch Gen Psychiatry 60(10):993–1000, 2003 14557144

Phan KL, Fitzgerald DA, Nathan PJ, et al: Association between amygdala hyperactivity to harsh faces and severity of social anxiety in generalized social phobia. Biol Psychiatry 59(5):424–429, 2006 16256956

Porto PR, Oliveira L, Mari J, et al: Does cognitive behavioral therapy change the brain? A systematic review of neuroimaging in anxiety disorders. J Neuropsychiatry Clin Neurosci 21(2):114–125, 2009 19622682

Roy-Byrne PP, Craske MG, Stein MB: Panic disorder. Lancet 368(9540):1023–1032, 2006 16980119

Sauer-Zavala S, Wilner JG, Barlow DH: Addressing neuroticism in psychological treatment. Pers Disord 8(3):191–198, 2017 29120218

Shin LM, Liberzon I: The neurocircuitry of fear, stress, and anxiety disorders. Neuropsychopharmacology 35(1):169–191, 2010 19625997

Steele SJ, Farchione TJ, Cassiello-Robbins C, et al: Efficacy of the Unified Protocol for transdiagnostic treatment of comorbid psychopathology accompanying emotional disorders compared to treatments targeting single disorders. J Psychiatr Res 104:211–216, 2018 30103069

Stewart RE, Chambless DL, Baron J: Theoretical and practical barriers to practitioners' willingness to seek training in empirically supported treatments. J Clin Psychol 68(1):8–23, 2012 21901749

Tsao JC, Lewin MR, Craske MG: The effects of cognitive-behavior therapy for panic disorder on comorbid conditions. J Anxiety Disord 12(4):357–371, 1998 9699119

Tsao JC, Mystkowski JL, Zucker BG, et al: Effects of cognitive-behavioral therapy for panic disorder on comorbid conditions: replication and extension. Behavior Therapy 33:493–509, 2002

Tsao JC, Mystkowski JL, Zucker BG, et al: Impact of cognitive-behavioral therapy for panic disorder on comorbidity: a controlled investigation. Behav Res Ther 43(7):959–970, 2005 15896289

Recommended Readings

Barlow DH, Farchione TJ: Applications of the Unified Protocol for Transdiagnostic Treatment of Emotional Disorders. New York, Oxford University Press, 2017

Barlow DH, Sauer-Zavala S, Carl JR, et al: The nature, diagnosis, and treatment of neuroticism: back to the future. Clin Psychol Sci 2:344–365, 2014

Barlow DH, Farchione TJ, Bullis JR, et al: The Unified Protocol for Transdiagnostic Treatment of Emotional Disorders compared with diagnosis-specific protocols for anxiety disorders: a randomized clinical trial. JAMA Psychiatry 74(9):875–884, 2017 28768327

Bullis JR, Boettcher H, Sauer-Zavala S, Farchione TJ, Barlow DH: What is an emotional disorder? A transdiagnostic mechanistic definition with implications for assessment, treatment, and prevention. Clin Psychol 26(2):e12278, 2019

CHAPTER 9

Combined Treatment of Anxiety Disorders

Jessica L. Maples-Keller, Ph.D.

Mark Burton, Ph.D.

Emily Mellen, B.A.

Julia Merker, B.S.

Kerry J. Ressler, M.D., Ph.D.

Barbara O. Rothbaum, Ph.D.

In this chapter, we examine the empirical literature on combined treatment for anxiety disorders. Of note, although OCD and PTSD are no longer considered anxiety disorders in the newest edition of DSM (DSM-5; American Psychiatric Association 2013), their inclusion in this chapter is rooted in the understanding that anxiety is a key feature of both disorders. By *combined treatment* we refer to some form of psychotherapy, most commonly short-term cognitive-behavioral therapy (CBT), combined with pharmacological treatment or novel combined approaches aimed to enhance therapeutic learning. The success of psychotherapy and medication individually in the treatment of anxiety disorders would reasonably indicate that the combination of both would be an even more effective treatment intervention. However, literature reviews and meta-analyses generally indicate that only incremental benefits are found for combination treatments over medication alone (Cuijpers et al. 2014) and that CBT alone is usually as effective as combination treatment (Black 2006; Foa et al. 2002; Otto et al. 2005). Notably, one meta-analysis of only randomized controlled trials (RCTs) that compared CBT plus medication treatments with CBT plus placebo treatments did find larger effect sizes for active combination treatments for panic disorder and generalized anxiety disorder (GAD) (Hofmann et al. 2009).

CBT has shown impressive efficacy in treating individuals with anxiety disorders and is a first-line treatment for anxiety. Many CBT treatments include some form of exposure therapy. Exposure therapy is based on emotional processing theory (Foa and Kozak 1986; Foa et al. 2006), which suggests that fear is a cognitive structure in memory that supports adaptive behavior when faced with a realistically threatening situation but becomes pathological when associations among stimulus, response, and meaning do not reflect reality (e.g., interpreting a safe environment as threatening). Exposure therapy is thought to activate and change this fear structure through confrontation with feared stimuli in a therapeutic manner (Rothbaum et al. 2007). Ways in which stimuli can be presented include imaginal (in imagination), in vivo (in real life), and in virtual reality. Additional CBT components include *cognitive restructuring* and *relaxation*. Cognitive restructuring teaches methods and skills for correcting errors in patients' thinking. Relaxation techniques often include breathing retraining or deep muscle relaxation. Relaxation has a smaller effect for some anxiety disorders compared with other components of CBT (Montero-Marin et al. 2018).

Review of the Literature

This chapter represents an updated review of the current state of the literature on combined treatment for anxiety disorders. The criteria selected for studies to be included in our review were that patients in the study had received a clinician-assessed diagnosis including panic disorder, OCD, social anxiety disorder, GAD, or PTSD and that the study included at least two groups, one treated with either pharmacotherapy or CBT and the other treated with a combination of CBT plus medication.

Panic Disorder

Panic disorder is characterized by repeated, unexpected, discrete episodes of intense fear and discomfort, accompanied by physical and cognitive changes (Allen and Barlow 2006). The benefits of CBT in the treatment of panic disorder are well documented (Barlow 2002). In panic disorder, individuals erroneously interpret the physiological responses associated with panic as dangerous, leading to anxiety and avoidance behaviors. CBT seeks to reduce panic symptoms by correcting these misinterpretations. Medications, including the selective serotonin reuptake inhibitors (SSRIs), tricyclic antidepressants, monoamine oxidase inhibitors (MAOIs), and benzodiazepines, have also been successful in treating this disorder (McHugh et al. 2009). For benzodiazepines, the short-term anxiolytic effects, as well as their potential impairment of fear extinction, may interfere with long-term anxiety reduction, and thus these agents are cautioned against in combination with CBT in the clinical literature (Cloos and Ferreira 2009; Dell'osso and Lader 2013). The American Psychiatric Association practice guidelines indicate that if a first-line treatment such as CBT, SSRIs, or the serotonin-norepinephrine reuptake inhibitors (SNRIs) has failed, adding a benzodiazepine to the first-line treatment is a common strategy to target enduring symptoms (American Psychiatric Association 2009). Guidelines also recommend a regular dosing schedule as opposed to as-needed use, with the goal of preventing panic attacks instead of reducing symptoms once a panic attack has occurred. With regard to combined approaches, the guidelines also note that as-needed benzodiazepine use may be inconsistent with CBT approaches because this might discourage patients from developing and using anxiety management skills.

Few studies have directly compared combination treatment with monotherapies for panic disorder specifically, but results from these studies suggest caution in simultaneously initiating benzodiazepines and CBT. One well-designed study of combination treatment with a benzodiazepine compared 8 weeks of alprazolam, exposure therapy, and alprazolam plus exposure therapy in the treatment of panic disorder with agoraphobia (Marks et al. 1993). Patients ($N=154$) were randomly assigned to exposure plus alprazolam, exposure plus placebo, relaxation plus alprazolam, or relaxation plus placebo. Both exposure conditions (with alprazolam or placebo) produced greater improvement at posttreatment on measures of phobic avoidance than did relaxation with either alprazolam or placebo. At 6-month follow-up, exposure treatment plus placebo outcome was reported as superior to all other conditions, suggesting that tapering off of alprazolam after the active treatment phase interfered with gains made in exposure therapy. Another study investigated two potential "next-step" options for patients with panic disorder who remained symptomatic after treatment with an SSRI at a moderate dosage for 6 weeks or standard panic pharmacotherapy (Simon et al. 2009). First, the SSRI dosage was increased for an additional 6 weeks. Then, patients who remained symptomatic were randomized to continued SSRI plus a 12-week course of CBT or medication optimization, with the SSRI at optimized dosage, plus clonazepam, a benzodiazepine. Results indicated that increased SSRI dosage did not result in greater benefit. At the second step, group differences were not identified, suggesting that both CBT and clonazepam augmentation of SSRI treatment are potentially appropriate next-step options for patients with treatment-refractory panic disorder.

Two studies have examined combination treatment with nonbenzodiazepine medications. The first included 77 patients with a diagnosis of panic disorder with agoraphobia who were randomly assigned to 16 weeks of either CBT plus buspirone or CBT plus placebo (Cottraux et al. 1995). Results indicated no treatment differences between groups at posttreatment and at follow-up, suggesting that the main effect in this study was the CBT and not the medication augmentation. The second study examined CBT, imipramine, and the combination of the two in the treatment of panic disorder. In this study, 312 patients were randomly assigned to CBT plus imipramine, CBT plus placebo, CBT alone, imipramine alone, or placebo alone (Barlow et al. 2000). CBT plus imipramine was found to be superior to CBT alone at both the 3- and 9-month assessments. However, at 6 months after treatment discontinuation, CBT groups without imipramine had a superior outcome compared with the group receiving the combined treatment.

Several meta-analyses have been conducted examining the effects of combination treatment for panic disorder. In a comprehensive study of psychological, pharmacological, and combined treatments for anxiety disorders, large pre/post effect sizes were found for CBT plus medication for panic disorder ($d=1.55$; Bandelow et al. 2015). A meta-analysis of studies directly comparing combination with monotherapy approaches showed that combined treatment for panic disorder was more effective than either psychological or pharmacological approaches alone (Bandelow et al. 2007). Finally, in a meta-analysis specifically focused on combination compared with medication-only treatments for a range of diagnoses, combination was again found to be superior to medication alone for the treatment of panic disorder (Cuijpers et al. 2014). These meta-analytical findings suggest a benefit for combining CBT and medication for the treatment of panic disorder. Furthermore, for those who have not responded to SSRI monotherapy, the addition of CBT may be helpful, whereas the combination of CBT and benzodiazepines is not indicated.

Obsessive-Compulsive Disorder

OCD is characterized by recurrent, intrusive, and distressing thoughts, images, and urges, along with ritualized behaviors or thoughts used to reduce related distress. Meta-analytic findings suggest that CBT is more effective compared with pharmacotherapy with serotonin reuptake inhibitors (SRIs) for OCD and that combined therapy is more effective than SRIs alone but not more effective than CBT alone (Romanelli et al. 2014). One trial compared exposure and ritual prevention (EX/RP) plus fluvoxamine, EX/RP plus placebo, and fluvoxamine alone in a 24-week treatment of 60 patients diagnosed with OCD (Cottraux et al. 1990). No group differences were detected at either posttreatment or follow-up.

Another trial compared EX/RP plus fluvoxamine with EX/RP plus placebo in the treatment of 58 patients (Hohagen et al. 1998). Both groups improved significantly from pretreatment to posttreatment, with no significant differences between groups. Percentage of responders, defined by 35% improvement in total Yale-Brown Obsessive Compulsive Scale score, indicated an advantage for the combined treatment. In a third study, cognitive therapy, EX/RP, fluvoxamine plus cognitive therapy, fluvoxamine plus EX/RP, and a waitlist condition were compared in 117 patients (van Balkom et al. 1998). All four active treatment conditions were found to be superior to waitlist at both midtreatment and posttreatment, with no significant differences revealed among active treatments.

In a double-blind, randomized trial, Foa et al. (2005) included a pill placebo condition when comparing clomipramine, EX/RP, and clomipramine plus EX/RP in the treatment of 122 adult outpatients with OCD. All active treatments were superior to placebo. EX/RP results did not differ from EX/RP plus clomipramine results, and both were superior to clomipramine alone.

Two trials have examined the effect of adding EX/RP for SRI-resistant OCD. In the first, individuals who had not responded to at least a 12-week course of SRI (i.e., adequate dosage of clomipramine, fluoxetine, paroxetine, sertraline, fluvoxamine, citalopram, or escitalopram) prior to the study were randomized to receive either EX/RP or stress management while continuing their current dosage of medication (Simpson et al. 2008). Results showed that those randomized to receive combination treatment with EX/RP responded better than those who received stress management. In a second trial with a similar design, individuals who had not responded to SRI treatment prior to starting the study were randomized to receive EX/RP or risperidone augmentation (Simpson et al. 2013). Again, those who received the additional EX/RP showed the highest reductions in symptoms, whereas the addition of risperidone did not lead to improvement. Although these studies showed benefit for adding EX/RP for SRI-resistant OCD, they did not directly compare a combination treatment with monotherapy and thus do not speak to the value of combination treatment specifically. The reviewed studies indicate no clear advantage for combined treatment with traditional antidepressant or anxiolytic medication over CBT alone in the treatment of OCD. Although some evidence suggests a benefit to adding CBT for those whose illness does not respond to SRIs, more research is needed comparing combination with medication monotherapy for this population.

Social Anxiety Disorder

Social anxiety disorder is characterized by persistent fear in social or performance situations. CBT treatment of social anxiety disorder has been largely based on the cognitive model (Rapee and Heimberg 1997), in which therapy is designed to challenge unrealistic thinking about social situations and evaluation from others. Validated pharmacotherapy for social anxiety disorder includes benzodiazepines, MAOIs, and SSRIs (Hood and Nutt 2001). SNRIs have also been found efficacious (Liebowitz et al. 2003). Meta-analytic findings suggest that CBT is more effective than medication treatment for social anxiety disorder and that combination treatment may yield larger effects compared with either CBT or medication treatment alone (Canton et al. 2012).

In a primary care study, sertraline, exposure therapy plus sertraline, exposure therapy plus placebo, and placebo alone were compared in the treatment of 387 patients diagnosed with social anxiety disorder (Blomhoff et al. 2001). Patients in all active treatment groups improved significantly more than placebo-treated patients at week 12, but at weeks 16 and 24, only improvement in the groups treated with sertraline remained significantly superior to placebo. However, no significant response differences were discovered between the active treatment groups. Notably, exposure was in the form of instructions for self-exposure and did not occur in sessions. A 1-year follow-up of these participants found that the exposure therapy plus placebo group demonstrated further improvement, whereas the exposure therapy plus sertraline group demonstrated a tendency toward symptom deterioration following treatment completion (Haug et al. 2003), suggesting that exposure therapy for social anxiety disorder without sertraline augmentation may be a more effective long-term treatment approach. In another study, 102 patients with social anxiety disorder were randomized to paroxetine, cognitive therapy, combined cognitive therapy and paroxetine, or placebo alone (Nordahl et al. 2016). At posttreatment, cognitive therapy was superior to the paroxetine and placebo groups but not to combined therapy plus paroxetine. At 12-month follow-up, outcome in the cognitive therapy group was superior to that of the placebo and paroxetine alone groups, with no significant differences between the combination, paroxetine alone, and placebo groups, again indicating that CBT-based psychotherapy alone may be an optimal approach long-term.

A randomized, placebo-controlled trial treating 60 patients with social anxiety disorder was conducted using cognitive therapy (weekly self-exposure assignments), fluoxetine plus self-exposure, or placebo plus self-exposure (Clark et al. 2003). Significant improvements were evidenced in all three treatment conditions, with cognitive therapy revealing superiority to fluoxetine plus self-exposure and placebo plus self-exposure at mid- and posttreatment.

In a randomized, double-blind, multisite, placebo-controlled trial, Davidson et al. (2004) compared fluoxetine, 14 weekly sessions of comprehensive group CBT, placebo, and combined fluoxetine and group CBT in the treatment of 295 outpatients diagnosed with generalized social anxiety disorder. All active treatments were found to show significantly better results than placebo but did not differ from each other posttreatment.

Finally, two studies have examined the effects of combination treatments with CBT and MAOIs. The first randomized 83 individuals to receive either group CBT with a medication placebo, medication treatment with an MAOI, moclobemide and a supportive therapy placebo, or the combination of group CBT plus moclobemide over a period of 6 months (Prasko et al. 2006). Results showed that although the combination group showed slightly better response in general anxiety at midtreatment, group CBT was superior to both the medication and combination groups for reducing social avoidance and generalized anxiety by the end of treatment. Another double-blind, placebo-controlled trial of 128 individuals with social anxiety disorder compared the combination of group CBT and the MAOI phenelzine sulfate with groups receiving either treatment alone and one receiving a medication placebo control (Blanco et al. 2010). Results showed that combination treatment was more effective than group CBT alone or phenelzine alone, with medication placebo demonstrating the smallest effects. A randomized trial combining escitalopram (an SSRI) or placebo with internet-delivered CBT for social anxiety disorder found significantly more responders and larger decreases in anticipatory speech anxiety at posttreatment in the escitalopram group (Gingnell et al. 2016).

Generalized Anxiety Disorder

The hallmark of GAD is excessive worry, along with chronic anxiety and multiple somatic symptoms. CBT for GAD focuses on the cognitive components of worry, such as intolerance of uncertainty, erroneous beliefs about worry, poor problem orientation, and cognitive avoidance (Behar and Borkovec 2006). Medication interventions that have been efficacious in the treatment of this disorder include benzodiazepines, SSRIs, and SNRIs. To our knowledge, only two RCTs of combined treatment for GAD have been published. The first randomly assigned 101 outpatients diagnosed with GAD to one of five conditions: diazepam alone, placebo alone, CBT, diazepam plus CBT, and placebo plus CBT (Power et al. 1990). All active treatments were evaluated as superior to placebo. Combined diazepam plus CBT produced the best results on almost all measures at posttreatment, but active treatment results did not significantly differ from one another. Initial treatment gains for all patients receiving CBT were maintained at follow-up. However, initial moderate treatment gains among patients in the group receiving diazepam were not well maintained at follow-up.

Another trial randomized 60 individuals diagnosed with GAD to receive anxiety management training with buspirone or a medication placebo or buspirone with a supportive therapy placebo (Bond et al. 2002). Results showed a reduction in GAD symptoms across groups, with no differences found between the groups. However, the type of therapy delivered in this treatment focused on relaxation, which may be less effective than more comprehensive CBT approaches (Montero-Marin et al. 2018). Although both studies reviewed here indicate a lack of an advantage for combined treatments for GAD, the evidence base is too small to identify true and generalizable effects.

Posttraumatic Stress Disorder

Evidence has shown effectiveness for both pharmacological and psychotherapeutic treatment interventions for PTSD. PTSD is characterized by exposure to a traumatic event, followed by symptoms of physiological arousal, avoidance, and reexperiencing of the trauma. CBT, and specifically *prolonged exposure* (PE), has the largest amount of empirical support in the literature (Powers et al. 2010). Studies have widely confirmed the efficacy of SSRIs as pharmacological treatment for PTSD (Davidson et al. 2001), and SNRIs have been found to be effective and well tolerated (Davidson et al. 2006).

Rothbaum et al. (2006) conducted a multicenter investigation of PE augmentation of sertraline in the treatment of PTSD. In the study, 88 male and female outpatients diagnosed with PTSD were treated with open-label sertraline for 10 weeks in phase I, and then were randomly assigned to receive either continuation with sertraline alone or augmentation with PE (10 twice-weekly sessions of 90–120 minutes) in phase II. Results indicated that 5 additional weeks of treatment with sertraline alone did not result in further improvement on measures of PTSD severity, depression, and general anxiety. Augmentation with PE did result in further reduction of PTSD severity but not of depression or general anxiety. Notably, the beneficial effect of PE augmentation was observed only among medication partial (weaker) responders.

A later study examined the effect of adding an SSRI (paroxetine) to PE for nonremitters after eight biweekly sessions of psychotherapy treatment (Simon et al. 2009). Forty-four individuals diagnosed with PTSD completed the first phase of monotherapy with PE, with significant reductions in PTSD symptoms on average. Twenty-five of these individuals did not meet remission status at the end of treatment and were subsequently randomized in a second phase of the trial to receive medication augmentation with either paroxetine or medication placebo for 10 weeks while also receiving an additional five sessions of PE. Results showed no difference between the paroxetine group and the placebo control group at the end of the second phase. Although this study suggested no added benefit of adjunctive SSRIs after low response to PE, findings are mixed regarding the effect of including SSRIs from the start of PE. Specifically, Schneier et al. (2012) randomized 37 individuals diagnosed with PTSD to receive PE in concert with paroxetine or with a medication placebo. Results showed significantly greater decreases in PTSD severity and higher remission rates for those receiving the combination of PE and active medication compared with those receiving PE with placebo; however, this effect was not maintained at follow-up. In another study, 179 motor vehicle crash survivors were randomized to PE alone, paroxetine alone, or combination treatment with both (Popiel et al. 2015). Results showed that remission rates were highest for the group receiving PE monotherapy and that combination treatment was not superior to either monotherapy approach.

A recent trial randomized 207 veterans to PE plus sertraline, PE plus placebo, or sertraline plus enhanced medication management (Rauch et al. 2019). PE involved 13 standard PE sessions, and sertraline dosing was adjusted between 50 and 100 mg and titrated upward through week 10 and subsequently maintained across the 24-week study time period. Enhanced medication management involved medical management as well as psychoeducation and active listening; trauma-related specifics and PTSD symptom intervention were not discussed in medication management sessions. Results indicated that PTSD symptoms decreased significantly overall for all participants, with no significant differences between study conditions. A second completed clinical trial compared combination PE and sertraline treatment with PE alone (without a placebo) in a civilian sample randomized to either choose their treatment or not (Feeny et al., in preparation). Results from this trial are not yet published but will add to the findings from previous work to identify whether choice plays a role in response to combination treatment with PE and sertraline (Feeny et al., in preparation).

Two trials have examined combination SSRI treatment with non-exposure-based approaches, also with mixed results. The first trial examined the effect of adding sertraline to Seeking Safety, a manualized treatment for PTSD and comorbid substance use disorder (Najavits 2002), and found in a sample of patients with subthreshold or full threshold PTSD that those receiving the sertraline combination showed greater reductions in PTSD symptom severity compared with those receiving placebo (Hien et al. 2015). The second trial examined the effect of combination treatment with either sertraline or the tetracyclic antidepressant mianserin added to a non-exposure-based "flexible" CBT treatment (Buhmann et al. 2016). Results showed no effect on PTSD symptoms for any treatment group, demonstrating the need to use manualized, exposure-based treatment as the foundation for monotherapeutic or combination treatments for PTSD.

This growing body of research suggests that PE is a robust treatment for PTSD with additive benefits over monotherapy with SSRIs and that an evidence-based, trauma-focused treatment should be the foundation for any combination approach. In addition, it may not be indicated to add an SSRI for patients with PTSD that is refractory to PE treatment. The Veterans Administration/Department of Defense's *Clinical Practice Guideline for the Management of Posttraumatic Stress Disorder and Acute Stress Disorder* does not provide specific recommendations on augmentation of pharmacotherapy for partial or nonresponders to trauma-focused therapy because of insufficient empirical evidence to guide clinical decision making; future research is needed in this area (Management of Posttraumatic Stress Disorder Work Group 2017). Using evidence-based psychotherapy is essential for combination approaches, as emphasized in an effectiveness trial that found "flexible" therapy for PTSD, in which most participants did not receive exposure, was not effective as a monotherapy or in combination with sertraline (Buhmann et al. 2016). More studies examining the combination of medications with evidence-based psychotherapy are needed to determine if and when adding medication is indicated for effective PTSD treatment.

Novel Treatments for Anxiety Disorders

In this section, we briefly assess nontraditional approaches to the treatment of anxiety disorders. Advances in animal research elucidating neurotransmitters involved in fear extinction (Davis and Myers 2002) have led to the exploration of combination treatment strategies for anxiety disorders, with a focus on the enhancement of *extinction learning* that occurs in CBT. In this model, pharmacotherapy is aimed at improving the learning that takes place during CBT (specifically exposure-based therapy) and not at treating the symptoms of anxiety (Davis et al. 2006). The glutamatergic NMDA receptor has been found to be critically involved in learning and memory (Newcomer and Krystal 2001), and this learning may be augmented by the NMDA partial agonist D-cycloserine (DCS). DCS has been shown in animal studies to facilitate the extinction of learned fear (Davis et al. 2006), with many additional replications thereafter.

The first clinical test of DCS combined it with exposure therapy for specific phobia (Ressler et al. 2004). The 28 participants diagnosed with acrophobia were randomly assigned to three treatment groups (double blind): placebo plus virtual reality exposure (VRE) therapy, 50 mg DCS plus VRE therapy, or 500 mg DCS plus VRE therapy. Participants who received DCS in conjunction with VRE therapy had significantly enhanced decreases in fear within the virtual environment and reported significantly more improvement than the placebo group in their overall acrophobic symptoms at 3-month follow-up, and skin conductance fluctuations were significantly decreased in this group (Ressler et al. 2004).

Subsequent investigations suggested that this approach demonstrated promise across the anxiety disorders. In a randomized, double-blind, placebo-controlled evaluation, 27 outpatients diagnosed with social anxiety disorder participated in a five-session exposure treatment and received 50 mg DCS or placebo 1 hour prior to each session (Hofmann et al. 2006). Participants who received DCS augmentation demonstrated significantly greater improvement at posttreatment and at follow-up evaluation. This finding was replicated in another sample of patients with social anxiety disorder that found that patients administered 50 mg DCS as an adjunct to exposure therapy reported greater improvement on measures of symptom severity, dysfunctional cognitions, and life impairment in comparison with patients given placebo (Guastella et al. 2008).

Initial trials in OCD also demonstrate promise. For instance, Kushner et al. (2007) examined the use of 125 mg DCS to accelerate reduction of obsession-related distress in patients diagnosed with OCD who were undergoing exposure therapy. Patients in the DCS group ($n=14$) reported a significantly greater decrease in obsession-related distress compared with those in the placebo group ($n=11$). In another randomized, double-blind, placebo-controlled trial of DCS (100 mg) compared with placebo augmentation of behavior therapy (10 sessions, twice per week) for 23 patients with OCD, the investigators found that OCD symptoms in the DCS group were significantly improved at midtreatment and that depressive symptoms were significantly further improved at posttreatment (Wilhelm et al. 2006). However, these results were not replicated in another study of 24 patients by Storch et al. (2007). The investigators reported no significant group differences across outcome variables, and the rate of improvement did not differ between groups. A double-blind RCT of internet-based CBT or OCD in which participants were randomized to 50 mg DCS or placebo also found no significant differences across groups (Andersson et al. 2015).

In a randomized, double-blind, placebo-controlled trial of DCS compared to placebo, 50 mg DCS prior to brief-exposure CBT for panic disorder was associated with better outcomes on a panic severity scale and a global outcome measure (Otto et al. 2010). Participants received two sessions of psychoeducation and cognitive restructuring followed by DCS or placebo prior to three exposure-based sessions. However, another RCT did not identify a significant difference between 50 mg DCS and placebo in patients with agoraphobia and panic, but a trend in more severe patients indicated that DCS may have accelerated symptom reduction (Siegmund et al. 2011).

Inconsistent findings have also been identified with regard to DCS augmentation of PTSD treatment across five RCTs (de Kleine et al. 2012; Difede et al. 2014, in preparation; Litz et al. 2012; Rothbaum et al. 2014). In a sample of sexual abuse survivors who received 50 mg DCS or placebo prior to PE, no significant difference was identified; however, exploratory session-by-session analyses revealed that DCS yielded higher symptom reduction in those who had more severe pretreatment PTSD and needed longer treatment (de Kleine et al. 2012). Litz et al. (2012) randomized 25 male combat veterans to either six-session manualized exposure therapy plus 50 mg DCS or therapy plus placebo. In contrast with previous findings, results indicated that those in the DCS combination group demonstrated *less* symptom reduction than the placebo combination group and were more likely to drop out. A small study of survivors of the World Trade Center attacks who received VRE and either 100 mg DCS or placebo found that remission rates were greater for the DCS group (Difede et al. 2014). Another study of 156 veterans compared the effects of DCS, alprazolam, or placebo prior to VRE. No significant differences were identified across the DCS and placebo groups. However, the DCS group demonstrated improved between-session extinction learning and lower cortisol and startle reactivity to virtual reality cues at posttreatment (Rothbaum et al. 2014). Finally, Difede et al. (in preparation) randomized 192 veterans to 50 mg DCS plus VRE or PE or placebo plus VRE or PE. The VRE intervention included nine weekly 90-minute sessions, with medication administered prior to sessions three through nine. All patients in all conditions improved significantly. The main effect of DCS was not significant, indicating that patients improved at a similar rate regardless of DCS or placebo grouping. Dropout rates in this study were 26.3% for the DCS groups and 36.1% in the placebo groups.

A meta-analytic review of randomized trials investigating DCS augmentation within exposure therapy across anxiety disorders suggests that overall, the DCS groups demonstrated lower symptom severity following exposure treatment compared with the placebo groups (Mataix-Cols et al. 2017), especially when dosed at least 60 minutes or more prior to treatment (Rosenfield et al. 2019), consistent with previous meta-analytic findings (Bontempo et al. 2012; Rodrigues et al. 2014). Results indicated that this effect is small overall ($d=-0.25$), and a significant difference was not identified in follow-up data. No patient or study moderators, including age, sex, primary diagnosis, number of sessions, dosage, timing, or number of DCS administrations, were found to be significantly associated with outcome. Trials have not targeted DCS augmentation in patients with extinction consolidation deficits who may require extinction enhancement. Our current understanding of these inconsistencies related to DCS is that cognitive enhancement with NMDA activation supports the most robust memory at the time of drug augmentation—which may either increase (sensitization or reconsolidation) or decrease (extinction) the trauma memory. Thus, to make use of this combined therapy approach, we need to understand better how to preferentially drive the extinction component of exposure therapy and to minimize sensitization or reconsolidation following cue reactivation.

Overall, this novel approach to combined psychotherapy proposes that a cognitive enhancer medication will specifically improve the efficacy of the emotional learning process that takes place in psychotherapy and possibly make these new emotional memories more robust, stable, and long-lasting. However, future research will have to consider timing of the dose, DCS dosage, and floor effects in addition to better understanding the effects of specific psychotherapies on the memory structures that are being altered or augmented by the pharmacotherapy.

Multiple additional agents are currently being examined for their potential to enhance exposure therapy for anxiety disorders, with most studies examining effects for PTSD treatment. Specifically, methylene blue was shown to enhance the effects of imaginal exposure for PTSD treatment in a sample of civilians (Zoellner et al. 2017), whereas yohimbine reduced depression and enhanced between-session habituation for veterans receiving PE but did not lead to a greater reduction in overall PTSD symptom severity (Tuerk et al. 2018). Several trials have examined the effect of a novel combination approach designed specifically for treatment-resistant PTSD that doses 3,4-methylenedioxymethamphetamine (MDMA) prior to a drug-assisted, 8-hour-long psychotherapy session (Bouso et al. 2008; Mithoefer et al. 2011, 2013, 2018; Oehen et al. 2013). These trials demonstrate strong effects for this combination treatment compared with treatment with placebo. Additional studies of MDMA, specifically in combination with evidence-based psychotherapy such as PE, are needed to determine whether it can enhance trauma-focused therapy for treatment-resistant PTSD.

Propranolol, which is theorized to enhance memory reconsolidation, led to significantly lower PTSD symptom severity compared with placebo for individuals undergoing brief memory reactivation sessions; however, this agent has not yet been tested as an adjunct to a full course of manualized treatment (Brunet et al. 2018). Corticosteroids have been tested in two trials examining augmentation of PE, with mixed results. The first showed that hydrocortisone provided prior to imaginal exposure led to greater retention in treatment and reduction in PTSD symptoms for a sample of veterans receiving PE (Yehuda et al. 2015). The second showed that dexamethasone led to greater dropout and may have increased reexperiencing symptoms following drug administration (Maples-Keller et al. 2019). Finally, the nonpharmacological adjunctive approach of combining repetitive transcranial magnetic stimulation (rTMS) with trauma-focused treatment was examined in a single trial that showed rTMS led to a greater reduction in PTSD symptom severity compared with sham treatment in combination with cognitive processing therapy (Kozel et al. 2018). These novel agents show promise for future research but currently do not have the evidence base to impact clinical recommendations for the treatment of PTSD and other anxiety disorders.

Conclusion

Given the lackluster performance of combination approaches and significant concerns about relapse following discontinuation of traditional medications, CBT has often been recommended as a first-line approach for the treatment of patients with anxiety disorders (American Psychiatric Association 2009; Management of Posttraumatic Stress Disorder Work Group 2017). However, if CBT is not readily available, SSRIs or SNRIs are a good first treatment. If these medications do not produce an adequate response, and if CBT is available, it is reasonable to augment treatment for partial medication responders with CBT. In addition, for patients presenting with anxiety and significant comorbid depression, combining medication treatment for depression with CBT for anxiety would be a logical approach. Future research should leverage our understanding of the neural mechanisms of anxiety, such as therapeutically targeting fear learning pathways with cognitive enhancers, to provide optimal pharmacological manipulation of the specific anxiety-related memories for a true precision medicine approach.

Key Points

- Several different strategies may be considered for combining pharmacotherapy and psychotherapy, and each presents challenges and advantages. The bulk of the studies reviewed did not find an advantage of combination therapy with traditional psychiatric medication over cognitive-behavioral therapy (CBT) alone.

- If antidepressant medication and psychotherapy are combined and are both begun at the same time, this presents the problem of time to response, generally about 4 weeks, for the medication. It may make more sense to combine these approaches sequentially, starting first with the antidepressant, so that the patient is receiving medication for at least 4 weeks before commencing psychotherapy.

- Anxiolytic medications other than antidepressants usually have a much quicker onset of action; therefore, they can be combined with psychotherapy from the outset. However, some evidence indicates that these medications, in particular benzodiazepines, may impede CBT, especially exposure therapy.

- In the case of the more novel medication approaches, such as D-cycloserine, the drug is not expected to afford any benefit in and of itself; medication is only effective in combination with exposure therapy, so both should be administered at the same time to specifically augment the emotional learning that underlies exposure therapy.

References

Allen LB, Barlow DH: Treatment of panic disorder, in Pathological Anxiety, Emotional Processing in Etiology and Treatment. New York, Guilford, 2006, pp 166–180

American Psychiatric Association: Practice Guideline for the Treatment of Patients With Panic Disorder. Washington, DC, American Psychiatric Association, 2009

American Psychiatric Association: Diagnostic and Statistical Manual of Mental Disorders, 5th Edition. Arlington, VA, American Psychiatric Association, 2013

Andersson E, Hedman E, Enander J, et al: d-Cycloserine vs placebo as adjunct to cognitive behavioral therapy for obsessive-compulsive disorder and interaction with antidepressants: a randomized clinical trial. JAMA Psychiatry 72(7):659–667, 2015 25970252

Bandelow B, Seidler-Brandler U, Becker A, et al: Meta-analysis of randomized controlled comparisons of psychopharmacological and psychological treatments for anxiety disorders. World J Biol Psychiatry 8(3):175–187, 2007 17654408

Bandelow B, Reitt M, Röver C, et al: Efficacy of treatments for anxiety disorders: a meta-analysis. Int Clin Psychopharmacol 30(4):183–192, 2015 25932596

Barlow DH: Anxiety and Its Disorders: The Nature and Treatment of Anxiety and Panic, 2nd Edition. New York, Guilford, 2002

Barlow DH, Gorman JM, Shear MK, et al: Cognitive-behavioral therapy, imipramine, or their combination for panic disorder: a randomized controlled trial. JAMA 283(19):2529–2536, 2000 10815116

Behar E, Borkovec TD: The nature and treatment of generalized anxiety disorder, in Pathological Anxiety: Emotional Processing in Etiology and Treatment. Edited by Rothbaum BO. New York, Guilford, 2006, pp 181–196

Black DW: Efficacy of combined pharmacotherapy and psychotherapy versus monotherapy in the treatment of anxiety disorders. CNS Spectr 11(10 suppl 12):29–33, 2006 17008828

Blanco C, Heimberg RG, Schneier FR, et al: A placebo-controlled trial of phenelzine, cognitive behavioral group therapy, and their combination for social anxiety disorder. Arch Gen Psychiatry 67(3):286–295, 2010 20194829

Blomhoff S, Haug TT, Hellström K, et al: Randomised controlled general practice trial of sertraline, exposure therapy and combined treatment in generalised social phobia. Br J Psychiatry 179:23–30, 2001 11435264

Bond AJ, Wingrove J, Valerie Curran H, et al: Treatment of generalised anxiety disorder with a short course of psychological therapy, combined with buspirone or placebo. J Affect Disord 72(3):267–271, 2002 12450644

Bontempo A, Panza KE, Bloch MH: d-Cycloserine augmentation of behavioral therapy for the treatment of anxiety disorders: a meta-analysis. J Clin Psychiatry 73(4):533–537, 2012 22579153

Bouso JC, Doblin R, Farré M, et al: MDMA-assisted psychotherapy using low doses in a small sample of women with chronic posttraumatic stress disorder. J Psychoactive Drugs 40(3):225–236, 2008 19004414

Brunet A, Saumier D, Liu A, et al: Reduction of PTSD symptoms with pre-reactivation propranolol therapy: a randomized controlled trial. Am J Psychiatry 175(5):427–433, 2018 29325446

Buhmann CB, Nordentoft M, Ekstroem M, et al: The effect of flexible cognitive-behavioural therapy and medical treatment, including antidepressants on post-traumatic stress disorder and depression in traumatised refugees: pragmatic randomised controlled clinical trial. Br J Psychiatry 208(3):252–259, 2016 26541687

Canton J, Scott KM, Glue P: Optimal treatment of social phobia: systematic review and meta-analysis. Neuropsychiatr Dis Treat 8:203–215, 2012 22665997

Clark DM, Ehlers A, McManus F, et al: Cognitive therapy versus fluoxetine in generalized social phobia: a randomized placebo-controlled trial. J Consult Clin Psychol 71(6):1058–1067, 2003 14622081

Cloos JM, Ferreira V: Current use of benzodiazepines in anxiety disorders. Curr Opin Psychiatry 22(1):90–95, 2009 19122540

Cottraux J, Mollard E, Bouvard M, et al: A controlled study of fluvoxamine and exposure in obsessive-compulsive disorder. Int Clin Psychopharmacol 5(1):17–30, 1990 2110206

Cottraux J, Note ID, Cungi C, et al: A controlled study of cognitive behaviour therapy with buspirone or placebo in panic disorder with agoraphobia. Br J Psychiatry 167(5):635–641, 1995 8564320

Cuijpers P, Sijbrandij M, Koole SL, et al: Adding psychotherapy to antidepressant medication in depression and anxiety disorders: a meta-analysis. World Psychiatry 13(1):56–67, 2014 24497254

Davidson JR, Rothbaum BO, van der Kolk BA, et al: Multicenter, double-blind comparison of sertraline and placebo in the treatment of posttraumatic stress disorder. Arch Gen Psychiatry 58(5):485–492, 2001 11343529

Davidson JR, Foa EB, Huppert JD, et al: Fluoxetine, comprehensive cognitive behavioral therapy, and placebo in generalized social phobia. Arch Gen Psychiatry 61(10):1005–1013, 2004 15466674

Davidson J, Baldwin D, Stein DJ, et al: Treatment of posttraumatic stress disorder with venlafaxine extended release: a 6-month randomized controlled trial. Arch Gen Psychiatry 63(10):1158–1165, 2006 17015818

Davis M, Myers KM: The role of glutamate and gamma-aminobutyric acid in fear extinction: clinical implications for exposure therapy. Biol Psychiatry 52(10):998–1007, 2002 12437940

Davis M, Ressler K, Rothbaum BO, et al: Effects of d-cycloserine on extinction: translation from preclinical to clinical work. Biol Psychiatry 60(4):369–375, 2006 16919524

de Kleine RA, Hendriks GJ, Kusters WJC, et al: A randomized placebo-controlled trial of d-cycloserine to enhance exposure therapy for posttraumatic stress disorder. Biol Psychiatry 71(11):962–968, 2012 22480663

Dell'osso B, Lader M: Do benzodiazepines still deserve a major role in the treatment of psychiatric disorders? A critical reappraisal. Eur Psychiatry 28(1):7–20, 2013 22521806

Difede J, Cukor J, Wyka K, et al: d-Cycloserine augmentation of exposure therapy for posttraumatic stress disorder: a pilot randomized clinical trial. Neuropsychopharmacology 39(5):1052–1058, 2014 24217129

Difede J, Rothbaum BO, Rizzo AS, et al: Enhancing exposure therapy for PTSD: virtual reality and imaginal exposure with a cognitive enhancer. Manuscript in preparation

Feeny NC, Mavissakalian M, Roy-Byrne PP, et al: Optimizing posttraumatic stress disorder treatment: prolonged exposure (PE) versus PE plus sertraline. Manuscript in preparation

Foa EB, Kozak MJ: Emotional processing of fear: exposure to corrective information. Psychol Bull 99(1):20–35, 1986 2871574

Foa EB, Franklin ME, Moser J: Context in the clinic: how well do cognitive-behavioral therapies and medications work in combination? Biol Psychiatry 52(10):987–997, 2002 12437939

Foa EB, Liebowitz MR, Kozak MJ, et al: Randomized, placebo-controlled trial of exposure and ritual prevention, clomipramine, and their combination in the treatment of obsessive-compulsive disorder. Am J Psychiatry 162(1):151–161, 2005 15625214

Foa EB, Huppert JD, Cahill SP: Emotional processing theory: an update, in Pathological Anxiety: Emotional Processing in Etiology and Treatment. Edited by Rothbaum BO. New York, Guilford, 2006, pp 3–24

Gingnell M, Frick A, Engman J, et al: Combining escitalopram and cognitive-behavioural therapy for social anxiety disorder: randomised controlled fMRI trial. Br J Psychiatry 209(3):229–235, 2016 27340112

Guastella AJ, Richardson R, Lovibond PF, et al: A randomized controlled trial of d-cycloserine enhancement of exposure therapy for social anxiety disorder. Biol Psychiatry 63(6):544–549, 2008 18179785

Haug TT, Blomhoff S, Hellstrøm K, et al: Exposure therapy and sertraline in social phobia: 1-year follow-up of a randomised controlled trial. Br J Psychiatry 182(4):312–318, 2003 12668406

Hien DA, Levin FR, Ruglass LM, et al: Combining seeking safety with sertraline for PTSD and alcohol use disorders: a randomized controlled trial. J Consult Clin Psychol 83(2):359, 2015

Hofmann SG, Meuret AE, Smits JA, et al: Augmentation of exposure therapy with d-cycloserine for social anxiety disorder. Arch Gen Psychiatry 63(3):298–304, 2006 16520435

Hofmann SG, Sawyer AT, Korte KJ, et al: Is it beneficial to add pharmacotherapy to cognitive-behavioral therapy when treating anxiety disorders? A meta-analytic review. Int J Cogn Ther 2(2):160–175, 2009 19714228

Hohagen F, Winkelmann G, Rashce-Rauchle H, et al: Combination of behavior therapy with fluvoxamine in comparison with behavior therapy and placebo: results of a multicentre study. Br J Psychiatry 173(S35):71–78, 1998

Hood SD, Nutt DJ: Psychopharmacological treatments: an overview, in International Handbook of Social Anxiety. Edited by Crozier WR, Alden LE. London, Wiley, 2001, pp 471–504

Kozel FA, Motes MA, Didehbani N, et al: Repetitive TMS to augment cognitive processing therapy in combat veterans of recent conflicts with PTSD: a randomized clinical trial. J Affect Disord 229:506–514, 2018 29351885

Kushner MG, Kim SW, Donahue C, et al: d-Cycloserine augmented exposure therapy for obsessive-compulsive disorder. Biol Psychiatry 62(8):835–838, 2007 17588545

Liebowitz MR, Allgulander C, Mangano R, et al: Comparison of venlafaxine-XR and paroxetine in the short-term treatment of SAD. Poster presented at the U.S. Psychiatric and Mental Health Congress, Orlando, FL, November 2003

Litz BT, Salters-Pedneault K, Steenkamp MM, et al: A randomized placebo-controlled trial of d-cycloserine and exposure therapy for posttraumatic stress disorder. J Psychiatr Res 46(9):1184–1190, 2012 22694905

Management of Posttraumatic Stress Disorder Work Group: VA/DOD Clinical Practice Guidelines for the Management of Posttraumatic Stress Disorder and Acute Stress Disorder. Washington, DC, Department of Veterans Affairs and Department of Defense, 2017

Maples-Keller JL, Jovanovic T, Dunlop BW, et al: When translational neuroscience fails in the clinic: dexamethasone prior to virtual reality exposure therapy increases drop-out rates. J Anxiety Disord 61:89–97, 2019 30502903

Marks IM, Swinson RP, Basoglu M, et al: Alprazolam and exposure alone and combined in panic disorder with agoraphobia. A controlled study in London and Toronto. Br J Psychiatry 162:776–787, 1993 8101126

Mataix-Cols D, De La Cruz LF, Monzani B, et al: d-Cycloserine augmentation of exposure-based cognitive behavior therapy for anxiety, obsessive-compulsive, and posttraumatic stress disorders: a systematic review and meta-analysis of individual participant data. JAMA Psychiatry 74:501–510, 2017

McHugh RK, Smits JAJ, Otto MW: Empirically supported treatments for panic disorder. Psychiatr Clin North Am 32(3):593–610, 2009 19716992

Mithoefer MC, Wagner MT, Mithoefer AT, et al: The safety and efficacy of ±3,4-methylenedioxy-methamphetamine-assisted psychotherapy in subjects with chronic, treatment-resistant posttraumatic stress disorder: the first randomized controlled pilot study. J Psychopharmacol 25(4):439–452, 2011 20643699

Mithoefer MC, Wagner MT, Mithoefer AT, et al: Durability of improvement in post-traumatic stress disorder symptoms and absence of harmful effects or drug dependency after 3,4-methylenedioxymethamphetamine-assisted psychotherapy: a prospective long-term follow-up study. J Psychopharmacol 27(1):28–39, 2013 23172889

Mithoefer MC, Mithoefer AT, Feduccia AA, et al: 3,4-methylenedioxymethamphetamine (MDMA)-assisted psychotherapy for post-traumatic stress disorder in military veterans, firefighters, and police officers: a randomised, double-blind, dose-response, phase 2 clinical trial. Lancet Psychiatry 5(6):486–497, 2018 29728331

Montero-Marin J, Garcia-Campayo J, López-Montoyo A, et al: Is cognitive-behavioural therapy more effective than relaxation therapy in the treatment of anxiety disorders? A meta-analysis. Psychol Med 48(9):1427–1436, 2018 29037266

Najavits L: Seeking Safety: A Treatment Manual for PTSD and Substance Abuse. New York, Guilford, 2002

Newcomer JW, Krystal JH: NMDA receptor regulation of memory and behavior in humans. Hippocampus 11(5):529–542, 2001 11732706

Nordahl HM, Vogel PA, Morken G, et al: Paroxetine, cognitive therapy or their combination in the treatment of social anxiety disorder with and without avoidant personality disorder: a randomized clinical trial. Psychother Psychosom 85(6):346–356, 2016 27744447

Oehen P, Traber R, Windmer V, et al: A randomized, controlled pilot study of MDMA (±3,4-methylenedioxymethamphetamine)-assisted psychotherapy for treatment of resistant, chronic post-traumatic stress disorder (PTSD). J Psychopharmacol 27(1):40–52, 2013 23118021

Otto MW, Smits JAJ, Reese HE: Combined psychotherapy and pharmacotherapy for mood and anxiety disorders in adults: review and analysis. Clin Psychol Sci Pract 12(1):72–86, 2005

Otto MW, Tolin DF, Simon NM, et al: Efficacy of d-cycloserine for enhancing response to cognitive-behavior therapy for panic disorder. Biol Psychiatry 67(4):365–370, 2010 19811776

Popiel A, Zawadzki B, Pragłowska E, et al: Prolonged exposure, paroxetine and the combination in the treatment of PTSD following a motor vehicle accident. A randomized clinical trial—The "TRAKT" study. J Behav Ther Exp Psychiatry 48:17–26, 2015 25677254

Power KG, Simpson RJ, Swanson V, et al: Controlled comparison of pharmacological and psychological treatment of generalized anxiety disorder in primary care. Br J Gen Pract 40(336):289–294, 1990 2081065

Powers MB, Halpern JM, Ferenschak MP, et al: A meta-analytic review of prolonged exposure for posttraumatic stress disorder. Clin Psychol Rev 30(6):635–641, 2010 20546985

Prasko J, Dockery C, Horacek J, et al: Moclobemide and cognitive behavioral therapy in the treatment of social phobia. A six-month controlled study and 24 months follow up. Neuro Endocrinol Lett 27(8):473–481, 2006 16891998

Rapee RM, Heimberg RG: A cognitive behavioral model of anxiety in social phobia. Behav Res Ther 35(8):741–756, 1997 9256517

Rauch SAM, Kim HM, Powell C, et al: Efficacy of prolonged exposure therapy, sertraline hydrochloride, and their combination among combat veterans with posttraumatic stress disorder: a randomized clinical trial. JAMA Psychiatry 76(2):117–126, 2019 30516797

Ressler KJ, Rothbaum BO, Tannenbaum L, et al: Cognitive enhancers as adjuncts to psychotherapy: use of d-cycloserine in phobic individuals to facilitate extinction of fear. Arch Gen Psychiatry 61(11):1136–1144, 2004 15520361

Rodrigues H, Figueira I, Lopes A, et al: Does d-cycloserine enhance exposure therapy for anxiety disorders in humans? A meta-analysis. PLoS One 9(7):e93519, 2014 24991926

Romanelli RJ, Wu FM, Gamba R, et al: Behavioral therapy and serotonin reuptake inhibitor pharmacotherapy in the treatment of obsessive-compulsive disorder: a systematic review and meta-analysis of head-to-head randomized controlled trials. Depress Anxiety 31(8):641–652, 2014 24390912

Rosenfield D, Hoffmann S, Mataix-Cols D, et al: Changes in dosing and dose timing of d-cycloserine explain its apparent declining efficacy for augmenting exposure therapy for anxiety-related disorders: an individual participant-data meta-analysis. J Anxiety Disord 2019 Epub ahead of print

Rothbaum BO, Cahill SP, Foa EB, et al: Augmentation of sertraline with prolonged exposure in the treatment of posttraumatic stress disorder. J Trauma Stress 19(5):625–638, 2006 17075912

Rothbaum BO, Foa EB, Hembree E: Reclaiming Your Life From a Traumatic Experience: Client Workbook. New York, Oxford University Press, 2007

Rothbaum BO, Price M, Jovanovic T, et al: A randomized, double-blind evaluation of d-cycloserine or alprazolam combined with virtual reality exposure therapy for posttraumatic stress disorder in Iraq and Afghanistan War veterans. Am J Psychiatry 171(6):640–648, 2014 24743802

Schneier FR, Neria Y, Pavlicova M, et al: Combined prolonged exposure therapy and paroxetine for PTSD related to the World Trade Center attack: a randomized controlled trial. Am J Psychiatry 169(1):80–88, 2012 21908494

Siegmund A, Golfels F, Finck C, et al: -Cycloserine does not improve but might slightly speed up the outcome of in-vivo exposure therapy in patients with severe agoraphobia and panic disorder in a randomized double blind clinical trial. J Psychiatr Res 45(8):1042–1047, 2011 21377691

Simon NM, Otto MW, Worthington JJ, et al: Next-step strategies for panic disorder refractory to initial pharmacotherapy: a 3-phase randomized clinical trial. J Clin Psychiatry 70(11):1563–1570, 2009 19814948

Simpson HB, Foa EB, Liebowitz MR, et al: A randomized, controlled trial of cognitive-behavioral therapy for augmenting pharmacotherapy in obsessive-compulsive disorder. Am J Psychiatry 165(5):621–630, 2008 18316422

Simpson HB, Foa EB, Liebowitz MR, et al: Cognitive-behavioral therapy vs risperidone for augmenting serotonin reuptake inhibitors in obsessive-compulsive disorder: a randomized clinical trial. JAMA Psychiatry 70(11):1190–1199, 2013 24026523

Storch EA, Merlo LJ, Bengtson M, et al: d-Cycloserine does not enhance exposure-response prevention therapy in obsessive-compulsive disorder. Int Clin Psychopharmacol 22(4):230–237, 2007 17519647

Tuerk PW, Wangelin BC, Powers MB, et al: Augmenting treatment efficiency in exposure therapy for PTSD: a randomized double-blind placebo-controlled trial of yohimbine HCl. Cogn Behav Ther 47(5):351–371, 2018 29448886

van Balkom AJ, de Haan E, van Oppen P, et al: Cognitive and behavioral therapies alone versus in combination with fluvoxamine in the treatment of obsessive compulsive disorder. J Nerv Ment Dis 186(8):492–499, 1998 9717867

Wilhelm S, Buhlmann U, Tolin D, et al: Augmentation of behavior therapy with d-cycloserine for obsessive-compulsive disorder. Paper presented at the 40th annual convention for the Association for Behavioral and Cognitive Therapies, Chicago, IL, November 2006

Yehuda R, Bierer LM, Pratchett LC, et al: Cortisol augmentation of a psychological treatment for warfighters with posttraumatic stress disorder: randomized trial showing improved treatment retention and outcome. Psychoneuroendocrinology 51:589–597, 2015 25212409

Zoellner LA, Telch M, Foa EB, et al: Enhancing extinction learning in posttraumatic stress disorder with brief daily imaginal exposure and methylene blue: a randomized controlled trial. J Clin Psychiatry78(7):e782–e789, 2017 28686823

Recommended Readings

Cuijpers P, Sijbrandij M, Koole SL, et al: Adding psychotherapy to antidepressant medication in depression and anxiety disorders: a meta-analysis. World Psychiatry 13(1):56–67, 2014 24497254

Hofmann SG, Sawyer AT, Korte KJ, et al: Is it beneficial to add pharmacotherapy to cognitive-behavioral therapy when treating anxiety disorders? A meta-analytic review. Int J Cogn Ther 2(2):160–175, 2009 19714228

Mataix-Cols D, De La Cruz LF, Monzani B, et al: d-Cycloserine augmentation of exposure-based cognitive behavior therapy for anxiety, obsessive-compulsive, and posttraumatic stress disorders: a systematic review and meta-analysis of individual participant data. JAMA Psychiatry 74:501–510, 2017

Montero-Marin J, Garcia-Campayo J, López-Montoyo A, et al: Is cognitive-behavioural therapy more effective than relaxation therapy in the treatment of anxiety disorders? A meta-analysis. Psychol Med 48(9):1427–1436, 2018 29037266

Otto MW, Smits JAJ, Reese HE: Combined psychotherapy and pharmacotherapy for mood and anxiety disorders in adults: review and analysis. Clin Psychol Sci Pract 12(1):72–86, 2005

CHAPTER 10

Core Principles in Pharmacotherapy of Anxiety Disorders

Valerie Rosen, M.D.
Charles B. Nemeroff, M.D., Ph.D.

The purpose of this chapter is to review the pharmacology of antianxiety agents. Because subsequent chapters deal with the treatment of individual anxiety syndromes, we review here agents with anxiolytic properties that cut across diagnostic categories and that by and large are FDA approved or have significant randomized controlled trial (RCT) data to support their use for the treatment of one or another anxiety disorder. These include benzodiazepines, buspirone and related compounds, selective serotonin reuptake inhibitors (SSRIs), the related serotonin-norepinephrine reuptake inhibitors (SNRIs), and antipsychotics.

The history of antianxiety agents is worthy of note. In comparison with animal models of depression, cognitive dysfunction, or schizophrenia, the animal screening tests for anxiolytic compounds such as the elevated plus maze have remarkable predictive value. This has been very helpful in the development of anxiolytic agents, although compounds that are effective after chronic but not after acute use are not always active in these tests. It is of paramount importance to note that several agents previously approved by the FDA and prescribed for the treatment of anxiety disorders are either no longer in our pharmacopoeia or are rarely used. These would include, for example, meprobamate, which was launched in the United States in 1955 and became the first blockbuster psychotropic drug in American history. By the mid-1960s, its abuse and dependence liability were recognized, as well as its low therapeutic index. It has been withdrawn from both the European and Canadian markets, and although still available in the United States, it is rarely prescribed because it is classified as a Schedule IV drug. Similarly, barbiturates possess clear antianxiety properties, but their lethality in overdose and other unfavorable side effects, including dependence liability, preclude their clinical utility for the treatment of anxiety disorders. Several drugs of abuse have well-documented anxiolytic properties, including alcohol and opiates, and this phenomenon undoubtedly underlies the common clinical presentation of patients with longstanding and severe anxiety who find themselves addicted to one of these agents in a futile attempt to treat their psychiatric disorder. Finally, several antipsychotic agents possess antianxiety properties. This was observed after the introduction of the typical antipsychotics, and low dosages of drugs such as thioridazine were often prescribed to patients with anxiety disorders. The emergence of tardive dyskinesia after chronic use of such agents quickly led to an end to this practice. However, second-generation antipsychotics with less likely side effect burden can be effective and safer for treatment-resistant anxiety disorders.

Antidepressants

Selective Serotonin Reuptake Inhibitors

SSRIs have demonstrated efficacy in all of the anxiety spectrum disorders as well as OCD and PTSD. SSRIs act primarily by increasing the synaptic concentrations of serotonin through inhibition of the presynaptic serotonin transporter (Table 10–1). However, this effect occurs immediately after administration, whereas the therapeutic effects are delayed for weeks. These drugs exert a myriad of other pharmacological effects that are beyond the scope of this chapter.

Side Effect Profile

Common initiation side effects for the first week or two include diarrhea, constipation, nausea, jitteriness, palpitations, sweating, and headaches. These may be similar to patients' anxiety symptoms and may lead to premature medication discontinuation before an effective dosage is reached (Ravindran and Stein 2010). Over time, sexual side effects, sleep disturbance, and weight gain are not uncommon and also often lead to treatment discontinuation. QTc prolongation is a rarer side effect; a meta-analysis (Beach et al. 2014) found SSRIs had a dose-dependent increase in QTc prolongation compared with placebo, with tricyclic antidepressants (TCAs) showing a significantly greater increase. Among SSRIs, citalopram had greater QTc increases than paroxetine, sertraline, and fluvoxamine. However, a large analysis of the Department of Veterans Affairs database revealed a very low rate of QTc prolongation with citalopram (Rector et al. 2016). Withdrawal symptoms upon discontinuation can be bothersome, particularly with paroxetine. However, careful, slow tapering or, when necessary, a change to a longer-acting SSRI while tapering can greatly mitigate these symptoms.

Advantages and Disadvantages

A large advantage of SSRIs is their efficacy in depression, which is a very common comorbidity with anxiety disorders. SSRIs have no addiction or abuse liability and therefore are deemed safe for patients with comorbid substance abuse or dependence. Disadvantages compared with benzodiazepines include longer onset of action and

TABLE 10–1.   **SSRIs and SNRIs with FDA indication for anxiety disorders**

Drug	FDA indications	Daily dosage range, *mg*	Half-life, *hours*	Protein binding	Metabolism
SSRIs					
Citalopram	None	20–40	24–48	80%	CYP3A4 and 2C19 (major) CYP2D6 (minor)
Escitalopram	GAD	10–20	27–32	56%	CYP2C19 and 3A4
Fluoxetine	OCD, PD	20–80	6 days; metabolite 4–16 days	95%	CYP2C19 and 2D6, to norfluoxetine
Fluvoxamine	OCD	50–300	14–16	80%	CYP1A2 and CYP2D6
Paroxetine	GAD, OCD, PD, PTSD, SAD	IR 10–60 CR 12.5–75	IR 21 CR 16–20	93%–95%	CYP2D6
Sertraline	OCD, PD, PTSD, SAD	50–200 PTSD≤250 OCD≤400	27.2	98%	CYP2C19 and CYP2D6
SNRIs					
Duloxetine	GAD	20–120	8–17	>90%	CYP1A2 (major) CYP2D6 (minor)
Venlafaxine	GAD, PD, SAD	XR 37.5–225 IR 37.5–375	IR 5±2 XR 10.7± 3.2	27%±2%	CYP2C19 (minor) CYP2C9 (minor) CYP2D6 (major) CYP3A4 (major)

Note.   CR=continuous release; GAD=generalized anxiety disorder; IR= immediate release; PD=panic disorder; SAD=social anxiety disorder; SNRI=serotonin-norepinephrine reuptake inhibitor; SSRI= selective serotonin reuptake inhibitor; XR=extended release.

sexual side effects (anorgasmia in women and delayed ejaculation in men). A recent meta-analysis by de Vries et al. (2016) indicated that the severity of anxiety disorders (mild, moderate, or severe) did not impact the efficacy of antidepressants, unlike recent findings in depression (Baumeister 2012) in which antidepressants were less efficacious in mild depression.

Serotonin-Norepinephrine Reuptake Inhibitors

SNRIs have demonstrated efficacy in anxiety disorders. Duloxetine has an FDA indication for generalized anxiety disorder (GAD), and venlafaxine has FDA indications for GAD, panic disorder, and social anxiety disorder (Table 10–1). A meta-analysis (Li et al. 2018) demonstrated that duloxetine improved symptoms of somatic and psychic anxiety and was well tolerated in the short-term treatment of GAD. Another meta-analysis (Li et al. 2017) examined 3,622 patients from 14 short-term randomized, double-blind, placebo-controlled trials who met DSM-IV criteria (American Psychiatric Association 1994) for GAD without other psychiatric or clinically serious medical

TABLE 10–2.   **TCAs with FDA indication for anxiety disorders**

Drug	FDA indication	Daily dosage range, mg	Half-life, hours	Protein binding	Metabolism
Clomipramine	OCD	150–300	15–60	97%	Primarily via CYP2D6, to some extent by CYP1A2
Doxepin	Anxiety	75–300	10–25	80%	CYP2C19 and CYP2D6, to a lesser extent by CYP1A2 and CYP2C9

Note. This table only includes FDA-approved TCAs; see text for TCAs with RCT efficacy data. RCT= randomized controlled trial; TCAs=tricyclic antidepressants.

conditions and found superior efficacy and tolerability for venlafaxine in the short-term treatment of GAD.

Both duloxetine and venlafaxine block serotonin reuptake at low dosages, and as the dosage is increased, norepinephrine reuptake blockade becomes increasingly more robust. Both share a similar side effect profile, with nausea, dizziness, dry mouth, headaches, and insomnia most commonly reported. Both can increase blood pressure and may confer a reduction in neuropathic pain.

Milnacipran is a dual-uptake inhibitor that shows preferential blockade of norepinephrine uptake over serotonin uptake (Vaishnavi et al. 2004). It acts very similarly to amitriptyline in terms of binding and uptake but has a more favorable side effect profile. It produces less nausea and less potential to increase anxiety compared with SSRIs. It has an elimination half-life of 8 hours, is not metabolized by cytochrome P450 isoenzymes but by phase II conjugation, and is renally excreted. Milnacipran is FDA approved for fibromyalgia but in a small open study (Tsukamoto et al. 2004) was effective in reducing the symptoms of GAD and was well tolerated. Levomilnacipran, approved by the FDA for treatment of major depression, has a similar pharmacological profile.

All of the SNRIs have side effects similar to SSRIs and can be associated with hypertension and withdrawal symptoms after acute cessation of treatment.

Tricyclic Antidepressants

The only TCAs that carry FDA indications for anxiety disorders are clomipramine (OCD) and doxepin (anxiety in general) (Table 10–2). Meta-analyses show larger effect sizes for clomipramine over SSRIs in the treatment of OCD, whereas head-to-head comparisons have shown equal efficacy (Fineberg and Gale 2005). Nortriptyline has been shown to be effective in panic disorder (Munjack et al. 1988), and imipramine has shown efficacy in treating agoraphobia (Zitrin et al. 1980). In fact, several RCTs have shown efficacy for this class of agents in panic and agoraphobia. Despite effectiveness in treating anxiety disorders, TCAs are considered a second-line treatment because SSRIs have a more favorable side effect profile and are safer in overdose.

TCAs block reuptake of norepinephrine and serotonin to varying degrees depending on the molecule. Thus, desipramine and nortriptyline are primarily norepinephrine reuptake inhibitors, whereas imipramine and amitriptyline inhibit both norepineph-

TABLE 10–3. **Affinity of selected antidepressants FDA indicated for anxiety disorders for neurotransmitter transporters/equilibrium dissociation constants**

Drug	Serotonin, *nM*	Norepinephrine, *nM*	Dopamine, *nM*
Citalopram	1.16	4,070	28,100
Clomipramine	0.28	38	2,190
Doxepin	68	29.5	12,100
Duloxetine	0.1	1.2	230
Fluoxetine	0.81	240	3,600
Fluvoxamine	2.2	1,300	9,200
Paroxetine	0.13	40	490
Sertraline	0.29	420	25
Venlafaxine	8.9	1,060	9,300

Source. Adapted from Tatsumi et al. 1997 and Vaishnavi et al. 2004.

rine and serotonin reuptake, especially at higher dosage ranges. Of the TCAs, clomipramine is the most potent and most selective inhibitor of serotonin (Table 10–3).

These first-generation antidepressants have considerable anticholinergic activity that may lead to dry mouth, tachycardia, constipation, urinary retention, confusion, and blurry vision. They can lead to ocular crisis in patients with narrow angle glaucoma. Orthostatic hypotension, QTc prolongation, and sedation are not uncommon and add to the less desirable side effect profile compared with SSRIs. TCAs are lethal in overdose and should therefore be used cautiously in patients with significant suicidal ideation. Monitoring blood levels can be helpful because therapeutic plasma levels have been established to avoid toxicity, to assess tolerability in the elderly, and to ensure lower initial levels when treating panic to avoid exacerbation of panic symptoms.

Monoamine Oxidase Inhibitors

Monoamine oxidase inhibitors (MAOIs) were first introduced as antidepressants in the 1950s and were also discovered to be effective in anxiety disorders. Irreversible MAOIs are estimated to have a response rate of 50%–60% for panic disorder (Schatzberg and Nemeroff 2017). Phenelzine, according to a National Institute for Health and Care Excellence (2013) study, was recommended for treatment-resistant social anxiety disorder in partial or nonresponders or those who declined SSRIs, SNRIs, individual cognitive-behavioral therapy (CBT), or a combination of these. Phenelzine is superior to placebo and, when combined with group CBT, was more efficacious than either alone in the acute treatment of social anxiety (Blanco et al. 2010). Phenelzine was more effective than placebo for panic disorder with agoraphobia (Sheehan et al. 1980). Despite their effectiveness, MAOIs are largely reserved for treatment-resistant depression and anxiety due to side effects, potential serious drug–drug interactions, and the lack of FDA indications for anxiety disorders.

MAOIs bind to monoamine oxidase, inhibiting its ability to deaminate neurotransmitters including serotonin, norepinephrine, and dopamine. In addition, after chronic treatment, MAOIs reduce the number of α_1 and α_2 adrenoceptors, β-adrenoceptors, and serotonin 5-HT$_1$ and 5-HT$_2$ receptors, similar to TCAs (DaPrada et al. 1989). In the United States, only irreversible MAOIs are on the pharmacopoeia, including phenelzine, tranylcypromine, and isocarboxazid. Moclobemide is a reversible inhibitor of monoamine oxidase A that is approved in Europe and Canada and shows promise for the treatment of anxiety disorders.

The limiting and potentially serious side effects of MAOIs are hypertensive crisis, which may occur when other sympathomimetic medications (stimulants, foods containing tyramine, anesthetics that contain epinephrine, and some decongestants) are combined with MAOIs, and serotonin syndrome due to combining them with other serotonergic agents (SSRIs, SNRIs, analgesics, or opiates that increase serotonin such as meperidine, tramadol, and methadone). However, these events are very rare and should not dissuade clinicians from prescribing these agents.

Benzodiazepines

In general, current practice guidelines suggest SSRIs and SNRIs as first-line treatment and benzodiazepines as second-line treatment for anxiety disorders. Several benzodiazepines are FDA indicated for anxiety disorders (Table 10–4). They often are prescribed as first-line by primary care providers (family physicians, internists, and nurse practitioners) and nonpsychiatric medical specialists, likely because of their quick onset of action. A well-intended desire to speed response may blind clinicians to the disadvantages of benzodiazepines, as discussed later, including a lack of efficacy in comorbid depression, more addictive liability, and possible dampening of psychotherapy treatment responses.

Benzodiazepines target anxiety by acting on the GABA$_A$ receptor complex. This complex mediates several actions of benzodiazepines, including their anxiolytic, muscle relaxant, sedative, and anticonvulsant effects. The α_2 and α_3 subunits of the GABA$_A$ receptor mediate the anxiolytic effects, while the α_1 subunit is responsible for the hypnotic effects (Schatzberg and Nemeroff 2017). Despite multiple attempts to develop subunit-specific benzodiazepine agonists with anxiolytic effects but without sedative or abuse liability, no such agents have been forthcoming.

Advantages and Disadvantages of Benzodiazepines

A major advantage of benzodiazepines is their quicker onset of action: same day, rather than the weeks required for antidepressants. However, an immediate response may also discourage patients from engaging in psychotherapy or attempting coping skills that may ultimately provide them more control over their symptoms. Choosing not to develop behavioral skills may increase the risk of medication dependence, even if only a psychological one. If benzodiazepines are used during CBT, especially in exposure and extinction learning, their numbing effect interferes with the critical component of experiencing and learning to tolerate distress. Most treatment guidelines for PTSD describe benzodiazepines as contraindicated or ineffective for core PTSD symptoms, and RCTs support this recommendation. In PTSD, trauma-focused psychotherapies, now considered to be first-line according to the 2017 U.S. Department of

TABLE 10–4. Benzodiazepines with FDA indications for anxiety disorders

Drug	FDA indications	Half-life, *hours*	Daily dosage range	Protein binding	Metabolism	K_i, *nM*
Alprazolam	Generalized anxiety disorder, panic disorder	IR 6.3–26.9 XR 10.7–15.8	IR 0.25–4 mg, divided tid XR 0.5–4 mg qd	80%	CYP3A4	4.8
Clorazepate	Anxiety	40–50	7.5–60 mg	97%–98%	Metabolized to oxazepam	NA
Chlordiazepoxide	Anxiety	24–48	5–100 mg	96%	CYP3A4	NA
Clonazepam	Panic disorder	24–56	0.25–4 mg	80%	CYP3A4	0.5
Diazepam	Anxiety	26–50	2–40 mg	98%	CYP2C19, 3A4	9.6
Lorazepam	Anxiety	10–20	1–10 mg	91%	Glucuronidation	3.8
Oxazepam	Anxiety	5–15	10–120 mg	96%–98%	Glucuronidation	17.2
Midazolam	Anxiety (use not recommended)	1–3	0.05–0.2 mg/kg IV	40%–50%	CYP3A4	0.4

Note. IR=immediate release; K_i=kinetic inhibition constant value; XR=extended release.
Source. Adapted from Sheehan DV: "Benzodiazepines," in *The American Psychiatric Association Publishing Textbook of Psychopharmacology*, 5th Edition. Edited by Schatzberg A, Nemeroff C. Washington, DC, American Psychiatric Association Publishing, 2017, p. 566. Copyright © 2017 American Psychiatric Association Publishing. Used with permission.

Veterans Affairs and Department of Defense clinical practice guidelines (Management of Posttraumatic Stress Disorder Work Group 2017), often include exposure to trauma-related emotions to support symptom reduction. The numbing effect of benzodiazepines may be one aspect that presents a barrier to emotional processing, because benzodiazepines can interfere with extinction learning. They may suppress the prefrontal cortex, which is required for cognitive flexibility in trauma recovery and is already hypofunctional in PTSD (Guina et al. 2015; Shalev et al. 1998).

Other advantages of benzodiazepines include muscle relaxant qualities that can reduce anxiety-related muscle tension. Their hypnotic effects can also be beneficial for anxiety-related insomnia. If a patient has mild anxiety and refuses recommendations for a daily medication regimen, benzodiazepines prescribed on an as-needed basis may be appropriate. Disadvantages include rebound anxiety and, particularly with the short-half-life agents, possible withdrawal or discontinuation symptoms, including seizure risk if abruptly stopped. However, slow titration can help minimize or avert such side effects. Several tapering recommendations exist, from no greater than a 25% reduction of dosage per week to a 10% reduction over 1–2 weeks. Switching to a longer-acting benzodiazepine for taper is a common strategy. Several medications, including SSRIs, SNRIs, buspirone, pregabalin, carbamazepine, and flumazenil, have been prescribed to reduce withdrawal symptoms during benzodiazepine tapers with varying success (Lader and Kyriacou 2016). No definitive consensus has been found for tapering guidelines; therefore, close monitoring of a patient's withdrawal symptoms is paramount in determining speed and length of tapering.

The risk of cognitive impairment is a downside that can manifest on a spectrum from lack of mental clarity to significant memory or psychomotor impairment. This is a serious problem in elderly patients, and recent studies suggest a possible connection to longer-term cognitive impairment, including dementia. In a case-control study in Quebec, Billioti de Gage et al. (2014) found the development of Alzheimer's disease was much more common in patients with more than 180 prescribed daily doses of benzodiazepines. The authors reported benzodiazepine use to be significantly associated with an increased risk of Alzheimer's disease, stronger for longer-acting than for shorter-acting agents. These results are controversial; others (Salzman and Shader 2015) have suggested that patients who develop Alzheimer's disease may have a prodromal syndrome characterized by anxiety or insomnia that responds well to benzodiazepines. Indeed, depression and anxiety syndromes themselves are risk factors for Alzheimer's disease (Burke et al. 2016). Moreover, other possible causal variables may play an important role, including alcohol or anticholinergic medication use. Salzman and Shader (2015) suggested the use of shorter-acting benzodiazepines in the elderly population. In a prospective study, Shash et al. (2016) found longer-acting benzodiazepine users had a 60% increased risk of developing dementia when variables such as anxiety, depression, and insomnia were controlled, but they found no direct causal link between benzodiazepine use and Alzheimer's disease. In addition, in another prospective study, Gray et al. (2016) found no link between Alzheimer's disease and the highest level of benzodiazepine use; however, those with lower levels of use had a small increase in risk of dementia. Shorter-acting benzodiazepines have less risk of cognitive impairment and sedation than longer-acting ones but unfortunately have more potential for abuse liability.

Addiction Liability

The risk of addiction varies widely for different patients; tolerance and dependency are not unsubstantial risks. Because of this potential, benzodiazepines should not be prescribed as first-line therapy for anxiety in patients with a current or past history of substance addiction. To avoid long-term dependence issues in lower-risk patients, benzodiazepines can be prescribed as a "bridge" until an antidepressant begins to take effect in the first 4–6 weeks of treatment. The benzodiazepine is then discontinued for SSRI/SNRI monotherapy. A recent meta-analysis (Gomez et al. 2018) showed benzodiazepines may be more efficacious than antidepressants for GAD, yielding a larger effect size (0.50) compared with SSRIs (0.34). Many patients with anxiety disorders such as GAD and social anxiety disorder receive a remarkable benefit from chronic treatment with low-dose benzodiazepines, usually long-acting agents such as clonazepam. Such patients rarely require an increase in dosage and do not go on to develop addiction.

In terms of drug–drug interactions, benzodiazepines should be used with caution in combination with medications that are also sedating because of the risk of respiratory depression. Medications that inhibit oxidation in the liver may alter or worsen benzodiazepine side effects because many are metabolized by oxidation. Hepatic enzyme inducers such as carbamazepine, phenytoin, phenobarbital, and rifampin may decrease the concentration and effectiveness of benzodiazepines. CYP3A4 inhibitors such as nefazodone, fluvoxamine, fluoxetine, erythromycin, diltiazem, and ritonavir may increase benzodiazepine concentrations, and a dosage reduction may be warranted. If such drugs must be used, or if liver impairment exists or is a presumed possibility, lorazepam, oxazepam, and temazepam should be chosen because they are metabolized by conjugation, not by oxidative pathways in the liver. In elderly patients, because of reduced liver function, a 50% decline in clearance resulted in a four- to ninefold increase in the half-lives of diazepam and chlordiazepoxide (Peppers 1996; Perry 2014), providing another reason to avoid their use in this population.

Buspirone

Buspirone is FDA approved for the treatment of GAD (Table 10–5). Buspirone is a full agonist at presynaptic 5-HT$_{1A}$ receptors in the dorsal raphe and a partial agonist at postsynaptic 5-HT$_{1A}$ receptors in the hippocampus and cortex (Eison and Eison 1994; Yocca 1990).

A Cochrane review from 2014 found buspirone to be less effective than placebo for panic disorder, but this review was limited by small sample sizes (Imai et al. 2014). DeMartinis et al. (2000) and Rickels and Schweizer (1990) found buspirone to be less effective for GAD in patients with previous recent exposure to benzodiazepines. Those with remote or no benzodiazepine exposure had more positive treatment results with buspirone, comparable to monotherapy benzodiazepine use. Recent prior use did not decrease outcomes for subsequent use—indicating prior use was not necessarily indicative of worse anxiety and treatment resistance in general. Some patients might experience benzodiazepine withdrawal worsened by buspirone because its metabolite has noradrenergic activity that may exacerbate withdrawal symptoms (Eng-

TABLE 10–5.   **Buspirone and selected alternate agents for the treatment of anxiety disorders**

Drug	FDA indication	Half-life, hours	Dosage range, mg	Metabolism
Buspirone	Generalized anxiety disorder	2–4	15–60 qd	CYP3A4
Gepirone	None	2–3	20 qd	CYP3A4
Gabapentin	None	5–7	IR 300–3,600 tid XR 300–1,800 qd	No hepatic metabolism
Pregabalin	None	IR 0.7–1.5 XR 5–12	IR up to 600 qd in divided doses XR up to 660 qd	Negligible hepatic metabolism
Hydroxyzine	Short-term treatment of anxiety	20–25	25–100 qid	CYP3A4

Note.   IR=immediate release; XR=extended release.

berg 1989; Giral et al. 1987; Lydiard 2000). Because patients grow accustomed to the rapid onset and sedative effects of benzodiazepines, explaining before starting buspirone that the reduction in anxiety will not feel the same may help set expectations. A recent Cochrane analysis confirmed that buspirone is less effective for the treatment of GAD in patients who had prior benzodiazepine treatment (Chessick et al. 2006).

The most common reported side effects include dizziness, lightheadedness, nausea, and nervousness. Buspirone is generally well tolerated and does not typically cause significant sedation or psychomotor impairment. It can be prescribed without concern for abuse, dependence, and withdrawal. Doses typically start at 7.5 mg twice a day and can be increased by 5 mg every 2–3 days, with a maximum recommended daily dosage of 60 mg. It is administered in multiple daily doses because of its short elimination half-life of 2–4 hours. It is metabolized by the liver and renally excreted. If hepatic or renal impairment is present, lower dosages are recommended. Evidence indicates that at higher dosages (90 mg/day) buspirone possesses antidepressant properties (Robinson et al. 1990).

Due to the risk of serotonin syndrome, buspirone is said to be contraindicated for use with MAOIs and cautioned if prescribed with SSRIs or SNRIs. Because it is metabolized by CYP3A4, any drug that inhibits 3A4 will lead to increased concentrations and inducers of 3A4 will reduce concentrations. It has few other significant drug–drug interactions.

Gepirone, an analogue of buspirone, is similarly a 5-HT_{1A} receptor partial agonist. Gepirone has a half-life of 2–3 hours and is metabolized via CYP3A4. For anxiety, it has been dosed at 20 mg/day. The extended-release version was found to be effective in anxious depression, with side effects of dizziness, nausea, and insomnia, and was similar to placebo in terms of weight gain and sexual side effects (Alpert et al. 2004). It has never been approved by the FDA (see Table 10–5).

Antipsychotics

Perhaps surprising to many, prochlorperazine has an FDA indication for nonpsychotic anxiety, and trifluperazine, 1–6 mg/day, is FDA approved for the short-term treatment of GAD, limited to 12 weeks or less because of risk of tardive dyskinesia with longer use. They are rarely prescribed because they carry a less favorable side effect profile than many other agents that have shown efficacy in treating anxiety. No other antipsychotics carry an FDA indication for anxiety disorders. However, studies have shown efficacy of second-generation antipsychotics for anxiety. Antipsychotics are believed to exert their anxiolytic effects as agonists at the $5\text{-}HT_{1A}$ receptor; in addition, histamine, $5\text{-}HT_2$, and dopamine D_2 receptor antagonism may also play a role. In a 2011 Cochrane review (Depping et al. 2010), seven RCTs evaluated the antipsychotics olanzapine, quetiapine, and risperidone in the treatment of GAD and social phobia. Quetiapine performed better than placebo for GAD but resulted in more dropouts due to metabolic side effects, extrapyramidal side effects, or sedation. The authors found no difference in efficacy between quetiapine and antidepressants, but quetiapine again incurred more dropouts. Olanzapine was without efficacy, and risperidone was not effective as an adjunctive medication.

Alternate Agents

Gabapentin

Gabapentin modulates calcium availability, acting at the $\alpha_2\delta$ subunit of voltage-gated calcium channels. Gabapentin is excreted unchanged in the urine and should be used with caution in renal impairment (see Table 10–5). It is generally well tolerated, with the most common side effects being dizziness and drowsiness and less common effects being blurry vision and peripheral edema. A small number of reports, mostly in patients with a history of substance abuse, have linked abuse liability to gabapentin; therefore, being mindful of repeated early refill requests is recommended. Conflicting reports exist on gabapentin as an efficacious treatment for alcohol withdrawal, but it has shown efficacy in associated sleep disturbances (Schatzberg and Nemeroff 2017). Evidence has shown that at higher doses gabapentin may be efficacious in reducing alcohol cravings.

Few RCTs of gabapentin use for the treatment of anxiety have been published. Gabapentin has been shown to reduce the symptoms of social phobia compared with placebo (Pande et al. 1999). Onder et al. (2008) demonstrated in a small RCT that adjunctive gabapentin may enhance the response to fluoxetine in patients with OCD. Pollack et al. (1998) demonstrated efficacy for gabapentin in two patient cases of social anxiety disorder and two cases of GAD. In a recent case report by Markota and Morgan (2017), a detailed description of gabapentin dose response effects on GAD symptoms demonstrated improvement and a reduction in benzodiazepine use. Despite a lack of robust evidence in the literature, gabapentin is used often in clinical practice because of its tolerability and anecdotal success for anxiety.

Pregabalin

Pregabalin modulates calcium similarly to gabapentin. It demonstrated clear efficacy in RCTs of GAD (Baldwin et al. 2013). Sleep disorders, which are common in patients with anxiety disorders, may improve earlier with pregabalin than with the SSRIs or SNRIs because pregabalin has sedating properties. Onset of efficacy is earlier with pregabalin than with antidepressants, and it is not subject to hepatic metabolism and hence does not interact with inhibitors or inducers of cytochrome P450 enzymes. Concerns have been raised about the abuse liability of pregabalin in individuals with substance abuse, and withdrawal syndromes have occurred after abrupt discontinuation (see Table 10–5).

Hydroxyzine

Although hydroxyzine does not have an FDA indication for anxiety disorders, it is often used as an as-needed medication because it confers no abuse or addiction potential and is relatively well tolerated. Hydroxyzine acts by blocking histamine and muscarinic receptors. Its main side effects include sedation or dry mouth. Hydroxyzine was shown to be superior to placebo in three RCTs for GAD (Ferreri and Hantouche 1998; Lader and Scotto 1998; Llorca et al. 2002). In Europe, it is restricted to 100 mg/day because of reports of ventricular arrhythmias (European Medicines Agency 2015; Schatzberg and Nemeroff 2017) (see Table 10–5).

Other Agents

Space constraints preclude discussion of novel agents, including ketamine, corticotropin-releasing hormone receptor antagonists, neurosteroid agonists such as brexanolone, glucocorticoid receptor antagonists such as mifepristone, and various compounds that purportedly act on opiate receptor subtypes. These and other novel treatments hold promise for future interventions. For a brief summary of the current most commonly utilized or studied medications for anxiety, see Table 10–6.

Treatment-Resistant Anxiety

Many comorbid psychiatric disorders can masquerade as an anxiety disorder. Significant overlap of symptoms often occurs among the major categories of psychiatric illness. For example, ADHD can lead to severe anxiety because of the inability to focus and complete tasks. Agitated mania or hypomania may be interpreted and described by the patient as anxiety; caution here is warranted because antidepressants, which are a first-line treatment for anxiety, have the propensity to worsen hypomania and induce rapid cycling. PTSD is the great mimicker and can look like virtually any other psychiatric disorder. Careful diagnosis is paramount, because if a practitioner is unaware of the root cause, an antianxiety medication may not address the core issue and symptoms may be erroneously labeled as "treatment resistant."

The literature is remarkably sparse and conflicting in terms of pharmacological treatment strategies for treatment-resistant anxiety disorders. In treatment-resistant OCD, up to 60% of patients do not respond to SSRI monotherapy. Because SSRIs are

TABLE 10–6.   **Pros and cons of the most commonly used and studied medication classes in the treatment of anxiety disorders**

Drug class	Pros	Cons
Selective serotonin reuptake inhibitors/serotonin-norepinephrine reuptake inhibitors	Safety profile, general tolerability, efficacy in comorbid depression	Longer onset of action, sexual side effects
Tricyclic antidepressants and monoamine oxidase inhibitors	Efficacy in comorbid depression	Poorer safety profile, less favorable side effect profile, more drug–drug interactions, may require additional burden of blood levels
Benzodiazepines	Speed of onset of action, patients may prefer as-needed dosing	Lack of efficacy in comorbid depression, addictive liability, cognitive impairment, discontinuation risk, drug–drug interactions, dampening of psychotherapy treatment responses

more easily tolerated and perhaps as effective as clomipramine, augmenting them with atypical antipsychotics often is warranted (Pallanti and Quercioli 2006). A 2015 meta-analysis (Dold et al. 2015) composed of 14 double-blind RCTs with a total of 491 participants found significant efficacy for adding antipsychotic drugs to SSRIs in treatment-resistant OCD. Aripiprazole, haloperidol, and risperidone were more efficacious than placebo, whereas olanzapine, paliperidone, and quetiapine were not. Ipser et al. (2006) reported similar results; 20 of 28 RCTs of treatment-resistant OCD demonstrated augmentation with antipsychotics and found they were beneficial for nonresponders of first-line pharmacological treatment. No difference in dropout rates was found between control and augmentation groups, and surprisingly, no additional side effect burden was found with augmentation. In contrast, Patterson and Van Ameringen (2016) completed a meta-analysis and found six placebo-controlled RCTs for treatment-resistant anxiety disorders that included three for GAD, one for social anxiety disorder, and two for panic disorder. For augmentation strategies, three involved atypical antipsychotics, two involved benzodiazepines, and one involved pregabalin. The authors reported a small reduction in symptoms for all six studies and no change in functional impairment, and they concluded that, overall, augmentation did not appear to be beneficial. This meta-analysis was limited by the small number of studies, partly due to the rigor of their inclusion criteria and the small sample sizes within the studies themselves. The authors also argued that GAD, social anxiety disorder, and panic disorder have high rates of placebo response, especially when compared with OCD, which may account for less of a difference with placebo. This may help explain why studies of treatment-resistant OCD have been more promising.

Conclusion

According to ClinCalc.com (2019), a website that calculates the Top 200 prescribed drugs annually, sertraline was the fourteenth most prescribed medication, with

37,105,238 prescriptions. Fluoxetine was twenty-ninth, citalopram twenty-first, escitalopram twenty-sixth, and paroxetine, duloxetine, venlafaxine, and amitriptyline were all in the top 100. Benzodiazepines were heavily represented; alprazolam was nineteenth with more than 27 million prescriptions, clonazepam was forty-second, and lorazepam was fifty-seventh. According to Grohol (2018), 11 of the top 25 most prescribed psychiatric medications in the United States for 2016 were antidepressants. Their research showed that more than 338 million prescriptions were written for antidepressants—enough for one for every man, woman, and child in the United States (total 2016 U.S. population 323.4 million). Sertraline was the number one prescribed psychotropic, alprazolam was the second-most prescribed, and lorazepam came in ninth. These statistics may be indicative of more people feeling comfortable seeking help for anxiety disorders, more lax prescribing, higher prevalence rates of anxiety due to societal stressors, or underutilization or unavailability of evidence-based psychosocial interventions. Regardless, these facts highlight the growing importance of careful diagnosis and evaluation to ensure such a large number of patients are being exposed to medications that are both necessary and beneficial for their symptoms.

Key Points

- Selective serotonin reuptake inhibitors (SSRIs) and serotonin-norepinephrine reuptake inhibitors (SNRIs) remain first-line pharmacological treatments for anxiety disorders despite multiple classes demonstrating strong efficacy.

- SSRIs, SNRIs, tricyclic antidepressants, and benzodiazepines remain the most commonly used classes of drugs for the treatment of anxiety disorders (see Table 10–6 for pros and cons).

- Some novel and adjunctive agents also may be helpful, particularly in the setting of lack of response to first-line interventions; however, more research is needed.

- Careful and accurate diagnosis is paramount to ensure patients receive the optimal treatment, with close consideration of patient preference for psychotherapy and medication options.

- Treatment selection should consider the needs of special populations, such as children, elderly patients, and those with co-occurring medical or substance use disorders, and patients' prior treatment tolerability and responses.

References

Alpert JE, Franznick DA, Hollander SB, et al: Gepirone extended-release treatment of anxious depression: evidence from a retrospective subgroup analysis in patients with major depressive disorder. J Clin Psychiatry 65(8):1069–1075, 2004 15323591

American Psychiatric Association: Diagnostic and Statistical Manual of Mental Disorders, 4th Edition. Washington, DC, American Psychiatric Association, 1994

Baldwin DS, Ajel K, Masdrakis V, et al: Pregabalin for the treatment of generalized anxiety disorder: an update. Neuropsychiatr Dis Treat 9:883–892, 2013 23836974

Baumeister H: Inappropriate prescriptions of antidepressant drugs in patients with subthreshold to mild depression: time for the evidence to become practice. J Affect Disord 139(3):240–243, 2012 21652081

Beach SR, Kostis WJ, Celano CM, et al: Meta-analysis of selective serotonin reuptake inhibitor-associated QTc prolongation. J Clin Psychiatry 75(5):e441–e449, 2014 24922496

Billioti de Gage S, Moride Y, Ducruet T, et al: Benzodiazepine use and risk of Alzheimer's disease: case-control study. BMJ 349:g5205, 2014 25208536

Blanco C, Heimberg RG, Schneier FR, et al: A placebo-controlled trial of phenelzine, cognitive behavioral group therapy and their combination for social anxiety disorder. Arch Gen Psychiatry 67(3):286–295, 2010 20194829

Burke SL, Maramaldi P, Cadet T, Kukull W: Associations between depression, sleep disturbance and apolipoprotein E in the development of Alzheimer's disease: dementia. Int Psychogeriatr 28(9):1409–1424, 2016 27020605

Chessick CA, Allen MH, Thase M, et al: Azapirones for generalized anxiety disorder. Cochrane Database Syst Rev (3):CD006115, 2006 16856115

ClinCalc.com: ClinCalc DrugStats Database, Version 19.0: The Top 200 of 2019. ClinCalc, August 2019. Available at: https://clincalc.com/DrugStats/Top200Drugs.aspx. Accessed June 14, 2019.

DaPrada M, Kettler R, Keller HH, et al: Neurochemical profile of moclobemide, a short-acting and reversible inhibitor of monoamine oxidase type A. J Pharmacol Exp Ther 248(1):400–414, 1989 2783611

de Vries YA, de Jonge P, van den Heuvel E, et al: Influence of baseline severity on antidepressant efficacy for anxiety disorders: meta-analysis and meta-regression. Br J Psychiatry 208(6):515–521, 2016 26989093

DeMartinis N, Runn M, Rickels K, et al: Prior benzodiazepine use and buspirone responses in the treatment of generalized anxiety disorder. J Clin Psychiatry 61(2):91–94, 2000 10732655

Depping AM, Komossa K, Kissling W, et al: Second-generation antipsychotics for anxiety disorders. Cochrane Database Syst Rev (12):CD008120, 2010 21154392

Dold M, Aigner M, Lanzenberger R, et al: Antipsychotic augmentation of serotonin reuptake inhibitors in treatment-resistant obsessive-compulsive disorder: an update meta-analysis of double-blind, randomized, placebo-controlled trials. Int J Neuropsychopharmacol 18(9):pyv047, 2015 25939614

Eison AS, Eison MS: Serotonergic mechanisms in anxiety. Prog Neuropsychopharmacol Biol Psychiatry 18(1):47–62, 1994 8115673

Engberg G: A metabolite of buspirone increases locus coeruleus activity via alpha 2-receptor blockade. J Neural Transm (Vienna) 76(2):91–98, 1989 2565361

European Medicines Agency: New Restrictions to Minimize the Risks of Effects on Heart Rhythm With Hydroxyzine-Containing Medicines (press release), March 27, 2015. Available at: https://www.ema.europa.eu/en/documents/referral/hydroxyzine-article-31-referral-new-restrictions-minimise-risks-effects-heart-rhythm-hydroxyzine_en.pdf. Accessed June 14, 2019.

Ferreri M, Hantouche EG: Recent clinical trials of hydroxyzine in generalized anxiety disorder. Acta Psychiatr Scand Suppl 393:102–108, 1998 9777055

Fineberg NA, Gale TM: Evidence-based pharmacotherapy of obsessive-compulsive disorder. Int J Neuropsychopharmacol 8(1):107–129, 2005 15450126

Giral P, Soubrie P, Puech AJ: Pharmacological evidence for the involvement of 1-(2-pyridinyl)-piperazine (1-PmP) in the interaction of buspirone or gepirone with noradrenergic systems. Eur J Pharmacol 134(1):113–116, 1987 2881793

Gomez AF, Barthel AL, Hofmann SG: Comparing the efficacy of benzodiazepines and serotonergic anti-depressants for adults with generalized anxiety disorder: a meta-analytic review. Expert Opin Pharmacother 19(8):883–894, 2018 1472767

Gray SL, Dublin S, Yu O, et al: Benzodiazepine use and risk of incident dementia or cognitive decline: prospective population based study. BMJ 352:i90, 2016 26837813

Grohol JM: Top 25 Psychiatric Medications for 2016. PsychCentral, July 8, 2018. Available at: https://psychcentral.com/blog/top-25-psychiatric-medications-for-2016. Accessed November 8, 2018.

Guina J, Rossetter SR, DeRhodes BJ, et al: Benzodiazepines for PTSD: a systematic review and meta-analysis. J Psychiatr Pract 21(4):281–303, 2015 26164054

Imai H, Tajika A, Chen P, et al: Azapirones versus placebo for panic disorder in adults. Cochrane Database Syst Rev (9):CD010828, 2014 25268297

Ipser JC, Carey P, Dhansay Y, et al: Pharmacotherapy augmentation strategies in treatment-resistant anxiety disorders. Cochrane Database Syst Rev (4):CD005473, 2006 17054260

Lader M, Kyriacou A: Withdrawing benzodiazepines in patients with anxiety disorders. Curr Psychiatry Rep 18(1):8, 2016 26733324

Lader M, Scotto JC: A multicentre double-blind comparison of hydroxyzine, buspirone and placebo in patients with generalized anxiety disorder. Psychopharmacology (Berl) 139(4):402–406, 1998 9809861

Li X, Zhu L, Su Y, et al: Short-term efficacy and tolerability of venlafaxine extended release in adults with generalized anxiety disorder without depression: a meta-analysis. PLoS One 12(10):e0185865, 2017 28982121

Li X, Zhu L, Zhou C, et al: Efficacy and tolerability of short-term duloxetine treatment in adults with generalized anxiety disorder: a meta-analysis. PLoS One 13(3):e0194501, 2018 29558528

Llorca PM, Spadone C, Sol O, et al: Efficacy and safety of hydroxyzine in the treatment of generalized anxiety disorder: a 3-month double-blind study. J Clin Psychiatry 63(11):1020–1027, 2002 12444816

Lydiard RB: An overview of generalized anxiety disorder: disease state–appropriate therapy. Clin Ther 22(suppl A):A3–A19, 2000 10815647

Management of Posttraumatic Stress Disorder Work Group: Clinical Practice Guideline for the Management of Posttraumatic Stress Disorder and Acute Stress Disorder. Washington, DC, Department of Veterans Affairs and Department of Defense, 2017. Available at: https://www.healthquality.va.gov/guidelines/MH/ptsd/VADoDPTSDCPGFinal.pdf. Accessed June 14, 2019.

Markota M, Morgan RJ: Treatment of generalized anxiety disorder with gabapentin. Case Rep Psychiatry 2017:6045017, 2017 29387502

Munjack DJ, Usigli R, Zulueta A, et al: Nortriptyline in the treatment of panic disorder and agoraphobia with panic attacks. J Clin Psychopharmacol 8(3):204–207, 1988 3379145

National Institute for Health and Care Excellence: Social Anxiety Disorder: Recognition, Assessment and Treatment (Clinical Guideline [CG159]). London, NICE, May 2013. Available at: https://www.nice.org.uk/guidance/cg159. Accessed June 14, 2019.

Onder E, Tural U, Gokbakan M: Does gabapentin lead to early symptom improvement in obsessive-compulsive disorder? Eur Arch Psychiatry Clin Neurosci 258(6):319–323, 2008 18297416

Pallanti S, Quercioli L: Treatment-refractory obsessive-compulsive disorder: methodological issues, operational definitions and therapeutic lines. Prog Neuropsychopharmacol Biol Psychiatry 30(3):400–412, 2006 16503369

Pande AC, Davidson JR, Jefferson JW et al: Treatment of social phobia with gabapentin: a placebo-controlled study. J Clin Psychopharmacol 19(4):341–348, 1999 10440462

Patterson B, Van Ameringen M: Augmentation strategies for treatment-resistant anxiety disorders: a systematic review and meta-analysis. Depress Anxiety 33(8):728–736, 2016 27175543

Peppers MP: Benzodiazepines for alcohol withdrawal in the elderly and in patients with liver disease. Pharmacotherapy 16(1):49–57, 1996 8700792

Perry EC: Inpatient management of acute alcohol withdrawal syndrome. CNS Drugs 28(5):401–410, 2014 24781751

Pollack, MH, Matthews J, Scott EL: Gabapentin as a potential treatment for anxiety disorders. Am J Psychiatry 155(7):992–993, 1998 9659873

Ravindran LN, Stein MB: The pharmacologic treatment of anxiety disorders. J Clin Psychiatry 71(7):839–854, 2010 20667290

Rector TS, Adabag S, Cunningham F, et al: Outcomes of citalopram dosage risk mitigation in a veteran population. Am J Psychiatry 173(9):896–902, 2016 27166093

Rickels K, Schweizer E: The clinical course and long-term management of generalized anxiety disorder. J Clin Psychopharmacol 10(3 suppl):101S–110S, 1990 1973934

Robinson DS, Rickels K, Feighner J, et al: Clinical effects of the 5-HT1A partial agonists in depression: a composite analysis of buspirone in the treatment of depression. J Clin Psychopharmacol 10(3 suppl):67S–76S, 1990 2198303

Salzman C, Shader RI: Benzodiazepine use and risk for Alzheimer disease. J Clin Psychopharmacol 35(1):1–3, 2015 25407694

Schatzberg A, Nemeroff C (eds): The American Psychiatric Association Publishing Textbook of Psychopharmacology, 5th Edition. Washington, DC, American Psychiatric Association Publishing, 2017

Shalev AY, Bloch M, Peri T, et al: Alprazolam reduces response to loud tones in panic disorder but not in posttraumatic stress disorder. Biol Psychiatry 44(1):64–68, 1998 9646885

Shash D, Kurth T, Bertrand M et al: Benzodiazepine, psychotropic medication, and dementia: a population-based cohort study. Alzheimers Dement 12(5):604–613, 2016 26602630

Sheehan DV, Ballenger J, Jacobsen G: Treatment of endogenous anxiety with phobic, hysterical, and hypochondriacal symptoms. Arch Gen Psychiatry 37(1):51–59, 1980 7352840

Tatsumi M, Groshan K, Blakely RD, et al: Pharmacological profile of antidepressants and related compounds at human monoamine transporters. Eur J Pharmacol 340(2–3):249–258, 1997 9537821

Tsukamoto T, Kondoh R, Ichikawa K: Efficacy and safety of milnacipran in the treatment of generalized anxiety disorder: an open study. Int J Psychiatry Clin Pract 8(4):255–258, 2004 24930555

Vaishnavi SN, Nemeroff CB, Plott SJ, et al: Milnacipran: a comparative analysis of human monoamine uptake and transporter binding affinity. Biol Psychiatry 55(3):320–322, 2004 14744476

Yocca FD: Neurochemistry and neurophysiology of buspirone and gepirone: interactions at presynaptic and postsynaptic 5-HT1A receptors. J Clin Psychpharmacol 10(3 suppl):6S–12S, 1990 1973941

Zitrin CM, Klein DF, Woerner MG: Treatment of agoraphobia with group exposure in vivo and imipramine. Arch Gen Psychiatry 37(1):63–72, 1980 6101535

Recommended Readings

Nemeroff C, Marmar C (eds): Post-Traumatic Stress Disorder. New York, Oxford University Press, 2018

Schatzberg A, Nemeroff C (eds): The American Psychiatric Association Publishing Textbook of Psychopharmacology, 5th Edition. Washington, DC, American Psychiatric Association Publishing, 2017

Stein DJ, Hollander E, Rothbaum B (eds): Textbook of Anxiety Disorders, 2nd Edition. Washington, DC, American Psychiatric Association Publishing, 2010

PART III

Generalized Anxiety Disorder

CHAPTER 11

Phenomenology of Generalized Anxiety Disorder

Katja Beesdo-Baum, Ph.D.

The hallmark feature of generalized anxiety disorder (GAD) is excessive and uncontrollable worry and anxiety about several activities or events. Individuals with GAD worry about or fear experiencing, for example, critical health, financial, occupational, or interpersonal issues. The symptoms accompanying the anxiety and worry are various and include restlessness, muscle tension, irritability, fatigue, and difficulties in concentration or sleep. Diagnostic criteria for GAD have remained largely unchanged from DSM-IV (American Psychiatric Association 1994) and its text revision (DSM-IV-TR; American Psychiatric Association 2000) to DSM-5 (American Psychiatric Association 2013), so previous research results employing DSM-IV criteria may be considered currently valid. However, given that prior to DSM-IV the diagnosis of GAD underwent considerable conceptual and criteria changes, this chapter largely omits results based on DSM-III (American Psychiatric Association 1980) and DSM-III-R (American Psychiatric Association 1987).

Epidemiology

GAD is a relatively common disorder in the general population. Lifetime prevalence estimates range between 3% and 6%, 12-month prevalence estimates between 2% and 4%, and point prevalence estimates between 1% and 2% (Beesdo et al. 2009b; Ruscio et al. 2017; Wittchen et al. 2011). The lifetime morbid risk has been estimated to be 9% as of age 75 (Kessler et al. 2012). GAD criteria do not include many overanxious children who would have formerly been diagnosed with overanxious disorder, which was subsumed under GAD in DSM-IV (Beesdo et al. 2009b). Among older adults (age

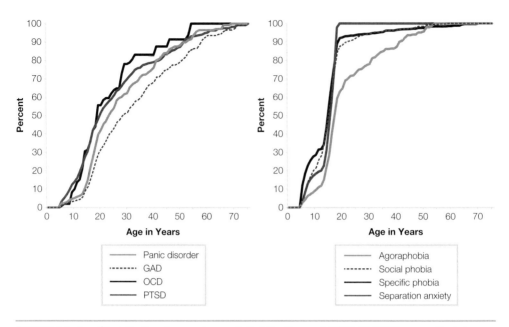

FIGURE 11–1.   Standardized age-at-onset distributions of DSM-IV-TR/Composite International Diagnostic Interview anxiety disorders with (*left*) later age at onset and (*right*) earlier age at onset from the National Comorbidity Survey (NCS) Replication and NCS Adolescent Supplement (*N*=12,175).

GAD=generalized anxiety disorder.

Source.   Reprinted from Kessler RC, Petukhova M, Sampson NA, et al: "Twelve-Month and Lifetime Prevalence and Lifetime Morbid Risk of Anxiety and Mood Disorders in the United States." *International Journal of Methods in Psychiatric Research* 21(3):169–184, 2012. Copyright © 2012 by John Wiley & Sons, Inc. Reprinted by permission of John Wiley & Sons, Inc.

≥55years), particularly high prevalence rates were found for GAD (Canuto et al. 2018; Gonçalves et al. 2011), but this is not a consistent finding because other studies indicate the highest prevalence of GAD in middle-aged adults (Kessler et al. 2012).

Individuals with GAD were shown to be high users of medical health care services. In primary care settings, a high point prevalence of about 4%–8% was found (Kroenke et al. 2007; Munk-Jørgensen et al. 2006; Wittchen 2002), accounting for 8%–9% of all mental disorder cases in this setting (Lieb et al. 2005). GAD also is prevalent in the specialized mental health care sector, with point prevalence rates greater than 10.0% (Bobes et al. 2011; Brown and Barlow 2002).

The first onset of GAD may occur at any time from childhood to late adulthood. Thus, the age-at-onset pattern of GAD differs from that of other anxiety disorders, with a relatively high proportion of individuals developing the condition after the age of 20 (Figure 11–1) (Kessler et al. 2012). The World Mental Health Survey (WMHS; Ruscio et al. 2017) showed that 25% of GAD cases emerge by age 25, 50% by age 39, and 75% by age 53. Studies among youth also show relatively few first-onset cases in childhood but show a sharp increase in incidence in adolescence (Beesdo et al. 2010b; Burstein et al. 2014; Copeland et al. 2014). Whereas the incidence curve for other anxiety disorders flattens after the age of 25, new GAD cases steadily emerge until old age (Kessler et al. 2012).

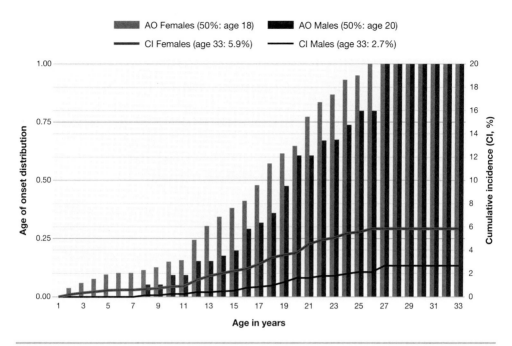

FIGURE 11–2. Estimated age-specific cumulative incidence and age-at-onset distribution of GAD by gender from the Early Developmental Stages of Psychopathology Study (*N*=3,021).

Source. Adapted from Beesdo-Baum K, Knappe S: "Developmental Epidemiology of Anxiety Disorders." *Child and Adolescent Psychiatric Clinics of North America* 21(3):457–478, 2012. Copyright © 2012. Used with permission from Elsevier.

Prevalence and incidence studies reveal that females are overall approximately 1.5–2 times as likely as males to develop GAD (Ruscio et al. 2017), with the female preponderance starting to emerge by early adolescence (Copeland et al. 2014) and increasing with age (Beesdo-Baum and Knappe 2012) (Figure 11–2). Whereas some studies suggest a slightly earlier age at onset and a preponderance of GAD among females at a very early age (Beesdo-Baum and Knappe 2012; Burstein et al. 2014; Steiner et al. 2005), other studies have not reported sex differences (Gonçalves and Byrne 2012; McLean et al. 2011).

Among others, the WMHS collaboration identified younger age (<60 years), being unmarried, having limited education, having a low household income, and being unemployed or disabled as demographic correlates of GAD (Ruscio et al. 2017). Worldwide, anxiety disorders are overall among the leading causes of global years lived with disability (James et al. 2018; Vos et al. 2017). The diagnosis also has been specifically associated with considerable personal burden as well as health care and societal costs (Gustavsson et al. 2011; Ruscio et al. 2017). The WMHS collaboration found that individuals with GAD reported 41 days out of role due to GAD in the past year, and half of the patients reported severe functional impairment (Ruscio et al. 2017). Even non-comorbid GAD cases showed considerable role impairment (37.5% severe impairment; Ruscio et al. 2017). Other studies revealed that the impairments in role functioning in GAD are comparable with those observed in individuals with major depression (Kessler et al. 2002b; Wittchen et al. 2002). Such impairments considerably reduce subjective health (Schonfeld et al. 1997), quality of life, and general well-being (Bobes et al. 2011) and are most intensive if comorbidity is present (Beesdo et al. 2009a; Hoffman et al. 2008).

GAD is also associated with considerable economic burden, not only because of direct costs associated with the high health care use by patients with GAD (Berger et al. 2009; Lieb et al. 2005; Wittchen et al. 2002) but also because of indirect costs associated with work impairment (e.g., sick leave, decreased productivity) (Andlin-Sobocki and Wittchen 2005; Hoffman et al. 2008). It is unfortunate that despite high associated health care use, the recognition of GAD is relatively low (Lieb et al. 2005). For example, general practitioners recognize the presence of a mental disorder in only about two-thirds of all GAD cases, and only one-third of these patients are specifically diagnosed with GAD (Munk-Jørgensen et al. 2006; Wittchen et al. 2002).

Clinical Features

DSM-5 Diagnostic Criteria

DSM-5 diagnostic criteria are shown in Box 11–1. The core clinical feature of GAD is excessive worry and anxiety about a number of events or activities. The worries mostly refer to everyday matters such as school or work performance and family or health issues, which makes it difficult to distinguish individuals with GAD from healthy individuals based on the content or focus of worry. Individuals with GAD anxiously anticipate bad things happening, such as an accident or severe illness in a loved one, a child being kidnapped or showing unfavorable development, a negative evaluation at school or work, getting fired and remaining unemployed, financial or environmentally related strains, or interpersonal difficulties. Such anxious expectations are indicative of GAD if they appear out of proportion to the actual likelihood of such events or the potential impact on the individual and if they occur on most days over a minimum of 6 months. The content may change over time, but in general, affected individuals have difficulty stopping the anxiety or worry. Anxious expectations and worry episodes are frequently triggered throughout the day by minor cues and are accompanied by symptoms of tension and hypervigilance as well as distress or impairment in everyday functioning. Although the diagnostic criteria require only one of six accompanying symptoms in children (compared with three in adults), research shows that children with GAD are mostly affected by multiple symptoms (Beesdo-Baum et al. 2011).

Box 11–1.   Diagnostic Criteria for Generalized Anxiety Disorder

---

A. Excessive anxiety and worry (apprehensive expectation), occurring more days than not for at least 6 months, about a number of events or activities (such as work or school performance).

B. The individual finds it difficult to control the worry.

C. The anxiety and worry are associated with three (or more) of the following six symptoms (with at least some symptoms having been present for more days than not for the past 6 months):

Note: Only one item is required in children.

1. Restlessness or feeling keyed up or on edge.
2. Being easily fatigued.
3. Difficulty concentrating or mind going blank.
4. Irritability.
5. Muscle tension.
6. Sleep disturbance (difficulty falling or staying asleep, or restless, unsatisfying sleep).

D. The anxiety, worry, or physical symptoms cause clinically significant distress or impairment in social, occupational, or other important areas of functioning.

E. The disturbance is not attributable to the physiological effects of a substance (e.g., a drug of abuse, a medication) or another medical condition (e.g., hyperthyroidism).

F. The disturbance is not better explained by another mental disorder (e.g., anxiety or worry about having panic attacks in panic disorder, negative evaluation in social anxiety disorder [social phobia], contamination or other obsessions in obsessive-compulsive disorder, separation from attachment figures in separation anxiety disorder, reminders of traumatic events in posttraumatic stress disorder, gaining weight in anorexia nervosa, physical complaints in somatic symptom disorder, perceived appearance flaws in body dysmorphic disorder, having a serious illness in illness anxiety disorder, or the content of delusional beliefs in schizophrenia or delusional disorder).

Source. Reprinted from American Psychiatric Association: *Diagnostic and Statistical Manual of Mental Disorders*, 5th Edition. Arlington, VA, American Psychiatric Association, 2013. Copyright © 2013 American Psychiatric Association. Used with permission.

Associated Features

Besides the hypervigilance and tension symptoms contained in the DSM-5 diagnostic criteria, pain symptoms (Beesdo et al. 2009a) as well as autonomous symptoms such as sweating, racing heart, diarrhea, or nausea also are common in individuals with GAD. Children with GAD often complain about stomachaches or headaches. Both in children and adults, complaints about physical symptoms often are not linked to their psychological cause, frequently resulting in incorrect diagnoses and inappropriate treatment (Wittchen et al. 2002).

A relevant feature in GAD is a pattern of fear of the unknown or unfamiliar, with interpretation of such situations as threatening, resulting in behaviors designed to avoid such situations (Carleton 2012). Individuals with GAD reveal a high intolerance toward uncertainty (Dugas et al. 1998; Gentes and Ruscio 2011) and therefore attempt to control their lives and emotions. Generally, awareness and acceptance of one's own emotions seems to be impaired in GAD, and more dysfunctional strategies of emotion regulation are used (Roemer et al. 2009). Among such inefficient and dysfunctional strategies are reassurance seeking (Cougle et al. 2012) and cognitive avoidance (Olatunji et al. 2010). These strategies aim at inhibiting or avoiding processing of aversive emotions. The popular Avoidance Model of Worry and GAD posits that the worry itself is a dysfunctional emotion regulation strategy that actually inhibits autonomic and somatic arousal and dampens aversive emotional states (Behar et al. 2009; Borkovec et al. 2004).

Thus, overall, individuals with GAD engage in various behaviors to reduce or prevent worry and anxiety. These behaviors have been suggested to be potentially useful for improved recognition and diagnosis (Andrews et al. 2010). Unfortunately, although clinically well known and targeted in cognitive-behavioral interventions for GAD (Hoyer et al. 2009; Rygh and Sanderson 2004), the empirical data basis on worry behaviors in GAD is relatively limited, with only a few studies published so far indicating its relevance (Beesdo-Baum et al. 2012a). Therefore, proposals to include a behavioral symptom criterion for GAD (Andrews et al. 2010) were not accepted, and GAD remains the only anxiety diagnosis in DSM-5 that does not contain a behavioral symptom criterion. More recent studies have begun to assess the classification accuracy when considering such a criterion for the diagnosis of GAD (Brown and Tung 2018) but have provided only fair interrater reliability for these behaviors thus far. Thus, considerably more research is needed, including the development of appropriate measures for worry behaviors (Mahoney et al. 2018).

Differential Diagnosis

Differential diagnosis in GAD may be difficult for three main reasons:

1. *Worry and anxiety—the core features of GAD—may be components of other mental disorders, but the focus of the worry may differ.* A diagnosis of GAD is appropriate if additional worries and symptoms are present that are not part of the another mental disorder. For example, worry and anxiety also occur in other anxiety disorders—with a focus on the specific content feared (e.g., fear of negative evaluation, embarrassment, and rejection in social anxiety disorder; fear of falling in height phobia; or fear of recurring panic attacks, losing control, or death in panic disorder). If additional excessive worries about activities or events relating to future real-life problems (e.g., ill health, financial ruin) are present, a GAD diagnosis is warranted.
2. *Some accompanying symptoms of GAD are also included in the diagnostic criteria sets of several other mental disorders.* For example, difficulties with concentration are also relevant for major depression and dysthymia, sleep problems for major depression and insomnia disorder, and irritability for major depression (at least in adolescents), premenstrual dysphoric disorder (in women), disruptive mood dysregulation disorder, bipolar disorder (in manic episodes), and PTSD.
3. *Comorbid conditions can develop as a consequence of GAD or independently at any point during the lifetime.* For example, major depression is a frequent comorbid condition in individuals with GAD. Depressive episodes may develop completely independent of the anxiety and worry (e.g., in response to the death of a loved one), or in the context or consequence of GAD (e.g., because of the distress and burden of anxiety and worry and the associated symptoms and impairments in functioning). Assessing the past history, onset, and course of co-occurring conditions usually helps with differential diagnosis or the decision to diagnose both or just one of these conditions (Figure 11–3).

Table 11–1 provides an overview on aspects of differential diagnoses to consider when deciding whether GAD or another mental disorder should be diagnosed, given the symptom presentation, or whether both disorders should be diagnosed as comorbid conditions.

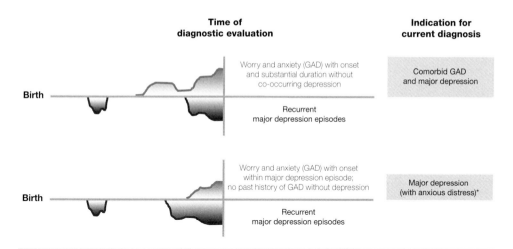

FIGURE 11–3. Differential diagnosis: generalized anxiety disorder (GAD) and major depression as comorbid diagnoses?

With regard to medical conditions and substances, the same applies to GAD as to other mental disorders. Given that medical conditions (e.g., hyperthyroidism) and substances (e.g., caffeine) may cause symptoms similar to those seen in GAD, it needs to be determined and ruled out whether the disturbance is attributable to the physiological effects of a substance or another medical condition. If the etiological factor is a medical condition or a substance, the diagnosis of an anxiety disorder due to another medical condition or a substance/medication-induced anxiety disorder is made.

Comorbidity

As with virtually all mental disorders, GAD reveals considerable comorbidity. Even in community samples, about 80%–90% of individuals with GAD are affected by at least one other mental disorder during their life course (Carter et al. 2001; Copeland et al. 2014; Ruscio et al. 2017). Conversely, GAD is often a comorbid condition in individuals with other mental disorders (Copeland et al. 2014; de Graaf et al. 2003). The strongest associations are commonly found for mood disorders and other anxiety disorders (particularly social anxiety disorder, panic disorder, and separation anxiety disorder), whereas associations with substance use disorders and impulse-control disorders as well as childhood externalizing or disruptive behavior disorders are weaker and less consistent (Burstein et al. 2014; Copeland et al. 2014; Grant et al. 2005; Ruscio et al. 2017). In addition, some studies show associations with dependent and avoidant personality disorders as well as with somatoform disorders and pain conditions (Beesdo et al. 2009a, 2010a; Faravelli et al. 2004). Eating disorders (anorexia and bulimia nervosa) have rarely been examined in general population samples but appear to also co-occur more frequently than expected by chance in individuals with GAD (Beesdo 2006; Carter et al. 2001; Faravelli et al. 2004).

Regarding the temporal order of onset, GAD may occur prior to, simultaneously with, or after the onset of any comorbid condition (Kessler et al. 2002a). With regard to any comorbid anxiety disorder (particularly specific phobia and social anxiety dis-

TABLE 11–1.   Differential diagnosis: distinguishing GAD from other mental disorders

DSM-5 disorder	Core feature	Differential diagnosis
Separation anxiety disorder	Anxiety concerning separation from attachment figures	Diagnosed if other worries (such as in GAD) occur but do not predominate the clinical picture. If separation is among other activities or events the person is worried about, GAD is diagnosed.
Social anxiety disorder	Worries focusing on social performance and others' evaluation	Social worries in GAD focus more on the nature of ongoing relationships than on fear of negative evaluations. Excessive worries about quality of social performance are accompanied by worries about nonsocial performance and at times when one is not being evaluated by others. Individuals with GAD may worry about whether they are being evaluated.
Agoraphobia	Marked fear or anxiety about situations such as using public transportation, being in open or enclosed spaces, standing in line or being in a crowd, or being outside of the home alone	GAD is characterized by worry and anxiety about events or activities relating to future real-life problems, not to particular situations (as in agoraphobia).
Specific phobia	Marked fear or anxiety about a specific object or situation (e.g., flying, heights, animals, injections, seeing blood)	GAD is characterized by worry and anxiety about events or activities relating to future real-life problems, not to particular objects or situations (as in specific phobia).
Panic disorder	Experience of recurrent unexpected panic attacks and worry about additional attacks or their consequences	If panic attacks are triggered only by worry, GAD alone is diagnosed. If unexpected panic attacks are experienced and worry or behavioral change persists because of the attacks, panic disorder should be considered.
OCD	Obsessions (recurrent and persistent intrusive or unwanted thoughts, urges, or images), compulsions (repetitive behaviors to prevent or reduce anxiety or distress), or both	Recurrent thoughts, avoidant behaviors, and repetitive requests for reassurance in GAD are excessive concerns about future real-life problems. Obsessions in OCD are usually inappropriate and intrusive ideas that may include odd or irrational content (e.g., contamination); they are frequently linked with rigid compulsions, behaviors, or mental acts the person feels driven to perform that are not connected realistically with what they are designed to prevent (e.g., washing hands, counting).

TABLE 11–1.   Differential diagnosis: distinguishing GAD from other mental disorders (continued)

DSM-5 disorder	Core feature	Differential diagnosis
Illness anxiety disorder	Preoccupation with having or acquiring a serious illness	Individuals with GAD worry about multiple events, situations, or activities, only one of which may involve health (fear of illness).
PTSD	Persistent intrusions, avoidance, and negative alterations in cognitions and mood, as well as arousal and reactivity, after the experience of a traumatic event	GAD may develop after a traumatic event, but avoidance, irritability, and anxiety in GAD are not (exclusively) linked to a specific trauma. GAD is not diagnosed if anxiety and worry are better explained as symptoms of PTSD. Recurrent intrusions in PTSD relate to past traumatic experience; worries in GAD usually refer to future real-life problems.
Adjustment disorder	Anxiety occurs in response to an identifiable stressor within 3 months of stressor onset and does not persist more than 6 months after termination of the stressor or its consequences	Adjustment disorder is a residual category that should be used only when the criteria for another disorder (including GAD) are not met.
Depressive disorders with anxious distress	Depressed mood accompanied by further symptoms (e.g., feelings of worthlessness, hopelessness, inappropriate guilt; recurrent thoughts of death or suicide; diminished ability to think or concentrate; difficulty making decisions); symptoms during most days of a major depressive episode or persistent depressive disorder (dysthymia) include feeling keyed up, tense, or unusually restless; having difficulty concentrating because of worry; or fearing something awful may happen or that one may lose control of oneself	Focus of worry in GAD is not on characteristic contents of rumination in depression but on activities or events related to future real-life problems. Symptoms of depression and GAD partly overlap; therefore, careful evaluation of past history and course is required to differentiate the diagnoses. Generalized anxiety symptoms or worries are a common associated feature in depressive episodes. If they exclusively occur during mood episodes and the severity does not warrant clinical attention, an anxious distress specifier should be recorded with the diagnosis of major depression or persistent depressive disorder.
Premenstrual dysphoric disorder (PMDD)	Symptoms linked to menstrual cycle (e.g., marked irritability, anxiety, tension, feeling keyed up or on edge)	Symptoms also are characteristic of GAD, but in PMDD they are of shorter duration and are linked to the menstrual cycle.
Bipolar disorder (mania)	Abnormally and persistently elevated, expansive, or irritable mood and increased goal-directed activity	Anxious ruminations in GAD may be mistaken for racing thoughts; efforts to minimize anxiety may be taken as impulsive behavior; irritability is a characteristic in both diagnoses. Careful evaluation of symptom history and course is needed to distinguish GAD from bipolar disorder.

TABLE 11–1.   Differential diagnosis: distinguishing GAD from other mental disorders *(continued)*

DSM-5 disorder	Core feature	Differential diagnosis
Disruptive mood dysregulation disorder (DMDD)	Severe recurrent temper outbursts, with persistently irritable mood between outbursts	Anxiety and worry are not characteristic features of DMDD. Irritability frequently occurs in GAD as a result of fear or worry.
Body dysmorphic disorder	Preoccupation with perceived defects or flaws in physical appearance that are not or are only slightly observable by others	GAD worries usually do not include perceived appearance flaws.
Somatic symptom disorder	Excessive thoughts and feelings or behaviors related to distressing somatic symptoms or associated health concerns	Main focus of worry in GAD is usually not on somatic symptoms.
Anorexia nervosa	Intense fear of gaining weight or becoming fat, leading to restriction of energy intake	GAD is characterized by worry and anxiety about events or activities relating to everyday matters, not particularly relating to weight, body shape, or food intake.
Insomnia disorder	Predominant complaint of dissatisfaction with sleep quantity or quality, linked to difficulty initiating or maintaining sleep	Sleep disturbances in GAD are often the result of hypervigilance, tension, and worrying. Insomnia disorder is not diagnosed if GAD adequately explains the insomnia.
Avoidant personality disorder	Feelings of general inadequacy, social inhibition, and hypersensitivity to negative evaluation	Fear of criticism or rejection and avoidance of situations or activities with interpersonal contact are present in both, but onset in avoidant personality disorder must occur by early adulthood.
Dependent personality disorder	Pervasive and excessive need to be taken care of that leads to submissive and clinging behavior and fears of separation	Dependency may arise as a consequence of GAD; individuals also may have difficulty making decisions and thus excessively seek reassurance from others. In dependent personality disorder, however, onset must occur by early adulthood and be present in various contexts.
Obsessive-compulsive personality disorder (OCPD)	Preoccupation with orderliness, perfectionism, and mental and interpersonal control	Individuals with GAD may be perfectionistic and rely on rules, lists, or schedules to reduce anxiety or worry. OCPD patients must be preoccupied with such tasks, and interference with task completion must be evident. OCPD onset occurs by early adulthood and is present in various contexts.

Note.   GAD=generalized anxiety disorder.
Source.   Adapted from American Psychiatric Association 2013.

order), GAD is usually a secondary-onset condition, because it tends to occur later compared with other anxiety conditions. However, GAD was still found to predict the secondary onset of other anxiety disorders (Beesdo et al. 2010b; Lee et al. 2009). Mood disorders, particularly depressive episodes, often emerge in the same year as GAD (in about 50% of comorbid cases) (Kessler et al. 2002a), which challenges differential diagnosis. Substance use disorders mostly occur secondary to the onset of GAD, and risk for secondary substance use disorders is particularly high in individuals with prolonged GAD episodes (Kessler et al. 2002a; Lee et al. 2009).

Besides comorbid psychiatric disorders, somatic complaints such as chest pain, irritable bowel syndrome, and chronic fatigue syndrome as well as medical illnesses (e.g., diabetes, hypertension, gastrointestinal and heart diseases) are associated with GAD (Lieb et al. 2005; Sareen et al. 2005). Generally, the presence of comorbid mental or physical disorders confers a greater level of disability in patients with GAD (Beesdo et al. 2009a; Sareen et al. 2005).

Course

Although patients in treatment settings report a long duration of GAD, suggesting considerable chronicity beyond the minimum duration of 6 months as specified in the diagnostic criteria, the natural course of GAD in affected individuals from the general population can be described as waxing and waning (Angst et al. 2009; Beesdo 2006; Wittchen et al. 2000). Recurring episodes lasting several months or years have been reported in community studies (Burstein et al. 2014; Grant et al. 2005; Kessler et al. 2005), with symptom-free intervals in about half of the cases (Angst et al. 2009). Nevertheless, individuals with GAD are affected by the condition in about 50%–60% of the years between first onset and last episode (Kessler et al. 2005). Persistence is similar among those with shorter and longer episode durations, indicating high recurrence among those with shorter episodes. For example, adults with GAD indicating a maximum episode duration of 6–11 months reported that episodes recurred for about 6.5 years after first onset; those with longer episodes were affected overall for 10.4 years (Kessler et al. 2005). The WMHS collaboration showed that individuals with GAD who had earlier onset and lower education and family income, as well as homemakers, revealed the highest persistence (Ruscio et al. 2017). In adolescents, the mean time in episodes since first disorder onset was 65 months (Burstein et al. 2014).

In clinical samples, a prolonged and chronic course of GAD is usually reported. For example, in an 8-year naturalistic follow-up study of patients with GAD, spontaneous remissions occurred (men 56%, women 46%) but were mostly not persisting (relapses in 43% of men and 36% of women) (Yonkers et al. 2003). In primary care patients with GAD, the cumulative probability of full or partial recovery within 2 years was 39% and 54%, respectively; roughly half of the fully remitted cases experienced a partial or full recurrence of symptoms (Rodriguez et al. 2006). No consistent indications have been found for sex differences in course patterns of GAD (Angst et al. 2009; Rodriguez et al. 2006; Yonkers et al. 2003), but comorbidity has been shown to negatively affect the course (Bruce et al. 2005; Ramsawh et al. 2009).

Regarding longitudinal course and comorbidity with other mental disorders, evidence clearly shows that the risk for onset of GAD is increased among those with other mental disorders, and vice versa (Beesdo et al. 2010b), even among those with subthreshold GAD (Ruscio et al. 2007). Among those with remission of GAD, diagnostic shifts are often observed, suggesting that complete remission from mental disorder over the long run is rare (Angst et al. 2009; Beesdo 2006; Rubio and López-Ibor 2007).

Evaluation

Diagnostic evaluation of GAD can be undertaken with structured or standardized clinical interviews. However, in clinical settings with restricted possibilities for conducting a time-intensive interview, screening measures also may be useful. Treatment processes ideally are monitored using repeated evaluations with symptom questionnaires tapping features of GAD.

A range of clinical interviews are available for the diagnosis of GAD, from semistructured to fully standardized (Table 11–2). Structured interviews give both interviewer and patient more freedom during the assessment but also require more intense training to successfully administer. These interviews are based on the DSM diagnostic criteria and can be used to diagnose GAD as well as a number of other mental disorders, which is useful with regard to differential diagnosis or assessment of comorbidity.

Standard measures for GAD symptom severity are typically self-report questionnaires. These have been relevant for many aspects of the diagnostic process (e.g., for supporting diagnosis or measuring progress during therapy), and such measures are likely to gain further importance because of the emphasis in DSM-5 on dimensional evaluation of disorders. During the development of DSM-5, a set of brief self-rating dimensional anxiety scales were developed for each of the anxiety diagnoses, including GAD. Good psychometric properties and classification performance were demonstrated for these scales in clinical and nonclinical samples (Beesdo-Baum et al. 2012b; Knappe et al. 2013, 2014; Lebeau et al. 2012; Möller et al. 2014), and the scales are now available for researchers and clinicians for further use (www.psychiatry.org/dsm5). Additional novel measures relate to the worry behaviors in GAD (Mahoney et al. 2018), which will be useful for further increasing understanding of the clinical presentation of the disorder as well as for monitoring treatment.

Beyond these novel scales, other, more traditional self-rated measures for GAD symptomatology are available (see Table 11–2). Reasonable to good psychometric properties have been reported for all of these questionnaires, including good specificity and sensitivity (Brown et al. 1992; Kroenke et al. 2007; Spitzer et al. 2006). In addition, several clinician-rated measures are available to rate the current severity of GAD.

Conclusion

GAD is one of the more prevalent anxiety disorders and has a comparatively late onset. Its defining feature of worries and anxiety focusing on various future real-life problems differentiates it from other mental disorders. However, recognition is difficult, and underdiagnosis leads to increased and prolonged individual and societal burden. More empirical data need to be obtained on how the diagnostic definition of GAD, and therefore recognition and diagnosis, could be further improved.

TABLE 11–2. Instruments for the diagnosis and evaluation of generalized anxiety disorder (GAD)

Type of instrument	Instruments	Remarks
Clinical interviews		
Standardized interview	Composite International Diagnostic Interview (CIDI; Kessler and Üstün 2004; Robins et al. 1988; World Health Organization 1990)	Available in paper-and-pencil and computer-assisted versions; assesses lifetime and current disorders; comprehensive (long duration). Internationally, the most commonly used interview in research—particularly in large-scale epidemiological studies
Structured interviews[a]	Structured Clinical Interview for DSM-5 Disorders—Clinician Version (SCID-5-CV; First et al. 2016)	Focuses on current diagnoses
	Mini-International Neuropsychiatric Interview (M.I.N.I.[b]; Sheehan et al. 1998)	Focuses on current diagnoses; short duration
	Anxiety Disorders Interview Schedule for DSM-5 (ADIS-5; Brown and Barlow 2014)	Available in a lifetime version and a version assessing current diagnoses
	Kiddie Schedule for Affective Disorders (K-SADS-PL[c]; Kaufman et al. 1997)	Interview for diagnosing children and adolescents; assesses lifetime and current disorders; besides information provided by child or adolescent, information from other sources (e.g., parents, teachers) considered
Severity and screening measures		
Self-report questionnaires	Dimensional anxiety scales for DSM-5 (American Psychiatric Association 2013)	Scale available specifically for GAD symptom severity
	Penn State Worry Questionnaire (PSWQ; Meyer et al. 1990)	Focuses on intensity, severity, and subjective controllability of worry; most widely used instrument for assessment of GAD symptom severity
	Generalized Anxiety Disorder–7 (GAD-7; Spitzer et al. 2006)	Screening for current presence of GAD
	Generalized Anxiety Questionnaire–IV (GAD-Q-IV; Newman et al. 2002)	Screening for current presence of GAD based on DSM-IV/DSM-5 criteria

TABLE 11–2.   Instruments for the diagnosis and evaluation of generalized anxiety disorder (GAD) (*continued*)

Type of instrument	Instruments	Remarks
Self-report questionnaires (*continued*)	Hospital Anxiety and Depression Scale (HADS; Zigmond and Snaith 1983)	Severity measure; also covers other anxiety disorders and depression
	Screen for Child Anxiety Related Emotional Disorders Scale (SCARED; Birmaher et al. 1997)	Screening measure; also covers other anxiety disorders
Clinician-rated scales	Hamilton Anxiety Rating Scale (HAM-A; Hamilton 1959)	Most widely used clinician-rated severity measure for GAD; for assessment, structured interview guide also available (GADSS; see next row)
	Generalized Anxiety Disorder Severity Scale (GADSS; Shear et al. 2006)	Consistent with DSM-IV/DSM-5 criteria
	DSM-IV GAD Severity Scale (DGSS; Stein 2013)	Consistent with DSM-IV/DSM-5 criteria; assesses both symptom severity and symptom frequency

Note.   [a]Both interviewer and patient have a greater degree of freedom with structured interviews during assessment; latter requires more intense training to successfully administer.
[b]For DSM-5 version see http://harmresearch.org/index.php/product/mini-international-neuropsychiatric-interview-mini-7-0-2-4.
[c]For DSM-5 version see https://osf.io/pqhxy/?action=download%26mode=render.

Key Points

- Generalized anxiety disorder (GAD) has developed since its first introduction in DSM-III from a residual category to an independent mental disorder. Thus, it can be diagnosed independently or as a comorbid condition whenever the diagnostic criteria are met, including that the presentation cannot be better explained by another mental disorder. Temporal co-occurrence of other mental disorders such as mood disorders (as in DSM-IV), psychotic disorders, or PTSD is no reason to rule out GAD.

- GAD is often accompanied by worry behaviors. Worry behaviors may include avoidance, such as not entering situations that might provoke worry, as well as more general safety behaviors including checking and reassurance seeking. Individuals with GAD often also are indecisive and procrastinate.

- Alcohol, tobacco, medications, or drugs may be used to cope with chronic anxiety and worry and associated symptoms such as problems sleeping and concentrating. This "self-medication" may lead to the development of independent comorbid substance use disorders.

References

American Psychiatric Association: Diagnostic and Statistical Manual of Mental Disorders, 3rd Edition. Washington, DC, American Psychiatric Association, 1980

American Psychiatric Association: Diagnostic and Statistical Manual of Mental Disorders, 3rd Edition, Revised. Washington, DC, American Psychiatric Association, 1987

American Psychiatric Association: Diagnostic and Statistical Manual of Mental Disorders, 4th Edition. Washington, DC, American Psychiatric Association, 1994

American Psychiatric Association: Diagnostic and Statistical Manual of Mental Disorders, 4th Edition, Text Revision. Washington, DC, American Psychiatric Association, 2000

American Psychiatric Association: Diagnostic and Statistical Manual of Mental Disorders, 5th Edition. Arlington, VA, American Psychiatric Association, 2013

Andlin-Sobocki P, Wittchen HU: Cost of anxiety disorders in Europe. Eur J Neurol 12(suppl 1):39–44, 2005 15877777

Andrews G, Hobbs MJ, Borkovec TD, et al: Generalized worry disorder: a review of DSM-IV generalized anxiety disorder and options for DSM-V. Depress Anxiety 27:134–147, 2010

Angst J, Gamma A, Baldwin DS, et al: The generalized anxiety spectrum: prevalence, onset, course and outcome. Eur Arch Psychiatry Clin Neurosci 259(1):37–45, 2009 18575915

Beesdo K: The Development of Generalized Anxiety: A Prospective-Longitudinal, Clinical-Epidemiologic Study Among Adolescents and Young Adults [in German]. Dresden, Germany, TUD Press, 2006

Beesdo K, Hoyer J, Jacobi F, et al: Association between generalized anxiety levels and pain in a community sample: evidence for diagnostic specificity. J Anxiety Disord 23(5):684–693, 2009a 19278819

Beesdo K, Knappe S, Pine DS: Anxiety and anxiety disorders in children and adolescents: developmental issues and implications for DSM-V. Psychiatr Clin North Am 32(3):483–524, 2009b 19716988

Beesdo K, Jacobi F, Hoyer J, et al: Pain associated with specific anxiety and depressive disorders in a nationally representative population sample. Soc Psychiatry Psychiatr Epidemiol 45(1):89–104, 2010a 19360362

Beesdo K, Pine DS, Lieb R, et al: Incidence and risk patterns of anxiety and depressive disorders and categorization of generalized anxiety disorder. Arch Gen Psychiatry 67(1):47–57, 2010b 20048222

Beesdo-Baum K, Knappe S: Developmental epidemiology of anxiety disorders. Child Adolesc Psychiatr Clin N Am 21(3):457–478, 2012 22800989

Beesdo-Baum K, Winkel S, Pine DS, et al: The diagnostic threshold of generalized anxiety disorder in the community: a developmental perspective. J Psychiatr Res 45(7):962–972, 2011 21227450

Beesdo-Baum K, Jenjahn E, Höfler M, et al: Avoidance, safety behavior, and reassurance seeking in generalized anxiety disorder. Depress Anxiety 29(11):948–957, 2012a 22581482

Beesdo-Baum K, Klotsche J, Knappe S, et al: Psychometric properties of the dimensional anxiety scales for DSM-V in an unselected sample of German treatment seeking patients. Depress Anxiety 29(12):1014–1024, 2012b 22933460

Behar E, DiMarco ID, Hekler EB, et al: Current theoretical models of generalized anxiety disorder (GAD): conceptual review and treatment implications. J Anxiety Disord 23(8):1011–1023, 2009 19700258

Berger A, Mychaskiw M, Dukes E, et al: Magnitude of potentially inappropriate prescribing in Germany among older patients with generalized anxiety disorder. BMC Geriatr 9(31):31, 2009 19635161

Birmaher B, Khetarpal S, Brent D, et al: The Screen for Child Anxiety Related Emotional Disorders (SCARED): scale construction and psychometric characteristics. J Am Acad Child Adolesc Psychiatry 36(4):545–553, 1997 9100430

Bobes J, Caballero L, Vilardaga I, et al: Disability and health-related quality of life in outpatients with generalised anxiety disorder treated in psychiatric clinics: is there still room for improvement? Ann Gen Psychiatry 10(1):7, 2011 21401940

Borkovec TD, Alcaine OM, Behar E: Avoidance theory of worry and generalized anxiety disorder, in Generalized Anxiety Disorder: Advances in Research and Practice. Edited by Heimberg R, Turk C, Mennin D. New York, Guilford, 2004, pp 77–108

Brown TA, Barlow DH: Classification of anxiety and mood disorders, in Anxiety and Its Disorders, 2nd Edition. Edited by Barlow DH. New York, Guilford, 2002, pp 292–329

Brown TA, Barlow DH: Anxiety and Related Disorders Interview Schedule for DSM-5 (ADIS-5)—Adult Version. New York, Oxford University Press, 2014

Brown TA, Tung ES: The contribution of worry behaviors to the diagnosis of generalized anxiety disorder. J Psychopathol Behav Assess 40(4):636–644, 2018 30739985

Brown TA, Antony MM, Barlow DH: Psychometric properties of the Penn State Worry Questionnaire in a clinical anxiety disorders sample. Behav Res Ther 30(1):33–37, 1992 1540110

Bruce SE, Yonkers KA, Otto MW, et al: Influence of psychiatric comorbidity on recovery and recurrence in generalized anxiety disorder, social phobia, and panic disorder: a 12-year prospective study. Am J Psychiatry 162(6):1179–1187, 2005 15930067

Burstein M, Beesdo-Baum K, He J-P, et al: Threshold and subthreshold generalized anxiety disorder among US adolescents: prevalence, sociodemographic, and clinical characteristics. Psychol Med 44(11):2351–2362, 2014 24384401

Canuto A, Weber K, Baertschi M, et al: Anxiety disorders in old age: psychiatric comorbidities, quality of life, and prevalence according to age, gender, and country. Am J Geriatr Psychiatry 26(2):174–185, 2018 29031568

Carleton RN: The intolerance of uncertainty construct in the context of anxiety disorders: theoretical and practical perspectives. Expert Rev Neurother 12(8):937–947, 2012 23002938

Carter RM, Wittchen H-U, Pfister H, et al: One-year prevalence of subthreshold and threshold DSM-IV generalized anxiety disorder in a nationally representative sample. Depress Anxiety 13(2):78–88, 2001 11301924

Copeland WE, Angold A, Shanahan L, et al: Longitudinal patterns of anxiety from childhood to adulthood: the Great Smoky Mountains Study. J Am Acad Child Adolesc Psychiatry 53(1):21–33, 2014 24342383

Cougle JR, Fitch KE, Fincham FD, et al: Excessive reassurance seeking and anxiety pathology: tests of incremental associations and directionality. J Anxiety Disord 26(1):117–125, 2012 22019424

de Graaf R, Bijl RV, Spijker J, et al: Temporal sequencing of lifetime mood disorders in relation to comorbid anxiety and substance use disorders—findings from the Netherlands Mental Health Survey and Incidence Study. Soc Psychiatry Psychiatr Epidemiol 38(1):1–11, 2003

Dugas MJ, Gagnon F, Ladouceur R, et al: Generalized anxiety disorder: a preliminary test of a conceptual model. Behav Res Ther 36(2):215–226, 1998 9613027

Faravelli C, Abrardi L, Bartolozzi D, et al: The Sesto Fiorentino study: background, methods and preliminary results. Lifetime prevalence of psychiatric disorders in an Italian community sample using clinical interviewers. Psychother Psychosom 73(4):216–225, 2004 15184716

First MB, Williams JBW, Karg RS, et al: Structured Clinical Interview for DSM-5 Disorders—Clinician Version (SCID-5-CV). Washington, DC, American Psychiatric Publishing, 2016

Gentes EL, Ruscio AM: A meta-analysis of the relation of intolerance of uncertainty to symptoms of generalized anxiety disorder, major depressive disorder, and obsessive-compulsive disorder. Clin Psychol Rev 31(6):923–933, 2011 21664339

Gonçalves DC, Byrne GJ: Sooner or later: age at onset of generalized anxiety disorder in older adults. Depress Anxiety 29(1):39–46, 2012 21898708

Gonçalves DC, Pachana NA, Byrne GJ: Prevalence and correlates of generalized anxiety disorder among older adults in the Australian National Survey of Mental Health and Well-Being. J Affect Disord 132(1–2):223–230, 2011 21429587

Grant BF, Hasin DS, Stinson FS, et al: Prevalence, correlates, co-morbidity, and comparative disability of DSM-IV generalized anxiety disorder in the USA: results from the National Epidemiologic Survey on Alcohol and Related Conditions. Psychol Med 35(12):1747–1759, 2005 16202187

Gustavsson A, Svensson M, Jacobi F, et al: Cost of disorders of the brain in Europe 2010. Eur Neuropsychopharmacol 21(10):718–779, 2011 21924589

Hamilton M: The assessment of anxiety states by rating. Br J Med Psychol 32(1):50–55, 1959 13638508

Hoffman DL, Dukes EM, Wittchen HU: Human and economic burden of generalized anxiety disorder. Depress Anxiety 25(1):72–90, 2008 17146763

Hoyer J, Beesdo K, Gloster AT, et al: Worry exposure versus applied relaxation in the treatment of generalized anxiety disorder. Psychother Psychosom 78(2):106–115, 2009 19218829

James SL, Abate D, Abate KH, et al: Global, regional, and national incidence, prevalence, and years lived with disability for 354 diseases and injuries for 195 countries and territories, 1990–2017: a systematic analysis for the Global Burden of Disease Study 2017. Lancet 392(10159):1789–1858, 2018 30496104

Kaufman J, Birmaher B, Brent D, et al: Schedule for Affective Disorders and Schizophrenia for School-Age Children–Present and Lifetime Version (K-SADS-PL): initial reliability and validity data. J Am Acad Child Adolesc Psychiatry 36(7):980–988, 1997 9204677

Kessler RC, Ustün TB: The World Mental Health (WMH) Survey Initiative Version of the World Health Organization (WHO) Composite International Diagnostic Interview (CIDI). Int J Methods Psychiatr Res 13(2):93–121, 2004 15297906

Kessler RC, Andrade LH, Bijl RV, et al: The effects of co-morbidity on the onset and persistence of generalized anxiety disorder in the ICPE surveys. Psychol Med 32(7):1213–1225, 2002a

Kessler RC, Berglund PA, Dewit DJ, et al: Distinguishing generalized anxiety disorder from major depression: prevalence and impairment from current pure and comorbid disorders in the US and Ontario. Int J Methods Psychiatr Res 11(3):99–111, 2002b 12459823

Kessler RC, Brandenburg N, Lane M, et al: Rethinking the duration requirement for generalized anxiety disorder: evidence from the National Comorbidity Survey Replication. Psychol Med 35(7):1073–1082, 2005 16045073

Kessler RC, Petukhova M, Sampson NA, et al: Twelve-month and lifetime prevalence and lifetime morbid risk of anxiety and mood disorders in the United States. Int J Methods Psychiatr Res 21(3):169–184, 2012 22865617

Knappe S, Klotsche J, Strobel A, et al: Dimensional anxiety scales for DSM-5: sensitivity to clinical severity. Eur Psychiatry 28(7):448–456, 2013 23541345

Knappe S, Klotsche J, Heyde F, et al: Test-retest reliability and sensitivity to change of the dimensional anxiety scales for DSM-5. CNS Spectr 19(3):256–267, 2014 24229639

Kroenke K, Spitzer RL, Williams JBW, et al: Anxiety disorders in primary care: prevalence, impairment, comorbidity, and detection. Ann Intern Med 146(5):317–325, 2007 17339617

Lebeau RT, Glenn DE, Hanover LN, et al: A dimensional approach to measuring anxiety for DSM-5. Int J Methods Psychiatr Res 21(4):258–272, 2012 23148016

Lee S, Tsang A, Ruscio AM, et al: Implications of modifying the duration requirement of generalized anxiety disorder in developed and developing countries. Psychol Med 39(7):1163–1176, 2009 19091158

Lieb R, Becker E, Altamura C: The epidemiology of generalized anxiety disorder in Europe. Eur Neuropsychopharmacol 15(4):445–452, 2005 15951160

Mahoney AEJ, Hobbs MJ, Newby JM, et al: Maladaptive behaviours associated with generalized anxiety disorder: an item response theory analysis. Behav Cogn Psychother 46(4):479–496, 2018 29553003

McLean CP, Asnaani A, Litz BT, et al: Gender differences in anxiety disorders: prevalence, course of illness, comorbidity and burden of illness. J Psychiatr Res 45(8):1027–1035, 2011

Meyer TJ, Miller ML, Metzger RL, et al: Development and validation of the Penn State Worry Questionnaire. Behav Res Ther 28(6):487–495, 1990 2076086

Möller EL, Majdandzic M, Craske MG, et al: Dimensional assessment of anxiety disorders in parents and children for DSM-5. Int J Methods Psychiatr Res 23(3):331–344, 2014 24943058

Munk-Jørgensen P, Allgulander C, Dahl AA, et al: Prevalence of generalized anxiety disorder in general practice in Denmark, Finland, Norway, and Sweden. Psychiatr Serv 57(12):1738–1744, 2006 17158488

Newman MG, Zuellig AR, Kachin KE, et al: Preliminary reliability and validity of the Generalized Anxiety Disorder Questionnaire–IV: a revised self-report diagnostic measure of generalized anxiety disorder. Behav Ther 33(2):215–233, 2002

Olatunji BO, Moretz MW, Zlomke KR: Linking cognitive avoidance and GAD symptoms: the mediating role of fear of emotion. Behav Res Ther 48(5):435–441, 2010 20096399

Ramsawh HJ, Raffa SD, Edelen MO, et al: Anxiety in middle adulthood: effects of age and time on the 14-year course of panic disorder, social phobia and generalized anxiety disorder. Psychol Med 39(4):615–624, 2009 18667095

Robins LN, Wing J, Wittchen HU, et al: The Composite International Diagnostic Interview: an epidemiologic instrument suitable for use in conjunction with different diagnostic systems and in different cultures. Arch Gen Psychiatry 45(12):1069–1077, 1988 2848472

Rodriguez BF, Weisberg RB, Pagano ME, et al: Characteristics and predictors of full and partial recovery from generalized anxiety disorder in primary care patients. J Nerv Ment Dis 194(2):91–97, 2006 16477186

Roemer L, Lee JK, Salters-Pedneault K, et al: Mindfulness and emotion regulation difficulties in generalized anxiety disorder: preliminary evidence for independent and overlapping contributions. Behav Ther 40(2):142–154, 2009 19433145

Rubio G, López-Ibor JJ: Generalized anxiety disorder: a 40-year follow-up study. Acta Psychiatr Scand 115(5):372–379, 2007 17430415

Ruscio AM, Chiu WT, Roy-Byrne P, et al: Broadening the definition of generalized anxiety disorder: effects on prevalence and associations with other disorders in the National Comorbidity Survey Replication. J Anxiety Disord 21(5):662–676, 2007 17118626

Ruscio AM, Hallion LS, Lim CCW, et al: Cross-sectional comparison of the epidemiology of DSM-5 generalized anxiety disorder across the globe. JAMA Psychiatry 74(5):465–475, 2017 28297020

Rygh JL, Sanderson WC: Treating Generalized Anxiety Disorder. New York, Guilford, 2004

Sareen J, Cox BJ, Clara I, et al: The relationship between anxiety disorders and physical disorders in the U.S. National Comorbidity Survey. Depress Anxiety 21(4):193–202, 2005 16075453

Schonfeld WH, Verboncoeur CJ, Fifer SK, et al: The functioning and well-being of patients with unrecognized anxiety disorders and major depressive disorder. J Affect Disord 43(2):105–119, 1997 9165380

Shear MK, Vander Bilt J, Rucci P, et al: Reliability and validity of a structured interview guide for the Hamilton Anxiety Rating Scale (SIGH-A). Depress Anxiety 13(4):166–178, 2001 11413563

Shear K, Belnap BH, Mazumdar S, et al: Generalized Anxiety Disorder Severity Scale (GADSS): a preliminary validation study. Depress Anxiety 23(2):77–82, 2006 16411185

Sheehan DV, Lecrubier Y, Sheehan KH, et al: The Mini-International Neuropsychiatric Interview (M.I.N.I.): the development and validation of a structured diagnostic psychiatric interview for DSM-IV and ICD-10. J Clin Psychiatry 59(suppl 20):22–33, quiz 34–57, 1998

Spitzer RL, Kroenke K, Williams JBW, et al: A brief measure for assessing generalized anxiety disorder: the GAD-7. Arch Intern Med 166(10):1092–1097, 2006 16717171

Stein DJ: Generalised anxiety disorder. S Afr J Psychiatry 19(3):175–179, 2013

Steiner M, Allgulander C, Ravindran A, et al: Gender differences in clinical presentation and response to sertraline treatment of generalized anxiety disorder. Hum Psychopharmacol 20(1):3–13, 2005 15551351

Vos T, Abajobir AA, Abbafati C, et al: Global, regional, and national incidence, prevalence, and years lived with disability for 328 diseases and injuries for 195 countries, 1990–2016: a systematic analysis for the Global Burden of Disease Study 2016. Lancet 390(10100):1211–1259, 2017 28919117

World Health Organization: Composite International Diagnostic Interview (CIDI). Geneva, World Health Organization, 1990

Wittchen HU: Generalized anxiety disorder: prevalence, burden, and cost to society. Depress Anxiety 16(4):162–171, 2002 12497648

Wittchen H-U, Lieb R, Pfister H, et al: The waxing and waning of mental disorders: evaluating the stability of syndromes of mental disorders in the population. Compr Psychiatry 41(2 suppl 1):122–132, 2000 10746914

Wittchen H-U, Kessler RC, Beesdo K, et al: Generalized anxiety and depression in primary care: prevalence, recognition, and management. J Clin Psychiatry 63(8 suppl 8):24–34, 2002

Wittchen HU, Jacobi F, Rehm J, et al: The size and burden of mental disorders and other disorders of the brain in Europe 2010. Eur Neuropsychopharmacol 21(9):655–679, 2011 21896369

Yonkers KA, Bruce SE, Dyck IR, et al: Chronicity, relapse, and illness—course of panic disorder, social phobia, and generalized anxiety disorder: findings in men and women from 8 years of follow-up. Depress Anxiety 17(3):173–179, 2003 12768651

Zigmond AS, Snaith RP: The Hospital Anxiety and Depression Scale. Acta Psychiatr Scand 67(6):361–370, 1983 6880820

Recommended Readings

Andrews G, Hobbs MJ, Borkovec TD, et al: Generalized worry disorder: a review of DSM-IV generalized anxiety disorder and options for DSM-V. Depress Anxiety 27:134–147, 2010

Beesdo K, Pine DS, Lieb R, et al: Incidence and risk patterns of anxiety and depressive disorders and categorization of generalized anxiety disorder. Arch Gen Psychiatry 67(1):47–57, 2010

Behar E, DiMarco ID, Hekler EB, et al: Current theoretical models of generalized anxiety disorder (GAD): conceptual review and treatment implications. J Anxiety Disord 23(8):1011–1023, 2009 19700258

Mahoney AEJ, Hobbs MJ, Newby JM, et al: Maladaptive behaviours associated with generalized anxiety disorder: an item response theory analysis. Behav Cogn Psychother 46(4):479–496, 2018 29553003

Ruscio AM, Hallion LS, Lim CCW, et al: Cross-sectional comparison of the epidemiology of DSM-5 generalized anxiety disorder across the globe. JAMA Psychiatry 74(5):465–475, 2017 28297020

CHAPTER 12

Pathogenesis of Generalized Anxiety Disorder

Amina Sutherland-Stolting, M.D.

Betty Liao, Ph.D.

Karen Kraus, M.D.

Craig Campbell, M.D.

Andrew W. Goddard, M.D.

Generalized anxiety disorder (GAD) is a chronic anxiety disorder characterized by a constellation of symptoms, including uncontrollable and excessive worrying, that influences behavior, mood, and overall functioning (see DSM-5; American Psychiatric Association 2013). Although worrying is a universal human experience, pathological worry is remarkable less for its content than for its severity and negative impact on functioning (Rabner et al. 2017). When compared with healthy subjects, individuals with a GAD diagnosis have more frequent negative intrusions and are more distressed by their anxious preoccupations (Hirsch et al. 2013). Associated symptoms of GAD, such as fatigue, restlessness, and irritability, also cause distress, are chronic, and are frequently underrecognized in general medical settings (Stein and Sareen 2015). Community surveys have observed a lifetime prevalence of GAD from 5.7% to 8.6% (Harvard Medical School 2007; Kessler et al. 2008), with lifetime estimates of experiencing any anxiety disorder up to 38% (Merikangas et al. 2010). Impairment in functioning and quality of life is a consistent finding among patients with GAD. In addition, patients with GAD had worse rates of remission than those with major depressive disorder (MDD), and the economic burden of illness, including costs of medical care and absenteeism, has been estimated to be even higher than for MDD or panic disorder (Bereza et al. 2012). Prognosis and treatment are frequently complicated by comorbid psychiatric disorders such as MDD, panic disorder, and substance use disorders. Thus, GAD is a significant public health concern.

In this chapter, we review multiple factors that have been implicated in the pathogenesis and maintenance of GAD. Biological factors we review include key findings from the fields of genetics, neurochemistry, neuropharmacology, functional brain imaging, neuroendocrinology, and immunology. Finally, we synthesize biological and psychosocial factors into several psychobiological models of GAD.

Biological Factors

Genetics

Genetic contributions to morbid anxiety have been an important focus of clinical investigation. Family studies data suggest a four- to fivefold lifetime risk increase of developing an anxiety disorder among first-degree relatives (Isomura et al. 2015), and recent twin studies examining anxious traits have observed heritability rates ranging from 0.32 to 0.42 (Gottschalk and Domschke 2017). Analysis of monozygotic twin data showed variability in phenotypic (anxiety) expression, despite identical DNA material, consistent with our understanding of anxiety as a complex human trait (Davies et al. 2015). Intergenerational analysis of children of twins demonstrated anxiety as a quality conveyed by environmental exposure more than by genetic heritability (Eley et al. 2015). Children of monozygotic twins had higher correlations of anxious and neurotic measures with their twin parent in comparison with an avuncular relative.

Polymorphisms of 5-HTTLPR, located in the promoter region of the serotonin transporter gene, have been identified as possible candidate genes for anxiety disorders because of their association with impaired serotonin reuptake (Lesch et al. 1996). Presence of these variants is more commonly seen in patients with GAD than in control subjects and may sensitize corticolimbic pathways to decreased stress resilience and increased anxiety (Hariri and Holmes 2006). More recent investigations into the candidacy of 5-HTTLPR have found that presence of the polymorphic short allele did not confer significant association with mood disorders in the context of stressful life events (Risch et al. 2009). Inconsistencies in these results may be due to possible gender difference, with male homozygous 5-HTTLPR short variant carriers reporting increased anxiety and neuroticism in comparison with heterozygotes and women (Chang et al. 2017). Additional studies have highlighted coding and noncoding regions as possible areas worthy of further investigation in the etiology of generalized anxiety, including a significant single-nucleotide polymorphism (SNP), RBFOX1, which was observed in twin subjects (Davies et al. 2015). Genome-wide association studies (GWASs) in a study of more than 12,000 Hispanic or Latino patients identified a region on chromosome 6, rs78602344, as a common finding in patients with GAD. However, this study was unable to reproduce significant findings in more refined analysis.

Despite data demonstrating familial clustering, localization of genes that may portend risk for development of anxiety disorders has yielded modest results. Information from the Brainstorm Consortium was analyzed by a compilation of GWASs with the goal of identifying patterns of heritability and genetic associations (Anttila et al. 2018). In comparison with neurological disorders such as epilepsy and Parkinson's disease, psychiatric disorders, including anxiety and MDD, were less genetically distinct and shared more common variant alleles representing risk factors. This calls into question the suitability of current nosological classifications of psychiatric disorders, given the genetic overlap among them.

Neurochemistry

Norepinephrine

Functioning as both hormone and neurotransmitter, norepinephrine is a catecholamine that activates the sympathetic nervous system (SNS), producing a physiological stress response. Somatic symptoms of SNS activation, including tachycardia and diaphoresis, are common presenting complaints for patients with GAD (Yamamoto et al. 2014). In prior preclinical studies, the relationship between norepinephrine system activation and anxiogenesis has been well documented. For example, electrical stimulation of the locus coeruleus (LC), a primary norepinephrine nucleus in the pons, promoted norepinephrine release, with attendant stress-related fear behaviors (McCall et al. 2017). Conversely, blockade of LC neuronal activity during conditions of stress decreased anxious behaviors. Chronic stress exposure also has yielded information regarding anxiety and norepinephrine system functioning. Norepinephrine plasma levels were increased in rodents with long-term stress exposure. Higher levels were correlated with increased α_2 receptor binding sites, suggesting that chronic anxiety resulted in norepinephrine system upregulation. Pathological states involving excessive norepinephrine production have been investigated to analyze possible causality. Interestingly, Starkman et al. (1990) reported that in patients with pheochromocytoma, high levels of norepinephrine and epinephrine were not associated with an additional diagnosis of GAD. In contrast, Paine et al. (2015), using urinary norepinephrine metabolite concentrations as a measure of sympathetic activation in hypertensive patients with self-reported anxiety, observed higher concentrations of epinephrine but not norepinephrine. However, monitoring of plasma levels of norepinephrine in anxiety states has yielded mixed results; thus, utilization of peripheral norepinephrine levels as a stress-sensitive biomarker has not been clinically applicable (Ryff et al. 2006).

Serotonin

Serotonin (5-HT), another monoamine neurotransmitter, is found widely throughout the body, including the CNS, intestines, and blood platelets. In the CNS, serotonin-producing neurons are grouped largely in the brainstem raphe nuclei. Furthermore, preclinical and human studies have highlighted the commonality of altered serotonin levels in GAD and anxious states, although it remains unclear if these findings are consistent with a prognostic or causal relationship. Transgenic murine models with disrupted serotonin activity repeatedly demonstrated increased anxiogenesis, decreased socialization, and decreased stress resilience (Stein and Sareen 2015). After administering a serotonin-specific depleting agent, *p*-chlorophenylalanine, to rats, investigators reported increased stress behaviors such as avoidance, sensitivity, and irritability.

In humans, increased serotonin neuronal activity, synthesis, and serotonin transporter availability were more prevalent in anxious-trait patients than healthy subjects (Furmark et al. 2016). Earlier studies using pharmacological challenge paradigms to probe serotonin system function reported both anxiolytic and anxiogenic effects and even anger (Germine et al. 1992; Handley et al. 1993). Such diverse emotional responses to serotonin system activation do not fit with the simple notion that excessive serotonin neurotransmission equates to heightened anxiousness. Rather, in anxiety and mood states, serotonin function may be dysregulated in different components of the fear circuit, with loss of the organism's stress-buffering capacity. In this scheme, serotonin fluctuations (decreased in some areas and excessive in others) may confer fear behaviors or mood disturbance. In addition, inconsistency in results may be due to diversity of serotonin receptor subtypes and their response to varying degrees of antagonism or agonism (Bourin 2015).

Activity of serotonin receptors and the serotonin transporter (5-HTT) has been studied in GAD. Early suppression or overexpression of serotonin receptors in mice led to variations in stress resilience, suggesting that early factors in receptor modulation may be responsible for lifelong proneness to exaggerated stress responses (Albert et al. 2014). In human studies, polymorphisms in 5-HTT alleles have been associated with trait anxiety (Murakami et al. 1999). Thus, the serotonin transporter and impairment of serotonin reuptake remain important targets for clinical drug development, as do serotonin receptor subtypes (e.g., $5-HT_4$ and $5-HT_6$) (Yohn et al. 2017).

Dopamine

Dopamine is synthesized in the brain and kidneys and functions as a neurotransmitter regulating several pathways, including those involved with reward and mood regulation. Deficits in dopamine, as related to the mesolimbic "reward" pathway, are implicated in anhedonia, a characteristic of MDD, a mood disorder frequently comorbid with GAD (Der-Avakian and Markou 2012). In animal studies, stressful stimuli activate dopaminergic systems as evidenced by increased release of dopamine. De La Garza and Mahoney (2004) reported increased dopamine metabolism after acute stress in the nucleus accumbens and amygdala in rats with anxious phenotypes versus control subjects. Preclinical studies also have revealed that altering dopamine excitation signaling correlated with generalized anxiety–like behaviors in mice confronted with aversive situations. These behaviors were resolved when abnormal dopamine signaling was corrected, further underscoring the relevance of the dopamine system in preventing the development of anxiety (Zweifel et al. 2011). Dopamine transport receptor knockout animal models produced increased extracellular dopamine and heightened anxiety-like behaviors; conversely, antagonism of the dopamine transporter led to anxiolysis (Kacprzak et al. 2017).

Human studies measuring dopamine release in patients with generalized social anxiety disorder were unable to detect a difference in receptor availability at baseline and after pharmacological stress with *d*-amphetamine (Schneier et al. 2009). To determine whether dopamine receptor polymorphisms played a role in the efficacy of medication management, Saung et al. (2014) stratified subjects based on dopamine transporter polymorphisms. However, using venlafaxine as the study treatment, they did not observe any significant difference between treatment responders and nonresponders. Of clinical relevance, anxiety disorders are common psychiatric comorbidities reported in Parkinson's disease, with an elevated GAD prevalence of up to 55% compared with control subjects (Broen et al. 2016); this suggests anxiety disorders are a risk factor for Parkinson's disease, given the prevalence of psychiatric symptoms prior to onset of movement disturbances. Sugama et al. (2016) illustrated that exposure to chronic stress resulted in statistically significant loss of neuronal tyrosine hydroxylase activity, an enzyme required for normal dopamine synthesis. Atrophy of substantia nigra pars compacta and the norepinephrine-containing LC confers specific risk for the development of Parkinson's disease.

GABA

The amino acid neurotransmitter GABA, the primary inhibitory CNS neurotransmitter, is present in most brain regions. Also, the benzodiazepine anxiolytics are well-described full agonists at the $GABA_A$ receptor complex, which increases the efficacy of native GABA at the receptor. Because of the compelling link between antianxiety treatments and GABA, the GABA neuronal system has been an important focus of research into the pathophysiology of human anxiety (Nutt and Malizia 2001).

Identification of GABA receptor genes that correlate with anxiety disorders has localized several possible candidate genes. Polymorphisms in the GABA transporter gene *SLC6A1* were associated with human anxiety disorders (Thoeringer et al. 2009). Additionally, two identified SNPs correlated with panic severity and were associated with an increase in disease odds ratio. This is of clinical relevance because tiagabine, a GABA transporter (GAT1)-selective inhibitor, has demonstrated effectiveness in decreasing anxious symptoms that is comparable to antidepressants (Rosenthal 2003). Conversely, Pham et al. (2009) did not find any statistically significant correlation between $GABA_A$ receptor gene SNPs and anxious phenotypes. Heldt and Ressler (2007) and Müller et al. (2015) examined the relationship between amygdalar GABA transmission, GABA isoenzyme glutamic acid decarboxylase 67 (GAD67) function, and anxious behaviors. In these studies, GAD67 knockout mice displayed increased anxiety and fear, impaired fear extinction, and diminished anxiolytic responses to benzodiazepine administration.

GABAergic neurons exert inhibitory control over pathways linked to the amygdala, where homeostasis between GABA and glutamate neurotransmission is thought to be responsible for appropriate emotional regulation. An analysis of motor cortical excitability used paired-pulse transcranial magnetic stimulation to monitor the influence of $GABA_A$ and $GABA_B$ transmission in drug-naive patients with GAD (Li et al. 2017). Data reported that deficits in intercortical facilitation, a process of neural communication regulated by $GABA_A$ and $GABA_B$ receptors, correlated with an abnormal increase in symptoms of anxiety in patients with GAD. These findings suggest that excitatory deficits instead of inhibition may be a processing characteristic in patients with GAD and a predictor of anxiety. Another study of the central benzodiazepine receptors found that benzodiazepine binding is significantly decreased in the left temporal pole of patients with GAD, and the density distribution of these cerebral benzodiazepine receptors is more homogeneous than in control subjects (Tiihonen et al. 1997), providing evidence for deficits in GABA function in GAD. Further assessment of the GABA neuronal system with molecular genetics and neuroimaging genetics techniques is warranted to determine the precise nature of GABA-related dysfunction in GAD.

Glutamate

Preclinical studies have demonstrated a key role for the amygdala/extended amygdala in the mammalian fear circuit, especially with respect to the acquisition and expression of conditioned fear (Garakani et al. 2006). The lateral amygdala seems to be responsible for key elements of fear conditioning (Shumyatsky et al. 2002), because disruptions of this area can interfere with the acquisition of conditioned fear and conditioned fear memories (Blair et al. 2005). Glutamate receptors, including NMDA and G protein–coupled metabotropic receptors (mGLur1–8), are distributed throughout the brain with increased density in mood-significant limbic and cortical regions such as the amygdala and dorsolateral prefrontal cortex, regions heavily implicated in emotional and fear processing. Cortese et al. (2010), inducing risk-taking behavior in rats via sleep deprivation, detected a significant decrease in prefrontal cortex measured glutamate activity. Additional studies have noted that decreased glutamate excitation results in anxiolytic responses, whereas inhibition of NMDA receptors in the amygdala can facilitate fear extinction (Bergink et al. 2004). Other preclinical studies of glutamate in anxiety have examined the synaptic protein (SAPAP/DLGAP), which modulates glutamate activity pre- and postsynaptically via regulation of glutamate receptor activity. Knockout DLGAP3 mice demonstrated increased fearful behaviors and OCD-like symptoms such as excessive grooming and hair removal (Welch et al. 2007). Furthermore, human imaging studies have observed a relationship between alterations in glutamate concentrations and level of anxiety. For instance, using magnetic resonance spectroscopy techniques, Modi et al. (2014) reported that in healthy subjects ($n=24$), elevated resting-state anterior cingulate glutamate and glutamine levels predicted high trait anxiety versus low trait anxiety.

Glutamate also may play an important role in the promotion of fear extinction via modulation of amygdaloid NMDA receptors. Memantine, a noncompetitive NMDA receptor antagonist used to enhance memory in patients with Alzheimer's disease, also has been found to have anxiolytic properties in some animal studies (Bertoglio and Carobrez 2003). Use of ketamine, a noncompetitive NMDA receptor antagonist, as a treatment for pathological anxiety is also now a growing area of research. Studies with intravenous ketamine thus far have noted its rapid anxiolytic effects, sustained action, and general tolerability (Feder et al. 2014; Glue et al. 2017). Riluzole, a glutamate modulator currently FDA approved for the treatment of amyotrophic lateral sclerosis, has been studied in the treatment of various affective and anxiety disorders, including GAD. Over an 8-week period, a sample of patients with GAD treated with riluzole showed discernible clinical improvement, with a significant percentage achieving remission (Mathew et al. 2005). Follow-up larger-scale GAD trials with riluzole-like agents are under way, including a multisite randomized controlled trial of BHV-4157, troriluzole (clinicaltrials.gov, NCT 03829241).

Neuropeptides/Orexins

Orexins, a pair of neuropeptides discovered in the late 1990s, are known to promote wakefulness and arousal. The posterior regions of the hypothalamus, where orexin-producing neurons are located, have been shown to influence circadian rhythms at rest and under conditions of stress (DiMicco et al. 2002). Acute stressors may result in higher cerebrospinal fluid and plasma orexins, whereas chronic stress states produce lower levels (Strawn et al. 2010). Chronic activation of the orexin system results in a positive feedback loop furthering release of orexin; persistent release could contribute to maintenance of an anxious state and influence other symptoms, including insomnia. Li et al. (2010) showed an increase in anxious behaviors in murine models given direct administration (via injection) of orexin receptor agonists, as well as decreased anxious behaviors after administration of orexin antagonists. Nollet et al. (2012) demonstrated decreases in both anxious behaviors and physiological stress responses in rodents after administration of an orexin antagonist. Anxiolytic effects were similar to administration of the antidepressant fluoxetine, although the antidepressant showed reversal of hypothalamic-pituitary-adrenal (HPA) axis stress-induced dysregulation. The mixed orexin receptor antagonist suvorexant is currently FDA approved for the treatment of insomnia. Nakamura and Nagamine (2017) administered suvorexant to inpatient psychiatric patients with varying diagnoses and reported significant improvement in anxiety and mood scores from baseline after 4 weeks of treatment. Thus, orexin antagonists have promise as a new class of anxiolytics; however, to date, no GAD trials have been conducted with them.

Neuropeptide Y

Neuropeptide Y (NPY) is a peptide neurotransmitter with a role in emotionality, appetite, and substance use. It is the most commonly found neuropeptide in the human brain, and activity of NPY systems has been linked to regulation of anxiety-related responses. Roseboom et al. (2014) measured NPY levels in primates and observed that increased NPY activity and metabolism in the amygdala was related to low trait anxiety. Investigations using homozygous NPY-negative knockout mice showed a significant increase in anxious behaviors (Bannon et al. 2000). Human studies have shown similar results, with NPY cerebrospinal fluid levels being abnormally low in individuals who developed PTSD after exposure to military combat (Sah et al. 2014). This further supports the hypothesis that proper NPY functioning confers resilience in anxiety-inducing situations and that an environment change may result in dynamic NPY expression. In preclinical studies, injection of NPY resulted in anxiolysis and suppression of physiological stress responses and behaviors as observed in Vogel conflict tests (Heilig and Murison 1987). Intranasal administration of NPY yielded anxiolytic effects in rats, and current human trials have shown tolerability and a dose-dependent decrease in anxiety compared with placebo (Sayed et al. 2018). As evidence continues to mount regarding the role of neuropeptides in anxiety and stress mediation, translational research studies will need to further explore the safety and clinical relevance of NPY as a therapeutic target.

Neuroendocrinology/Immunology

Generalized anxiety may occur in the presence of endocrine disorders and following exogenous hormone administration. Furthermore, the HPA axis is an important feedback circuit that triggers the release of multiple hormones during stress, eventually resulting in the release of cortisol from the adrenal glands.

Although the HPA system is activated by stressors, results of studies investigating cortisol levels in GAD have been mixed: hypercortisolemia has been reported at baseline in patients with GAD (Mantella et al. 2008). However, evidence of hypocortisolemia has also been noted in hair samples of patients with GAD in comparison with control subjects, suggestive of undersecretion of cortisol during states of chronically heightened stress (Steudte et al. 2011). Diurnal patterns of adults and adolescents with GAD versus control subjects were also variable (Tafet et al. 2001). However, endocrine biomarkers have demonstrated utility for correlating traditional measures of anxiety in dynamic settings and for monitoring response. Adrenocorticotropin hormone and cortisol are some of the key stress hormones that have been investigated as important biomarkers in evaluation of stress and anxiety.

Additionally, the HPA axis plays a role in regulating immune processes. Abnormal levels of hormones, including cortisol, are associated with either proinflammatory or suppressed immunological responses. The Netherlands Study of Depression and Anxiety, which evaluated data from more than 2,800 adult participants, reported statistically significant elevations in C-reactive protein (CRP), interleukin-6, and tumor necrosis factor alpha (TNF-α) in subjects with increased cognitive and somatic symptoms of anxiety (Duivis et al. 2013). Men, but not women, with an anxiety disorder had higher levels of CRP, potentially due to hormonal differences and variation in lifetime stressor exposure. Furthermore, the study also detected correlations between medications and biomarkers, with decreased CRP noted in individuals receiving selective serotonin reuptake inhibitors and increased TNF-α in those receiving tricyclic antidepressants. Psychoneuroimmunology as a field suggests many avenues of clinical importance for novel anxiolytic treatment development. For example, Yang et al. (2016) demonstrated that injection of a lipopolysaccharide in mice triggered an inflammatory chemokine response and induced anxiety. In the presence of these inflammatory agents, animals that received chemokine receptor antagonists had reduced anxiety-like behaviors. A similar animal study examined post-lipopolysaccharide exposure inflammatory responses and reported decreases in both behavioral and physiological anxiety-related characteristics in the population treated with the antibiotic minocycline (Majidi et al. 2016).

Further research examining pro- and anti-inflammatory proteins may yield promising immunotherapy targets for anxiety in the future. Inhibition of production of cytokines and other inflammatory entities such as prostaglandins has led to the evaluation of cyclooxygenase (COX-2) inhibitors for the treatment of mood disorders. In animal/mouse models, administration of COX-2 inhibitors and substrate-selective COX-2 inhibitors resulted in decreases in onset of both stress-induced symptoms and fear behaviors (Gamble-George et al. 2016). In a randomized placebo-controlled trial, Müller et al. (2006) noted decreased depressive symptoms with the addition of celecoxib, a COX-2 inhibitor, in combination with the antidepressant reboxetine. These findings have implications for future GAD treatment strategies.

Functional Neuroanatomy

The functional neuroanatomy of GAD is being explicated via increasingly sophisticated preclinical and clinical study methods. Experimental study of fear responses to threats has generated information regarding areas of the brain that are activated during fear processing (e.g., amygdala, hippocampus, hypothalamus, prefrontal cortex) (LeDoux 2000). Biological distinctions between GAD and other mood and anxiety disorders are becoming more feasible as novel CNS biomarkers distinguish between diagnostic groups, even when symptom presentations overlap.

Analysis of brain connectivity and circuitry was performed on subjects with either GAD, MDD, or comorbid GAD and MDD using resting-state functional MRI (fMRI) (Oathes et al. 2015). During task-independent brain activity, anxiety and distress were correlated with increasing signaling in limbic and paralimbic regions and increased connectivity in the anterior cingulate cortex and ventral striatum, an area of the brain associated with behavioral processes such as motivation and reward conditioning. Connectivity data for patients with MDD had a profile distinct from patients with GAD, further supporting claims that our current classification of affective and anxiety disorders has significant limitations. Aberrant signaling in these areas also is supported by anatomical studies. For example, investigators demonstrated abnormally increased gray matter volume in the basal ganglia and decreased white matter in the dorsolateral prefrontal cortex in GAD (Hilbert et al. 2015). Lower white matter volumes in this region correlated with findings of impairment in working memory due to stress exposure, which is of clinical functional significance. However, in healthy subjects, administration of anxiety-inducing cholecystokinin-4 did not produce a distinct pattern of neural activation (Eser et al. 2009). Higher amygdalar activation was seen in subjects who reported higher ratings of fear, but differences were not statistically significant. Fear activation in healthy subjects may occur without a predictable neural pattern, which contrasts with a more uniform activation for patients with an anxiety disorder. Although amygdalar activation is a consistent end result, this finding suggests an adaptation of processing in anxiety disorders, which is established prior to introduction of an acute threat.

The limbic system includes the hippocampus, which is involved in behavioral monitoring, understanding, and conflict processing. Resting and task-activated changes in hippocampal circuit activity were assessed in GAD, PTSD, and healthy comparison subjects (Chen and Etkin 2013). fMRI findings noted nonsignificant decreased anterior and posterior hippocampal connectivity in GAD (and PTSD) subjects in comparison with healthy control subjects, although no volumetric differences in gray matter were found. Connectivity patterns were also able to differentiate between GAD and PTSD, suggesting that fear extinction and fear recall mechanisms are under distinct regulation. Hippocampal dysfunction, via interaction with other brain regions including the prefrontal cortex, amygdala, and basal ganglia, can result in altered communication in the mood regulation network. Additional volumetric studies reported decreased hippocampal volumes in GAD as well as dysfunctional connectivity to the orbitofrontal cortex (Hettema et al. 2012). These findings implicate disrupted hippocampo-cortical communication in the pathogenesis of generalized anxiety.

To determine if a specific abnormality in connectivity could be associated with GAD, other investigators examined connectivity patterns in GAD at several areas within the amygdala (Etkin et al. 2009). Evaluation of the amygdalar basolateral complex, associated with encoding fear and threat memories, was examined using fMRI and voxel-based morphometry. Findings from animal connectivity models were confirmed; in GAD the basolateral complex was connected to cortical regions associated with recall of fear, including the prefrontal cortex. Decreased severity of anxiety was correlated with increasing connectivity, which suggested that this activity was an adaptive strategy to offset dysfunction. Similarly, Bishop et al. (2004) reported decreased activity in the prefrontal cortex in subjects with higher trait anxiety. These results support the theory of loss of "top down" control in GAD, because the prefrontal cortex is associated with regulation of excessive anxiety.

In addition, dysfunction in decision making and reinforcement has been reported in GAD. White et al. (2017) conducted a task activation fMRI study and observed increased activity in healthy subjects versus patients with GAD that correlated with enhanced error correction. Decreased modulation of activity at the cingulate cortex/dorsomedial prefrontal cortex, anterior insular cortex, and posterior cingulate cortex correlated with increased uncertainty in decision making for subjects with GAD. This disruption in feedback may further sustain poor decision making and continued worry in GAD.

Importantly, fear-circuit neural connections may be malleable and responsive to treatment. For example, after a 7-week treatment trial with citalopram, patients ($n=6$) with GAD had decreased fMRI amygdala activation in response to anxiety-inducing and neutral stimuli (Hoehn-Saric et al. 2004). Other groups have evaluated activation of regions of interest during anticipatory tasks in healthy control subjects (Aupperle et al. 2011). With prescan administration of pregabalin, a dose-dependent blunting of activation occurred in the amygdala and insula, which represented a moderation of emotional response with anticipation of negative stimuli. Thus, functional imaging may be useful in determining the anxiolytic potential of new pharmacological treatments and in assessing responses in patients, in addition to self-report.

Psychobiological Models

Both biological and psychosocial factors appear to contribute to the development and maintenance of GAD. However, a single explanatory model for GAD has yet to emerge. Its primary features can be considered dimensions of vulnerability in etiological models (Clark et al. 1994). In considering a risk/diathesis model, Kendler (1996) suggested that events involving danger are distinctly associated with developing anxiety; in contrast, facing profound loss (especially early loss) is associated with developing clinical depression. Other earlier theories integrating this information posited a CNS behavioral inhibition system (Gray 1988). This theory proposed that the septohippocampal area is responsible for processing threat-relevant stimuli. The presence of danger activates the behavioral inhibition system, resulting in increased arousal and inhibition of all regular behaviors. Noradrenergic and serotonergic stimulation of the septohippocampal region further activates this system. Gray (1988) proposed that this increased state of vigilance is analogous to the GAD syndrome. More recent iterations of Gray's model also include the amygdala and prefrontal cortex as components of the behavioral inhibition system. Alternatively, Cloninger (1986) proposed a model in which inherited abnormalities in neurotransmitter systems cause personality traits that could manifest as GAD. He focused on three aspects of personality—novelty seeking, harm avoidance, and reward dependence, which he argued are determined by monoamine activity. Several studies support the idea that novelty seeking is associated with low basal dopaminergic activity, harm avoidance is seen in individuals with high serotonergic activity, and reward dependence results from low basal noradrenergic activity (Cloninger 1986). More modern theories consider GAD to be a fear network disorder with potential dysregulation between fear-circuit structures contributing to symptomatology. For example, as noted earlier, investigators have found fMRI evidence of intra-amygdala dysfunction and frontoparietal network (executive control) overcompensation in GAD, which could account for cognitive and physiological symptoms (Etkin et al. 2009). Other groups have posited that clinical features of GAD such as chronic stress and hyperarousal may be due to overactivation and long-term changes in a structure near the amygdala, the bed nucleus of the stria terminalis, an important node in sustained threat monitoring (Avery et al. 2016). Thus, in the Research Domain Criteria framework, dimensions of GAD psychopathology may prove to be due to circuits subserving the negative valence domain and the sustained threat construct within that domain. Moreover, evolving neurodevelopmental theories provide accounts of how early adversity and experience may affect long-term fear-circuit function and risk for adult mood and anxiety spectrum disorders (Meyer and Lee 2019).

Key Points

- Generalized anxiety disorder (GAD) is a high-prevalence, chronic anxiety syndrome with morbidity and illness burdens that approximate levels seen in major depressive disorder.

- Comprehensive assessment and classification of GAD should include biological and behavioral domains.

- Biological factors have been implicated in the pathogenesis of GAD. Neurochemical studies have implicated dysregulation in the serotonin, norepinephrine, dopamine, GABA, glutamatergic, and peptide (orexin, neuropeptide Y) transmitter systems. Endocrine and immunological targets are under current investigation as potential biomarkers and treatment strategies. Conclusive candidate genes have yet to be identified; however, family and twin studies imply a strong component of heritability.

- Functional neuroanatomy has illuminated brain regions of interest and dysfunction in neural connectivity in GAD. Components of the human fear circuit that may be of particular relevance include the prefrontal cortex (subserving fear extinction processes), the amygdala (risk assessment processing), and the hippocampus (fear conditioning recall).

- GAD characteristics include overestimation of threat stimuli, behavioral inhibition, and disproportionately high arousal and worry.

- Cognitive factors that portend the emergence and maintenance of GAD include maladaptive recall bias and avoidance strategies.

- Genesis of the anxious temperament is supported by early environment exposure and subsequent neurobiological feedback and adaptation.

References

Albert PR, Vahid-Ansari F, Luckhart C: Serotonin-prefrontal cortical circuitry in anxiety and depression phenotypes: pivotal role of pre- and post-synaptic 5-HT1A receptor expression. Front Behav Neurosci 8:199, 2014 24936175

American Psychiatric Association: Diagnostic and Statistical Manual of Mental Disorders, 5th Edition. Arlington, VA, American Psychiatric Association, 2013

Anttila V, Bulik-Sullivan B, Finucane HK, et al: Analysis of shared heritability in common disorders of the brain. Science 360(6395):1–12, 2018 29930110

Aupperle RL, Ravindran L, Tankersley D, et al: Pregabalin influences insula and amygdala activation during anticipation of emotional images. Neuropsychopharmacology 36(7):1466–1477, 2011 21430645

Avery SN, Clauss JA, Blackford JU: The human BNST: functional role in anxiety and addiction. Neuropsychopharmacology 41(1):126–141, 2016 26105138

Bannon AW, Seda J, Carmouche M, et al: Behavioral characterization of neuropeptide Y knockout mice. Brain Res 868(1):79–87, 2000 10841890

Bereza BG, Machado M, Papadimitropoulos M, et al: A Markov model approach assessing the cost of illness of generalized anxiety disorder in Canada. Neurol Ther 1(1):1, 2012 26000207

Berginck V, van Megen HJ, Westenberg HG: Glutamate and anxiety. Eur Neuropsychopharmacol 14(3):175–183, 2004

Bertoglio LJ, Carobrez AP: Anxiolytic-like effects of NMDA/glycine-B receptor ligands are abolished during the elevated plus-maze trial 2 in rats. Psychopharmacology (Berl) 170(4):335–342, 2003 13680083

Bishop S, Duncan J, Brett M, et al: Prefrontal cortical function and anxiety: controlling attention to threat-related stimuli. Nat Neurosci 7(2):184–188, 2004 14703573

Blair HT, Sotres-Bayon F, Moita MA, et al: The lateral amygdala processes the value of conditioned and unconditioned aversive stimuli. Neuroscience 133(2):561–569, 2005 15878802

Bourin M: Animal models for screening anxiolytic-like drugs: a perspective. Dialogues Clin Neurosci 17(2):295–303, 2015 15878802

Broen MP, Narayen NE, Kuijf ML, et al: Prevalence of anxiety in Parkinson's disease: a systematic review and meta-analysis. Mov Disord 31(8):1125–1133, 2016 27125963

Chang CC, Chang HA, Fang WH, et al: Gender-specific association between serotonin transporter polymorphisms (5-HTTLPR and rs25531) and neuroticism, anxiety and depression in well-defined healthy Han Chinese. J Affect Disord 207:422–428, 2017 27788383

Chen AC, Etkin A: Hippocampal network connectivity and activation differentiates post-traumatic stress disorder from generalized anxiety disorder. Neuropsychopharmacology 38(10):1889–1898, 2013 23673864

Clark LA, Watson D, Mineka S: Temperament, personality, and the mood and anxiety disorders. J Abnorm Psychol 103(1):103–116, 1994 8040472

Cloninger CR: A unified biosocial theory of personality and its role in the development of anxiety states. Psychiatr Dev 4(3):167–226, 1986 3809156

Cortese BM, Mitchell TR, Galloway MP, et al: Region-specific alteration in brain glutamate: possible relationship to risk-taking behavior. Physiol Behav 99(4):445–450, 2010 20006966

Davies MN, Verdi S, Burri A, et al: Generalised anxiety disorder—a twin study of genetic architecture, genome-wide association and differential gene expression. PLoS One 10(8):e0134865, 2015 26274327

De La Garza R 2nd, Mahoney JJ 3rd: A distinct neurochemical profile in WKY rats at baseline and in response to acute stress: implications for animal models of anxiety and depression. Brain Res 1021(2):209–218, 2004 15342269

Der-Avakian A, Markou A: The neurobiology of anhedonia and other reward-related deficits. Trends Neurosci 35(1):68–77, 2012 22177980

DiMicco JA, Samuels BC, Zaretskaia MV, et al: The dorsomedial hypothalamus and the response to stress: part renaissance, part revolution. Pharmacol Biochem Behav 71(3):469–480, 2002 11830181

Duivis HE, Vogelzangs N, Kupper N, et al: Differential association of somatic and cognitive symptoms of depression and anxiety with inflammation: findings from the Netherlands Study of Depression and Anxiety (NESDA). Psychoneuroendocrinology 38(9):1573–1585, 2013 23399050

Eley TC, McAdams TA, Rijsdijk FV, et al: The intergenerational transmission of anxiety: a children-of-twins study. Am J Psychiatry 172(7):630–637, 2015 25906669

Eser D, Leicht G, Lutz J, et al: Functional neuroanatomy of CCK-4-induced panic attacks in healthy volunteers. Hum Brain Mapp 30(2):511–522, 2009 18095276

Etkin A, Prater KE, Schatzberg AF, et al: Disrupted amygdalar subregion functional connectivity and evidence of a compensatory network in generalized anxiety disorder. Arch Gen Psychiatry 66(12):1361–1372, 2009 19996041

Feder A, Parides MK, Murrough JW, et al: Efficacy of intravenous ketamine for treatment of chronic posttraumatic stress disorder: a randomized clinical trial. JAMA Psychiatry 71(6):681–688, 2014 24740528

Furmark T, Marteinsdottir I, Frick A, et al: Serotonin synthesis rate and the tryptophan hydroxylase-2: G-703T polymorphism in social anxiety disorder. J Psychopharmacol 30(10):1028–1035, 2016 27189957

Gamble-George JC, Baldi R, Halladay L, et al: Cyclooxygenase-2 inhibition reduces stress-induced affective pathology. eLife 5:e14137, 2016 27162170

Garakani A, Mathew SJ, Charney DS: Neurobiology of anxiety disorders and implications for treatment. Mt Sinai J Med 73(7):941–949, 2006 17195879

Germine M, Goddard AW, Woods SW, et al: Anger and anxiety responses to m-chlorophenylpiperazine in generalized anxiety disorder. Biol Psychiatry 32(5):457–461, 1992 1486151

Glue P, Medlicott NJ, Harland S, et al: Ketamine's dose-related effects on anxiety symptoms in patients with treatment refractory anxiety disorders. J Psychopharmacol 31(10):1302–1305, 2017 28441895

Gottschalk MG, Domschke K: Genetics of generalized anxiety disorder and related traits. Dialogues Clin Neurosci 19(2):159–168, 2017 28867940

Gray JA: The neurobiological basis of anxiety, in Handbook of Anxiety Disorder. Edited by Last CG, Hersen M. New York, Pergamon, 1988, pp 10–37

Handley SL, McBlane JW, Critchley MA, et al: Multiple serotonin mechanisms in animal models of anxiety: environmental, emotional and cognitive factors. Behav Brain Res 58(1–2):203–210, 1993 8136047

Hariri AR, Holmes A: Genetics of emotional regulation: the role of the serotonin transporter in neural function. Trends Cogn Sci 10(4):182–191, 2006 16530463

Harvard Medical School: Lifetime prevalence of DSM-IV/WMH-CIDI disorders by sex and cohort (table). National Comorbidity Survey, July 19, 2007. Available at: https://www.hcp.med.harvard.edu/ncs/ftpdir/NCS-R_Lifetime_Prevalence_Estimates.pdf. Accessed June 18, 2019.

Heilig M, Murison R: Intracerebroventricular neuropeptide Y suppresses open field and home cage activity in the rat. Regul Pept 19(3–4):221–231, 1987 3432602

Heldt SA, Ressler KJ: Training-induced changes in the expression of GABAA-associated genes in the amygdala after the acquisition and extinction of Pavlovian fear. Eur J Neurosci 26(12):3631–3644, 2007 18088283

Hettema JM, Kettenmann B, Ahluwalia V, et al: Pilot multimodal twin imaging study of generalized anxiety disorder. Depress Anxiety 29(3):202–209, 2012 21994092

Hilbert K, Pine DS, Muehlhan M, et al: Gray and white matter volume abnormalities in generalized anxiety disorder by categorical and dimensional characterization. Psychiatry Res 234(3):314–320, 2015 26490569

Hirsch CR, Mathews A, Lequertier B, et al: Characteristics of worry in generalized anxiety disorder. J Behav Ther Exp Psychiatry 44(4):388–395, 2013 23651607

Hoehn-Saric R, Schlund MW, Wong SHY: Effects of citalopram on worry and brain activation in patients with generalized anxiety disorder. Psychiatry Res 131(1):11–21, 2004 15246451

Isomura K, Boman M, Rück C, et al: Population-based, multi-generational family clustering study of social anxiety disorder and avoidant personality disorder. Psychol Med 45(8):1581–1589, 2015 25215596

Kacprzak V, Patel NA, Riley E, et al: Dopaminergic control of anxiety in young and aged zebrafish. Pharmacol Biochem Behav 157:1–8, 2017 28408289

Kendler KS: Major depression and generalised anxiety disorder. Same genes, (partly) different environments—revisited. Br J Psychiatry Suppl 30(30):68–75, 1996 8864151

Kessler RC, Gruber M, Hettema JM, et al: Co-morbid major depression and generalized anxiety disorders in the National Comorbidity Survey follow-up. Psychol Med 38(3):365–374, 2008 18047766

LeDoux JE: Emotion circuits in the brain. Annu Rev Neurosci 23:155–184, 2000 10845062

Lesch KP, Bengel D, Heils A, et al: Association of anxiety-related traits with a polymorphism in the serotonin transporter gene regulatory region. Science 274(5292):1527–1531, 1996 8929413

Li CT, Lu CF, Lin HC, et al: Cortical inhibitory and excitatory function in drug-naive generalized anxiety disorder. Brain Stimul 10(3):604–608, 2017 28040450

Li Y, Li S, Wei C, et al: Orexins in the paraventricular nucleus of the thalamus mediate anxiety-like responses in rats. Psychopharmacology (Berl) 212(2):251–265, 2010

Majidi J, Kosari-Nasab M, Salari AA: Developmental minocycline treatment reverses the effects of neonatal immune activation on anxiety- and depression-like behaviors, hippocampal inflammation, and HPA axis activity in adult mice. Brain Res Bull 120:1–13, 2016 26521068

Mantella RC, Butters MA, Amico JA, et al: Salivary cortisol is associated with diagnosis and severity of late-life generalized anxiety disorder. Psychoneuroendocrinology 33(6):773–781, 2008 18407426

Mathew SJ, Amiel JM, Coplan JD, et al: Open-label trial of riluzole in generalized anxiety disorder. Am J Psychiatry 162(12):2379–2381, 2005 16330605

McCall JG, Siuda ER, Bhatti DL, et al: Locus coeruleus to basolateral amygdala noradrenergic projections promote anxiety-like behavior. eLife 6:e18247, 2017 28708061

Merikangas KR, He JP, Burstein M, et al: Lifetime prevalence of mental disorders in U.S. adolescents: results from the National Comorbidity Survey Replication—Adolescent Supplement (NCS-A). J Am Acad Child Adolesc Psychiatry 49(10):980–989, 2010 20855043

Meyer HC, Lee FS: Translating developmental neuroscience to understand risk for psychiatric disorders. Am J Psychiatry 176(3):179–185, 2019 30818985

Modi S, Rana P, Kaur P, et al: Glutamate level in anterior cingulate predicts anxiety in healthy humans: a magnetic resonance spectroscopy study. Psychiatry Res 224(1):34–41, 2014 25156662

Müller N, Schwarz MJ, Dehning S, et al: The cyclooxygenase-2 inhibitor celecoxib has therapeutic effects in major depression: results of a double-blind, randomized, placebo controlled, add-on pilot study to reboxetine. Mol Psychiatry 11(7):680–684, 2006 16491133

Müller I, Çalıskan G, Stork O: The GAD65 knock out mouse—a model for GABAergic processes in fear- and stress-induced psychopathology. Genes Brain Behav 14(1):37–45, 2015 25470336

Murakami F, Shimomura T, Kotani K, et al: Anxiety traits associated with a polymorphism in the serotonin transporter gene regulatory region in the Japanese. J Hum Genet 44(1):15–17, 1999 9929970

Nakamura M, Nagamine T: Neuroendocrine, autonomic, and metabolic responses to an orexin antagonist, suvorexant, in psychiatric patients with insomnia. Innov Clin Neurosci 14(3–4):30–37, 2017 28584695

Nollet M, Gaillard P, Tanti A, et al: Neurogenesis-independent antidepressant-like effects on behavior and stress axis response of a dual orexin receptor antagonist in a rodent model of depression. Neuropsychopharmacology 37(10):2210–2221, 2012 22713907

Nutt DJ, Malizia AL: New insights into the role of the GABA(A)-benzodiazepine receptor in psychiatric disorder. Br J Psychiatry 179:390–396, 2001 11689393

Oathes DJ, Patenaude B, Schatzberg AF, et al: Neurobiological signatures of anxiety and depression in resting-state functional magnetic resonance imaging. Biol Psychiatry 77(4):385–393, 2015 25444162

Paine NJ, Watkins LL, Blumenthal JA, et al: Association of depressive and anxiety symptoms with 24-hour urinary catecholamines in individuals with untreated high blood pressure. Psychosom Med 77(2):136–144, 2015 25647750

Pham X, Sun C, Chen X, et al: Association study between GABA receptor genes and anxiety spectrum disorders. Depress Anxiety 26(11):998–1003, 2009 19842164

Rabner J, Mian ND, Langer DA, et al: The relationship between worry and dimensions of anxiety symptoms in children and adolescents. Behav Cogn Psychother 45(2):124–138, 2017 27852349

Risch N, Herrell R, Lehner T, et al: Interaction between the serotonin transporter gene (5-HTTLPR), stressful life events, and risk of depression: a meta-analysis. JAMA 301(23):2462–2471, 2009 19531786

Roseboom PH, Nanda SA, Fox AS, et al: Neuropeptide Y receptor gene expression in the primate amygdala predicts anxious temperament and brain metabolism. Biol Psychiatry 76(11):850–857, 2014 24342924

Rosenthal M: Tiagabine for the treatment of generalized anxiety disorder: a randomized, open-label, clinical trial with paroxetine as a positive control. J Clin Psychiatry 64(10):1245–1249, 2003 14658975

Ryff CD, Dienberg Love G, Urry HL, et al: Psychological well-being and ill-being: do they have distinct or mirrored biological correlates? Psychother Psychosom 75(2):85–95, 2006 16508343

Sah R, Ekhator NN, Jefferson-Wilson L, et al: Cerebrospinal fluid neuropeptide Y in combat veterans with and without posttraumatic stress disorder. Psychoneuroendocrinology 40:277–283, 2014 24485499

Saung WT, Narasimhan S, Lohoff FW: Lack of influence of DAT1 and DRD2 gene variants on antidepressant response in generalized anxiety disorder. Hum Psychopharmacol 29(4):316–321, 2014 24723432

Sayed S, Van Dam NT, Horn SR, et al: A randomized dose-ranging study of neuropeptide Y in patients with posttraumatic stress disorder. Int J Neuropsychopharmacol 21(1):3–11, 2018 29186416

Schneier FR, Abi-Dargham A, Martinez D, et al: Dopamine transporters, D2 receptors, and dopamine release in generalized social anxiety disorder. Depress Anxiety 26(5):411–418, 2009 19180583

Shumyatsky GP, Tsvetkov E, Malleret G, et al: Identification of a signaling network in lateral nucleus of amygdala important for inhibiting memory specifically related to learned fear. Cell 111(6):905–918, 2002 12526815

Starkman MN, Cameron OG, Nesse RM, et al: Peripheral catecholamine levels and the symptoms of anxiety: studies in patients with and without pheochromocytoma. Psychosom Med 52(2):129–142, 1990 2330387

Stein MB, Sareen J: Clinical practice. Generalized anxiety disorder. N Engl J Med 373(21):2059–2068, 2015 26580998

Steudte S, Stalder T, Dettenborn L, et al: Decreased hair cortisol concentrations in generalised anxiety disorder. Psychiatry Res 186(2–3):310–314, 2011 20889215

Strawn JR, Pyne-Geithman GJ, Ekhator NN, et al: Low cerebrospinal fluid and plasma orexin-A (hypocretin-1) concentrations in combat-related posttraumatic stress disorder. Psychoneuroendocrinology 35(7):1001–1007, 2010 20116928

Sugama S, Sekiyama K, Kodama T, et al: Chronic restraint stress triggers dopaminergic and noradrenergic neurodegeneration: possible role of chronic stress in the onset of Parkinson's disease. Brain Behav Immun 51:39–46, 2016 26291405

Tafet GE, Idoyaga-Vargas VP, Abulafia DP, et al: Correlation between cortisol level and serotonin uptake in patients with chronic stress and depression. Cogn Affect Behav Neurosci 1(4):388–393, 2001 12467090

Thoeringer CK, Ripke S, Unschuld PG, et al: The GABA transporter 1 (SLC6A1): a novel candidate gene for anxiety disorders. J Neural Transm 116(6):649–657, 2009 18607529

Tiihonen J, Kuikka J, Räsänen P, et al: Cerebral benzodiazepine receptor binding and distribution in generalized anxiety disorder: a fractal analysis. Mol Psychiatry 2(6):463–471, 1997 9399689

Welch JM, Lu J, Rodriguiz RM, et al: Cortico-striatal synaptic defects and OCD-like behaviours in Sapap3-mutant mice. Nature 448(7156):894–900, 2007 17713528

White SF, Geraci M, Lewis E, et al: Prediction error representation in individuals with generalized anxiety disorder during passive avoidance. Am J Psychiatry 174(2):110–117, 2017 27631963

Yamamoto K, Shinba T, Yoshii M: Psychiatric symptoms of noradrenergic dysfunction: a pathophysiological view. Psychiatry Clin Neurosci 68(1):1–20, 2014 24372896

Yang L, Wang M, Guo YY, et al: Systemic inflammation induces anxiety disorder through CXCL12/CXCR4 pathway. Brain Behav Immun 56:352–362, 2016 26952745

Yohn CN, Gergues MM, Samuels BA: The role of 5-HT receptors in depression. Mol Brain 10(1):28, 2017 28646910

Zweifel LS, Fadok JP, Argilli E, et al: Activation of dopamine neurons is critical for aversive conditioning and prevention of generalized anxiety. Nat Neurosci 14(5):620–626, 2011 21499253

Recommended Readings

Etkin A, Prater KE, Schatzberg AF, et al: Disrupted amygdalar subregion functional connectivity and evidence of a compensatory network in generalized anxiety disorder. Arch Gen Psychiatry 66(12):1361–1372, 2009 19996041

LeDoux JE, Pine DS: Using neuroscience to help understand fear and anxiety: a two system framework. Am J Psychiatry 173(11):1083–1093, 2016

Patriquin MA, Mathew SJ: The neurobiological mechanisms of generalized anxiety disorder and chronic stress. Chronic Stress (Thousand Oaks) Jan–Dec:1, 2017 29503978

Stein MB, Sareen J: Clinical practice. Generalized anxiety disorder. N Engl J Med 373(21):2059–2068, 2015 26580998

CHAPTER 13

Pharmacotherapy for Generalized Anxiety Disorder

Michael Van Ameringen, M.D., FRCPC

Beth Patterson, B.Sc.N., B.Ed., M.Sc.

Grishma Dabas, B.Sc.

Isobel Sharpe, B.Sc.

Daniel Marrello, B.Sc.

The diagnostic classification of generalized anxiety disorder (GAD) has changed significantly over time, from psychoanalytic theories of neurosis to a more research-based concept that anxiety results from the interaction of neurobiology, psychological factors, and environmental stressors (Rickels and Rynn 2001). The evaluation of pharmacological treatments for GAD has spanned a broad range of drug classes. Industry has turned to GAD as proof of concept of the anxiolytic properties of a drug; virtually every class of psychotropic agent has been tested for GAD efficacy. Although benzodiazepines were long the mainstay of GAD treatment, selective serotonin reuptake inhibitors (SSRIs) and serotonin-norepinephrine reuptake inhibitors (SNRIs) have emerged as the gold standard treatment. Anticonvulsants also have been widely used, and agents from classes such as azapirones, atypical antipsychotics, antihistamines, and β-blockers have been evaluated in GAD. This chapter reviews current evidence for the pharmacotherapy of GAD, specifically focusing on first- and second-line treatments, treatment-refractory conditions, combined treatments, and comorbidity-related issues.

First-Line Treatments

A broad range of pharmacotherapeutic agents are supported by evidence from randomized controlled trials (RCTs) and meta-analyses in GAD. Study details can be found in Table 13–1. First- and second-line treatments were determined using levels of evidence as described in the Canadian Clinical Practice Guidelines (Katzman et al. 2014). Level 1 (the highest) is achieved with a meta-analysis or at least two RCTs that included a placebo condition; level 2 is at least one RCT with placebo or active comparison condition; level 3 is achieved with an uncontrolled trial with at least 10 subjects; level 4 is for anecdotal reports or expert opinion. First-line treatment was considered level-1 or level-2 evidence plus clinical support for efficacy and safety; second-line treatment was level-3 evidence or higher plus clinical support for efficacy and safety.

Antidepressants

Selective Serotonin Reuptake Inhibitors and Serotonin-Norepinephrine Reuptake Inhibitors

Based on their strong efficacy in RCTs and their broad spectrum of action on comorbid conditions, as well as their safety and tolerability profiles, SSRIs and SNRIs are considered first-line agents in the treatment of GAD. Specifically, the SSRIs escitalopram, sertraline, and paroxetine are supported by strong and consistent evidence, with effect sizes ranging from 0.3 to 1.0. The SNRIs duloxetine and venlafaxine extended release (XR) are also supported by multiple RCTs and meta-analyses. Effect sizes for both agents are large: venlafaxine mean deviation 3.31, 95% CI 1.44–5.18 (Li et al. 2017); duloxetine mean deviation 2.32, 95% CI 1.77–2.88 (Li et al. 2018).

In general, head-to-head comparisons show similar efficacy of SSRIs and SNRIs (Qian et al. 2017; Kim et al. 2006), although one study found venlafaxine XR superior to escitalopram (Bose et al. 2008), and one study found venlafaxine XR superior to fluoxetine (Silverstone and Salinas 2001).

Other Antidepressants

Agomelatine has a novel mechanism of action, primarily affecting the hormone melatonin, which is involved in the maintenance of circadian rhythms (Zupancic and Guilleminault 2006). Agomelatine has demonstrated efficacy over placebo in three 12-week double-blind RCTs, with large effect sizes (0.53–1.31), and was found equal in efficacy to escitalopram (Stein et al. 2014). Agomelatine is not currently available in Canada or the United States but has been available in Europe since 2009 and in Australia since 2010.

Vilazodone is a relatively new agent approved by the FDA as an antidepressant in 2011. Three large positive RCTs as well as two meta-analyses have supported its use in GAD, although the effect sizes are relatively low (0.22–0.31) (see Table 13–1).

TABLE 13–1.　Short-term randomized controlled trials

Drug and class	Study	N	Weeks	Design*	Results*	Notes
Selective serotonin reuptake inhibitors (SSRIs)						
Escitalopram RCTs	Davidson et al. 2004	307	8	ESC (10–20) vs. PBO	ESC>PBO	
	Goodman et al. 2005	856	8	ESC (10–20) vs. PBO	ESC>PBO	
	Baldwin et al. 2006	681	12	ESC (5, 10, 20) vs. PAR (20) vs. PBO	ESC (10, 20) > PAR (20) = ESC (5) > PBO	
	Mikami et al. 2014	176	52	ESC (5–10) vs. PBO vs. PST	ESC=PST>PBO	Assessed prevention of poststroke GAD
	Qian et al. 2017	226	8	ESC vs. VEN	ESC=VEN	Brief report
Paroxetine RCTs	Rocca et al. 1997	81	8	PAR (20) vs. IMP (50–100) vs. DIA (3–6)	PAR=IMP=DIA	
	Hewett et al. 2001	364	8	PAR (20–50) vs. PBO	PAR=PBO	
	Pollack et al. 2001	324	8	PAR (20–50) vs. PBO	PAR>PBO	
	Rickels et al. 2003	566	8	PAR (20, 40) vs. PBO	PAR>PBO	
	Feltner et al. 2009	169	4	PAR (20) vs. LOR (1.5 mg tid) vs. PBO	PAR=LOR>PBO	Primarily assessing sensitivity of 15-item DAS-A questionnaire
Sertraline RCTs	Morris et al. 2003	188	12	SER (50–150) vs. PBO	SER>PBO	
	Allgulander et al. 2004	330	12	SER (50–150) vs. PBO	SER> PBO	
	Ball et al. 2005	55	8	SER (25–100) vs. PAR (10–40) vs. PBO	SER=PAR>PBO	
	Steiner et al. 2005	370	12	SER (50–150) vs. PBO	SER>PBO	

TABLE 13–1.   Short-term randomized controlled trials *(continued)*

Drug and class	Study	N	Weeks	Design*	Results*	Notes
Selective serotonin reuptake inhibitors (SSRIs) *(continued)*						
	Brawman-Mintzer et al. 2006a	326	10	SER (50–200) vs. PBO	SER>PBO	
	Schuurmans et al. 2006	84	12	15 sessions CBT vs. SSRI (max dosage 150 mg) vs. PBO	SER>PBO	
Post hoc analyses	Sjodin et al. 2003	188	12	SER (50–150) vs. PBO	SER>PBO	
	Dahl et al. 2005	373	12	SER (50–100) vs. PBO	SER>PBO	
Serotonin norepinephrine reuptake inhibitors (SNRIs)						
Venlafaxine						
RCTs	Davidson et al. 1999	365	8	VEN (75, 150) vs. BUS (30) vs. PBO	VEN>PBO and BUS > PBO on some measures	
	Rickels et al. 2000b	377	8	VEN-XR (75, 150, 225) vs. PBO	VEN-XR (225) > PBO (four of four primary outcome) VEN-XR (150) > PBO (two of four)	Primary outcome was quality of life assessment
	Hackett et al. 2003	540	8	VEN-XR (75 or 150) vs. DIA (15) vs. PBO	VEN=DIA=PBO	High PBO response rate Secondary analysis Subdivided study centers according to ability to detect difference between DIA and PBO on HAM-A total score and showed VEN-XR = DIA>PBO
	Nimatoudis et al. 2004	46	8	VEN (75, 150) vs. PBO	VEN>PBO	
	Kim et al. 2006	60	8	VEN (37.5–225) vs. PAR (10–40)	VEN=PAR	

TABLE 13–1. Short-term randomized controlled trials *(continued)*

Drug and class	Study	N	Weeks	Design*	Results*	Notes
	Bose et al. 2008	392	8	ESC (10–20) vs. VEN-XR (75–225) vs. PBO	VEN=ESC>PBO	
Meta-analysis	Li et al. 2017	3,622	6–10	10 VEN vs. PBO RCTs	VEN >PBO	Effect size: MD 3.31; 95% CI 1.44–5.18
Duloxetine RCTs	Hartford et al. 2007	487	10	DUL (60–120) vs. VEN-XR (75–225) vs. PBO	DUL=VEN >PBO	Greater AE-related discontinuation in DUL+VEN-XR
	Koponen et al. 2007	513	9	DUL (60) vs. DUL (120) vs. PBO	DUL>PBO	
	Rynn et al. 2008	327	10	DUL (60–120 mg) vs. PBO	DUL>PBO	Significantly higher discontinuation due to AEs in DUL vs. PBO
	Nicolini et al. 2009	581	10	DUL (60–120; mean 90± 31.4) vs. DUL(20) vs. VEN (75–225; mean 151.3± 69.5) vs. PBO (2:1:2:2)	DUL=VEN>PBO	
Post hoc analysis	Pollack et al. 2008b	1,163	9–10	Combined data from three RCTs of DUL vs. PBO	DUL>PBO	
Meta-analyses	Allgulander et al. 2007	1,100	9–10	Pooled analysis of three studies DUL (60–120) vs. PBO DUL (60, 120) vs. PBO DUL (60–120) vs. VEN (75–225) vs. PBO	 DUL>PBO DUL>PBO DUL=VEN>PBO	Effect size: DUL vs. PBO (overall): 0.399
	Allgulander et al. 2008	984	10	Pooled analysis of two studies; DUL (60–120) vs. VEN-XR (75–225) vs. PBO	DUL=VEN>PBO	
	Zhang et al. 2016	2,674	9–15	Seven DUL RCTs	DUL>PBO	Effect size: RR 1.48; 95% CI 1.34–1.63
	Li et al. 2018	2,399	9–15	Eight DUL RCTs	DUL>PBO	Effect size: MD 2.32; 95% CI 1.77–2.88

TABLE 13–1.   Short-term randomized controlled trials *(continued)*

Drug and class	Study	N	Weeks	Design*	Results*	Notes
Tricyclic antidepressants (TCAs)						
Imipramine						
RCTs	Hoehn-Saric et al. 1988	52	6	IMP (25–300) vs. ALP (1.5–6)	IMP=ALP	
	Rickels et al. 1993	230	8	IMP (25–200) vs. TRA (50–400) vs. DIA (5–40) vs. PBO	IMP=TRA=DIA>PBO	
Opipramol						
RCT	Möller et al. 2001	310	4	OPI (200) vs. ALP (2) vs. PBO	OPI=ALP>PBO	ICD-10 criteria
Other antidepressants						
Vortioxetine						
RCTs	Bidzan et al. 2012	301	8	VOR (5) vs. PBO	VOR>PBO	Less than half of sample had been previously treated for GAD, mostly with SSRI
	Mahableshwarkar et al. 2014a	457	8	VOR (2.5) vs. VOR (10) vs. PBO	VOR=PBO	
	Rothschild et al. 2012	304	8	VOR (5) vs. PBO	VOR=PBO	
	Mahableshwarkar et al. 2014b	781	8	VOR (2.5) vs. VOR (5) vs. VOR (10) vs. DUL (60) vs. PBO	DUL>PBO VOR=PBO	
Post hoc analysis	Christensen et al. 2019	988	8–12	One VOR acute study and one VOR relapse study	VOR>PBO	Analysis of the efficacy of VOR in working patients
Meta-analyses	Pae et al. 2015	1,831	8	Four VOR RCTs (listed above)	VOR>PBO	Effect size: SMD −0.118; 95% CI −0.203 to −0.033

TABLE 13–1. Short-term randomized controlled trials *(continued)*

Drug and class	Study	N	Weeks	Design*	Results*	Notes
	Fu et al. 2016	1,843	8	Four VOR RCTs (listed above)	VOR=PBO	Effect size: VOR 2.5 vs. PBO: OR 1.16; 95% CI 0.84–1.60 VOR 5 vs. PBO: OR 1.41; 95% CI 0.82–2.41 VOR 10 vs. PBO: OR 1.05; 95% CI 0.76–1.46
Bupropion XL RCT	Bystritsky et al. 2008	32	12	BUP-XL(300) vs. ESC (20) vs. PBO	BUP>ESC>PBO	
Agomelatine RCTs	Stein et al. 2008	121	12	AGO (20–50) vs. PBO	AGO>PBO	
	Stein et al. 2014	412	12	AGO (25–50) vs. ESC (10–20) vs. PBO	AGO=ESC>PBO	Higher incidence of AEs in ESC
	Stein et al. 2017	412	12	AGO (10) vs. AGO (25) vs. PBO	AGO>PBO	
Anticonvulsants						
Pregabalin RCTs	Feltner et al. 2003	271	4	PRE (150) vs. PRE (600) vs. LOR (6)	PRE (600)>PBO LOR>PBO	
	Pande et al. 2003	276	6	PRE (150, 600) vs. LOR (6) vs. PBO	PRE (600)=LOR>PBO	
	Pohl et al. 2005	341	6	PRE (200, 400, 450) vs. PBO	PRE>PBO	
	Rickels et al. 2005	454	4	PRE (300, 450, 600) vs. ALP (1.5) vs. PBO	PRE=ALP>PBO	

TABLE 13–1. Short-term randomized controlled trials (continued)

Drug and class	Study	N	Weeks	Design*	Results*	Notes
Anticonvulsants (continued)						
	Montgomery et al. 2006	421	6	PRE (400, 600) vs. VEN (75) vs. PBO	PRE=VEN>PBO	
	Kasper et al. 2009	374	8	PRE (300–600 bid; mean 424±118) vs. VEN (75–225; mean 155±60) vs. PBO	PRE>VEN=PBO	
	Hadley et al. 2012	106	12	Patients stabilized on ALZ given PRE (300–600) vs. PBO, while tapering ALZ for first 6 weeks	PRE>PBO	Switching from BDZ to PRE (PRE began during BDZ taper)
Post hoc analyses	Lydiard et al. 2010	1,854	4–6	Six PRE RCTs	PRE>PBO	
	Boschen 2012	1,766	4–6	Five PRE RCTs	PRE (450 mg) > other dosages; PRE (450 mg) > PRE (600 mg+)	Primarily analyzing the dose-response relationship using HAM-A scores
	Baldwin et al. 2013	1,354	4–8	Four PRE RCTs	PRE>PBO	
	Ruiz et al. 2015	1,546	~24	ADAN study—prospective non-interventional trial; PRE vs. usual care	PRE>usual care	PRE group includes those who are PRE naive and starting or adding PRE to existing therapy at baseline for 6 months; usual-care group includes those changing prior treatment to anything other than PRE
	Montgomery et al. 2017	2,155	4–8	Nine PRE RCTs	PRE>PBO	
Meta-analyses	Boschen 2011	1,352	4–8	Seven PRE RCTs	PRE>PBO	
	Zaccara et al. 2011	11,918	4–14	38 PRE RCTs for neurological or psychiatric conditions (7 for GAD)	39 AEs occurred with PRE treatment; highest RR for balance disorder, then euphoria, incoordination, ataxia, edema	
	Generoso et al. 2017	2,299	4–8	Eight PRE RCTs	PRE>PBO	

TABLE 13–1. **Short-term randomized controlled trials** *(continued)*

Drug and class	Study	N	Weeks	Design*	Results*	Notes
Tiagabine						
RCT	Pollack et al. 2005	272	8	TIA (mean 10.5) vs. PBO	TIA=PBO	
Meta-analyses	Pollack et al. 2008c	1,790	10	Three TIA RCTs		
				TIA (4, 8, 12) vs. PBO	TIA=PBO	
				TIA (4–16) vs. PBO	TIA=PBO	
				TIA (4–16) vs. PBO	TIA=PBO	
Divalproex chrono						
RCT	Aliyev and Aliyev 2008	80	6	DPX-C (1,500) vs. PBO	DPX-C >PBO	All-male sample
Benzodiazepines						
Alprazolam						
RCTs	Chouinard et al. 1983	50	8	ALP (0.25–3) vs. PBO	ALP>PBO	Mixed anxiety sample (30 GAD, 20 panic disorder); 18 patients began behavior therapy at week 5
	Elie and Lamontagne 1984	48	4	DIA (10–25) vs. ALP (1–3)	DIA>ALP	
	Lydiard et al. 1997	180	4	ABE vs. ALP vs. PBO	ABE=ALP>PBO	
	Brown et al. 2015	32	4	ALP (0.5–1 mg) vs. PBO [2:1]	ALP>PBO	Primary goal to assess brain activity during emotion face matching task
Bromazepam, diazepam, and lorazepam						
RCTs	Fontaine et al. 1984	48	4	BRO (18) vs. DIA (15) vs. PBO	BRO>DIA>PBO	
	Fontaine et al. 1986	60	4	BRO (12, 18) vs. LOR (4, 6) vs. PBO	BRO=LOR>PBO	
	Rickels et al. 1988	62	4	CLO (15–30) vs. LOR (2–4)	CLO=LOR	

TABLE 13–1.   Short-term randomized controlled trials (continued)

Drug and class	Study	N	Weeks	Design*	Results*	Notes
Benzodiazepines (continued)						
	Rickels et al. 1997	198	8	GEP (10–45) vs. DIA (10–45) vs. PBO	GEP=DIA>PBO	Primarily examining efficacy of GEP
	Fresquet et al. 2000	161	6	LES (40–80) vs. LOR (2–4) vs. PBO	LES=LOR>PBO	
	Rickels et al. 2000a	310	6–24	ABE (mean 12) vs. DIA (mean 22) vs. PBO	DIA=ABE>PBO (after 1 week of treatment) DIA>ABE=PBO (after 6 weeks of treatment)	DIA caused temporary discontinuation symptoms in patients treated ≥12 weeks
Meta-analyses	Mitte 2005			48 studies investigating 26 drugs	BDZ=AZA	Evaluating efficacy of pharmacotherapy in GAD, especially comparing BDZ and AZA. Effect size (weighted Hedges' g): BDZ 0.32 (ALP 0.33; DIA 0.3; LOR 0.17; AZA 0.3; BUS 0.34; VEN 0.33
	Martin et al. 2007	2,326	2–24	23 double-blind RCTs: BDZ vs. PBO	BDZ>PBO	
Antipsychotics						
Quetiapine RCTs	Brawman-Mintzer et al. 2006b	38	6	QUE (25–300) vs. PBO	QUE=PBO	
	Chouinard et al. 2007	873	8	QUE (50,150) vs. PAR (20) vs. PBO	QUE (50, 150)>PBO PAR>PBO	
	Joyce et al. 2008	951	8	QUE (50, 150, 300) vs. PBO	QUE (50, 150)>PBO QUE (300)=PBO	
	Merideth et al. 2008	854	10	QUE-XR (150, 300) vs. ESC (10) vs. PBO	QUE (150, 300)>PBO ESC>PBO	

TABLE 13–1. Short-term randomized controlled trials *(continued)*

Drug and class	Study	N	Weeks	Design*	Results*	Notes
	Bandelow et al. 2010	873	8	QUE-XR (50) vs. QUE-XR (150) vs. PAR (20) vs. PBO	QUE-XR=PAR>PBO	
	Khan et al. 2011	951	8	QUE-XR (50) vs. QUE-XR (150) vs. QUE (300) vs. PBO	QUE-XR (50, 150) > PBO QUE-XR (300)=PBO	
	Merideth et al. 2012	854	8	QUE-XR (150) vs. QUE-XR (300) vs. ESC (10) vs. PBO	QUE=ESC>PBO	
Post hoc analyses	Stein et al. 2011	2,248	8	Three QUE-XR RCTs	QUE-XR>PBO	
	Endicott et al. 2012	2,248	8	Three QUE RCTs and one relapse study	QUE (150)>PBO QUE (50, 300)=PBO	
	Montgomery et al. 2014	2,171	8	Three QUE RCTs	QUE>PBO	
Meta-analyses	Maneeton et al. 2016	2,248	8	Three QUE RCTs	QUE (50, 150 mg)>PBO QUE (300 mg)=PBO	
Trifluoperazine RCT	Mendels et al. 1986	415	4	TRI (2–6) vs. PBO	TRI>PBO	Effect size: WMD −2.19; 95% CI −2.94 to −1.45
Azapirones						
Buspirone RCTs	Cohn and Rickels 1989	367	4	BUS (10–60) vs. DIA (10–60) vs. PBO	BUS=DIA>PBO	
	Ansseau et al. 1991	26	6	BUS (15) vs. OXA (45)	OXA>BUS	
	Enkelmann 1991	94	6	BUS (15–40) vs. ALP (1.5–4) vs. PBO	ALP>BUS>PBO	
	Sramek et al. 1996	162	6	BUS (15–45) vs. PBO	BUS>PBO	

TABLE 13–1.   Short-term randomized controlled trials *(continued)*

Drug and class	Study	N	Weeks	Design*	Results*	Notes
Azapirones *(continued)*						
	Sramek et al. 1997	119	8	BUS (15 mg bid) vs. BUS (10 mg tid) vs. PBO	BUS>PBO BUS bid=BUS tid	
	Laakmann et al. 1998	125	10	BUS (15) vs. LOR (3) vs. PBO	BUS=LOR>PBO	
Gepirone						
RCT	Rickels et al. 1997	198	8	GEP (10–45) vs. DIA (10–45) vs. PBO	GEP=DIA>PBO	
Antihistamines						
Hydroxyzine						
RCTs	Darcis et al. 1995	100	4	HYD (50) vs. PBO	HYD>PBO	
	Lader and Scotto 1998	214	4	HYD (50) vs. BUS (20) vs. PBO	HYD>BUS=PBO	
	Llorca et al. 2002	334	12	HYD (50) vs. BRO (6) vs. PBO	HYD=BRO>PBO	
Meta-analyses	Guaiana et al. 2010	884	4–12	Five HYD studies	HYD>PBO	
β-Blockers						
Atenolol						
RCT	Rickels et al. 1986	63	3	ATN (100) vs. PBO	ATN=PBO	
Propranolol						
RCT	Meibach et al. 1987	212	3	PRO (80, 160, 320) vs. CHL (30, 45, 75) vs. PBO	PRO=CHL=PBO	

TABLE 13–1.   Short-term randomized controlled trials *(continued)*

Drug and class	Study	N	Weeks	Design*	Results*	Notes
Other agents						
Vilazodone						
RCTs	Gommoll et al. 2015a	402	8	VIL (20–40) vs. PBO	VIL>PBO	
	Gommoll et al. 2015b	680	8	VIL (20) vs. VIL (40) vs. PBO	VIL (20)=PBO, VIL (40)>PBO	
	Durgam et al. 2016	415	8	VIL (20–40) vs. PBO	VIL>PBO	
Post hoc analyses	Clayton et al. 2017	1,373	8	Three VIL RCTs	VIL=PBO	Analysis of sexual function
	Khan et al. 2016	1,462	8	Three VIL RCTs	VIL>PBO	
Meta-analyses	Zareifopoulos and Dylja 2017	1,462	8	Three VIL RCTs	VIL>PBO	Effect size: Cohen's d=0.26
Ocinaplon						
RCT	Czobor et al. 2010	60	4	OCI (90 mg tid) vs. PBO	OCI>PBO	
Pexacerfont						
RCT	Coric et al. 2010	260	8	PEX (100; first week 300 loading dose) vs. PBO vs. ESC (20) (2:2:1)	PEX=PBO, ESC>PBO	

Note.   ABE=abecarnil; ADAN=Amplification of Definition of Anxiety; AE=adverse event; AGO=agomelatine; ALP=alprazolam; ALZ=Alzheimer's disease; ATN=atenolol; AZA=azapirones; BDZ=benzodiazepines; BRO=bromazepam; BUP-XL=bupropion XL; BUS=buspirone; CBT=cognitive-behavioral therapy; CHL=chlordiazepoxide; CLO=clorazepate; DAS-A=Daily Assessment of Symptoms-Anxiety; DIA=diazepam; DPX-C=divalproex chrono; DUL=duloxetine; ESC=escitalopram; GAD=generalized anxiety disorder; GEP=gepirone; HAM-A=Hamilton Anxiety Scale; HYD=hydroxyzine; IMP=imipramine; LES=lesopitron; LOR=lorazepam; MD=mean deviation; OCI=ocinaplon; OPI=opipramol; OXA=oxazepam; PAR=paroxetine; PBO=placebo; PEX=pexacerfont; PRE=pregabalin; PRO=propranolol; PST=problem-solving therapy; QUE=quetiapine; RCT=randomized controlled trial; SER=sertraline; SMD=standard mean difference; TIA=tiagabine; TRA=trazodone; TRI=trifluoperazine; VEN=venlafaxine; VIL=vilazodone; VOR=vortioxetine; WMD=weighted mean difference; XR=extended release.
*Dosages are mg/day unless otherwise indicated.

Anticonvulsants

Pregabalin

Abnormalities in the inhibitory neurotransmitter GABA and glutamatergic (excitatory) systems have been associated with GAD. Pregabalin is a structural analogue to GABA, with a novel mechanism of action, binding to the delta subunit of voltage-dependent calcium channels in the CNS and acting as a presynaptic modulator of several excitatory neurotransmitters. Pregabalin has demonstrated consistent superiority to placebo in RCTs and meta-analyses (see Table 13–1). It has been found equally as effective as the benzodiazepines lorazepam (Feltner et al. 2003) and alprazolam (Rickels et al. 2005), with a similar speed of therapeutic onset. Pregabalin was more effective than venlafaxine XR in one RCT (Kasper et al. 2009) and equivalent to it in another (Montgomery et al. 2006).

Second-Line Treatments

Benzodiazepines

Benzodiazepines have a long history of use in GAD and continue to be the most commonly prescribed anxiolytic medications. The GAD treatment literature includes positive placebo-controlled RCTs of clorazepate, lorazepam, bromazepam, diazepam, and alprazolam. Although many of these results were obtained in patient populations defined by DSM-III GAD criteria (American Psychiatric Association 1980), they are likely still relevant for patients defined by DSM-5 criteria (American Psychiatric Association 2013). Despite their demonstrated efficacy and level-1 evidence, benzodiazepines have several disadvantages. Some benzodiazepines (e.g., alprazolam, lorazepam) have a relatively short half-life, requiring frequent dosing and sometimes resulting in interdose rebound anxiety. These agents also are associated with discontinuation symptoms, high rates of relapse, and toxicity in overdose, as well as potential for abuse, especially in patients with a predisposition toward substance abuse. Other potential side effects of benzodiazepines include attentional, psychomotor, cognitive, and memory impairments. Furthermore, benzodiazepines lack the broad-spectrum efficacy of antidepressants for common comorbid conditions such as depression, which limits their utility. Therefore, these agents, although effective, are considered second-line treatments for GAD.

Atypical Antipsychotics

Quetiapine

The second-generation or atypical antipsychotics are less likely to cause extrapyramidal effects or tardive dyskinesia than first-generation agents and have various effects on serotonin receptors. This, coupled with their known efficacy in bipolar and refractory depression, has encouraged the investigation of their use in GAD, particularly when GAD is refractory to first-line agents. Acute monotherapy studies of quetiapine for nonrefractory GAD have been primarily positive using 150 mg/day, although results are less positive for 300 mg/day. Quetiapine monotherapy was also found to be significantly superior to placebo and equivalent to antidepressants in several GAD meta-analyses but was associated with more weight gain, sedation, and higher dropout rates due to adverse events compared with placebo or antidepressants (Depping et al. 2010). Because of tolerability and long-term safety concerns with atypical antipsychotics, such as weight gain, hyperglycemia, diabetes, hyperlipidemia, and other manifestations of metabolic syndrome, this treatment is recommended as a second-line option for patients who do not respond to or tolerate antidepressants or benzodiazepines.

Tricyclic Antidepressants and Other Antidepressants

In RCTs, imipramine has established efficacy for GAD and has also been reported to be as effective as benzodiazepines (Hoehn-Saric et al. 1988; Rickels et al. 1993). The tricyclic antidepressant (TCA) opipramol is widely prescribed in Germany and has demonstrated greater efficacy than placebo and equivalent efficacy to alprazolam (Möller et al. 2001). Other TCAs also may be effective but have little systematic data. However, TCAs are associated with significant side effects including sedation, weight gain, orthostasis, and antimuscarinic effects attributable to blockade at the histamine (H_1) receptor, α_1-adrenoceptors, and muscarinic receptors. In addition, they are potentially lethal in overdose. Thus, despite its efficacy and limited potential for abuse, imipramine is recommended as a second-line option.

Bupropion XL is an antidepressant that acts as a norepinephrine and dopamine reuptake inhibitor as well as a nicotinic agonist (Ascher et al. 1995). Although it was found to have comparable efficacy to escitalopram in one small RCT (Bystritsky et al. 2008), it has not been examined further in GAD and is therefore considered a second-line treatment.

Other Second-Line Agents

Buspirone

Buspirone, an azapirone derivative, is a partial agonist at postsynaptic 5-HT_{1A} receptors in the limbic system and was approved by the FDA for GAD in 1986 (Gammans et al. 1992). It has anxiolytic efficacy similar to benzodiazepines (Rickels 1982), with a better safety profile (Rakel 1990). Despite its tolerability and demonstrable efficacy in clinical trials, it has been considered inconsistently effective in clinical practice, limiting its use as antianxiety monotherapy. It may be helpful as an augmentation agent.

Hydroxyzine

Hydroxyzine is an H_1 receptor antagonist, as well as a mild serotonin-2 (5-HT_2) receptor antagonist, and has been shown to possess some anxiolytic properties (Kubo et al. 1987). A handful of RCTs have demonstrated efficacy of hydroxyzine in GAD with similar efficacy to benzodiazepines and buspirone. Although its evidence would place hydroxyzine as a second-line treatment, its sedating properties have limited its use in clinical practice. Hydroxyzine typically is used as an augmentation or alternative strategy for patients whose illness is treatment refractory or who are intolerant of standard interventions.

Other Treatments

Antidepressants

Although other SSRIs are classified as first-line GAD treatment, the current literature on citalopram and fluoxetine provides only level-3 evidence for these agents. Both citalopram (Varia and Rauscher 2002) and fluoxetine (Simon et al. 2006b) were found to be efficacious in open-label studies.

Vortioxetine

Vortioxetine is a multimodal agent. Although results are mixed, RCTs are largely negative for GAD; one large post hoc analysis as well as one meta-analysis found vortioxetine superior to placebo in GAD, but another meta-analysis was negative (see Table 13–1). It is notable that the dosages used in the short-term studies of GAD (2.5–10 mg vortioxetine daily) were lower than those used in the more positive studies of major depressive disorder (MDD) (dosages up to 20 mg/day). The current conflicting evidence suggests that vortioxetine should be considered a third-line treatment.

Typical Antipsychotics

Trifluoperazine has an early onset of action and a relatively long duration of activity, while producing minimal autonomic and endocrine side effects (Ayd 1959; Moyer and Conner 1958). An early, short-term RCT provided support for its efficacy (Mendels et al. 1986). However, typical antipsychotics are associated with significant side effects following prolonged use, such as extrapyramidal symptoms and tardive dyskinesia, limiting their clinical utility (Seeman 2002).

Anticonvulsants

Tiagabine is a selective GABA reuptake inhibitor (Borden et al. 1994); however, evidence from four RCTs was negative for GAD (see Table 13–1). It is therefore not a recommended treatment. However, the anticonvulsant divalproex (chrono) was effective in a small RCT, but because it is not widely available, this agent has little use in clinical practice (see Table 13–1; Katzman et al. 2014).

Beta-Blockers

Although the antianxiety effects of β-blockers have been identified in other disorders, the current evidence does not support the use of propranolol or atenolol in GAD (see Table 13–1).

Other

Gepirone, an azapirone and a partial 5-HT$_{1A}$ agonist, produced significant anxiolytic effects in one RCT (see Table 13–1). However, it also showed a significant delay in therapeutic onset with relatively low patient retention, thus limiting its clinical use. The efficacy of ocinaplon, a positive allosteric modulator of GABA$_A$ receptors, is supported by a small RCT (see Table 13–1). The current literature does not support the use of either pexacerfont or memantine for GAD.

Long-Term Efficacy and Relapse Prevention Studies

Given that GAD is commonly a chronic condition associated with significant functional impairment, treatments that demonstrate long-term benefits are essential. GAD treatments have been examined in both long-term and relapse prevention studies with a duration of greater than 12 weeks.

Long-Term Studies

Venlafaxine, escitalopram, paroxetine, buspirone, clorazepate, and diazepam all have been examined in long-term studies. Four studies evaluated the long-term efficacy of venlafaxine, with one study of duloxetine, ranging in duration from 24 to 28 weeks (Table 13–2). All of these studies demonstrated the efficacy of SNRIs over placebo for most dosages. In addition, buspirone was found superior to placebo in two 24-week studies (Tollefson et al. 1992) and equal in efficacy to clorazepate (Rickels et al. 1988). Diazepam demonstrated superior efficacy to placebo in one 22-week study (Rickels et al. 1993). Comparative efficacy was examined in a small 24-week study comparing escitalopram with paroxetine; both drugs showed significant reduction in GAD symptoms (Bielski et al. 2005). Another study examined discontinuation effects of long-term pregabalin treatment compared with lorazepam or placebo (Kasper et al. 2014b). All groups had low rates of rebound anxiety following treatment discontinuation at week 14 (1.9%–5.2%) and week 26 (0–6%). Furthermore, improvements in anxiety and global impression scores were recorded for both pregabalin and lorazepam treatment within the first 12 weeks, which was maintained in all groups in the second phase (24 weeks) of the study, including placebo.

Relapse Prevention Studies

The long-term benefits of paroxetine, escitalopram, duloxetine, venlafaxine XR, pregabalin, quetiapine XR, vortioxetine, and agomelatine have been evaluated in GAD relapse prevention studies. Typically, these studies involve 12 weeks or more of open-label or single-blind treatment, with responders randomized to double-blind treatment for an additional 24–26 weeks or more. The SSRIs paroxetine and escitalopram have demonstrated significantly lower rates of relapse (11%–33%) compared with placebo (40%–64%), with placebo-treated participants being two to four times more likely to relapse compared with those receiving an SSRI (Table 13–3). Similarly, relapse rates were significantly lower for the SNRIs duloxetine and venlafaxine XR compared with placebo; relapse rates were also significantly lower in study participants who were initially treated for 12 months with open-label venlafaxine XR versus those initially treated for only 6 months (Rickels et al. 2010). A post hoc analysis of these data revealed that individuals displaying residual anxiety symptoms prior to the continuation phase were at greater risk of relapse, with anxious mood (HR 1.648,

TABLE 13–2.   **Long-term studies of GAD pharmacotherapy**

Study	N	Weeks	Design*	Results*	Notes
Rickels 1982	180	6–22	6 weeks DIA (15–40) then 18 weeks PBO vs. 14 weeks DIA (15–40) then 10 weeks PBO vs. 22 weeks DIA (15–40) then 2 weeks PBO	DIA > PBO	
Rickels et al. 1988	150	24	BUS (10–40) vs. LOR (15–60)	BUS = LOR	Mixed anxiety sample (134 with GAD, 16 with PD)
Hackett et al. 1999	544	24	VEN-XR (37.5, 75, 150) vs. PBO	VEN (150) > VEN (37.5) > PBO	
Gelenberg et al. 2000	251	28	VEN-XR (75, 150, 225) vs. PBO	VEN > PBO	
Allgulander et al. 2001	541	24	VEN-XR (37.5) vs. VEN-XR (75) vs. VEN-XR (150) vs. PBO	VEN > PBO	
Lenox-Smith and Reynolds 2003	244	24	VEN-XR (75–150) vs. PBO	VEN > PBO	GAD ± comorbid depression (MADRS ≥ 23)
Bielski et al. 2005	121	24	ESC (10–20) vs. PAR (20–50)	ESC = PAR	Significantly fewer patients withdrew from ESC than PAR due to adverse events
Wu et al. 2011	210	15	DUL (60–120) vs. PBO	DUL > PBO	

Note.   BUS=buspirone; DIA=diazepam; DUL=duloxetine; ESC=escitalopram; GAD=generalized anxiety disorder; LOR=lorazepam; MADRS=Montgomery-Åsberg Depression Rating Scale; PAR=paroxetine; PBO=placebo; PD=panic disorder; VEN=venlafaxine; XR=extended release.
*Dosages are mg/day unless otherwise indicated.

$P=0.009$) and pain while awake (HR 2.813, $P<0.001$) found to be the strongest predictors of relapse (Bodkin et al. 2011). Pregabalin was found to be efficacious in reducing rates of and time to relapse in one study ($P=0.0001$); relapse criteria by study endpoint were met for 65.3% receiving placebo compared with 42.3% of those receiving pregabalin (see Table 13–3).

Quetiapine XR was found to significantly decrease time to an anxiety event, with the risk of an event reduced by 81% (HR=0.19, $P<0.001$) compared with placebo (see Table 13–3). A post hoc analysis found that relative to placebo, quetiapine XR was significantly better at maintaining improvements in disability (Sheehan Disability Scale; $P=0.017$) and sleep (Pittsburgh Sleep Quality Index; $P<0.001$).The antidepressants vortioxetine and agomelatine have both demonstrated efficacy in preventing relapse

TABLE 13–3. Relapse prevention studies

Randomized controlled trials

Drug (Study)	Study	Dosage, mg/day	N	Open label, weeks	RCT extension, weeks	Relapse
Agomelatine	Stein et al. 2012	25 or 50	477	16	26	AGO: 19.5%; PBO: 13.7%
Duloxetine	Davidson et al. 2008	60–120	887	26	26	DUL: 13.7%; PBO: 41.8%
Escitalopram	Allgulander et al. 2006	20	491	12	24–76	ESC: 19%; PBO: 56%
	Bakish et al. 2006	20	72	12	24	ESC: 33%; PBO: 64%
Paroxetine	Stocchi et al. 2003	20–50	652	8	24	PAR: 10.9%; PBO: 39.9%
Pregabalin	Feltman et al. 2008	450	338	8	24	PRE: 42.3%; PBO: 65.3%
Quetiapine XR	Katzman et al. 2011	50–300	433	16–24	Up to 52	QUE-XR: 10.2%, PBO: 38.9%
Venlafaxine XR	Rickels et al. 2010	75–225	268	24	48	VEN: 6.7%; PBO: 53.7%
Vortioxetine	Baldwin et al. 2012	5 or 10	687	20	24–56	VOR: 15%; PBO: 34%

Post hoc analyses

Study	N	Weeks	Design	Results
Bodkin et al. 2011	429	26+26	Data from Davidson et al. 2008, analyzed predictors of time to relapse	DUL> PBO
Sheehan et al. 2013	432	16–24+52	Data from Katzman et al. 2011, analyzed for long-term functioning and sleep quality	QUE> PBO

Meta-analyses

Study	N	Weeks	Design	Results
Donovan et al. 2010	1,342	8–26	Three studies (ESC, PAR, DUL vs. PBO)	ESC=PAR=DUL> PBO

Note. AGO=agomelatine; DUL=duloxetine; ESC=escitalopram; PAR=paroxetine; PBO=placebo; PRE=pregabalin; QUE=quetiapine; VEN=venlafaxine; VOR=vortioxetine; XR=extended release.

compared with placebo, with agomelatine also demonstrating more pronounced anxiety reductions in severely anxious participants (baseline Hamilton Anxiety Rating Scale [HAM-A] score≥25 and Clinical Global Impression–Severity [CGI-S] scale score ≥5). Finally, in a meta-analysis of 22 studies examining the comparative efficacy of antidepressants in relapse prevention for anxiety disorders, including GAD (three studies), continued antidepressant treatment was noted to have a substantial and consistent effect on relapse, with the greatest treatment effect observed in GAD (pooled OR 0.20; 95% CI 0.15–0.26). These findings highlight the importance of sustaining antidepressant treatment beyond acute therapy (see Table 13–3).

Treatment-Refractory Generalized Anxiety Disorder

Relatively few systematic data are available concerning next-step treatments and strategies for GAD that is refractory to standard treatment. Based on the available literature, the strongest evidence appears to be for pregabalin augmentation, because it has demonstrated efficacy in two RCTs and two post hoc analyses, but not in a third post hoc analysis (Table 13–4). Open-label studies of aripiprazole augmentation (Hoge et al. 2008; Menza et al. 2007) and risperidone (Simon et al. 2006a) have shown significant reduction in GAD symptoms. Small RCTs of olanzapine and risperidone also have demonstrated efficacy as augmentation agents for the treatment of patients with GAD who remain symptomatic despite standard anxiolytic therapy, although a larger RCT with risperidone augmentation was negative (see Table 13–4). Augmentation studies of quetiapine and ziprasidone for refractory GAD were also negative. Therefore, with the exception of open-label evidence, atypical antipsychotics have little support for use in treatment-refractory GAD. This conclusion is supported by two meta-analyses (LaLonde and Van Lieshout 2011; Patterson and Van Ameringen 2016). One found that augmentation using atypical antipsychotics was not superior to placebo for response or remission (response: RR 1.14, 95% CI 0.92–1.41; remission: RR 1.28, 95% CI 0.96–1.71) and that patients treated with second-generation antipsychotics were 43% more likely to discontinue treatment compared with those receiving placebo (RR 1.43, 95% CI 1.04–1.96) (LaLonde and Van Lieshout 2011). In the other analysis, which included three studies of treatment-refractory GAD, no significant treatment effect was found for response (CGI-I≤2) or HAM-A change with quetiapine, olanzapine, or pregabalin augmentation (Patterson and Van Ameringen 2016).

In clinical experience, the combination of two first-line, evidence-based agents—pregabalin or benzodiazepines (in particular)—with an SSRI/SNRI has been the most beneficial strategy for patients with treatment-refractory GAD. In addition, selecting agents with the lowest adverse event profile is very important, given the propensity for somatic distress in patients with GAD (Van Ameringen et al. 2017).

Combined Treatments

A few studies have examined pharmacotherapy in combination with psychotherapy for the treatment of GAD. Overall, combining psychotherapy with pharmacotherapy does not appear to yield benefits above either treatment alone (Table 13–5), although mindfulness-based cognitive therapy combined with alprazolam and paroxetine or escitalopram was found to be more efficacious than the same medications delivered

TABLE 13–4. Treatment-refractory GAD

Randomized controlled trials

Drug	Study	N	Weeks	Design[a]	Results	Notes
Olanzapine	Pollack et al. 2006	24	6	Adjunctive OLAN (5–20) vs. PBO	OLAN>PBO	Primary medication fluoxetine
Pregabalin	Miceli et al. 2009	358	8	Adjunctive PRE (150–600) vs. PBO	PRE>PBO	Primary medications ESC, PAR, VEN-XR
	Rickels et al. 2012	356	8+8	8-week open-label dosing with ESC, PAR, or VEN, then partial responders randomized to 8-week augmentation with PRE (150–600) vs. PBO	PRE>PBO	
Quetiapine	Simon et al. 2008	22	8	Adjunctive QUE (25–400) vs. PBO	QUE=PBO	Primary medication PAR-CR
	Altamura et al. 2011	20	8	Adjunctive QUE (25–150; mean 50) vs. PBO	QUE>PBO	Primary medications SSRIs; patients had already undergone SSRI treatment for 8 weeks, showing partial or no response
Quetiapine XR	Khan et al. 2013	409	8	Adjunctive QUE-XR (50–300 mg; mean 174.3 mg) vs. PBO	QUE=PBO	Primary medications SSRI or SNRI; patients had history of partial or no response to DUL, ESC, PAR, VEN-XR
Risperidone	Brawman-Mintzer et al. 2005	40	5	Adjunctive RISP (0.5–1.5) vs. PBO	RISP>PBO	Mixed primary medications
	Pandina et al. 2007	417	4	Adjunctive RISP vs. PBO	RISP=PBO	Mixed primary medications
Ziprasidone	Lohoff et al. 2010	62	8	ZIP (20–80) vs. PBO (2:1, patients either augmented or nonaugmented, both groups)	ZIP=PBO	Patients with treatment failure of at least one trial of SSRI, SNRI, BDZ, or combination

TABLE 13–4.   Treatment-refractory GAD (continued)

Post hoc analyses

Drug	Study	N	Weeks	Design[a]	Results	Notes
Pregabalin	De Salas-Cansado et al. 2012	282	24	PRE (monotherapy or adjunctive, mean 163) vs. PBO (continuation with SSRI/SNRI)	PRE=PBO	Cost-effectiveness analysis of ADAN study[b]; cases refractory to previous BDZ therapy
	Álvarez et al. 2015	725	24	Adjunctive PRE (150–600) vs. UC	PRE+SSRI > UC	Analysis of ADAN study[b] for clinical and economic outcomes; patients who had partial response to SSRI monotherapy
	Olivares et al. 2015	133	24	Adjunctive PRE (mean 222)	PRE = sign improvement	Analysis of ADAN study[b], patients who had inadequate response to previous antidepressant treatment

Meta-analysis

Drug	Study	N	Weeks	Design[a]	Results	Notes
	LaLonde and Van Lieshout 2011	2,459	2–12	12 studies on SGA augmentation for refractory GAD (6 RCTs, 6 open label), 6 studies on SGA monotherapy (4 RCTs, 2 open label)	Augmentation RCTs: SGA= PBO Monotherapy RCTs: SGA> PBO	Augmentation RCTs: SGAs not superior to PBO for response or remission Monotherapy RCTs: SGAs superior to PBO for response and remission Effect sizes: Augmentation: response RR 1.14, 95% CI 0.92–1.41; remission RR 1.28, 95% CI 0.96–1.71 Monotherapy: response RR 1.31, 95% CI 1.20–1.44; remission RR 1.44, 95% CI 1.23–1.68

Note.   ADAN=Amplification of Definition of Anxiety; BDZ=benzodiazepine; CR=continuous release; DUL=duloxetine; ESC=escitalopram; GAD=generalized anxiety disorder; OLAN=olanzapine; PAR=paroxetine; PBO=placebo; PRE=pregabalin; QUE=quetiapine; RCT=randomized controlled trial; RISP=risperidone; SGA=second-generation antipsychotic; SNRI=serotonin norepinephrine reuptake inhibitor; SSRI=selective serotonin reuptake inhibitor; UC=usual care; VEN=venlafaxine; XR=extended release; ZIP=ziprasidone.

[a]Dosages are mg/day unless otherwise indicated.
[b]Álvarez et al. 2012.

TABLE 13–5.			Randomized controlled trials of combined treatment		
Study	**N**	**Weeks**	**Design***	**Results**	**Notes**
Power et al. 1990	101	10	DIA (15) vs. CBT vs. PBO vs. DIA (15)+ CBT vs. CBT+ PBO	DIA= CBT= DIA+ CBT= CBT+ PBO > PBO	
Ferrero et al. 2007	87	13 sessions	MED vs. B-APP vs. MED+B-APP	MED=B-APP=MED+ B-APP	MED group: SSRI or SNRI; BDZ if necessary
Kim et al. 2009	46	8	PAR (mean 21) or ESC (mean 15) or VEN (mean 150)+ALP (mean 0.52) + MBCT vs. PAR (mean 22) or ESC (mean 16) or VEN (mean 160)+ ALP (mean 0.48)+ ADE	MBCT>ADE	GAD or panic disorder
Crits-Christoph et al. 2011	268	24	VEN (75–225) vs. VEN (75–225)+ CBT vs. open-label VEN (75–225)	VEN=CBT= open label	Participants randomly asked if they wanted to include CBT in their treatment

Note. ADE=anxiety disorder education; ALP=alprazolam; B-APP=brief Alderian psychodynamic psychotherapy; BDZ=benzodiazepine; CBT=cognitive-behavioral therapy; DIA=diazepam; ESC=escitalopram; GAD=generalized anxiety disorder; MBCT= mindfulness-based cognitive therapy; MED= pharmacotherapy; PAR=paroxetine; PBO=placebo; SNRI=serotonin-norepinephrine reuptake inhibitor; SSRI=selective serotonin uptake inhibitor; VEN= venlafaxine.
*Dosages are mg/day unless otherwise indicated.

with anxiety disorder education (Kim et al. 2009). Additionally, cognitive-behavioral therapy (CBT) is an effective facilitator of benzodiazepine tapering and discontinuation up to 12 months following CBT treatment compared with nonspecific psychological treatment (Gosselin et al. 2006). Given the dearth of literature, additional research on combined treatments is needed.

Natural Integrative Therapies

Kava Kava

Kava kava (*Piper methysticum)* is a popular herbal medicine sometimes used in the naturopathic treatment of anxiety (Singh and Singh 2002). It has been evaluated in several RCTs in GAD, yielding mixed results. Although two RCTs found kava kava superior to placebo (Sarris et al. 2009, 2013a), findings from a pooled analysis of three trials (Sarris et al. 2013b) as well as a meta-analysis (Ooi et al. 2018) did not. In another randomized, double-blind, reference-controlled trial, kava kava was found to be equally as efficacious as buspirone and opipramol (Boerner et al. 2003), and in another RCT was found to be equally as efficacious as venlafaxine XR (Connor et al. 2006).

Passionflower

Passionflower (*Passiflora incarnata*) has traditionally been used for its sedative, sleep-inducing properties (Bergner 1995). Passionflower was found to be equally efficacious compared with oxazepam in one RCT (Akhondzadeh et al. 2001) and was found to be significantly superior to placebo in reducing anxiety symptoms when used adjunctively with sertraline (Nojoumi et al. 2016).

Chamomile

Chamomile (*Chamomilla recutita*) has traditionally been used for its relaxing and calming effects. One open-label trial (Keefe et al. 2016) and a small, randomized, double-blind, placebo-controlled trial (Amsterdam et al. 2009) found that chamomile was an effective treatment for individuals with GAD. A small relapse prevention study by Mao et al. (2016) demonstrated that although relapse rates using chamomile were low, results were not significant compared with placebo.

Lavender

Lavender (*Lavandula angustifolia*) essences are widely known for their relaxing, calming, and mood-alleviating effects (Cavanagh and Wilkinson 2002). A small RCT found lavender to be equal in efficacy to lorazepam (Woelk and Schläfke 2010), whereas a larger RCT found it superior to placebo (Kasper et al. 2014a). Overall, lavender may have some potential as a possible future treatment option for GAD.

Ketamine

Potential evidence for the use of ketamine to treat anxiety comes from subanalyses of studies in other disorders. However, a cross-sectional study (Shadli et al. 2018), as well as a number of case studies, measured the effect of ketamine in patients with GAD and found significant improvement in anxiety symptoms (HAM-A and Fear Questionnaire scores).

Other Traditional Therapies

Many traditional medications and therapies have been examined for their utility as either monotherapy or augmentation in treating GAD. Of these, balneotherapy, which consists of spa therapy with mineral water and other somatic care, was found to be more efficacious than paroxetine in treating GAD (Dubois et al. 2010). In addition, *Galphimia glauca*, a Mexican plant traditionally used as a tranquilizer for mental disorders, was found to be a more efficacious GAD treatment than lorazepam (Herrera-Arellano et al. 2012). In terms of adjunctive therapy, an Iranian herb used for mood enhancement, *Echium amoenum*, was found to be effective in augmenting fluoxetine treatment compared with placebo augmentation (Sayyah et al. 2012). A Chinese medication, yiqiyangxin, was found to be an equally efficacious adjunct to CBT as paroxetine (Wang et al. 2012). Several other traditional therapies have been studied, but their effectiveness has not yet been proven (Gupta and Mamidi 2014; Park et al. 2014; Song et al. 2017; Tubaki et al. 2012; Wang et al. 2018).

Addressing Comorbidity

Comorbidity would be considered the norm rather than the exception in patients with GAD, because a high rate of both psychiatric and medical comorbidity is common. About 90% of adults with GAD are estimated to have other co-occurring psychiatric disorders, the most common being MDD (61%) (Reinhold and Rickels 2015). GAD also is associated with various medical illnesses, including pain (migraines, rheumatoid arthritis, back pain), gastrointestinal (peptic ulcer disease, irritable bowel syndrome), cardiovascular (coronary heart disease), endocrine (hyperthyroidism, diabetes), and respiratory conditions (asthma, chronic obstructive pulmonary disease) (Culpepper 2009). These comorbidities can negatively affect GAD treatment response and remission (Yonkers et al. 1996) and obfuscate GAD diagnosis (Wittchen et al. 2002). Conversely, the early identification of GAD comorbidity may reduce the development of secondary psychiatric comorbidity, such as depression (Goodwin and Gorman 2002).

The literature examining the efficacy of GAD pharmacotherapy in individuals with co-occurring psychiatric and medical conditions is meager, because comorbidity is a common exclusion criteria in clinical trials. In fact, 70% of individuals with GAD would be excluded from typical pharmacological trials because of issues of comorbidity (Hoertel et al. 2012). Nevertheless, although GAD with psychiatric comorbidity has not been prospectively examined, several post hoc analyses have explored the pharmacotherapeutic response of GAD with co-occurring disorders. For example, venlafaxine XR has demonstrated efficacy in individuals with GAD and secondary MDD, whereas fluoxetine has not (Silverstone and Salinas 2001). Preliminary evidence indicates mirtazapine reduces depressive and anxiety symptoms in individuals with GAD-MDD comorbidity (Goodnick et al. 1999), and pregabalin was efficacious in a sample with treatment-resistant GAD and severe depressive symptoms (Olivares et al. 2015). Quetiapine XR was found to be effective in one controlled trial, either as a monotherapy or in conjunction with an antidepressant (Li et al. 2016), suggesting that atypical antipsychotics may be effective for GAD-MDD comorbidity.

Few other psychiatric comorbidities have been examined in the context of GAD; however, preliminary evidence indicates that buspirone reduces both anxiety symptoms and the desire for alcohol in comorbid GAD and alcohol dependence or abuse (Tollefson et al. 1992). Quetiapine XR as monotherapy or as an adjunctive therapy to a mood stabilizer was not efficacious in GAD-bipolar comorbidity (Gao et al. 2014). Individuals with GAD and bipolar disorder are often treated with benzodiazepines, which have demonstrated benefit in both disorders separately (Preti et al. 2016). However, benzodiazepines may exacerbate depressive symptoms, making them an unfavorable treatment option for this comorbidity (Ferreira-Garcia et al. 2017). Comorbid GAD and personality disorders have shown poor response to escitalopram and duloxetine, suggesting first-line SSRI and SNRI treatments may not be efficacious in this subset of individuals (Pierò and Locati 2011).

Short-term insomnia symptoms have been improved in adults with GAD by using the sedating antidepressants trazodone and mirtazapine, and SSRIs and SNRIs have demonstrated long-term enhancements in sleep (Mayers and Baldwin 2005). Combined administration of escitalopram and eszopiclone improved sleep-related issues and anxiety symptoms to a greater extent than escitalopram alone in individuals with GAD and insomnia (Pollack et al. 2008a). Sleep disturbances and anxiety symptoms in individuals with GAD and insomnia also improve with pregabalin (Bollu et al. 2010; Montgomery et al. 2009) and the benzodiazepines lorazepam and alprazolam (Montgomery et al. 2009). Duloxetine has demonstrated efficacy in reducing painful physical symptoms, including headaches, body pain, and overall pain (Beesdo et al. 2009; Hartford et al. 2007; Nicolini et al. 2009; Russell et al. 2008) and symptoms of irritable bowel syndrome (Kaplan et al. 2014) in comorbid GAD. In individuals with GAD and prominent gastrointestinal symptoms, 300–600 mg pregabalin improved both conditions; however, benzodiazepines did not improve either anxiety or gastrointestinal symptoms (Stein et al. 2009). Preliminary evidence indicates that the benzodiazepine fludiazepam may reduce anxiety symptoms in individuals with diabetes (Okada et al. 1994); however, benzodiazepines should be avoided in comorbid respiratory conditions given their potential to suppress respiratory drive and compromise lung function (Brenes 2003). Furthermore, both buspirone (Argyropoulou et al. 1993) and duloxetine (Papp et al. 1995) have been shown to reduce anxiety symptoms in individuals with chronic obstructive pulmonary disease. Finally, in a study comparing the addition of fluoxetine to propranolol compared with propranolol alone in patients with mitral valve prolapse and GAD, the addition of fluoxetine aggravated chest pain, had no effect on electrocardiography, and worsened anxiety symptoms (Esfehani et al. 2017).

Conclusions and Future Directions

A broad range of pharmacotherapeutic agents have been examined and found to be efficacious in the short- and long-term treatment of GAD, enabling clinicians some flexibility when selecting a first- or second-line treatment. Given this broad range, it would be helpful to have predictors of response to better guide clinicians. The burgeoning field of genetics and the identification of genetic polymorphisms may contribute to more effective clinical treatment of GAD, such as has begun to occur for depression and social anxiety disorder (Stein et al. 2006). Furthermore, considering that 90% of individuals with GAD also have a comorbid condition and that comorbidity can have significant treatment implications, future trials should incorporate comorbid populations to better guide treatment selection.

Key Points

- A broad range of pharmacotherapeutic agents have been examined and found to be efficacious in the short- and long-term treatment of generalized anxiety disorder (GAD) as well as in the prevention of relapse.

- Although benzodiazepines have long been the mainstay of GAD treatment, selective serotonin reuptake inhibitors and serotonin-norepinephrine reuptake inhibitors have emerged as the gold standard treatment.

- Roughly 90% of individuals who have GAD also have a co-occurring psychiatric condition, and GAD also is associated with high rates of medical comorbidity. Unfortunately, most clinical research has been conducted in noncomorbid populations.

- Few evidence-based strategies for treatment-refractory GAD are available; however, augmentation with pregabalin or benzodiazepines may be helpful.

References

Akhondzadeh S, Naghavi HR, Vazirian M, et al: Passionflower in the treatment of generalized anxiety: a pilot double-blind randomized controlled trial with oxazepam. J Clin Pharm Ther 26(5):363–367, 2001 11679026

Aliyev NA, Aliyev ZN: Valproate (depakine-chrono) in the acute treatment of outpatients with generalized anxiety disorder without psychiatric comorbidity: randomized, double-blind placebo-controlled study. Eur Psychiatry 23(2):109–114, 2008 17945470

Allgulander C, Hackett D, Salinas E: Venlafaxine extended release (ER) in the treatment of generalised anxiety disorder: twenty-four-week placebo-controlled dose-ranging study. Br J Psychiatry 179(1):15–22, 2001 11435263

Allgulander C, Dahl AA, Austin C, et al: Efficacy of sertraline in a 12-week trial for generalized anxiety disorder. Am J Psychiatry 161(9):1642–1649, 2004 15337655

Allgulander C, Florea I, Huusom AK: Prevention of relapse in generalized anxiety disorder by escitalopram treatment. Int J Neuropsychopharmacol 9(5):495–505, 2006 16316482

Allgulander C, Hartford J, Russell J, et al: Pharmacotherapy of generalized anxiety disorder: results of duloxetine treatment from a pooled analysis of three clinical trials. Curr Med Res Opin 23(6):1245–1252, 2007 17559726

Allgulander C, Nutt D, Detke M, et al: A non-inferiority comparison of duloxetine and venlafaxine in the treatment of adult patients with generalized anxiety disorder. J Psychopharmacol 22(4):417–425, 2008 18635722

Altamura AC, Serati M, Buoli M, et al: Augmentative quetiapine in partial/nonresponders with generalized anxiety disorder: a randomized, placebo-controlled study. Int Clin Psychopharmacol 26(4):201–205, 2011 21403524

Álvarez E, Carrasco JL, Olivares JM, et al: Broadening of generalized anxiety disorders definition does not affect the response to psychiatric care: findings from the observational ADAN study. Clin Pract Epidemiol Ment Health 8:158–168, 2012 23173012

Álvarez E, Olivares JM, Carrasco JL, et al: Clinical and economic outcomes of adjunctive therapy with pregabalin or usual care in generalized anxiety disorder patients with partial response to selective serotonin reuptake inhibitors. Ann Gen Psychiatry 14(1):2, 2015 25632294

American Psychiatric Association: Diagnostic and Statistical Manual of Mental Disorders, 3rd Edition. Washington, DC, American Psychiatric Association, 1980

American Psychiatric Association: Diagnostic and Statistical Manual of Mental Disorders, 5th Edition. Arlington, VA, American Psychiatric Association, 2013

Amsterdam JD, Li Y, Soeller I, et al: A randomized, double-blind, placebo-controlled trial of oral Matricaria recutita (chamomile) extract therapy for generalized anxiety disorder. J Clin Psychopharmacol 29(4):378–382, 2009 19593179

Ansseau M, Papart P, Gérard MA, et al: Controlled comparison of buspirone and oxazepam in generalized anxiety. Neuropsychobiology 24(2):74–78, 1991 2134114

Argyropoulou P, Patakas D, Koukou A, et al: Buspirone effect on breathlessness and exercise performance in patients with chronic obstructive pulmonary disease. Respiration 60(4):216–220, 1993 8265878

Ascher JA, Cole JO, Colin JN, et al: Bupropion: a review of its mechanism of antidepressant activity. J Clin Psychiatry 56(9):395–401, 1995 7665537

Ayd FJ Jr: Trifluoperazine therapy for everyday psychiatric problems. Curr Ther Res Clin Exp 1:17–25, 1959 13795347

Bakish D, Huusom AKT, Legault M: Escitalopram prevents relapse in generalized anxiety disorder: an analysis of data from Canadian patients participating in a multinational clinical study. Int J Neuropsychopharmacol 9:S185–S186, 2006

Baldwin DS, Huusom AK, Maehlum E: Escitalopram and paroxetine in the treatment of generalised anxiety disorder: randomised, placebo-controlled, double-blind study. Br J Psychiatry 189:264–272, 2006 16946363

Baldwin DS, Loft H, Florea I: Lu AA21004, a multimodal psychotropic agent, in the prevention of relapse in adult patients with generalized anxiety disorder. Int Clin Psychopharmacol 27(4):197–207, 2012 22475889

Baldwin DS, Ajel K, Masdrakis VG, et al: Pregabalin for the treatment of generalized anxiety disorder: an update. Neuropsychiatr Dis Treat 9:883–892, 2013 23836974

Ball SG, Kuhn A, Wall D, et al: Selective serotonin reuptake inhibitor treatment for generalized anxiety disorder: a double-blind, prospective comparison between paroxetine and sertraline. J Clin Psychiatry 66(1):94–99, 2005 15669894

Bandelow B, Chouinard G, Bobes J, et al: Extended-release quetiapine fumarate (quetiapine XR): a once-daily monotherapy effective in generalized anxiety disorder. Data from a randomized, double-blind, placebo- and active-controlled study. Int J Neuropsychopharmacol 13(3):305–320, 2010 19691907

Beesdo K, Hartford J, Russell J, et al: The short- and long-term effect of duloxetine on painful physical symptoms in patients with generalized anxiety disorder: results from three clinical trials. J Anxiety Disord 23(8):1064–1071, 2009 19643572

Bergner P: Passionflower. Medical Herbalism 7:13–14, 1995

Bidzan L, Mahableshwarkar AR, Jacobsen P, et al: Vortioxetine (Lu AA21004) in generalized anxiety disorder: results of an 8-week, multinational, randomized, double-blind, placebo-controlled clinical trial. Eur Neuropsychopharmacol 22(12):847–857, 2012 22898365

Bielski RJ, Bose A, Chang CC: A double-blind comparison of escitalopram and paroxetine in the long-term treatment of generalized anxiety disorder. Ann Clin Psychiatry 17(2):65–69, 2005

Bodkin JA, Allgulander C, Llorca PM, et al: Predictors of relapse in a study of duloxetine treatment for patients with generalized anxiety disorder. Hum Psychopharmacol 26(3):258–266, 2011 21678494

Boerner RJ, Sommer H, Berger W, et al: Kava-kava extract LI 150 is as effective as opipramol and buspirone in generalised anxiety disorder: an 8-week randomized, double-blind multicentre clinical trial in 129 out-patients. Phytomedicine 10(suppl 4):38–49, 2003 12807341

Bollu V, Bushmakin AG, Cappelleri JC, et al: Pregabalin reduces sleep disturbance in patients with generalized anxiety disorder via both direct and indirect mechanisms. Eur J Psychiatry 24(1):18–27, 2010

Borden LA, Murali Dhar TG, Smith KE, et al: Tiagabine, SK&F 89976-A, CI-966, and NNC-711 are selective for the cloned GABA transporter GAT-1. Eur J Pharmacol 269(2):219–224, 1994

Boschen MJ: A meta-analysis of the efficacy of pregabalin in the treatment of generalized anxiety disorder. Can J Psychiatry 56(9):558–566, 2011 21959031

Boschen MJ: Pregabalin: dose-response relationship in generalized anxiety disorder. Pharmacopsychiatry 45(2):51–56, 2012 22086745

Bose A, Korotzer A, Gommoll C, Li D: Randomized placebo-controlled trial of escitalopram and venlafaxine XR in the treatment of generalized anxiety disorder. Depress Anxiety 25(10):854–861, 2008 18050245

Brawman-Mintzer O, Knapp RG, Nietert PJ: Adjunctive risperidone in generalized anxiety disorder: a double-blind, placebo-controlled study. J Clin Psychiatry 66(10):1321–1325, 2005

Brawman-Mintzer O, Knapp RG, Rynn M, et al: Sertraline treatment for generalized anxiety disorder: a randomized, double-blind, placebo-controlled study. J Clin Psychiatry 67(6):874–881, 2006a 16848646

Brawman-Mintzer O, Nietert PJ, Rynn MA, et al: Quetiapine monotherapy in patients with GAD. Paper presented at the annual meeting of the American Psychiatric Association, Toronto, Canada, May 2006b

Brenes GA: Anxiety and chronic obstructive pulmonary disease: prevalence, impact, and treatment. Psychosom Med 65(6):963–970, 2003 14645773

Brown GG, Ostrowski S, Stein MB, et al: Temporal profile of brain response to alprazolam in patients with generalized anxiety disorder. Psychiatry Res Neuroimaging 233(3):394–401, 2015

Bystritsky A, Kerwin L, Feusner JD, et al: A pilot controlled trial of bupropion XL versus escitalopram in generalized anxiety disorder. Psychopharmacol Bull 41(1):46–51, 2008

Cavanagh HM, Wilkinson JM: Biological activities of lavender essential oil. Phytother Res 16(4):301–308, 2002 12112282

Chouinard G, Labonte A, Fontaine R, et al: New concepts in benzodiazepine therapy: rebound anxiety and new indications for the more potent benzodiazepines. Prog Neuropsychopharmacol Biol Psychiatry 7(4–6):669–673, 1983 6141609

Chouinard G, Bandelow B, Ahokas A, et al: Once-daily extended release quetiapine fumarate (quetiapine XR) monotherapy in generalized anxiety disorder: a phase III, double-blind, placebo-controlled study. Poster presented at the annual meeting of the American College of Neuropsychopharmacology, Boca Raton, FL, December 2007

Christensen MC, Loft H, Florea I, et al: Efficacy of vortioxetine in working patients with generalized anxiety disorder. CNS Spectr 24(2):249–257, 2019 29081307

Clayton AH, Durgam S, Li D, et al: Effects of vilazodone on sexual functioning in healthy adults: results from a randomized, double-blind, placebo-controlled, and active-controlled study. Int Clin Psychopharmacol 32(1):27–35, 2017 27643885

Cohn JB, Rickels K: A pooled, double-blind comparison of the effects of buspirone, diazepam and placebo in women with chronic anxiety. Curr Med Res Opin 11(5):304–320, 1989 2649317

Connor KM, Payne V, Davidson JRT: Kava in generalized anxiety disorder: three placebo-controlled trials. Int Clin Psychopharmacol 21(5):249–253, 2006 16877894

Coric V, Feldman HH, Oren DA, et al: Multicenter, randomized, double-blind, active comparator and placebo-controlled trial of a corticotropin-releasing factor receptor-1 antagonist in generalized anxiety disorder. Depress Anxiety 27(5):417–425, 2010 20455246

Crits-Christoph P, Newman MG, Rickels K, et al: Combined medication and cognitive therapy for generalized anxiety disorder. J Anxiety Disord 25(8):1087–1094, 2011 21840164

Culpepper L: Generalized anxiety disorder and medical illness. J Clin Psychiatry 70(suppl 2):20–24, 2009 19371503

Czobor P, Skolnick P, Beer B, et al: A multicenter, placebo-controlled, double-blind, randomized study of efficacy and safety of ocinaplon (DOV 273,547) in generalized anxiety disorder. CNS Neurosci Ther 16(2):63–75, 2010 20041911

Dahl AA, Ravindran A, Allgulander C, et al: Sertraline in generalized anxiety disorder: efficacy in treating the psychic and somatic anxiety factors. Acta Psychiatr Scand 111(6):429–435, 2005

Darcis T, Ferreri M, Natens J: A multicentre double-blind placebo controlled study investigating the anxiolytic efficacy of hydroxyzine in patients with generalized anxiety disorder. Hum Psychopharmacol 10(3):181–187, 1995

Davidson JR, DuPont RL, Hedges D, et al: Efficacy, safety, and tolerability of venlafaxine extended release and buspirone in outpatients with generalized anxiety disorder. J Clin Psychiatry 60(8):528–535, 1999 10485635

Davidson JR, Bose A, Korotzer A, et al: Escitalopram in the treatment of generalized anxiety disorder: double-blind, placebo controlled, flexible-dose study. Depress Anxiety 19(4):234–240, 2004 15274172

Davidson JR, Wittchen HU, Llorca PM, et al: Duloxetine treatment for relapse prevention in adults with generalized anxiety disorder: a double-blind placebo-controlled trial. Eur Neuropsychopharmacol 18(9):673–681, 2008 18559291

De Salas-Cansado M, Olivares JM, Alvarez E, et al: Pregabalin versus SSRIs and SNRIs in benzodiazepine-refractory outpatients with generalized anxiety disorder: a post hoc cost-effectiveness analysis in usual medical practice in Spain. Clinicoecon Outcomes Res 4:157–168, 2012 22745564

Depping AM, Komossa K, Kissling W, et al: Second-generation antipsychotics for anxiety disorders. Cochrane Database Syst Rev (12):CD008120, 2010 21154392

Donovan MR, Glue P, Kolluri S, et al: Comparative efficacy of antidepressants in preventing relapse in anxiety disorders—a meta-analysis. J Affect Disord 123(1–3):9–16, 2010 19616306

Dubois O, Salamon R, Germain C, et al: Balneotherapy versus paroxetine in the treatment of generalized anxiety disorder. Complement Ther Med 18(1):1–7, 2010 20178872

Durgam S, Gommoll C, Forero G, et al: Efficacy and safety of vilazodone in patients with generalized anxiety disorder: a randomized double-blind, placebo controlled, flexible-dose trial. J Clin Psychiatry 77(12):1687–1694, 2016 27232052

Elie R, Lamontagne Y: Alprazolam and diazepam in the treatment of generalized anxiety. J Clin Psychopharmacol 4(3):125–129, 1984 6145726

Endicott J, Svedsäter H, Locklear JC: Effects of once-daily extended release quetiapine fumarate on patient-reported outcomes in patients with generalized anxiety disorder. Neuropsychiatr Dis Treat 8:301–311, 2012 22848184

Enkelmann R: Alprazolam versus buspirone in the treatment of outpatients with generalized anxiety disorder. Psychopharmacology (Berl) 105(3):428–432, 1991 1798836

Esfehani RJ, Kamranian H, Jalalyazdi M: Effect of fluoxetine administration on clinical and echocardiographic findings in patients with mitral valve prolapse and generalized anxiety disorder: randomized clinical trial. Electron Physician 9(1):3483–3491, 2017 28243397

Feltner DE, Crockatt JG, Dubovsky SJ, et al: A randomized, double-blind, placebo-controlled, fixed-dose, multicenter study of pregabalin in patients with generalized anxiety disorder. J Clin Psychopharmacol 23(3):240–249, 2003 12826986

Feltner D, Wittchen HU, Kavoussi R, et al: Long-term efficacy of pregabalin in generalized anxiety disorder. Int Clin Psychopharmacol 23(1):18–28, 2008 18090504

Feltner DE, Harness J, Brock J, et al: Clinical evaluation of the Daily Assessment of Symptoms–Anxiety (DAS-A): a new instrument to assess the onset of symptomatic improvement in generalized anxiety disorder. CNS Neurosci Ther 15(1):12–18, 2009 19228175

Ferreira-Garcia R, Mochcovitch M, Costa do Cabo M, et al: Predictors of pharmacotherapy response in generalized anxiety disorder: a systematic review. Harv Rev Psychiatry 25(2):65–79, 2017 28272131

Ferrero A, Pierò A, Fassina S, et al: A 12-month comparison of brief psychodynamic psychotherapy and pharmacotherapy treatment in subjects with generalised anxiety disorders in a community setting. Eur Psychiatry 22(8):530–539, 2007 17900875

Fontaine R, Chouinard G, Annable L: Rebound anxiety in anxious patients after abrupt withdrawal of benzodiazepine treatment. Am J Psychiatry 141(7):848–852, 1984 6145363

Fontaine R, Mercier P, Beaudry P, et al: Bromazepam and lorazepam in generalized anxiety: a placebo-controlled study with measurement of drug plasma concentrations. Acta Psychiatr Scand 74(5):451–458, 1986 2880459

Fresquet A, Sust M, Lloret A, et al: Efficacy and safety of lesopitron in outpatients with generalized anxiety disorder. Ann Pharmacother 34(2):147–153, 2000 10676820

Fu J, Peng L, Li X: The efficacy and safety of multiple doses of vortioxetine for generalized anxiety disorder: a meta-analysis. Neuropsychiatr Dis Treat 12:951–959, 2016 27143896

Gammans RE, Stringfellow JC, Hvizdos AJ, et al: Use of buspirone in patients with generalized anxiety disorder and coexisting depressive symptoms. A meta-analysis of eight randomized, controlled studies. Neuropsychobiology 25(4):193–201, 1992 1454160

Gao K, Wu R, Kemp DE, et al: Efficacy and safety of quetiapine-XR as monotherapy or adjunctive therapy to a mood stabilizer in acute bipolar depression with generalized anxiety disorder and other comorbidities: a randomized, placebo-controlled trial. J Clin Psychiatry 75(10):1062–1068, 2014 25007003

Gelenberg AJ, Lydiard RB, Rudolph RL, et al: Efficacy of venlafaxine extended-release capsules in nondepressed outpatients with generalized anxiety disorder: a 6-month randomized controlled trial. JAMA 283(23):3082–3088, 2000 10865302

Generoso MB, Trevizol AP, Kasper S, et al: Pregabalin for generalized anxiety disorder: an updated systematic review and meta-analysis. Int Clin Psychopharmacol 32(1):49–55, 2017 27643884

Gommoll C, Durgam S, Mathews M, et al: A double-blind, randomized, placebo-controlled, fixed-dose phase III study of vilazodone in patients with generalized anxiety disorder. Depress Anxiety 32(6):451–459, 2015a 25891440

Gommoll C, Forero G, Mathews M, et al: Vilazodone in patients with generalized anxiety disorder: a double-blind, randomized, placebo-controlled, flexible-dose study. Int Clin Psychopharmacol 30(6):297–306, 2015b 26291335

Goodman WK, Bose A, Wang Q: Treatment of generalized anxiety disorder with escitalopram: pooled results from double-blind, placebo-controlled trials. J Affect Disord 87(2–3):161–167, 2005 15982747

Goodnick PJ, Puig A, DeVane CL, et al: Mirtazapine in major depression with comorbid generalized anxiety disorder. J Clin Psychiatry 60(7):446–448, 1999 10453798

Goodwin RD, Gorman JM: Psychopharmacologic treatment of generalized anxiety disorder and the risk of major depression. Am J Psychiatry 159(11):1935–1937, 2002 12411233

Gosselin P, Ladouceur R, Morin CM, et al: Benzodiazepine discontinuation among adults with GAD: a randomized trial of cognitive-behavioral therapy. J Consult Clin Psychol 74(5):908–919, 2006 17032095

Guaiana G, Barbui C, Cipriani A: Hydroxyzine for generalised anxiety disorder. Cochrane Database Syst Rev (12):CD006815, 2010 21154375

Gupta K, Mamidi P: Efficacy of Saraswata choorna on quality of life and manasika pariksha bhava's in generalized anxiety disorder—ancillary findings. Int J Res Ayurveda Pharm 6(2):216–220, 2014

Hackett D, Desmet A, Salinas EO: Dose-response efficacy of venlafaxine XR in GAD. Poster presented at 11th World Congress of Psychiatry, Hamburg, Germany, August 1999

Hackett D, Haudiquet V, Salinas E: A method for controlling for a high placebo response rate in a comparison of venlafaxine XR and diazepam in the short-term treatment of patients with generalised anxiety disorder. Eur Psychiatry 18(4):182–187, 2003 12814852

Hadley SJ, Mandel FS, Schweizer E: Switching from long-term benzodiazepine therapy to pregabalin in patients with generalized anxiety disorder: a double-blind, placebo-controlled trial. J Psychopharmacol 26(4):461–470, 2012 21693549

Hartford J, Kornstein S, Liebowitz M, et al: Duloxetine as an SNRI treatment for generalized anxiety disorder: results from a placebo and active-controlled trial. Int Clin Psychopharmacol 22(3):167–174, 2007 17414743

Herrera-Arellano A, Jiménez-Ferrer JE, Zamilpa A, et al: Therapeutic effectiveness of Galphimia glauca vs. lorazepam in generalized anxiety disorder. A controlled 15-week clinical trial. Planta Med 78(14):1529–1535, 2012 22828921

Hewett K, Adams A, Bryson H, et al: Generalized anxiety disorder: efficacy of paroxetine. Paper presented at the 7th World Congress of Biological Psychiatry, Berlin, Germany, July 2001

Hoehn-Saric R, McLeod DR, Zimmerli WD: Differential effects of alprazolam and imipramine in generalized anxiety disorder: somatic versus psychic symptoms. J Clin Psychiatry 49(8):293–301, 1988 3045099

Hoertel N, Le Strat Y, Blanco C, et al: Generalizability of clinical trial results for generalized anxiety disorder to community samples. Depress Anxiety 29(7):614–620, 2012 22495990

Hoge EA, Worthington JJ 3rd, Kaufman RE, et al: Aripiprazole as augmentation treatment of refractory generalized anxiety disorder and panic disorder. CNS Spectr 13(6):522–527, 2008

Joyce M, Khan A, Atkinson S, et al: Efficacy and safety of extended release quetiapine fumarate (quetiapine XR) monotherapy in patients with generalized anxiety disorder (GAD). Poster presented at the 161st annual meeting of the American Psychiatric Association, Washington, DC, May 3–8, 2008

Kaplan A, Franzen MD, Nickell PV, et al: An open-label trial of duloxetine in patients with irritable bowel syndrome and comorbid generalized anxiety disorder. Int J Psychiatry Clin Pract 18(1):11–15, 2014 23980534

Kasper S, Herman B, Nivoli G, et al: Efficacy of pregabalin and venlafaxine-XR in generalized anxiety disorder: results of a double-blind, placebo-controlled 8-week trial. Int Clin Psychopharmacol 24(2):87–96, 2009 21456104

Kasper S, Gastpar M, Müller WE, et al: Lavender oil preparation Silexan is effective in general-ized anxiety disorder—a randomized, double-blind comparison to placebo and paroxe-tine. Int J Neuropsychopharmacol 17(6):859–869, 2014a 24456909

Kasper S, Iglesias-García C, Schweizer E, et al: Pregabalin long-term treatment and assessment of discontinuation in patients with generalized anxiety disorder. Int J Neuropsychophar-macol 17(5):685–695, 2014b 24351233

Katzman MA, Brawman-Mintzer O, Reyes EB, et al: Extended release quetiapine fumarate (que-tiapine XR) monotherapy as maintenance treatment for generalized anxiety disorder: a long-term, randomized, placebo-controlled trial. Int Clin Psychopharmacol 26(1):11–24, 2011

Katzman MA, Bleau P, Blier P, et al: Canadian clinical practice guidelines for the management of anxiety, posttraumatic stress and obsessive-compulsive disorders. BMC Psychiatry 14(suppl 1):S1, 2014 25081580

Keefe JR, Mao JJ, Soeller I, et al: Short-term open-label chamomile (Matricaria chamomilla L.) therapy of moderate to severe generalized anxiety disorder. Phytomedicine 23(14):1699–1705, 2016 27912871

Khan A, Joyce M, Atkinson S, et al: A randomized, double-blind study of once-daily extended release quetiapine fumarate (quetiapine XR) monotherapy in patients with generalized anxiety disorder. J Clin Psychopharmacol 31(4):418–428, 2011 21694613

Khan A, Atkinson S, Mezhebovsky I, et al: Extended-release quetiapine fumarate (quetiapine XR) as adjunctive therapy in patients with generalized anxiety disorder and a history of inadequate treatment response: a randomized, double-blind study. Ann Clin Psychiatry 25(4):E7–E22, 2013 24199224

Khan A, Durgam S, Tang X, et al: Post hoc analyses of anxiety measures in adult patients with generalized anxiety disorder treated with vilazodone. Prim Care Companion CNS Disord 18(2), 2016 27486544

Kim TS, Pae CU, Yoon SJ, et al: Comparison of venlafaxine extended release versus paroxetine for treatment of patients with generalized anxiety disorder. Psychiatry Clin Neurosci 60(3):347–351, 2006 16732752

Kim YW, Lee SH, Choi TK, et al: Effectiveness of mindfulness-based cognitive therapy as an adjuvant to pharmacotherapy in patients with panic disorder or generalized anxiety dis-order. Depress Anxiety 26(7):601–606, 2009 19242985

Koponen H, Allgulander C, Erickson J, et al: Efficacy of duloxetine for the treatment of gener-alized anxiety disorder: implications for primary care physicians. Prim Care Companion J Clin Psychiatry 9(2):100–107, 2007 17607331

Kubo N, Shirakawa O, Kuno T, et al: Antimuscarinic effects of antihistamines: quantitative evaluation by receptor-binding assay. Jpn J Pharmacol 43(3):277–282, 1987 2884340

Laakmann G, Schüle C, Lorkowski G, et al: Buspirone and lorazepam in the treatment of gen-eralized anxiety disorder in outpatients. Psychopharmacology (Berl) 136(4):357–366, 1998

Lader M, Scotto JC: A multicentre double-blind comparison of hydroxyzine, buspirone and placebo in patients with generalized anxiety disorder. Psychopharmacology (Berl) 139(4):402–406, 1998 9809861

LaLonde CD, Van Lieshout RJ: Treating generalized anxiety disorder with second generation antipsychotics: a systematic review and meta-analysis. J Clin Psychopharmacol 31(3):326–333, 2011 21508847

Lenox-Smith AJ, Reynolds A: A double-blind, randomised, placebo controlled study of venla-faxine XL in patients with generalised anxiety disorder in primary care. Br J Gen Pract 53(495):772–777, 2003 14601352

Li R, Wu R, Chen J, et al: A randomized, placebo-controlled pilot study of quetiapine-XR mono-therapy or adjunctive therapy to antidepressant in acute major depressive disorder with current generalized anxiety disorder. Psychopharmacol Bull 46(1):8–23, 2016 27738370

Li X, Zhu L, Su Y, Fang S: Short-term efficacy and tolerability of venlafaxine extended release in adults with generalized anxiety disorder without depression: a meta-analysis. PLoS One 12(10):e0185865, 2017 28982121

Li X, Zhu L, Zhou C, et al: Efficacy and tolerability of short-term duloxetine treatment in adults with generalized anxiety disorder: a meta-analysis. PLoS One 13(3):e0194501, 2018 29558528

Llorca PM, Spadone C, Sol O, et al: Efficacy and safety of hydroxyzine in the treatment of generalized anxiety disorder: a 3-month double-blind study. J Clin Psychiatry 63(11):1020–1027, 2002 12444816

Lohoff FW, Etemad B, Mandos LA, et al: Ziprasidone treatment of refractory generalized anxiety disorder: a placebo-controlled, double-blind study. J Clin Psychopharmacol 30(2):185–189, 2010 20520293

Lydiard RB, Ballenger JC, Rickels K, et al: A double-blind evaluation of the safety and efficacy of abecarnil, alprazolam, and placebo in outpatients with generalized anxiety disorder. J Clin Psychiatry 58(11 suppl 11):11–18, 1997 9363043

Lydiard RB, Rickels K, Herman B, et al: Comparative efficacy of pregabalin and benzodiazepines in treating the psychic and somatic symptoms of generalized anxiety disorder. Int J Neuropsychopharmacol 13(2):229–241, 2010 19737439

Mahableshwarkar AR, Jacobsen PL, Chen Y, et al: A randomised, double-blind, placebo-controlled, duloxetine-referenced study of the efficacy and tolerability of vortioxetine in the acute treatment of adults with generalized anxiety disorder. Int J Clin Pract 68(1):49–59, 2014a 24341301

Mahableshwarkar AR, Jacobsen PL, Serenko M, et al: A randomized, double-blind, fixed-dose study comparing the efficacy and tolerability of vortioxetine 2.5 and 10 mg in acute treatment of adults with generalized anxiety disorder. Hum Psychopharmacol 29(1):64–72, 2014b 24424707

Maneeton N, Maneeton B, Woottiluk P, et al: Quetiapine monotherapy in acute treatment of generalized anxiety disorder: a systematic review and meta-analysis of randomized controlled trials. Drug Des Devel Ther 10:259–276, 2016 26834458

Mao JJ, Xie SX, Keefe JR, et al: Long-term chamomile (Matricaria chamomilla L.) treatment for generalized anxiety disorder: a randomized clinical trial. Phytomedicine 23(14):1735–1742, 2016 27912875

Martin JL, Sainz-Pardo M, Furukawa TA, et al: Benzodiazepines in generalized anxiety disorder: heterogeneity of outcomes based on a systematic review and meta-analysis of clinical trials. J Psychopharmacol 21(7):774–782, 2007 17881433

Mayers AG, Baldwin DS: Antidepressants and their effect on sleep. Hum Psychopharmacol 20(8):533–559, 2005 16229049

Meibach RC, Dunner D, Wilson LG, et al: Comparative efficacy of propranolol, chlordiazepoxide, and placebo in the treatment of anxiety: a double-blind trial. J Clin Psychiatry 48(9):355–358, 1987 3305488

Mendels J, Krajewski TF, Huffer V, et al: Effective short-term treatment of generalized anxiety disorder with trifluoperazine. J Clin Psychiatry 47(4):170–174, 1986 3514583

Menza MA, Dobkin RD, Marin H: An open-label trial of aripiprazole augmentation for treatment-resistant generalized anxiety disorder. J Clin Psychopharmacol 27(2):207–210, 2007

Merideth C, Cutler A, Neijber A, et al: Efficacy and tolerability of extended release quetiapine fumarate monotherapy in the treatment of GAD. Eur Neuropsychopharmacol 18:S499–S500, 2008

Merideth C, Cutler AJ, She F, et al: Efficacy and tolerability of extended release quetiapine fumarate monotherapy in the acute treatment of generalized anxiety disorder: a randomized, placebo controlled and active-controlled study. Int Clin Psychopharmacol 27(1):40–54, 2012 22045039

Miceli JJ, Ramey TS, Weaver JJ, et al: Adjunctive pregabalin treatment after partial response in generalized anxiety disorder: results of a double-blind, placebo-controlled trial. Presented at the 162nd annual meeting of the American Psychiatric Association, San Francisco, CA, May 16–21, 2009

Mikami K, Jorge RE, Moser DJ, et al: Prevention of post-stroke generalized anxiety disorder, using escitalopram or problem-solving therapy. J Neuropsychiatry Clin Neurosci 26(4):323–328, 2014 24457590

Mitte K: Meta-analysis of cognitive-behavioral treatments for generalized anxiety disorder: a comparison with pharmacotherapy. Psychol Bull 131(5):785–795, 2005 16187860

Möller HJ, Volz HP, Reimann IW, et al: Opipramol for the treatment of generalized anxiety disorder: a placebo-controlled trial including an alprazolam-treated group. J Clin Psychopharmacol 21(1):59–65, 2001 11199949

Montgomery SA, Tobias K, Zornberg GL, et al: Efficacy and safety of pregabalin in the treatment of generalized anxiety disorder: a 6-week, multicenter, randomized, double-blind, placebo-controlled comparison of pregabalin and venlafaxine. J Clin Psychiatry 67(5):771–782, 2006 16841627

Montgomery SA, Herman BK, Schweizer E, et al: The efficacy of pregabalin and benzodiazepines in generalized anxiety disorder presenting with high levels of insomnia. Int Clin Psychopharmacol 24(4):214–222, 2009 19542983

Montgomery SA, Locklear JC, Svedsäter H, et al: Efficacy of once-daily extended release quetiapine fumarate in patients with different levels of severity of generalized anxiety disorder. Int Clin Psychopharmacol 29(5):252–262, 2014 24394383

Montgomery SA, Lyndon G, Almas M, et al: Early improvement with pregabalin predicts endpoint response in patients with generalized anxiety disorder: an integrated and predictive data analysis. Int Clin Psychopharmacol 32(1):41–48, 2017 27583543

Morris PLP, Dahl AA, Kutcher SP, et al: Efficacy of sertraline for the acute treatment of generalized anxiety disorder (GAD). Eur Neuropsychopharmacol 13:S375, 2003

Moyer JH, Conner PK: Clinical and laboratory observations on two trifluoromethyl phenothiazine derivatives. J Lab Clin Med 51(2):185–197, 1958 13514224

Nicolini H, Bakish D, Duenas H, et al: Improvement of psychic and somatic symptoms in adult patients with generalized anxiety disorder: examination from a duloxetine, venlafaxine extended-release and placebo-controlled trial. Psychol Med 39(2):267–276, 2009 18485261

Nimatoudis I, Zissis NP, Kogeorgos J, et al: Remission rates with venlafaxine extended release in Greek outpatients with generalized anxiety disorder. A double-blind, randomized, placebo controlled study. Int Clin Psychopharmacol 19(6):331–336, 2004 15486518

Nojoumi M, Ghaeli P, Salimi S, et al: Effects of passion flower extract, as an add-on treatment to sertraline, on reaction time in patients with generalized anxiety disorder: a double-blind placebo-controlled study. Iran J Psychiatry 11(3):191–197, 2016 27928252

Okada S, Ichiki K, Tanokuchi S, et al: Effect of an anxiolytic on lipid profile in non-insulin-dependent diabetes mellitus. J Int Med Res 22(6):338–342, 1994 7895897

Olivares JM, Álvarez E, Carrasco JL, et al: Pregabalin for the treatment of patients with generalized anxiety disorder with inadequate treatment response to antidepressants and severe depressive symptoms. Int Clin Psychopharmacol 30(5):265–271, 2015 26111356

Ooi SL, Henderson P, Pak SC: Kava for generalized anxiety disorder: a review of current evidence. J Altern Complement Med 24(8):770–780, 2018 29641222

Pae CU, Wang SM, Han C, et al: Vortioxetine, a multimodal antidepressant for generalized anxiety disorder: a systematic review and meta-analysis. J Psychiatr Res 64:88–98, 2015 25851751

Pande AC, Crockatt JG, Feltner DE, et al: Pregabalin in generalized anxiety disorder: a placebo-controlled trial. Am J Psychiatry 160(3):533–540, 2003 12611835

Pandina GJ, Canuso CM, Turkoz I, et al: Adjunctive risperidone in the treatment of generalized anxiety disorder: a double-blind, prospective, placebo-controlled, randomized trial. Psychopharmacol Bull 40(3):41–57, 2007 18007568

Papp LA, Weiss JR, Greenberg HE, et al: Sertraline for chronic obstructive pulmonary disease and comorbid anxiety and mood disorders. Am J Psychiatry 152(10):1531, 1995 7573598

Park DM, Kim SH, Park YC, et al: The comparative clinical study of efficacy of Gamisoyo-San (Jiaweixiaoyaosan) on generalized anxiety disorder according to differently manufactured preparations: multicenter, randomized, double blind, placebo controlled trial. J Ethnopharmacol 158(Pt A):11–17, 2014 25456420

Patterson B, Van Ameringen M: Augmentation strategies for treatment-resistant anxiety disorders: a systematic review and meta-analysis. Depress Anxiety 33(8):728–736, 2016 27175543

Pierò A, Locati E: An open, non-randomised comparison of escitalopram and duloxetine for the treatment of subjects with generalized anxiety disorder. Hum Psychopharmacol 26(1):63–71, 2011 21305612

Pohl RB, Feltner DE, Fieve RR, et al: Efficacy of pregabalin in the treatment of generalized anxiety disorder: double-blind, placebo-controlled comparison of bid versus tid dosing. J Clin Psychopharmacol 25(2):151–158, 2005 15738746

Pollack MH, Zaninelli R, Goddard A, et al: Paroxetine in the treatment of generalized anxiety disorder: results of a placebo-controlled, flexible-dosage trial. J Clin Psychiatry 62(5):350–357, 2001 11411817

Pollack MH, Roy-Byrne PP, Van Ameringen M, et al: The selective GABA reuptake inhibitor tiagabine for the treatment of generalized anxiety disorder: results of a placebo-controlled study. J Clin Psychiatry 66(11):1401–1408, 2005 16420077

Pollack MH, Simon NM, Zalta AK, et al: Olanzapine augmentation of fluoxetine for refractory generalized anxiety disorder: a placebo controlled study. Biol Psychiatry 59(3):211–215, 2006

Pollack M, Kinrys G, Krystal A, et al: Eszopiclone coadministered with escitalopram in patients with insomnia and comorbid generalized anxiety disorder. Arch Gen Psychiatry 65(5):551–562, 2008a 18458207

Pollack MH, Kornstein SG, Spann ME, et al: Early improvement during duloxetine treatment of generalized anxiety disorder predicts response and remission at endpoint. J Psychiatr Res 42(14):1176–1184, 2008b 18348888

Pollack MH, Tiller J, Xie F, et al: Tiagabine in adult patients with generalized anxiety disorder: results from 3 randomized, double-blind, placebo-controlled, parallel-group studies. J Clin Psychopharmacol 28(3):308–316, 2008c 18480688

Power KG, Simpson RJ, Swanson V, et al: Controlled comparison of pharmacological and psychological treatment of generalized anxiety disorder in primary care. Br J Gen Pract 40(336):289–294, 1990 2081065

Preti A, Vrublevska J, Veroniki AA, et al: Prevalence, impact and treatment of generalised anxiety disorder in bipolar disorder: a systematic review and meta-analysis. Evid Based Ment Health 19(3):73–81, 2016 27405742

Qian M, Shen Z, Lin M, et al: Early improvement predicts 8-week treatment outcome in patients with generalized anxiety disorder treated with escitalopram or venlafaxine. Asia-Pac Psychiatry 9(4):e12270, 2017 29193711

Rakel RE: Long-term buspirone therapy for chronic anxiety: a multicenter international study to determine safety. South Med J 83(2):194–198, 1990 2406933

Reinhold JA, Rickels K: Pharmacological treatment for generalized anxiety disorder in adults: an update. Expert Opin Pharmacother 16(11):1669–1681, 2015 26159446

Rickels K: Benzodiazepines in the treatment of anxiety. Am J Psychother 36(3):358–370, 1982

Rickels K, Rynn M: Overview and clinical presentation of generalized anxiety disorder. Psychiatr Clin North Am 24(1):1–17, 2001 11225502

Rickels K, Csanalosi IB, Chung HR, et al: The beta-blocker atenolol in anxiety: a controlled study. Curr Ther Res Clin Exp 40(1):149–155, 1986

Rickels K, Fox IL, Greenblatt DJ, et al: Clorazepate and lorazepam: clinical improvement and rebound anxiety. Am J Psychiatry 145(3):312–317, 1988 2894175

Rickels K, Downing R, Schweizer E, et al: Antidepressants for the treatment of generalized anxiety disorder. A placebo-controlled comparison of imipramine, trazodone, and diazepam. Arch Gen Psychiatry 50(11):884–895, 1993 8215814

Rickels K, Schweizer E, DeMartinis N, et al: Gepirone and diazepam in generalized anxiety disorder: a placebo-controlled trial. J Clin Psychopharmacol 17(4):272–277, 1997 9241006

Rickels K, DeMartinis N, Aufdembrinke B: A double-blind, placebo-controlled trial of abecarnil and diazepam in the treatment of patients with generalized anxiety disorder. J Clin Psychopharmacol 20(1):12–18, 2000a 10653203

Rickels K, Pollack MH, Sheehan DV, et al: Efficacy of extended-release venlafaxine in nondepressed outpatients with generalized anxiety disorder. Am J Psychiatry 157(6):968–974, 2000b

Rickels K, Zaninelli R, McCafferty J, et al: Paroxetine treatment of generalized anxiety disorder: a double-blind, placebo-controlled study. Am J Psychiatry 160(4):749–756, 2003 12668365

Rickels K, Pollack MH, Feltner DE, et al: Pregabalin for treatment of generalized anxiety disorder: a 4-week, multicenter, double-blind, placebo-controlled trial of pregabalin and alprazolam. Arch Gen Psychiatry 62(9):1022–1030, 2005 16143734

Rickels K, Etemad B, Khalid-Khan S, et al: Time to relapse after 6 and 12 months' treatment of
generalized anxiety disorder with venlafaxine extended release. Arch Gen Psychiatry
67(12):1274–1281, 2010 21135327

Rickels K, Shiovitz TM, Ramey TS, et al: Adjunctive therapy with pregabalin in generalized
anxiety disorder patients with partial response to SSRI or SNRI treatment. Int Clin Psychopharmacol 27(3):142–150, 2012 22302014

Rocca P, Fonzo V, Scotta M, et al: Paroxetine efficacy in the treatment of generalized anxiety
disorder. Acta Psychiatr Scand 95(5):444–450, 1997 9197912

Rothschild AJ, Mahableshwarkar AR, Jacobsen P, et al: Vortioxetine (Lu AA21004) 5 mg in generalized anxiety disorder: results of an 8-week randomized, double-blind, placebo-controlled
clinical trial in the United States. Eur Neuropsychopharmacol 22(12):858–866, 2012 22901736

Ruiz MA, Álvarez E, Carrasco JL, et al: Modeling the longitudinal latent effect of pregabalin on
self-reported changes in sleep disturbances in outpatients with generalized anxiety disorder managed in routine clinical practice. Drug Des Devel Ther 9:4329–4340, 2015 26273194

Russell JM, Weisberg R, Fava M, et al: Efficacy of duloxetine in the treatment of generalized
anxiety disorder in patients with clinically significant pain symptoms. Depress Anxiety
25(7):E1–E11, 2008 17587217

Rynn M, Russell J, Erickson J, et al: Efficacy and safety of duloxetine in the treatment of generalized anxiety disorder: a flexible-dose, progressive-titration, placebo-controlled trial. Depress Anxiety 25(3):182–189, 2008 17311303

Sarris J, Kavanagh DJ, Byrne G, et al: The Kava Anxiety Depression Spectrum Study (KADSS):
a randomized, placebo-controlled crossover trial using an aqueous extract of Piper
methysticum. Psychopharmacology (Berl) 205(3):399–407, 2009 19430766

Sarris J, Stough C, Bousman CA, et al: Kava in the treatment of generalized anxiety disorder: a
double-blind, randomized, placebo-controlled study. J Clin Psychopharmacol 33(5):643–
648, 2013a 23635869

Sarris J, Stough C, Teschke R, et al: Kava for the treatment of generalized anxiety disorder RCT:
analysis of adverse reactions, liver function, addiction, and sexual effects. Phytother Res
27(11):1723–1728, 2013b 23348842

Sayyah M, Siahpoosh A, Khalili H, et al: A double-blind, placebo-controlled study of the aqueous extract of echium amoenum for patients with general anxiety disorder. Iran J Pharm
Res 11(2):697–701, 2012 24250495

Schuurmans J, Comijs H, Emmelkamp PM, et al: A randomized, controlled trial of the effectiveness of cognitive-behavioral therapy and sertraline versus a waitlist control group for anxiety disorders in older adults. Am J Geriatr Psychiatry 14(3):255–263, 2006 16505130

Seeman P: Atypical antipsychotics: mechanism of action. Can J Psychiatry 47(1):27–38, 2002
11873706

Shadli SM, Kawe T, Martin D, et al: Ketamine effects on EEG during therapy of treatment-
resistant generalized anxiety and social anxiety. Int J Neuropsychopharmacol 21(8):717–724,
2018

Sheehan DV, Svedsäter H, Locklear JC, et al: Effects of extended-release quetiapine fumarate
on long-term functioning and sleep quality in patients with generalized anxiety disorder
(GAD): data from a randomized-withdrawal, placebo-controlled maintenance study. J Affect Disord 151(3):906–913, 2013 24135509

Silverstone PH, Salinas E: Efficacy of venlafaxine extended release in patients with major depressive disorder and comorbid generalized anxiety disorder. J Clin Psychiatry 62(7):523–
529, 2001 11488362

Simon NM, Hoge EA, Fischmann D, et al: An open-label trial of risperidone augmentation for
refractory anxiety disorders. J Clin Psychiatry 67(3):381–385, 2006a 16649823

Simon NM, Zalta AK, Worthington JJ 3rd, et al: Preliminary support for gender differences in
response to fluoxetine for generalized anxiety disorder. Depress Anxiety 23(6):373–376,
2006b 17068858

Simon NM, Connor KM, LeBeau RT, et al: Quetiapine augmentation of paroxetine CR for the treatment of refractory generalized anxiety disorder: preliminary findings. Psychopharmacology (Berl) 197(4):675–681, 2008 18246327

Singh YN, Singh NN: Therapeutic potential of kava in the treatment of anxiety disorders. CNS Drugs 16(11):731–743, 2002 12383029

Sjodin I, Kutcher SP, Ravindran A, et al: Efficacy of sertraline in improving quality of life and functioning in generalized anxiety disorder (GAD). Eur Neuropsychopharmacol 13:S365–S366, 2003

Song MF, Hu LL, Liu WJ, et al: Modified suanzaorentang had the treatment effect for generalized anxiety disorder for the first 4 weeks of paroxetine medication: a pragmatic randomized controlled study. Evid Based Complement Alternat Med 2017:8391637, 2017 28553362

Sramek JJ, Tansman M, Suri A, et al: Efficacy of buspirone in generalized anxiety disorder with coexisting mild depressive symptoms. J Clin Psychiatry 57(7):287–291, 1996 8666569

Sramek JJ, Frackiewicz EJ, Cutler NR: Efficacy and safety of two dosing regimens of buspirone in the treatment of outpatients with persistent anxiety. Clin Ther 19(3):498–506, 1997 9220214

Stein MB, Seedat S, Gelernter J: Serotonin transporter gene promoter polymorphism predicts SSRI response in generalized social anxiety disorder. Psychopharmacology (Berl) 187(1):68–72, 2006 16525856

Stein DJ, Ahokas AA, de Bodinat C: Efficacy of agomelatine in generalized anxiety disorder: a randomized, double-blind, placebo-controlled study. J Clin Psychopharmacol 28(5):561–566, 2008 18794654

Stein DJ, Bruce Lydiard R, Herman BK, et al: Impact of gastrointestinal symptoms on response to pregabalin in generalized anxiety disorder: results of a six-study combined analysis. Int Clin Psychopharmacol 24(3):126–132, 2009 19352198

Stein DJ, Bandelow B, Merideth C, et al: Efficacy and tolerability of extended release quetiapine fumarate (quetiapine XR) monotherapy in patients with generalised anxiety disorder: an analysis of pooled data from three 8-week placebo-controlled studies. Hum Psychopharmacol 26(8):614–628, 2011 22143997

Stein DJ, Ahokas A, Albarran C, et al: Agomelatine prevents relapse in generalized anxiety disorder: a 6-month randomized, double-blind, placebo-controlled discontinuation study. J Clin Psychiatry 73(7):1002–1008, 2012 22901350

Stein DJ, Ahokas A, Márquez MS, et al: Agomelatine in generalized anxiety disorder: an active comparator and placebo-controlled study. J Clin Psychiatry 75(4):362–368, 2014 24569045

Stein DJ, Ahokas A, Jarema M, et al: Efficacy and safety of agomelatine (10 or 25 mg/day) in non-depressed out-patients with generalized anxiety disorder: a 12-week, double-blind, placebo-controlled study. Eur Neuropsychopharmacol 27(5):526–537, 2017 28298261

Steiner M, Allgulander C, Ravindran A, et al: Gender differences in clinical presentation and response to sertraline treatment of generalized anxiety disorder. Hum Psychopharmacol 20(1):3–13, 2005 15551351

Stocchi F, Nordera G, Jokinen RH, et al: Efficacy and tolerability of paroxetine for the long-term treatment of generalized anxiety disorder. J Clin Psychiatry 64(3):250–258, 2003 12716265

Tollefson GD, Montague-Clouse J, Tollefson SL: Treatment of comorbid generalized anxiety in a recently detoxified alcoholic population with a selective serotonergic drug (buspirone). J Clin Psychopharmacol 12(1):19–26, 1992 1552035

Tubaki BR, Chandrashekar CR, Sudhakar D, et al: Clinical efficacy of Manasamitra vataka (an Ayurveda medication) on generalized anxiety disorder with comorbid generalized social phobia: a randomized controlled study. J Altern Complement Med 18(6):612–621, 2012

Van Ameringen M, Patterson B, Turna J, et al: The treatment of refractory generalized anxiety disorder. Curr Treat Options Psychiatry 4(4):407–417, 2017

Varia I, Rauscher F: Treatment of generalized anxiety disorder with citalopram. Int Clin Psychopharmacol 17(3):103–107, 2002 11981350

Wang S, Zhao LL, Qiu XJ, et al: Efficacy and safety of a formulated herbal granula, jiu wei zhen xin, for generalized anxiety disorder: a meta-analysis. Evid Based Complement Alternat Med 2018:9090181, 2018 29707037

Wang T, Ding JY, Xu GX, et al: Efficacy of yiqiyangxin Chinese medicine compound combined with cognitive therapy in the treatment of generalized anxiety disorders. Asian Pac J Trop Med 5(10):818–822, 2012 23043923

Wittchen HU, Kessler RC, Beesdo K, et al: Generalized anxiety and depression in primary care: prevalence, recognition, and management. J Clin Psychiatry 63(suppl 8):24–34, 2002 12044105

Woelk H, Schläfke S: A multi-center, double-blind, randomised study of the lavender oil preparation Silexan in comparison to lorazepam for generalized anxiety disorder. Phytomedicine 17(2):94–99, 2010 19962288

Wu WY, Wang G, Ball SG, et al: Duloxetine versus placebo in the treatment of patients with generalized anxiety disorder in China. Chin Med J (Engl) 124(20):3260–3268, 2011 22088518

Yonkers KA, Warshaw MG, Massion AO, et al: Phenomenology and course of generalised anxiety disorder. Br J Psychiatry 168(3):308–313, 1996 8833684

Zaccara G, Gangemi P, Perucca P, et al: The adverse event profile of pregabalin: a systematic review and meta-analysis of randomized controlled trials. Epilepsia 52(4):826–836, 2011 21320112

Zareifopoulos N, Dylja I: Efficacy and tolerability of vilazodone for the acute treatment of generalized anxiety disorder: a meta-analysis. Asian J Psychiatr 26:115–122, 2017 28483071

Zhang Y, Huang G, Yang S, et al: Duloxetine in treating generalized anxiety disorder in adults: a meta-analysis of published randomized, double-blind, placebo-controlled trials. Asia-Pac Psychiatry 8(3):215–225, 2016 26238298

Zupancic M, Guilleminault C: Agomelatine: a preliminary review of a new antidepressant. CNS Drugs 20(12):981–992, 2006 17140278

Recommended Readings

Kasper S, Herman B, Nivoli G, et al: Efficacy of pregabalin and venlafaxine-XR in generalized anxiety disorder: results of a double-blind, placebo-controlled 8-week trial. Int Clin Psychopharmacol 24(2):87–96, 2009 21456104

Kim YW, Lee SH, Choi TK, et al: Effectiveness of mindfulness-based cognitive therapy as an adjuvant to pharmacotherapy in patients with panic disorder or generalized anxiety disorder. Depress Anxiety 26(7):601–606, 2009 19242985

Qian M, Shen Z, Lin M, et al: Early improvement predicts 8-week treatment outcome in patients with generalized anxiety disorder treated with escitalopram or venlafaxine. Asia-Pac Psychiatry 9(4), 2017 29193711

Reinhold JA, Rickels K: Pharmacological treatment for generalized anxiety disorder in adults: an update. Expert Opin Pharmacother 16(11):1669–1681, 2015 26159446

Stein MB, Seedat S, Gelernter J: Serotonin transporter gene promoter polymorphism predicts SSRI response in generalized social anxiety disorder. Psychopharmacology (Berl) 187(1):68–72, 2006 16525856

CHAPTER 14

Psychotherapy for Generalized Anxiety Disorder

Jonathan D. Huppert, Ph.D.
William C. Sanderson, Ph.D.

Nature of Generalized Anxiety Disorder

Until the advent of DSM-III-R in 1987 (American Psychiatric Association 1987), the development of treatment for generalized anxiety disorder (GAD) was aimed at treating "anxious neurotics." Two primary techniques were used: relaxation or biofeedback to address physiological tension (Rice and Blanchard 1982) and cognitive therapy to address the anxious thoughts associated with GAD (Beck 1976). Most cognitive-behavioral therapy (CBT) treatment protocols developed until the mid-1990s continued to integrate these two major strategies. However, as a result of greater precision in the definition of GAD and an increased understanding of the nature of worry and anxiety (DSM-IV, DSM-5; American Psychiatric Association 1994, 2013), newer treatment protocols also include strategies to address these recently identified components, such as techniques to minimize experiential avoidance, techniques to enhance problem solving, and techniques involving metacognitive processing.

Worry

Diagnosis of GAD depends on the existence of two core symptoms: worry (i.e., preoccupation with negative events occurring in the future) and physiological hyperarousal (e.g., muscle tension, sleep disturbance, feeling keyed up). Worry is frequently the most prominent symptom and considered the cardinal feature of GAD. It is a cognitive activity often referred to as "anxious apprehension" and is elicited by the perception of *potential* future danger (Hirsch and Mathews 2012), such as "What if I fail the licensing exam I am taking next week, and as a result I am not able to get a job?" Worry is often accompanied by behavior directed at gaining control to avoid the occurrence of the negative event (Rapee 1991).

Individuals with GAD experience excessive worry, reporting worry most of the day, nearly every day (Brown et al. 1993; Dupuy et al. 2001). Even though worry often activates attempts at problem solving in nearly everyone, individuals with GAD lack confidence in their solutions, thereby leading to continued worry (Davey 1994). Worriers report five major functions of worry: 1) superstitious avoidance of catastrophes, 2) actual avoidance of catastrophes, 3) avoidance of deeper emotional topics, 4) coping preparation, and 5) motivating devices (Borkovec 1994).

Worry appears to inhibit autonomic arousal, thereby avoiding certain affective states and the reduction of anxious states (see Borkovec et al. 2004 for a review). Similarly, more recent theories suggest that worry is a choice to feel bad now instead of feeling much worse later or being surprised by negative feelings (Newman and Llera 2011). Counterintuitively, relaxation has been shown to increase the amount of worry in some patients with GAD (Borkovec et al. 1991).

As with most anxiety disorders, worry in GAD is related to increased attentional biases, decreased attentional control, and biased processing of emotional information (Hirsch and Mathews 2012). In addition, individuals with GAD often have a heightened sense of the likelihood of negative events happening (i.e., increased risk perception) and often exaggerate the negative consequences that would result (Brown et al. 1993). Patients with GAD tend to worry frequently about minor matters (Brown et al. 1994).

Physiological Hyperarousal

In addition to worry, patients with GAD experience unpleasant somatic sensations associated with their chronic physiological hyperarousal or stress. Although both the cognitive and somatic sensations usually increase during the course of a "worry episode," for the most part these symptoms are relatively chronic and are not limited to episodes of worry. The most common somatic symptom reported by patients with GAD is muscle tension.

Cognitive-Behavioral Therapy Techniques

As the following discussion makes clear, CBT is the main psychotherapeutic approach for GAD, with strong empirical support from controlled research studies. Although some subtle differences in the treatment packages employed within these studies may exist, for the most part, several common "essential" elements are contained in CBT treatments for GAD. These components include psychoeducation, self-monitoring, cognitive restructuring, relaxation, worry exposure, worry behavior control, and problem solving. Of course, these techniques should be delivered within the context of a good psychotherapeutic atmosphere that includes all of the nonspecific elements of therapy (e.g., a good therapeutic relationship, positive expectancy, warmth). Each technique is briefly described in sections that follow.

Psychoeducation

Psychoeducation about GAD is an important aspect of therapy. Many patients who come in for treatment have never been told their diagnosis and frequently have misconceptions about their disorder (e.g., that anxiety will lead to psychosis) and misunderstandings about common responses (e.g., physiological, emotional) to worry and stress (e.g., that all worry is bad). Psychoeducation includes informing the patient about the biopsychosocial model of anxiety (Borkovec et al. 2004; Newman and Llera 2011; Rygh and Sanderson 2004). Many patients experience great relief in knowing that their experiences are not uncommon, that scientific knowledge exists, and that effective treatments are available. Providing psychoeducation is also a way to review the treatment rationale and thus facilitate treatment compliance. Psychoeducation should be provided in written form (or online) and followed up in session.

Self-Monitoring

Self-monitoring is one of the most basic yet essential parts of CBT. Monitoring is used as both an assessment procedure and a treatment strategy. Each time patients feel worried or anxious, they should record when and where the anxiety began and the intensity of the experience, including symptoms that were present. Avoidance of monitoring is detrimental to treatment because the patient is likely avoiding anxiety. Thus, one should simplify and problem solve to attain compliance rather than eliminate the monitoring. To enhance compliance, therapists should inform the patients of the reasoning behind the monitoring. The basic aspects of worry monitoring to record are date, time began, time ended, place, event (trigger), average anxiety (from 1 [minimal] to 10 [extremely distressing]), peak anxiety (1–10), average depression (1–10), and topics of worry. Once cognitive restructuring is introduced, monitoring the specific thought process involving worries is added to this list.

Cognitive Therapy: Restructuring the Worry

Patients with anxiety disorders, and with GAD in particular, overestimate the likelihood of negative events and underestimate their ability to cope with difficult situations (Beck et al. 1985). These "cognitive distortions" can play a major role in the vicious circle of anxiety, and they accentuate the patient's feelings of danger and threat. Threaded throughout the biopsychosocial model is the theme that cognition plays a major role in eliciting and perpetuating the cycle of anxiety. Cognitive restructuring is introduced in detail by discussing the concepts of automatic thoughts, anxious predictions, and the maintenance of anxiety through unchallenged/unchecked negative predictions about the future. *Automatic thoughts* are described as learned responses to cues that can occur so quickly that they may be outside of one's awareness. Thus, patients are taught to observe their own thoughts at the moment of anxiety (or immediately after), to assess what cues may have triggered the feeling, and to elaborate on what thoughts were going through their minds. Initially, the thoughts are not immediately challenged but collected as data to determine common thoughts that occur during worry. In addition to self-monitoring, anxious cognitions are accessed within the therapy session through Socratic questioning, roleplaying, and imagery. It is often helpful to warn patients that monitoring thoughts can provoke anxiety because they are focusing on anxious cognitions and to explain that exposure to such thoughts, while uncomfortable, is necessary for change.

Relaxation

Relaxation exercises are an important component of most CBT-oriented treatments for GAD. The function of these exercises is to reduce physiological arousal, broaden the focus of attention, and increase patients' ability to consider alternatives. In addition, relaxation may facilitate getting unstuck from perseverating thoughts or divide attention to other foci. Finally, in contrast to the aforementioned effects, relaxation may at times facilitate the activation of anxious thoughts that are otherwise not being processed (Borkovec and Whisman 1996), thereby assisting in exposure to the anxious thoughts. GAD typically includes muscle tension and problems sleeping. Relaxation often helps patients with GAD. Most recent methods of teaching relaxation have adapted a flexible concept rather than insisting on any particular approach. Thus, although progressive muscle relaxation techniques are emphasized for most patients and have the most empirical support, if a patient prefers another method and is able to use it effectively, then we recommend continued use of that strategy.

Worry Exposure

As noted, the perpetuation of worry in patients with GAD may be caused by incomplete processing of the worry, which may be a result of avoiding focusing on the worry itself. Instead of focusing on a worry that will increase anxiety in the short run, patients attempt to avoid fully processing the worry through various behaviors (discussed in the next section), as well as through constant shifting of worries. For this reason, Brown et al. (1993) described a technique in which patients purposely expose themselves both to worry and to images associated with the worry for an extended period. The concept is to have patients activate the worst possible outcome in order to process it and habituate to the anxiety associated with it. Borkovec et al. (1983) developed a similar technique referred to as *stimulus control*. In this approach, patients are asked to postpone worrying when it begins to happen, make a list of the worries that occur, and then set aside an hour in the evening to focus exclusively on the worries. Recent research showed that writing such exposures and reading the same content repeatedly can reduce GAD symptoms (Fracalanza et al. 2014).

Worry Behavior Control

Many patients who worry may behave in certain ways to try to avoid it. Although it is an aversive experience, uncontrollable worry may serve the function of avoiding an even more intolerable experience (i.e., by focusing on the worry instead of the other experience). Behaviors that facilitate the avoidance of the worry itself may then result in avoidance of both the anxiety created by worry and the experience avoided through worrying. According to this explanation, patients' preoccupation with worry distracts them from the original source of the negative state (e.g., fear, depression). Therefore, eliminating worry behaviors allows patients to fully experience and process the worry. To prevent worry behaviors, patients carefully monitor what they do when they notice the onset of worry, and they are asked to refrain from these behaviors. If many behaviors are involved, or if a patient is too anxious to just give up the behaviors, hierarchies are created to assist the patient in systematically giving up the behaviors, starting with easier ones and moving on to more difficult behaviors, making the task considerably less overwhelming.

Problem Solving

Teaching problem solving is a classic CBT approach for many disorders. Dugas et al. (1998, 2003, 2010) outlined two main problems for individuals with GAD. They suggested that the core problem of GAD is the intolerance of uncertainty and that this has an impact on two types of problems that GAD patients face. The first type is "unrealistic problems." These problems cannot be solved rationally and must be dealt with via *worry exposure*. The second type of problem is "catastrophic thinking" about real issues. Problem solving includes identifying the problem, setting goals, generating alternative solutions, selecting and implementing a solution, and evaluating the results. The goal in introducing these steps is not only to solve the problem being focused on but also to help patients develop better problem-solving skills and learn that problems often have multiple solutions.

Reviews of Treatment Outcome Studies

Treatment Guidelines

Many treatment guidelines throughout the world recommend CBT as a first-line treatment for GAD. These includes reviews by the National Institute for Clinical Excellence in the United Kingdom (Baker et al. 2015) and the International Consensus Group on Anxiety and Depression (Ballenger et al. 2001), as well as Dutch guidelines (van Dijk et al. 2012). These treatment recommendations are based on accumulated literature demonstrating the efficacy of CBT for GAD as well as support for the cost-effectiveness of such treatments (Ophuis et al. 2017). Therefore, consistent with the empirical literature, our review emphasizes CBT. More recent analyses have focused on cost-effectiveness analyses and found that CBT tends to be more cost-effective than medications and that internet-based interventions tend to be the most cost-effective (Ophuis et al. 2017). In most cases, comorbid anxiety disorders may not need to be addressed directly. This may be largely a result of the fact that the treatment for GAD may be useful in reducing other anxiety symptoms as well (Steele et al. 2018).

Meta-Analytic Reviews

In a recent meta-analysis, Cuijpers et al. (2014) reviewed 41 studies of psychotherapy for GAD (including internet-based interventions) and concluded that CBT for GAD is more effective than control conditions in terms of both primary symptoms and depression. Interestingly, they found that self-report measures yielded larger effects than interviewer ratings. Nonspecific treatments (e.g., supportive psychotherapy) were reported to have large within-group effect sizes, but smaller than with CBT. The authors also found that long-term follow-up suggested smaller, but sustained, advantages of CBT over other treatments. A meta-analysis by Mitte (2005) in which CBT was compared to medications revealed that, overall, CBT was superior to no treatment or to placebo control conditions and was similar in effectiveness to medications (benzodiazepines and antidepressants). However, further analyses suggested that medications for GAD may be somewhat more effective than CBT, even though CBT may be more tolerable than medications (based on lower dropout rates). Most reviews concluded that approximately 50% of patients receiving CBT are categorized as responders and that approximately 17% drop out of treatment (Gersh et al. 2017).

Recent Studies of Cognitive-Behavioral Therapy

Given the number of reviews and studies of CBT alone, we choose here to focus on studies that include novel findings that go beyond the efficacy of CBT for GAD alone. This is not to de-emphasize the efficacy of CBT but rather to describe more novel methods and findings. Newman et al. (2011) conducted a trial of CBT alone compared with an integrated CBT plus interpersonal and emotion-focused therapy. Results suggest that CBT alone was as effective as the integrated treatment at posttreatment and at 1-year follow-up. However, patients who had a more dismissive or avoidant attachment style demonstrated advantages with the integrated treatment for anxiety symptom reduction at 2-year follow-up (Newman et al. 2015). In addition, an examination of CBT with a focus on intolerance of uncertainty versus relaxation therapy versus a waitlist condition found that CBT was superior to the waitlist condition, whereas relaxation therapy was less so, but the differences between CBT and relaxation failed to reach significance, likely due to the underpowered nature of the study (Dugas et al. 2010). Similarly, a randomized controlled trial of acceptance and commitment therapy versus relaxation found little difference between the two conditions (Hayes-Skelton et al. 2013). On the other hand, metacognitive therapy has demonstrated promising results, including superiority to treatment focusing on intolerance of uncertainty (Nordahl et al. 2018; van der Heiden et al. 2012). In addition, some studies have demonstrated that adding motivational interviewing to traditional CBT may enhance motivation to reduce worry and thereby enhance long-term outcomes (Westra et al. 2016). Adding well-being therapy also has been shown to improve outcomes (Fava et al. 2005). Finally, addressing emotion regulation deficits has shown promise (Mennin et al. 2018).

One question that has received little attention is whether CBT can improve outcomes in individuals receiving optimal dosages of medications. In the context of a venlafaxine extended-release (XR) study, 77 patients were offered adjunctive CBT (Crits-Christoph et al. 2011). Only 37% agreed, and no difference was found between those who received CBT and those who received medication alone, raising questions regarding the efficacy of adding CBT to optimal medication treatments. Overall, acceptance and mindfulness-based approaches appear similarly effective to traditional CBT or relaxation, whereas metacognitive CBT has shown some promise for improved outcomes. Finally, although much of this review has focused on GAD-specific treatments, data are accumulating that transdiagnostic protocols that focus on general emotion regulation deficits, reduction of safety behaviors, and increasing use of cognitive reappraisal have shown equivalent outcomes to those that examine GAD-specific procedures (Barlow et al. 2017).

Internet-Based Interventions

Since 2009, substantial progress has been made in development and study of internet-based interventions, including interventions for GAD; more than 15 randomized controlled trials have been published. These interventions can either be standalone or guided self-help, with the latter tending to yield better adherence and completion rates, although neither the intensity of therapist interaction nor therapist experience/expertise was related to outcomes (Domhardt et al. 2019). The interventions vary in the level of activity from text-only or pdf downloads of the techniques recommended (typically CBT as described earlier, but not only) to interactive websites with videos, multiple exercises, enabled chats, and more. These interventions can be either disorder focused or transdiagnostic, and they appear to yield similar results (Domhardt et al. 2019). The interventions appear to yield results similar to face-to-face treatments (Richards et al. 2015) and have effect sizes that are larger than those for either active online control treatments or peer support groups. In addition to the literature establishing the efficacy of internet-based CBT, one study has examined internet-based psychodynamic treatment versus internet-based CBT and found that these treatments were not statistically superior to a waitlist control, although some analyses demonstrated superiority of CBT and psychodynamic treatment to waitlist (Andersson et al. 2012). Overall, both treatments look promising, and given that this is the only trial of internet-based psychodynamic treatment, more study is needed.

Psychodynamic Treatment Studies

Several studies have examined the efficacy of psychodynamic treatments for GAD by using different types of psychodynamic therapy: psychoanalytic/classical Freudian, neo-Freudian interpersonal, Adlerian, intensive short-term dynamic psychotherapy, and supportive-expressive psychotherapy. Although some reports have been uncontrolled naturalistic studies, treatments are reported to yield significant improvements in symptoms. One study reported similar outcomes to medications in the same clinic (Ferrero et al. 2007), and another study reported reduced health care costs (Lilliengren et al. 2017). Many of these treatments posit that anxiety is related to conflictual interpersonal attachment patterns and incomplete processing of past traumatic or other emotional events. Relationships explored included current and past relationships as well as the therapeutic relationship. Durham et al. (1994, 1999, 2003) were the first investigators to examine both cognitive and psychodynamic therapies for GAD in a randomized trial and found CBT to be superior. Crits-Christoph et al. (1996, 2004, 2005) conducted an uncontrolled open trial of short-term psychodynamic therapy for GAD with 1-year follow-up as well as a randomized trial that failed to show superiority to supportive therapy. Finally, Leichsenring et al. (2009) conducted a randomized trial of CBT versus supportive-expressive psychotherapy and found that the two yielded good outcomes on symptom measures of GAD, with CBT being moderately more effective, but CBT was clearly superior on measures of worry and depression. In sum, evidence suggests short-term psychodynamic treatments for GAD may be more effective than waitlist or no treatment. However, data are equivocal in terms of their superiority over simpler supportive therapy, with more than one study suggesting some advantages of CBT over psychodynamic therapy for GAD (Durham et al. 1999;

Leichsenring et al. 2009). However, some of the foci in dynamic therapies have been adopted or integrated in newer CBT treatments.

Conclusion

Considerable progress has been made in understanding GAD and its treatment. With a focus on the nature and function of worry, clinical researchers have been able to develop treatments that specifically target the putative underlying psychopathological mechanisms. Investigators have not been satisfied with treatment results from standard CBT packages that appear to help approximately 50% of patients. Some promising directions include integration of motivational interviewing or emotional processing with CBT techniques. Work also is advancing on scaling these interventions via the internet to provide access to more individuals. These continuing research efforts suggest a promising future in the treatment of GAD.

Key Points

- Substantial evidence suggests that cognitive-behavioral therapy (CBT) for generalized anxiety disorder (GAD) is effective, helping approximately 50% of patients with GAD achieve significant symptom reduction and high end-state functioning.

- CBT typically consists of psychoeducation, self-monitoring, relaxation, and cognitive restructuring.

- Additional techniques such as worry exposure, problem solving, emotional processing, motivational interviewing, addressing metacognitive beliefs about worry, and focusing on improving positive aspects of one's life also are potentially helpful.

References

American Psychiatric Association: Diagnostic and Statistical Manual of Mental Disorders, 3rd Edition, Revised. Washington, DC, American Psychiatric Association, 1987

American Psychiatric Association: Diagnostic and Statistical Manual of Mental Disorders, 4th Edition. Washington, DC, American Psychiatric Association, 1994

American Psychiatric Association: Diagnostic and Statistical Manual of Mental Disorders, 5th Edition. Arlington, VA, American Psychiatric Association, 2013

Andersson G, Paxling B, Roch-Norlund P, et al: Internet-based psychodynamic versus cognitive behavioral guided self-help for generalized anxiety disorder: a randomized controlled trial. Psychother Psychosom 81(6):344–355, 2012 22964540

Baker M, Willet S, Sharp S: Generalised Anxiety Disorder and Panic Disorder (With or Without Agoraphobia) in Adults: Management in Primary, Secondary and Community Care (CG113). London, National Institute for Health and Care Excellence: Centre for Clinical Practice—Surveillance Programme, July 2015. Available at: https://www.nice.org.uk/guidance/cg113/evidence/surveillance-review-decision-july 2015-pdf-2482902685. Accessed June 19, 2019.

Ballenger JC, Davidson JRT, Lecrubier Y, et al: Consensus statement on generalized anxiety disorder from the International Consensus Group on Depression and Anxiety. J Clin Psychiatry 62(suppl 11):53–58, 2001 11414552

Barlow DH, Farchione TJ, Bullis JR, et al: The unified protocol for transdiagnostic treatment of emotional disorders compared with diagnosis-specific protocols for anxiety disorders: a randomized clinical trial. JAMA Psychiatry 74(9):875–884, 2017 28768327

Beck AT: Cognitive Therapy and the Emotional Disorders. New York, New American Library, 1976

Beck AT, Emery G, Greenberg RL: Anxiety Disorders and Phobias: A Cognitive Perspective. New York, Basic Books, 1985

Borkovec TD: The nature, functions, and origins of worry, in Worrying: Perspectives on Theory, Assessment and Treatment. Edited by Davey GCL, Tallis F. New York, Wiley, 1994, pp 5–33

Borkovec TD, Whisman MA: Psychosocial treatment for generalized anxiety disorder, in Long-Term Treatments of Anxiety Disorders. Edited by Mavissakalian MR, Prien RF. Washington, DC, American Psychiatric Press, 1996, pp 171–199

Borkovec TD, Wilkinson L, Folensbee R, et al: Stimulus control applications to the treatment of worry. Behav Res Ther 21(3):247–251, 1983 6615390

Borkovec TD, Shadick RN, Hopkins M: The nature of normal and pathological worry, in Chronic Anxiety: Generalized Anxiety Disorder and Mixed Anxiety-Depression. Edited by Rapee RM, Barlow DH. New York, Guilford, 1991, pp 29–51

Borkovec TD, Alcaine O, Behar E: Avoidance theory of worry and generalized anxiety disorder, in Generalized Anxiety Disorder: Advances in Research and Practice. Edited by Heimberg RG, Turk CL, Mennin DS. New York, Guilford, 2004, pp 77–108

Brown TA, O'Leary TA, Barlow DH: Generalized anxiety disorder, in Clinical Handbook of Psychological Disorders, 2nd Edition. Edited by Barlow DH. New York, Guilford, 1993, pp 137–188

Brown TA, Barlow DH, Liebowitz MR: The empirical basis of generalized anxiety disorder. Am J Psychiatry 151(9):1272–1280, 1994 8067480

Crits-Christoph PC, Connolly MB, Azarian K, et al: An open trial of brief supportive-expressive psychotherapy in the treatment of generalized anxiety disorder. Psychotherapy 33:418–430, 1996

Crits-Christoph PC, Gibbons MBC, Crits-Christoph K: Supportive-expressive psychodynamic therapy, in Generalized Anxiety Disorder: Advances in Research and Practice. Edited by Heimberg RG, Turk CL, Mennin DS. New York, Guilford, 2004, pp 293–319

Crits-Christoph PC, Gibbons MBC, Narducci J, et al: Interpersonal problems and the outcome of interpersonally oriented psychodynamic treatment of GAD. Psychotherapy 42:211–224, 2005

Crits-Christoph P, Newman MG, Rickels K, et al: Combined medication and cognitive therapy for generalized anxiety disorder. J Anxiety Disord 25(8):1087–1094, 2011 21840164

Cuijpers P, Sijbrandij M, Koole S, et al: Psychological treatment of generalized anxiety disorder: a meta-analysis. Clin Psychol Rev 34(2):130–140, 2014 24487344

Davey GCL: Pathological worrying as exacerbated problem-solving, in Worrying: Perspectives on Theory, Assessment and Treatment. Edited by Davey GCL, Tallis F. New York, Wiley, 1994, pp 35–59

Domhardt M, Geßlein H, von Rezori RE, et al: Internet- and mobile-based interventions for anxiety disorders: a meta-analytic review of intervention components. Depress Anxiety 36(3):213–224, 2019 30450811

Dugas MJ, Gagnon F, Ladouceur R, et al: Generalized anxiety disorder: a preliminary test of a conceptual model. Behav Res Ther 36(2):215–226, 1998 9613027

Dugas MJ, Ladouceur R, Léger E, et al: Group cognitive-behavioral therapy for generalized anxiety disorder: treatment outcome and long-term follow-up. J Consult Clin Psychol 71(4):821–825, 2003 12924687

Dugas MJ, Brillon P, Savard P, et al: A randomized clinical trial of cognitive-behavioral therapy and applied relaxation for adults with generalized anxiety disorder. Behav Ther 41(1):46–58, 2010 20171327

Dupuy J-B, Beaudoin S, Rhéaume J, et al: Worry: daily self-report in clinical and non-clinical populations. Behav Res Ther 39(10):1249–1255, 2001 11579992

Durham RC, Murphy T, Allan T, et al: Cognitive therapy, analytic psychotherapy and anxiety management training for generalised anxiety disorder. Br J Psychiatry 165(3):315–323, 1994 7994500

Durham RC, Fisher PL, Treliving LR, et al: One year follow-up of cognitive therapy, analytic psychotherapy and anxiety management training for generalized anxiety disorder: symptom change, medication usage and attitudes to treatment. Behav Cogn Psychother 27:19–35, 1999

Durham RC, Chambers JA, MacDonald RR, et al: Does cognitive-behavioural therapy influence the long-term outcome of generalized anxiety disorder? An 8–14 year follow-up of two clinical trials. Psychol Med 33(3):499–509, 2003 12701670

Fava GA, Ruini C, Rafanelli C, et al: Well-being therapy of generalized anxiety disorder. Psychother Psychosom 74(1):26–30, 2005 15627853

Ferrero A, Pierò A, Fassina S, et al: A 12-month comparison of brief psychodynamic psychotherapy and pharmacotherapy treatment in subjects with generalised anxiety disorders in a community setting. Eur Psychiatry 22(8):530–539, 2007 17900875

Fracalanza K, Koerner N, Antony MM: Testing a procedural variant of written imaginal exposure for generalized anxiety disorder. J Anxiety Disord 28(6):559–569, 2014 24983797

Gersh E, Hallford DJ, Rice SM, et al: Systematic review and meta-analysis of dropout rates in individual psychotherapy for generalized anxiety disorder. J Anxiety Disord 52:25–33, 2017 29028610

Hayes-Skelton SA, Roemer L, Orsillo SM: A randomized clinical trial comparing an acceptance-based behavior therapy to applied relaxation for generalized anxiety disorder. J Consult Clin Psychol 81(5):761–773, 2013 23647281

Hirsch CR, Mathews A: A cognitive model of pathological worry. Behav Res Ther 50(10):636–646, 2012 22863541

Leichsenring F, Salzer S, Jaeger U, et al: Short-term psychodynamic psychotherapy and cognitive-behavioral therapy in generalized anxiety disorder: a randomized, controlled trial. Am J Psychiatry 166(8):875–881, 2009 19570931

Lilliengren P, Johansson R, Town JM, et al: Intensive short-term dynamic psychotherapy for generalized anxiety disorder: a pilot effectiveness and process-outcome study. Clin Psychol Psychother 24(6):1313–1321, 2017 28675661

Mennin DS, Fresco DM, O'Toole MS, et al: A randomized controlled trial of emotion regulation therapy for generalized anxiety disorder with and without co-occurring depression. J Consult Clin Psychol 86(3):268–281, 2018 29504794

Mitte K: Meta-analysis of cognitive-behavioral treatments for generalized anxiety disorder: a comparison with pharmacotherapy. Psychol Bull 131(5):785–795, 2005 16187860

Newman MG, Llera SJ: A novel theory of experiential avoidance in generalized anxiety disorder: a review and synthesis of research supporting a contrast avoidance model of worry. Clin Psychol Rev 31(3):371–382, 2011 21334285

Newman MG, Castonguay LG, Borkovec TD, et al: A randomized controlled trial of cognitive-behavioral therapy for generalized anxiety disorder with integrated techniques from emotion-focused and interpersonal therapies. J Consult Clin Psychol 79(2):171–181, 2011 21443321

Newman MG, Castonguay LG, Jacobson NC, et al: Adult attachment as a moderator of treatment outcome for generalized anxiety disorder: comparison between cognitive-behavioral therapy (CBT) plus supportive listening and CBT plus interpersonal and emotional processing therapy. J Consult Clin Psychol 83(5):915–925, 2015

Nordahl HM, Borkovec TD, Hagen R, et al: Metacognitive therapy versus cognitive-behavioural therapy in adults with generalised anxiety disorder. BJPsych Open 4(5):393–400, 2018 30294448

Ophuis RH, Lokkerbol J, Heemskerk SC, et al: Cost-effectiveness of interventions for treating anxiety disorders: a systematic review. J Affect Disord 210:1–13, 2017 27988373

Rapee RM: Psychological factors involved in generalized anxiety, in Chronic Anxiety: Generalized Anxiety Disorder and Mixed Anxiety-Depression. Edited by Rapee RM, Barlow DH. New York, Guilford, 1991, pp 76–94

Rice KM, Blanchard EB: Biofeedback in the treatment of anxiety disorders. Clin Psychol Rev 2:557–577, 1982

Richards D, Richardson T, Timulak L, et al: The efficacy of internet-delivered treatment for generalized anxiety disorder: a systematic review and meta-analysis. Internet Interv 2:272–282, 2015

Rygh JL, Sanderson WC: Treating Generalized Anxiety Disorder: Evidence-Based Strategies, Tools, and Techniques. New York, Guilford, 2004

Steele SJ, Farchione TJ, Cassiello-Robbins C, et al: Efficacy of the Unified Protocol for transdiagnostic treatment of comorbid psychopathology accompanying emotional disorders compared to treatments targeting single disorders. J Psychiatr Res 104:211–216, 2018 30103069

van der Heiden C, Muris P, van der Molen HT: Randomized controlled trial on the effectiveness of metacognitive therapy and intolerance-of-uncertainty therapy for generalized anxiety disorder. Behav Res Ther 50(2):100–109, 2012 22222208

van Dijk MK, Verbraak MJ, Oosterbaan DB, et al: Implementing practice guidelines for anxiety disorders in secondary mental health care: a case study. Int J Ment Health Syst 6(1):20, 2012 22995737

Westra HA, Constantino MJ, Antony MM: Integrating motivational interviewing with cognitive-behavioral therapy for severe generalized anxiety disorder: an allegiance-controlled randomized clinical trial. J Consult Clin Psychol 84(9):768–782, 2016 26985729

Recommended Readings

Antony MM, Norton PJ: The Anti-Anxiety Workbook: Proven Strategies to Overcome Worry, Phobias, Panic, and Obsessions. New York, Guilford, 2015

Clark DA, Beck AT: The Anxiety and Worry Workbook: The Cognitive Behavioral Solution. New York, Guilford, 2011

Cuijpers P, Sijbrandij M, Koole S, et al: Psychological treatment of generalized anxiety disorder: a meta-analysis. Clin Psychol Rev 34(2):130–140, 2014 24487344

Domhardt M, Geßlein H, von Rezori RE, et al: Internet- and mobile-based interventions for anxiety disorders: a meta-analytic review of intervention components. Depress Anxiety 36(3):213–224, 2019 30450811

Newman MG, Llera SJ: A novel theory of experiential avoidance in generalized anxiety disorder: a review and synthesis of research supporting a contrast avoidance model of worry. Clin Psychol Rev 31(3):371–382, 2011 21334285

Rygh JL, Sanderson WC: Treating Generalized Anxiety Disorder: Evidence-Based Strategies, Tools, and Techniques. New York, Guilford, 2004

van Dijk MK, Verbraak MJ, Oosterbaan DB, et al: Implementing practice guidelines for anxiety disorders in secondary mental health care: a case study. Int J Ment Health Syst 6(1):20, 2012 22995737

PART IV

Obsessive-Compulsive and
Related Disorders

CHAPTER 15

Phenomenology of OCD

Christina L. Boisseau, Ph.D.

Brianna Prichett, B.S.

Steven A. Rasmussen, M.D.

Jane L. Eisen, M.D.

Obsessive-compulsive disorder, an intriguing and often-debilitating disorder characterized by the presence of obsessions and compulsions, is not a newly observed condition. Indeed, descriptions of obsessions and compulsions can be found from sources dating back hundreds of years (Berrios 1995). In 1621, Robert Burton wrote in *The Anatomy of Melancholy* of an individual who

> dared not go over a bridge, come near a pool, rock, steep hill, lie in a chamber where cross beams were, for fear he be tempted to hang, drawn or precipitate himself. In a silent auditorium as at a sermon, he [was] afraid he shall speak aloud at unawares, something indecent, unfit to be said. (Burton 1883, p. 253)

Another example, written in 1791, is Boswell's description of Dr. Johnson's

> peculiarity…it appeared to me some superstitious habit, which [he] had contracted early…that was his anxious care to go out or in at a door or passage, by a certain number of steps from a certain point, or at least so that either his right or his left foot (I am not certain which) should constantly make the first actual movement when he came close to the door or passage. (Boswell 1791, quoted in Berrios 1995, p. 141)

Described since antiquity, obsessive-compulsive behaviors were often explained in social and religious terms (Berrios 1995; Mora 1969). The evolution from *behavior* to *disorder* originated in France and Germany during the second half of the nineteenth century. OCD was first classified as insanity, as a "reasoning or instinctive monomania …an involuntary, irresistible, and instinctive activity" where the subject was "chained to actions that neither reason nor emotion have originated, that conscience rejects, and will cannot suppress" (Esquirol 1838). Several decades later, Morel (1866) classified OCD as a *délire emotif* (disease of the emotions), which he considered to be a neurosis, an illness that originated in the autonomic nervous system.

At the beginning of the twentieth century, Janet (1903) described OCD symptoms in terms that are clearly recognizable to clinicians more than 100 years later (translated by Pitman 1987). He described the development of frank obsessions and compulsions as being preceded by a period he termed the *psychasthenic state*, characterized by a sense that actions are performed incompletely and by a strong focus on order and uniformity, indecisiveness, and restricted emotional expression. At the same time that Janet contributed to our conceptualization of OCD, Freud wrote groundbreaking observations of individuals struggling with obsessions and compulsions (Freud 1895/1962, 1909/1955).

Spurred by findings from several epidemiological surveys conducted in the 1980s that documented surprisingly high prevalence rates of OCD, tremendous interest and a rapid growth in the understanding of the clinical features and treatment of this disorder have occurred. Since the mid-1980s, specialized treatment centers have succeeded in enrolling large cohorts of patients with OCD, allowing a more sophisticated analysis of the disorder's heterogeneity and comorbidity as well as the relationship of these variables to treatment outcome. Prospective longitudinal studies have contributed further insights into the clinical characteristics, course, and prognosis of the illness. In this chapter, we review the current state of knowledge of the epidemiology, clinical features, and evaluation of OCD.

Epidemiology

OCD is a psychiatric disorder characterized by distressing intrusive thoughts, urges, or images (*obsessions*) and repetitive behaviors and mental acts aimed at reducing anxiety or distress (*compulsions*) (American Psychiatric Association 2013). Although it was once considered an extremely rare condition, the 12-month prevalence of OCD was estimated at 1.0% in the National Comorbidity Survey Replication (Kessler et al. 2005a, 2005b). Early cross-national epidemiological studies found similar prevalence of OCD in several countries (Weissman et al. 1994); however, more recent systematic reviews highlight considerable cross-cultural differences in the lifetime prevalence of OCD (0.3%–2.7%) (Adam et al. 2012; Andrade et al. 2012; Fontenelle et al. 2006). Epidemiological studies with children and adolescents suggest similar lifetime prevalence rates to adult studies. Based on the current world population (U.S. Census Bureau 2018), it can be estimated that 115 million people worldwide struggle with OCD during their lifetime. Adult females appear to develop OCD slightly more frequently than do adult males (Pinto et al. 2006; Rasmussen and Eisen 1988), whereas a 2:1 male-to-female ratio has been observed in pediatric clinical samples (Swedo et al. 1989). OCD typically emerges in adolescence or young adulthood, with earlier onset in males; modal onset is ages 13–15 in males and ages 20–24 in females (Rasmussen and Eisen 1990). Symptom onset is typically gradual, and most patients describe minor symptoms (i.e., obsessions or compulsions that do not cause significant distress or impairment) prior to development of full criteria for OCD (Grant et al. 2007). Although OCD usually begins in late adolescence, prepubertal onset is not rare: 34% report onset of OCD before age 14, and 23% report onset before age 12 (Grant et al. 2007). In some cases of prepubertal onset, acute attack associated with group A β-hemolytic streptococcal infections is followed by an episodic course with intense exacerbations (Swedo et al. 1998). These patients also frequently have comorbid tic and other movement disorders including choreiform movements and behavioral dysregulation. Research highlights that this syndrome, now known as pediatric autoimmune neuropsychiatric disorder associated with streptococcal infections (PANDAS), may be associated with a less chronic course than other presentations of childhood-onset OCD and tics (Leon et al. 2018; Murphy et al. 2012). To facilitate more rapid diagnosis and treatment, recent clinical consensus places more attention on the distinctive features of this acute-onset presentation rather than the association with streptococcal infection. Thus, a broader syndrome, pediatric acute-onset neuropsychiatric syndrome (PANS), is used to describe the group of acute-onset cases of OCD, whereas PANDAS denotes cases with a documented association with streptococcal infection.

OCD is associated with significant morbidity, high rates of functional impairment, and markedly decreased quality of life (Boisseau et al. 2017). Impairment is often broad and manifests across many areas, including family and interpersonal relationships, work, and general ability to function in daily life. Prospective, longitudinal studies suggest that nearly one out of every seven treatment-seeking adults with OCD reports receiving disability benefits because of their illness (Eisen et al. 2006). Many individuals have OCD for years without receiving treatment; studies suggest that patients first present for treatment on average 7 years after OCD symptom onset (Altamura et al. 2010).

Clinical Features

Diagnosis

Diagnosis of OCD (Box 15–1) requires a psychiatric examination and history. DSM-5 defines OCD as the presence of either obsessions or compulsions (Criterion A) that are time consuming or cause significant distress or functional impairment (Criterion B) (American Psychiatric Association 2013). Symptoms may not be attributable to the physiological effects of a substance or medical condition (Criterion C). Although other psychiatric disorders may be present, the obsessive/compulsive symptoms must not be secondary to another disorder (Criterion D). Patients' level of insight (awareness of the senselessness or unreasonableness of obsessions) varies, with 15%–36% of the OCD population classified as having poor insight (Catapano et al. 2010; Marazziti et al. 2002; Matsunaga et al. 2002). DSM-5 contains specifiers to denote *with good or fair insight* or *with poor insight* (see Box 15–1). The second specifier in DSM-5, whether or not OCD is *tic related*, reflects the high degree of lifetime comorbidity between OCD and tic disorders (Leckman et al. 1993) as well as phenomenological differences between patients with OCD with and without a history of tics (Holzer et al. 1994).

Box 15–1.   Diagnostic criteria for obsessive-compulsive disorder

---

A. Presence of obsessions, compulsions, or both:

Obsessions are defined by (1) and (2):

1. Recurrent and persistent thoughts, urges, or images that are experienced, at some time during the disturbance, as intrusive and unwanted, and that in most individuals cause marked anxiety or distress.
2. The individual attempts to ignore or suppress such thoughts, urges, or images, or to neutralize them with some other thought or action (i.e., by performing a compulsion).

Compulsions are defined by (1) and (2):

1. Repetitive behaviors (e.g., hand washing, ordering, checking) or mental acts (e.g., praying, counting, repeating words silently) that the individual feels driven to perform in response to an obsession or according to rules that must be applied rigidly.
2. The behaviors or mental acts are aimed at preventing or reducing anxiety or distress, or preventing some dreaded event or situation; however, these behaviors or mental acts are not connected in a realistic way with what they are designed to neutralize or prevent, or are clearly excessive.

    Note: Young children may not be able to articulate the aims of these behaviors or mental acts.

B. The obsessions or compulsions are time-consuming (e.g., take more than 1 hour per day) or cause clinically significant distress or impairment in social, occupational, or other important areas of functioning.

C. The obsessive-compulsive symptoms are not attributable to the physiological effects of a substance (e.g., a drug of abuse, a medication) or another medical condition.

D. The disturbance is not better explained by the symptoms of another mental disorder (e.g., excessive worries, as in generalized anxiety disorder; preoccupation with appearance, as in body dysmorphic disorder; difficulty discarding or parting with possessions, as in hoarding disorder; hair pulling, as in trichotillomania [hair-pulling disorder]; skin picking, as in excoriation [skin-picking] disorder; stereotypies, as in stereotypic movement disorder; ritualized eating behavior, as in eating disorders; preoccupation with substances or gambling, as in substance-related and addictive disorders; preoccupation with having an illness, as in illness anxiety disorder; sexual urges or fantasies, as in paraphilic disorders; impulses, as in disruptive, impulse-control, and conduct disorders; guilty ruminations, as in major depressive disorder; thought insertion or delusional preoccupations, as in schizophrenia spectrum and other psychotic disorders; or repetitive patterns of behavior, as in autism spectrum disorder).

Specify if:

   With good or fair insight: The individual recognizes that obsessive-compulsive disorder beliefs are definitely or probably not true or that they may or may not be true.

   With poor insight: The individual thinks obsessive-compulsive disorder beliefs are probably true.

   With absent insight/delusional beliefs: The individual is completely convinced that obsessive-compulsive disorder beliefs are true.

Specify if:

   Tic-related: The individual has a current or past history of a tic disorder.

Source.   Reprinted from American Psychiatric Association: *Diagnostic and Statistical Manual of Mental Disorders,* 5th Edition. Arlington, VA, American Psychiatric Association, 2013, p. 237. © 2013 American Psychiatric Association. Used with permission.

TABLE 15–1. **Frequency of current obsessions and compulsions among Brown Longitudinal Obsessive Compulsive Study participants**

	Children (N=20), n (%)	Adolescents (N=44), n (%)	Adults (N=293), n (%)
Obsessions			
Contamination	11 (55.0)	30 (68.2)	169 (57.7)
Overresponsibility for harm	9 (45.0)	25 (56.8)	164 (56.0)
Symmetry	13 (65.0)	26 (59.1)	140 (47.8)
Aggressive	3 (15.0)	21 (47.7)	133 (45.4)
Hoarding	8 (40.0)	12 (27.3)	86 (29.4)
Somatic	5 (25.0)	8 (18.2)	77 (26.3)
Religious	4 (20.0)	12 (27.3)	77 (26.3)
Sexual	1 (5.0)	11 (25.0)	39 (13.3)
Miscellaneous	5 (25.0)	13 (29.5)	167 (57.0)
Compulsions			
Checking	14 (70.0)	26 (59.1)	202 (68.9)
Washing/Cleaning	7 (35.0)	24 (54.5)	176 (60.1)
Repeating	13 (65.0)	26 (59.1)	165 (56.3)
Ordering	12 (60.0)	26 (59.1)	127 (43.3)
Hoarding	8 (40.0)	9 (20.5)	83 (28.3)
Counting	2 (10.0)	5 (11.4)	76 (25.9)
Miscellaneous	18 (90.0)	40 (90.9)	176 (60.1)

Source. Pinto et al. 2006.

Symptoms

Investigators have systematically characterized obsessions and compulsions based on the content of the obsession or the specific compulsive behavior. Data from the Brown Longitudinal Obsessive Compulsive Study, a National Institute of Mental Health–funded observational study of OCD course, are presented in Table 15–1 (Pinto et al. 2006). In adults with primary OCD, the most common obsession is fear of contamination, followed by overresponsibility for harm (e.g., fire or accidents), aggressive obsessions, and need for symmetry. The most common compulsion is checking, followed by washing, repeating routine activities, and ordering/arranging. Children and adolescents with OCD present with similar OCD symptoms but may show some developmental differences (Geller et al. 2001). For example, sexual, religious, and aggressive obsessions appear to emerge in adolescence. "Miscellaneous" types of compulsions, such as rituals involving other people (usually family members) and tic-like compulsions (touching, tapping, or rubbing), are common among children and adolescents and among adults with a juvenile-onset of OCD (Geller et al. 2001; Rosario-Campos et al. 2001).

Most adults and children with OCD have multiple obsessions and compulsions over time, with a particular fear or concern dominating the clinical picture at any one time. The presence of pure obsessions without compulsions is unusual. Indeed, patients who appear to have obsessions alone frequently have reassurance rituals or unrecognized mental compulsions in addition to their obsessions (Williams et al. 2011). Pure compulsions are extremely rare in adult populations (Foa et al. 1995); however, they do occur in children with OCD, especially in the very young (e.g., ages 6–8 years) (Swedo et al. 1989).

Approaches to OCD Subtyping

To advance our understanding of the clinical, neurobiological, and genetic features of OCD, an effort has been made to identify meaningful subtypes of this heterogeneous disorder (Mataix-Cols et al. 2005). Proposed strategies for subtyping include by symptom dimensions (Baer 1994; Pinto et al. 2007), by core underlying motivation (e.g., harm avoidance and incompleteness; Rasmussen and Eisen 1992; Summerfeldt 2004), or by patterns of comorbidity (e.g., tic disorders; Leckman et al. 2009).

Common Clinical Presentations

The following descriptions of contamination, overresponsibility for harm; symmetry, somatic, sexual, and aggressive obsessions; and mental compulsions illustrate common clinical presentations of OCD.

Contamination

Contamination obsessions, the most frequently encountered obsessions in OCD, typically are characterized by a fear of dirt or germs. Contamination fears also may involve toxins or environmental hazards (e.g., asbestos or lead) or bodily waste or secretions. Patients usually describe a feared consequence from contacting a contaminated object (e.g., spreading disease or contracting an illness themselves). However, the fear occasionally is based on a fear of the sensory experience of not being clean or feelings of disgust (Cisler et al. 2009). The content of the obsession and the feared consequence commonly change over time—for example, a fear of cancer may be replaced by a fear of venereal disease. Washing is the compulsion most commonly associated with contamination obsessions. This behavior usually occurs after contact with the feared object; however, proximity to the feared stimulus often is sufficient to engender severe anxiety and washing compulsions, even though the contaminated object has not been touched. Most patients with washing compulsions perform these rituals in response to a fear of contamination, but these behaviors occasionally occur in response to a drive for perfection or a need for symmetry. Many patients with contamination fears use avoidance to prevent contact with contaminants, in addition to excessive washing. The fear structure for contamination is similar to that seen in specific phobias: precipitation by a specific external trigger, high level of anxiety, and a well-developed and coherent cognitive framework. In some cases, a specific feared object and associated avoidance become more generalized, a pattern also described in specific phobias. Unlike specific phobias, patients with contamination obsessions often worry that they will inadvertently cause others to be harmed or become ill.

Overresponsibility for Harm

Patients with overresponsibility for harm are plagued by the concern that they will be responsible for a dire event as a result of their carelessness. They may, for example, worry that they will start a fire because they neglected to turn off the stove before leaving the house. Such patients often describe doubting their own perceptions. Excessive doubt and associated feelings of excessive responsibility frequently lead to checking rituals. Patients may spend several hours checking their home before they leave. As is the case for contamination obsessions, overresponsibility for harm also can lead to marked avoidance behavior. Some patients become housebound to avoid the responsibility of leaving the house potentially unlocked. Overresponsibility for harm also is embedded in the cognitive framework of several other obsessions. Patients with aggressive obsessions may be plagued by the doubt that they inadvertently harmed someone without knowing that they did so.

Need for Symmetry

Need for symmetry is a drive to order or arrange things "perfectly," to do and undo certain motor actions in an exact sequence, or to perform certain behaviors symmetrically or in a balanced way. Patients describe an urge to repeat motor acts until they achieve a "just right" feeling that the act has been completed perfectly. These patients can be divided into two groups: 1) those with primary magical thinking and 2) those with primary obsessive slowness. Individuals with primary magical thinking report obsessional worries about feared consequences to their loved ones. They perform certain ordering and arranging compulsions to prevent harm to loved ones from occurring. Patients who have primary obsessive slowness take an inordinate amount of time to complete the simplest of tasks (Rachman and Hodgson 1980). Unlike most patients with OCD, those with obsessive slowness may not experience their symptoms as ego-dystonic. Instead, they seem to have lost their goal directedness in favor of completing a given subroutine perfectly.

Patients with symmetry obsessions and compulsions often describe feeling uneasy or unsettled rather than fearful or anxious when things are not lined up "just so"' or "perfectly." In that sense, these patients can be seen as being at the extreme end of the spectrum of compulsive personality, in which the need for every detail to be perfect or just so is greatest. The desire to "even up" or balance movements may be present in patients with tapping or touching rituals. Patients may, for example, feel that the right side of the chair must be tapped after the left side has been tapped. Their description of rising tension followed by relief after the act is more similar to the subjective sensory experience of patients with tics than to the anxiety experienced by other patients with OCD without comorbid tic disorders (Leckman et al. 1994; Miguel et al. 1995). Investigators have used terms such as "sensory phenomena" (Miguel et al. 1995, 2000), "just right" perceptions (Leckman et al. 1994), and "not just right" experiences (Coles et al. 2003) to describe these sensations (see "Harm Avoidance and Incompleteness" section). Patients with obsessional slowness or extreme perfectionism may not respond as well to behavior therapy interventions, which may be related to this lack of subjective anxiety (Summerfeldt 2004).

Somatic Obsessions

Somatic obsessions (i.e., the irrational and persistent fears of developing a serious life-threatening illness) may be seen in various disorders, including OCD, illness anxiety disorder, major depressive disorder (MDD), and panic disorder. Several features may be useful in distinguishing OCD with somatic obsessions from illness anxiety or somatoform presentations. Patients with OCD usually have other past or current classic

OCD obsessions; are more likely to engage in classic OCD compulsions, such as checking and reassurance seeking; and generally do not experience somatic and visceral symptoms of illness. Somatic obsessions are more easily distinguished from somatization disorder, because patients with somatic obsessions usually focus on one illness at a time and are not preoccupied with a diverse, apparently unrelated array of somatic symptoms. In contrast to many patients with contamination obsessions, patients with somatic obsessions usually are worried about their own health rather than the well-being of others. Common somatic obsessions include fear of cancer or venereal disease or of developing AIDS. Compulsions to check and recheck the body part of concern, as well as reassurance seeking, are commonly associated with this fear.

Sexual and Aggressive Obsessions

Patients with sexual or aggressive obsessions are plagued by fears that they might commit a sexually unacceptable act, such as molestation, or harm others. They often fear not only that they will commit a dreadful act in the future but also that they have already committed such an act. Patients usually are horrified by the content of their obsessions and are reluctant to divulge them. It is quite striking that the content of these obsessions tends to consist of ideas that patients find particularly abhorrent. Individuals with these obsessions frequently have checking and confession or reassurance rituals. They may report themselves to the police or repeatedly seek out priests to confess their imagined crimes. An unsolved murder case in the media may cause tremendous anxiety and lead to extensive reassurance rituals. Patients may repeatedly tell their therapist, spouse, or close friend some terrible thought or deed that they feel they have committed as a way of seeking reassurance that they really are not capable of doing what they are worried about. Guilt and anxiety are the dominant affective symptoms. Patients may think that they should be jailed for their thoughts (both to protect them from what they think they might do and because they feel they deserve to be punished). Patients also may use extensive avoidance to prevent obsessions (e.g., removing all sharp implements, such as scissors and knives, from the home or avoiding all television programs with references to violence, such as the news).

Mental Compulsions

Traditionally, obsessions have been considered mental events (e.g., thoughts, images), whereas compulsions were thought of as observable behaviors (e.g., washing or checking). More recently, this view has shifted to the prevailing concept that obsessions are mental events that cause distress, and compulsions are either behavioral or mental acts that are performed to neutralize or reduce obsessional distress. Mental compulsions, therefore, are neutralizing thoughts such as mental counting or praying that decrease anxiety or discomfort caused by obsessions. Indeed, mental rituals were the third most common type of compulsion after hand washing and checking in the DSM-IV field trial (American Psychiatric Association 1994; Foa et al. 1995). The presence of mental rituals is associated with a more chronic course of illness, greater illness severity, and decreased functional impairment (Sibrava et al. 2011).

Harm Avoidance and Incompleteness

Rasmussen and Eisen (1992) proposed a conceptual model of two core constructs of OCD, harm avoidance and incompleteness, that integrated symptom subtypes, temperament, and neurocircuitry to explain the marked comorbidity between OCD, the obsessive-compulsive spectrum disorders, and the anxiety disorders. Over the past two decades, interest in incompleteness has been increasing, with other researchers also actively investigating this putative core feature, using related terms such as "just right experiences" (Coles et al. 2003; Leckman et al. 1994) and "sensory phenomena" (Miguel et al. 2000). Research suggests that these core features cut across phenomenological subtypes, such as checking, washing, and the need for symmetry, although some symptom subtypes appear to be more closely associated with one core feature than another—for example, overresponsibility for harm and aggressive and sexual obsessions are more associated with harm avoidance, and symmetry and hoarding are more associated with incompleteness (Sibrava et al. 2016). Patterns of comorbidity in OCD also support this distinction, with harm avoidance in OCD associated with comorbid anxiety disorders and incompleteness associated with hoarding and obsessive-compulsive personality disorder (OCPD) features, specifically perfectionism and preoccupation with details (Sibrava et al. 2016). Further empirical validation of this proposed subtyping according to core features is necessary and may have important implications for diagnosis and treatment.

Comorbidity

Early psychiatric literature documented the presence of obsessive-compulsive symptoms among mood disorders, anxiety disorders, and premorbid personality traits (Kringlin 1965; Pollitt 1957), and large-scale OCD studies have replicated the high prevalence of these comorbidities in more recent years (Brakoulias et al. 2017; Pinto et al. 2006). For example, a large international collaboration studying 3,711 adults with OCD found that 28% had comorbid MDD and 69% had a comorbid anxiety disorder, most commonly generalized anxiety disorder, social phobia, and specific phobia (Brakoulias et al. 2017). When OCD co-occurs with other anxiety disorders, it is usually the disorder of greatest severity (Antony et al. 1998). The high frequency of current and lifetime anxiety disorders suggests that patients with OCD are vulnerable to many types of anxiety that may be caused by common developmental and temperamental traits whose phenotypic expression is secondary to shared genotypic and psychosocial factors.

Lifetime prevalence of MDD occurs at a rate upward of 50% in OCD populations (Pinto et al. 2006; Yap et al. 2012). Although it may be difficult to distinguish a primary from a secondary diagnosis, some patients with OCD view their depressive symptoms as occurring secondary to the demoralization and hopelessness accompanying their OCD symptoms. Meanwhile, others view their MDD symptoms as occurring independently of their OCD symptoms, with some patients reporting their OCD symptoms either lessening or intensifying as they cycle into a depressive episode. Regarding the temporal relation between development of depression and OCD, depressive symptoms developing long after OCD onset remains the predominant pattern (Ruscio et al. 2010).

Attention also has been focused on the relation between tic disorders and OCD. Leckman et al. (1993) found that patients with Tourette syndrome had high rates of comorbid OCD and obsessive-compulsive symptoms (30%–40% reporting obsessive-compulsive symptoms). Conversely, approximately 20% of patients with OCD have a lifetime history of multiple tics, and 5%–10% have a lifetime history of Tourette syndrome (Leckman et al. 1994). In addition to genetic comorbidity data linking OCD and tic disorders, some evidence suggests that these disorders are linked phenomenologically; certain obsessions and compulsions such as symmetry and ordering are more common in patients with these two disorders than in patients with OCD alone (Labad et al. 2008). Individuals with tic-related OCD also are more likely to be male and have an earlier age of OCD onset (Diniz et al. 2006). DSM-5 draws attention to differences between OCD patients with and without a history of tics by incorporating a tic-related specifier into the diagnostic criteria for OCD.

Approximately one-quarter of patients with OCD present with comorbid OCPD (Coles et al. 2008). Compared with those with OCD alone, patients with both OCD and OCPD have distinct clinical characteristics (e.g., age at onset of initial obsessive-compulsive symptoms, the types of obsessions and compulsions they experience, and psychiatric comorbidity). The presence of comorbid OCPD is a significant risk factor for OCD relapse (Eisen et al. 2013). Whether OCPD comorbid with OCD is a specific subtype (Coles et al. 2008; Garyfallos et al. 2010) or a marker of severity in OCD (Lochner et al. 2011) remains an area for future research.

Differential Diagnosis

Patients with OCD frequently have comorbid depression, and these patients may be difficult to distinguish from patients with depression who have concurrent obsessive symptoms. The distinction between primary and secondary obsessions rests on the order of occurrence. In addition, depressive rumination may present similarly to pure obsessions. Ruminations, in contrast to obsessions, are usually focused on a past incident rather than a current or future event and are rarely resisted (Hollander and Simeon 2003).

OCD and anxiety disorders may present very similarly. All are characterized by avoidant behavior, excessive fear, and intense subjective and autonomic responses to focal stimuli and appear to respond to similar behavioral interventions. Patients with OCD who experience high levels of anxiety may describe panic-like episodes, but these are secondary to obsessions and do not arise spontaneously, unlike in panic disorder. Individuals with OCD can never avoid the obsession entirely, whereas patients with specific phobia have more focal, external stimuli that they can successfully avoid (Hollander and Simeon 2003). The content of worry in generalized anxiety disorder usually focuses on everyday concerns. In contrast to ego-syntonic worry, obsessions tend to involve less commonly held fears, are more likely to be unrealistic or magical, and are more likely to be perceived by the individual as inappropriate or nonsensical (ego-dystonic).

Prior to DSM-5, compulsive hoarding, which is characterized by persistent difficulty discarding items and excessive saving of items, was considered a symptom subtype in OCD. However, differences in onset, course, and phenomenology led to it being considered a distinct and separate disorder in DSM-5 (Mataix-Cols et al. 2010). In addition to the clinical differences between OCD and hoarding disorder, neuropsychological task differences, such as decision making, have been more recently identified (Pushkarskaya et al. 2017). The distinction between these disorders has significant treatment implications. The treatment approaches used for OCD have not been nearly as effective in hoarding disorder (Tolin et al. 2015), leading to more effective cognitive-behavioral therapy approaches designed specifically for hoarding (Steketee et al. 2010). Despite these differences, some overlap occurs between these disorders; 20% of individuals with hoarding disorder also meet criteria for OCD (Frost et al. 2011).

OCD must be distinguished from schizophrenia and other psychotic disorders. The natural history of both OCD and schizophrenia may involve chronic debilitation and functional (e.g., social and occupational) decline. Subtle distinctions between an obsession and a delusion may be difficult to identify. In general, an obsession is egodystonic, resisted, and recognized as having an internal origin; a delusion is not resisted and is believed to be external, although rare exceptions have been found where individuals with obsessions lack insight into the irrationality of their concerns. In OCD, obsessions of delusional intensity also tend to be accompanied by compulsive behavior (Eisen et al. 1998).

The literature supports a distinction between OCPD and OCD (Baer 1998). The classic distinction of compulsions being ego-syntonic in OCPD as opposed to egodystonic in OCD is useful but not absolute. Some patients with cleaning compulsions and those with the need for symmetry or obsessive slowness who strive for perfection or completeness find their rituals ego-syntonic until they begin to impair social and occupational function. Whether these patients should be classified as having OCPD or subthreshold OCD is a subject for further empirical study.

Course

DSM-5 describes the course of OCD as typically chronic, with some fluctuation in symptom severity over time (American Psychiatric Association 2013). Prospective observational studies of treatment-seeking adults with OCD conducted since the 1990s have found varying rates of full remission (no OCD symptoms) and partial remission (subclinical noninterfering symptoms) ranging from 43% to 76% (Eisen et al. 2013; Nakajima et al. 2018; Steketee et al. 1999). Differences in rates of remission may be due to different methodology across studies and the heterogeneity of OCD. Several studies have investigated predictors of OCD course in adults. In general, greater functional impairment and longer duration of illness predict decreased probability of OCD remission (Eisen et al. 2013; Steketee et al. 1999). Comorbid MDD has also been associated with a more chronic course (Marcks et al. 2011; Steketee et al. 1999), as has comorbid OCPD (Eisen et al. 2013). Although nascent, some evidence suggests that different OCD symptom categories (e.g., overresponsibility for harm) may be associated with greater probability of remission (Eisen et al. 2013).

Whereas studies of adults have generally supported the hypothesis that OCD is a chronic lifelong disorder, child and adolescent studies have found a surprisingly high percentage of patients with an episodic course. Across pediatric OCD studies, remission rates range from 32% to 79% depending on methodology and sample studied (Stewart et al. 2004). More recent follow-up studies of children and adolescents have supported high rates of remission in pediatric OCD (Bloch et al. 2009; Micali et al. 2010). Prospective, longitudinal studies following both children and adults have found that youth remit from OCD at a significantly faster rate than adults (Mancebo et al. 2014). Only a few studies have examined predictors of course in pediatric OCD. Similar to adult studies, a greater burden of comorbidity is generally associated with protracted course (Bloch et al. 2009; Leonard et al. 1993). Shorter latency to treatment and lower levels of functional impairment are associated with a better prognosis, highlighting the importance of early detection and intervention (Mancebo et al. 2014).

Evaluation

Rating Scales

Like most psychiatric disorders, the diagnosis of OCD rests on purely clinical grounds (i.e., psychiatric examination and history). Yet formal assessments, in the form of structured interviews, self- and significant other report questionnaires, and clinical rating scales, play an important role in research, administration, and clinical settings. We review the most frequently used instruments relevant to OCD here.

Several semistructured diagnostic interviews include OCD modules. Among the most extensively used in adults are the Structured Clinical Interview for DSM-5 (First et al. 2016) and the more circumscribed Anxiety Disorders Interview Schedule for DSM-5 (Brown and Barlow 2014); the Kiddie Schedule for Affective Disorders and Schizophrenia (Kaufman et al. 2016) provides a semistructured diagnostic interview for children and adolescents. OCD-specific symptom severity measures include the Yale-Brown Obsessive Compulsive Scale (Y-BOCS; Goodman et al. 1989a, 1989b) and its child version (Scahill et al. 1997). Widely used in observational and treatment outcome studies and considered the gold standard in OCD assessment, both rater-administered assessments include a symptom checklist of common obsessions and compulsions followed by a 10-item severity scale. Insight into OCD symptoms can be assessed using the Brown Assessment of Beliefs Scale (Eisen et al. 1998), a seven-item semistructured interview that measures the degree and presence of delusional thinking. Supplementing these interviews are self-report measures designed to assess OCD symptoms and severity, including the Y-BOCS self-report (Steketee et al. 1996), the Obsessive-Compulsive Inventory–Revised (Foa et al. 2002), and the Dimensional Obsessive-Compulsive Scale (Abramowitz et al. 2010). Corresponding child- and parent-report versions exist for many of these self-report measures.

Conclusion

The past 35 years have seen tremendous strides in our knowledge about the etiology, epidemiology, and treatment of OCD. We now know that OCD is a common psychiatric disorder not only in the United States but also globally. Research regarding phenomenological aspects of OCD has focused on various areas, including identifying meaningful subtypes and investigating patterns of comorbidity. Continued refinement of our thinking about the heterogeneity of OCD is necessary to unravel important questions about etiology and to develop more personalized treatments for this often-debilitating disorder.

Key Points

- OCD is a clinically heterogeneous disorder that is characterized by multiple symptom dimensions.

- Individuals with OCD frequently present with comorbid conditions.

- The course of OCD is typically chronic, with some fluctuation in symptom severity over time.

References

Abramowitz JS, Deacon BJ, Olatunji BO, et al: Assessment of obsessive-compulsive symptom dimensions: development and evaluation of the Dimensional Obsessive-Compulsive Scale. Psychol Assess 22(1):180–198, 2010 20230164

Adam Y, Meinlschmidt G, Gloster AT, et al: Obsessive-compulsive disorder in the community: 12-month prevalence, comorbidity and impairment. Soc Psychiatry Psychiatr Epidemiol 47(3):339–349, 2012 21287144

Altamura AC, Buoli M, Albano A, et al: Age at onset and latency to treatment (duration of untreated illness) in patients with mood and anxiety disorders: a naturalistic study. Int Clin Psychopharmacol 25(3):172–179, 2010 20305566

American Psychiatric Association: Diagnostic and Statistical Manual of Mental Disorders, 4th Edition. Washington, DC, American Psychiatric Association, 1994

American Psychiatric Association: Diagnostic and Statistical Manual of Mental Disorders, 5th Edition. Arlington, VA, American Psychiatric Association, 2013

Andrade LH, Wang YP, Andreoni S, et al: Mental disorders in megacities: findings from the São Paulo megacity mental health survey, Brazil. PLoS One 7(2):e31879, 2012 22348135

Antony MM, Downie F, Swinson RP: Diagnostic issues and epidemiology in obsessive-compulsive disorder, in Obsessive-Compulsive Disorder: Theory, Research, and Treatment. Edited by Swinson RP, Antony MM, Rachman AS, et al. New York, Guilford, 1998, pp 3–32

Baer L: Factor analysis of symptom subtypes of obsessive compulsive disorder and their relation to personality and tic disorders. J Clin Psychiatry 55(suppl):18–23, 1994 8077163

Baer L: Personality disorders in obsessive-compulsive disorder, in Obsessive-Compulsive Disorders: Practical Management, 3rd Edition. Edited by Jenike MA, Baer L, Minichiello WE. St Louis, MO, Mosby, 1998, pp 65–83

Berrios GE: Obsessive-compulsive disorder, in History of Clinical Psychiatry: The Origin and History of Psychiatric Disorders. Edited by Berrios GE, Porter RA. London, Athlone Press, 1995, pp 573–592

Bloch MH, Craiglow BG, Landeros-Weisenberger A, et al: Predictors of early adult outcomes in pediatric-onset obsessive-compulsive disorder. Pediatrics 124(4):1085–1093, 2009 19786445

Boisseau CL, Schwartzman CM, Rasmussen SA: Quality of life and psychosocial functioning of OCD, in Obsessive-Compulsive Disorder: Phenomenology, Pathophysiology, and Treatment. Edited by Pittenger C. New York, Oxford University Press, 2017, pp 57–64

Boswell J: The Life of Samuel Johnson. London, Dent, 1791

Brakoulias V, Starcevic V, Belloch A, et al: Comorbidity, age of onset and suicidality in obsessive-compulsive disorder (OCD): an international collaboration. Compr Psychiatry 76:79–86, 2017 28433854

Brown TA, Barlow DH: Anxiety and Related Disorders Interview Schedule for DSM-5, Adult Version. New York, Oxford University Press, 2014

Burton R: The Anatomy of Melancholy. London, Chatto and Windus, 1883

Catapano F, Perris F, Fabrazzo M, et al: Obsessive-compulsive disorder with poor insight: a three-year prospective study. Prog Neuropsychopharmacol Biol Psychiatry 34(2):323–330, 2010 20015461

Cisler JM, Olatunji BO, Lohr JM: Disgust, fear, and the anxiety disorders: a critical review. Clin Psychol Rev 29(1):34–46, 2009 18977061

Coles ME, Frost RO, Heimberg RG, et al: "Not just right experiences": perfectionism, obsessive-compulsive features and general psychopathology. Behav Res Ther 41(6):681–700, 2003

Coles ME, Pinto A, Mancebo MC, et al: OCD with comorbid OCPD: a subtype of OCD? J Psychiatr Res 42(4):289–296, 2008 17382961

Diniz JB, Rosario-Campos MC, Hounie AG, et al: Chronic tics and Tourette syndrome in patients with obsessive-compulsive disorder. J Psychiatr Res 40(6):487–493, 2006 16289552

Eisen JL, Phillips KA, Baer L, et al: The Brown Assessment of Beliefs Scale: reliability and validity. Am J Psychiatry 155(1):102–108, 1998 9433346

Eisen JL, Mancebo MA, Pinto A, et al: Impact of obsessive-compulsive disorder on quality of life. Compr Psychiatry 47(4):270–275, 2006 16769301

Eisen JL, Sibrava NJ, Boisseau CL, et al: Five-year course of obsessive-compulsive disorder: predictors of remission and relapse. J Clin Psychiatry 74(3):233–239, 2013 23561228

Esquirol JED: Des Maladies Mentales Considérées Sous les Rapports Médical, Hygienique et Médico-legal. Paris, Baillière, 1838

First MB, Williams JBW, Karg RS, et al: Structured Clinical Interview for DSM-5 Axis I Disorders–Clinician Version (SCID-5-CV). Washington, DC, American Psychiatric Association, 2016

Foa EB, Kozak MJ, Goodman WK, et al: DSM-IV field trial: obsessive-compulsive disorder. Am J Psychiatry 152(1):90–96, 1995 7802127

Foa EB, Huppert JD, Leiberg S, et al: The Obsessive-Compulsive Inventory: development and validation of a short version. Psychol Assess 14(4):485–496, 2002 12501574

Fontenelle LF, Mendlowicz MV, Versiani M: The descriptive epidemiology of obsessive-compulsive disorder. Prog Neuropsychopharmacol Biol Psychiatry 30(3):327–337, 2006

Freud S: Notes upon a case of obsessional neurosis (1909), in The Standard Edition of the Complete Psychological Works of Sigmund Freud, Vol 10. Translated and edited by Strachey J. London, Hogarth, 1955, pp 151–318

Freud S: On the grounds for detaching a particular syndrome from neurasthenia under the description "anxiety neurosis" (1895), in The Standard Edition of the Complete Psychological Works of Sigmund Freud, Vol 3. Translated and edited by Strachey J. London, Hogarth, 1962, pp 90–117

Frost RO, Steketee G, Tolin DF: Comorbidity in hoarding disorder. Depress Anxiety 28(10):876–884, 2011 21770000

Garyfallos G, Katsigiannopoulos K, Adamopoulou A, et al: Comorbidity of obsessive-compulsive disorder with obsessive-compulsive personality disorder: does it imply a specific subtype of obsessive-compulsive disorder? Psychiatry Res 177(1–2):156–160, 2010 20163876

Geller DA, Biederman J, Faraone S, et al: Developmental aspects of obsessive compulsive disorder: findings in children, adolescents, and adults. J Nerv Ment Dis 189(7):471–477, 2001 11504325

Goodman WK, Price LH, Rasmussen SA, et al: The Yale-Brown Obsessive Compulsive Scale. I. Development, use, and reliability. Arch Gen Psychiatry 46(11):1006–1011, 1989a 2684084

Goodman WK, Price LH, Rasmussen SA, et al: The Yale-Brown Obsessive Compulsive Scale. II. Validity. Arch Gen Psychiatry 46(11):1012–1016, 1989b 2510699

Grant JE, Mancebo MC, Pinto A, et al: Late-onset obsessive compulsive disorder: clinical characteristics and psychiatric comorbidity. Psychiatry Res 152(1):21–27, 2007 17363071

Hollander E, Simeon D: Anxiety disorders, in The American Psychiatric Publishing Textbook of Clinical Psychiatry, 4th Edition. Edited by Hales R, Yudofsky S. Washington, DC, American Psychiatric Publishing, 2003, pp 543–630

Holzer JC, Goodman WK, McDougle CJ, et al: Obsessive-compulsive disorder with and without a chronic tic disorder. A comparison of symptoms in 70 patients. Br J Psychiatry 164(4):469–473, 1994 8038934

Janet P: Les Obsessions et la Psychasthénie. Paris, Alcan, 1903

Kaufman J, Birmaher B, Axelson D, et al: K-SADS-PL-DSM-5, November 2016. Available at: https://www.kennedykrieger. org/sites/default/files/library/documents/faculty/ksads-dsm-5-screener.pdf. Accessed June 20, 2019.

Kessler RC, Berglund P, Demler O, et al: Lifetime prevalence and age-of-onset distributions of DSM-IV disorders in the National Comorbidity Survey Replication. Arch Gen Psychiatry 62(6):593–602, 2005a 15939837

Kessler RC, Chiu WT, Demler O, et al: Prevalence, severity, and comorbidity of 12-month DSM-IV disorders in the National Comorbidity Survey Replication. Arch Gen Psychiatry 62(6):617–627, 2005b 15939839

Kringlin E: Obsessional neurotics: a long-term follow-up. Br J Psychiatry 111:709–722, 1965

Labad J, Menchon JM, Alonso P, et al: Gender differences in obsessive-compulsive symptom dimensions. Depress Anxiety 25(10):832–838, 2008 17436312

Leckman JF, Walker DE, Cohen DJ: Premonitory urges in Tourette's syndrome. Am J Psychiatry 150(1):98–102, 1993 8417589

Leckman JF, Walker DE, Goodman WK, et al: "Just right" perceptions associated with compulsive behavior in Tourette's syndrome. Am J Psychiatry 151(5):675–680, 1994 8166308

Leckman JF, Bloch MH, King RA: Symptom dimensions and subtypes of obsessive-compulsive disorder: a developmental perspective. Dialogues Clin Neurosci 11(1):21–33, 2009 19432385

Leon J, Hommer R, Grant P, et al: Longitudinal outcomes of children with pediatric autoimmune neuropsychiatric disorder associated with streptococcal infections (PANDAS). Eur Child Adolesc Psychiatry 27(5):637–643, 2018 29119300

Leonard HL, Swedo SE, Lenane MC, et al: A 2- to 7-year follow-up study of 54 obsessive-compulsive children and adolescents. Arch Gen Psychiatry 50(6):429–439, 1993 8498877

Lochner C, Serebro P, van der Merwe L, et al: Comorbid obsessive-compulsive personality disorder in obsessive-compulsive disorder (OCD): a marker of severity. Prog Neuropsychopharmacol Biol Psychiatry 35(4):1087–1092, 2011 21411045

Mancebo MC, Boisseau CL, Garnaat SL, et al: Long-term course of pediatric obsessive-compulsive disorder: 3 years of prospective follow-up. Compr Psychiatry 55(7):1498–1504, 2014 24952937

Marazziti D, Dell'Osso L, Di Nasso E, et al: Insight in obsessive-compulsive disorder: a study of an Italian sample. Eur Psychiatry 17(7):407–410, 2002 12547307

Marcks BA, Weisberg RB, Dyck I, et al: Longitudinal course of obsessive-compulsive disorder in patients with anxiety disorders: a 15-year prospective follow-up study. Compr Psychiatry 52(6):670–677, 2011 21349511

Mataix-Cols D, Rosario-Campos MC, Leckman JF: A multidimensional model of obsessive-compulsive disorder. Am J Psychiatry 162(2):228–238, 2005 15677583

Mataix-Cols D, Frost RO, Pertusa A, et al: Hoarding disorder: a new diagnosis for DSM-V? Depress Anxiety 27(6):556–572, 2010 20336805

Matsunaga H, Kiriike N, Matsui T, et al: Obsessive-compulsive disorder with poor insight. Compr Psychiatry 43(2):150–157, 2002 11893994

Micali N, Heyman I, Perez M, et al: Long-term outcomes of obsessive-compulsive disorder: follow-up of 142 children and adolescents. Br J Psychiatry 197(2):128–134, 2010 20679265

Miguel EC, Coffey BJ, Baer L, et al: Phenomenology of intentional repetitive behaviors in obsessive-compulsive disorder and Tourette's disorder. J Clin Psychiatry 56(6):246–255, 1995

Miguel EC, do Rosário-Campos MC, Prado HS, et al: Sensory phenomena in obsessive-compulsive disorder and Tourette's disorder. J Clin Psychiatry 61(2):150–156, quiz 157, 2000 10732667

Mora G: The scrupulosity syndrome. Int Psychiatry Clin 5(4):163–174, 1969 4892138

Morel BA: Du délire emotif. Nevrose du systeme nerveus ganglionaire visceral. Archives Générales de Médecine 7:385–402, 1866

Murphy TK, Storch EA, Lewin AB, et al: Clinical factors associated with pediatric autoimmune neuropsychiatric disorders associated with streptococcal infections. J Pediatr 160(2):314–319, 2012 21868033

Nakajima A, Matsuura N, Mukai K, et al: Ten-year follow-up study of Japanese patients with obsessive-compulsive disorder. Psychiatry Clin Neurosci 72(7):502–512, 2018 29652103

Pinto A, Mancebo MC, Eisen JL, et al: The Brown Longitudinal Obsessive Compulsive Study: clinical features and symptoms of the sample at intake. J Clin Psychiatry 67(5):703–711, 2006

Pinto A, Eisen JL, Mancebo MC, et al: Taboo thoughts and doubt/checking: a refinement of the factor structure for obsessive-compulsive disorder symptoms. Psychiatry Res 151(3):255–258, 2007 17368563

Pitman RK: Pierre Janet on obsessive-compulsive disorder (1903). Review and commentary. Arch Gen Psychiatry 44(3):226–232, 1987 3827518

Pollitt J: Natural history of obsessional states; a study of 150 cases. BMJ 1(5012):194–198, 1957

Pushkarskaya H, Tolin D, Ruderman L, et al: Value-based decision making under uncertainty in hoarding and obsessive-compulsive disorders. Psychiatry Res 258:305–315, 2017 28864119

Rachman S, Hodgson R: Obsessions and Compulsions. Englewood Cliffs, NJ, Prentice-Hall, 1980

Rasmussen SA, Eisen JL: Clinical and epidemiologic findings of significance to neuropharmacologic trials in OCD. Psychopharmacol Bull 24(3):466–470, 1988 3153510

Rasmussen SA, Eisen JL: Epidemiology of obsessive compulsive disorder. J Clin Psychiatry 51(suppl):10–13, discussion 14, 1990 2404965

Rasmussen SA, Eisen JL: The epidemiology and clinical features of obsessive-compulsive disorder. Psychiatr Clin North Am 15(4):742–758, 1992 1461792

Rosario-Campos MC, Leckman JF, Mercadante MT, et al: Adults with early onset obsessive-compulsive disorder. Am J Psychiatry 158(11):1899–1903, 2001 11691698

Ruscio AM, Stein DJ, Chiu WT, et al: The epidemiology of obsessive-compulsive disorder in the National Comorbidity Survey Replication. Mol Psychiatry 15(1):53–63, 2010 18725912

Scahill L, Riddle MA, McSwiggin-Hardin M, et al: Children's Yale-Brown Obsessive Compulsive Scale: reliability and validity. J Am Acad Child Adolesc Psychiatry 36(6):844–852, 1997 9183141

Sibrava NJ, Boisseau CL, Mancebo MC, et al: Prevalence and clinical characteristics of mental rituals in a longitudinal clinical sample of obsessive-compulsive disorder. Depress Anxiety 28(10):892–898, 2011 21818825

Sibrava NJ, Boisseau CL, Eisen JL, et al: An empirical investigation of incompleteness in a large clinical sample of obsessive compulsive disorder. J Anxiety Disord 42:45–51, 2016 27268401

Steketee G, Frost R, Bogart K: The Yale-Brown Obsessive Compulsive Scale: interview versus self-report. Behav Res Ther 34(8):675–684, 1996 8870295

Steketee G, Eisen J, Dyck I, et al: Predictors of course in obsessive-compulsive disorder. Psychiatry Res 89(3):229–238, 1999 10708269

Steketee G, Frost RO, Tolin DF, et al: Waitlist-controlled trial of cognitive behavior therapy for hoarding disorder. Depress Anxiety 27(5):476–484, 2010 20336804

Stewart SE, Geller DA, Jenike M, et al: Long-term outcome of pediatric obsessive-compulsive disorder: a meta-analysis and qualitative review of the literature. Acta Psychiatr Scand 110(1):4–13, 2004 15180774

Summerfeldt LJ: Understanding and treating incompleteness in obsessive-compulsive disorder. J Clin Psychol 60(11):1155–1168, 2004 15389620

Swedo SE, Rapoport JL, Leonard H, et al: Obsessive-compulsive disorder in children and adolescents. Clinical phenomenology of 70 consecutive cases. Arch Gen Psychiatry 46(4):335–341, 1989 2930330

Swedo SE, Leonard HL, Garvey M, et al: Pediatric autoimmune neuropsychiatric disorders associated with streptococcal infections: clinical description of the first 50 cases. Am J Psychiatry 155(2):264–271, 1998 9464208

Tolin DF, Frost RO, Steketee G, et al: Cognitive behavioral therapy for hoarding disorder: a meta-analysis. Depress Anxiety 32(3):158–166, 2015 25639467

U.S. Census Bureau: World Population Day: July 11, 2018. Available at: https://www.census.gov/newsroom/stories/2018/world-population.html. Accessed June 20, 2019.

Weissman MM, Bland RC, Canino GJ, et al: The cross national epidemiology of obsessive compulsive disorder. J Clin Psychiatry 55(suppl):5–10, 1994 8077177

Williams MT, Farris SG, Turkheimer E, et al: Myth of the pure obsessional type in obsessive-compulsive disorder. Depress Anxiety 28(6):495–500, 2011 21509914

Yap K, Mogan C, Kyrios M: Obsessive-compulsive disorder and comorbid depression: the role of OCD-related and non-specific factors. J Anxiety Disord 26(5):565–573, 2012 22495108

CHAPTER 16

Pathophysiology of Obsessive-Compulsive and Related Disorders

Darin D. Dougherty, M.D.

Scott L. Rauch, M.D.

Benjamin D. Greenberg, M.D., Ph.D.

In this chapter, we review neurochemical models, neuroendocrine factors, and immunological etiology as putative mechanisms leading to striatal pathology in OCD. We present a brief heuristic model of obsessive-compulsive and related disorders (OCRD) based on phenomenological characteristics and informed by neuroanatomical considerations. We outline the relevant functional anatomy of cortico-striato-thalamo-cortical (CSTC) circuitry and review data that implicate various elements of this system in different subtypes of OCD and in other candidate obsessive-compulsive spectrum disorders. The genetics of OCRD are covered in Chapter 2, "Genetic Contributions to Anxiety and Related Disorders." We attempt to provide an integrated view of pathogenetic models as they pertain to OCRD, and we conclude by foreshadowing future research directions in this field.

Neurochemistry and Neuropharmacology

Serotonin and the Pathogenesis of OCD and Related Disorders

Serotonin (5-HT) is a neurotransmitter released from neurons whose cell bodies are located within the raphe nuclei of the midbrain. Serotonergic projections from the raphe are widespread. Moreover, numerous different serotonergic receptor subtypes exist, each with its own profile in terms of distribution in the brain, location on neurons, effector mechanisms (e.g., second messengers), and influences on neuronal firing (Hoyer et al. 1994). Consequently, dissection of the serotonergic system is a complex and challenging enterprise.

A serotonergic hypothesis of OCD was originally prompted by the observed differential efficacy of serotonin reuptake inhibitors (SRIs) in alleviating OCD symptoms (Thorén et al. 1980; Zohar and Insel 1987). The concept that SRIs might be producing their antiobsessional effects by correcting some fundamental abnormality in the serotonergic system was instantly appealing. However, the fact that medications with serotonergic action serve as effective antiobsessionals does not necessarily mean that the serotonergic system is fundamentally dysfunctional in OCD. Rather, SRIs may act via modulation of an intact system to compensate for underlying pathophysiology in OCD that is otherwise unrelated to serotonin function. Therefore, it is critical to distinguish between these different concepts; although some research efforts may speak to the hypothesis that a primary serotonergic abnormality exists in patients with OCD, others more directly address how and where SRIs confer their beneficial antiobsessional effects.

A considerable literature has accrued that is based on indirect measurements of serotonergic function in OCD. Numerous studies of peripheral receptor binding in the blood or concentrations of serotonin metabolites in the cerebrospinal fluid have been performed, but these studies have yielded disappointingly inconsistent results (for reviews, see Barr et al. 1992 and Marazziti et al. 1994). Furthermore, these measures do not necessarily represent accurate indicators of serotonergic function within the brain. Pharmacological challenge studies provide another indirect approach. By administering serotonergic agents and measuring endocrine or behavioral variables, investigators have attempted to assess central serotonergic sensitivities. For example, meta-chlorophenylpiperazine was found to exacerbate OCD symptoms in four studies (Hollander et al. 1992; Khanna et al. 2001; Pigott et al. 1991; Zohar et al. 1987) but not in two others (Goodman et al. 1995; Ho Pian et al. 1998). However, in pharmacological challenge studies, use of lactate (Gorman et al. 1985), carbon dioxide (Perna et al. 1995), yohimbine (Rasmussen et al. 1987), cholecystokinin receptor agonists (de Leeuw et al. 1996), and tryptophan depletion (Corchs et al. 2015) for anxiogenic purposes has not exacerbated OCD symptoms. These findings suggest that specific serotonergic dysfunction is associated with OCD.

Methods for probing the serotonergic system in the brain are necessary for directly testing a serotonergic hypothesis of OCD pathophysiology. With the advent of functional imaging receptor characterization techniques, such studies are now feasible. Thus far, most such studies have focused on the role of the serotonin transporter in the pathophysiology of OCD. Using single-photon emission computed tomography (SPECT) and [^{123}I]-β-CIT, two studies (Hesse et al. 2005; Zitterl et al. 2007) have found a reduction in serotonin transporter binding in the thalamus/hypothalamus that correlated with symptom severity in OCD cohorts. One of these studies also found decreased serotonin transporter binding in the midbrain and brain stem (Hesse et al. 2005). However, another study using SPECT and [^{123}I]-β-CIT found increased serotonin transporter binding in the midbrain (Pogarell et al. 2003). Lastly, one SPECT study using [^{123}I]-β-CIT failed to find any difference between subjects with OCD and psychiatrically healthy control subjects (van der Wee et al. 2004). One study (Simpson et al. 2003) using PET scanning and the serotonin transporter ligand [^{11}C]McN5652 failed to show a difference between subjects with OCD and psychiatrically healthy control subjects, whereas a study using PET and the serotonin transporter ligand [^{11}C]DASB showed reduced binding in the thalamus and midbrain of subjects with OCD when compared with psychiatrically healthy control subjects (Reimold et al. 2007). Another PET study using the serotonin transporter ligand [^{11}C]DASB showed higher binding in the putamen of subjects with early onset OCD than in subjects with late-onset OCD (no control subjects were included) (Lee et al. 2018).

Finally, considerable pharmacological research has begun to clarify the therapeutic mechanisms of SRIs. Animal studies indicate that antidepressants can potentiate serotonergic transmission (Blier and de Montigny 1994). In SRIs, potentiation of serotonergic transmission appears to be mediated by autoreceptor desensitization (Blier and Bouchard 1994; Blier et al. 1988). The time course of these receptor changes parallels the observed delay between initiation of SRIs and onset of therapeutic response. In an important study, el Mansari et al. (1995) showed that SRI-induced changes in serotonergic transmission occur more quickly in the lateral frontal cortex than in the medial frontal cortex of rodents. This finding corresponds beautifully with the observation that the antidepressant effects of SRIs tend to occur sooner than antiobsessional effects (Fineberg et al. 1992). Furthermore, current models of mediating anatomy suggest that lateral prefrontal areas are involved in the pathophysiology of major depression, whereas the medial frontal (i.e., orbitofrontal) cortex has been implicated in the pathophysiology of OCD. The ultimate neuropharmacological effects of SRIs on the frontal cortex and other relevant territories remain to be fully delineated. Likewise, the relative role of different receptor subtypes (Piñeyro et al. 1994), as well as downstream effects on second messengers and genetic transcription factors (Lesch et al. 1993), requires further study.

In summary, although some evidence supports a serotonergic hypothesis of OCD pathophysiology, modulation of serotonergic systems clearly plays a role in the effective pharmacotherapy of OCD with serotonergic agents. Emerging data suggest that SRIs might produce their beneficial effects several weeks after treatment initiation by downregulating terminal autoreceptors (5-HT$_{1D}$) in the orbitofrontal cortex, thereby facilitating serotonergic transmission in that region (el Mansari et al. 1995). Advances in radiochemistry and pharmacology, together with contemporary in vivo neuroimaging methods, should soon provide an opportunity to directly test the serotonergic hypothesis of OCD pathophysiology. Additional studies are necessary to clarify the precise mechanisms that underlie the antiobsessional effects of SRIs as well as those of other effective treatments, including nonpharmacological modalities.

It is not clear how this information generalizes to other obsessive-compulsive spectrum disorders. SRIs appear to be of modest therapeutic benefit for body dysmorphic disorder (BDD) and trichotillomania but are not typically effective for reducing the tics of Tourette syndrome (TS), although they can be helpful in addressing other associated affective or behavioral manifestations. Thus, a model of SRI action in OCRD must explain the observed differential efficacy across this spectrum of disorders. Given the data at hand, it may be that SRIs exert their effects by modulating corticostriatal systems at the level of the cortex and with prominent effects within the medial and lateral prefrontal zones. Therefore, spectrum disorders that entail dysfunction within the cognitive and affective corticostriatal circuits might be preferentially responsive to SRIs, whereas chronic tics involving the sensorimotor cortex may be unresponsive to such interventions.

Dopaminergic Systems and the Pathogenesis of OCD and Related Disorders

Transgenic mice expressing a neuropotentiating cholera toxin transgene in dopamine D_1 receptor–expressing neurons have been found to engage in biting and in perseverative locomotor and behavioral abnormalities consistent with animal models of OCD (Campbell et al. 1999a, 1999b). The researchers suggested that the chronic potentiation of cortical and limbic D_1 neurons might be responsible for these obsessive-compulsive behaviors (Campbell et al. 2000; McGrath et al. 2000). In addition, rats chronically treated with quinpirole (a D_2/D_3 receptor agonist) exhibited ritualistic behavior resembling checking behavior (Ben-Pazi et al. 2001; Einat and Szechtman 1995; Szechtman et al. 1998, 2001). Other studies have failed to demonstrate a link between D_2 receptors and OCD (Novelli et al. 1994).

In humans, few peripheral measures of dopamine in OCD cohorts have been performed, and none has yielded positive results. Likewise, few pharmacological probes to assess the role of dopaminergic function in the pathophysiology of OCD have been conducted. However, agents that affect dopaminergic function, such as cocaine (Koizumi 1985) and methylphenidate/amphetamine (Frye and Arnold 1981), have been reported to exacerbate or induce OCD symptoms. In addition, augmentation of SRIs with dopamine antagonists constitutes an effective strategy for treating patients with OCD who do not respond to SRIs alone (for review, see Dougherty et al. 2007). Multiple in-vivo neuroimaging studies focusing on dopaminergic function in OCD have also been conducted. Two such studies found increased dopamine transporter binding in the basal ganglia of OCD cohorts (Kim et al. 2003; van der Wee et al. 2004), whereas another failed to detect a difference (Pogarell et al. 2003). Another study demonstrated decreased D_2 receptor binding in the basal ganglia of an OCD cohort (Denys et al. 2004). Finally, one study demonstrated a decrease in binding potential to the D_2/D_3 receptor in subjects with OCD and showed that chronic stimulation of the striatum using deep brain stimulation increased plasma homovanillic acid levels, suggesting that this approach induces striatal dopamine release in subjects with OCD (Figee et al. 2014). Taken together, these findings suggest higher synaptic concentrations of dopamine in the basal ganglia of patients with OCD.

Complementing the previous discussion of serotonin and its role in OCD, dopamine antagonists are effective for reducing the tics of TS as well as the manifestations of other hyperkinetic movement disorders. Conversely, dopamine agonists are known to exacerbate tics and other adventitial movements. Considerable data implicate primary dopaminergic abnormalities in TS.

The cell bodies of dopamine-containing neurons are principally concentrated in the midbrain and tegmentum and project rostrally, forming the nigrostriatal pathway as well as the mesolimbic and mesocortical systems. It has long been presumed that the therapeutic effects of dopamine antagonists in hyperkinetic movement disorders follow logically from the well-established role of dopamine in mediating motor control via the nigrostriatal system. A comparison of postmortem tissue from people with TS revealed higher binding rates for a dopamine transporter site ligand in the striatum compared with control subjects (Singer et al. 1991). A recent meta-analysis of PET studies using dopaminergic ligands found increased striatal dopamine transporter binding (but this difference did not remain significant when corrected for age differences among the cohorts) and a trend toward lower D_2/D_3 receptor binding in the striatum in subjects with TS (Hienert et al. 2018). Taken together, the findings from these studies suggest that patients with TS exhibit abnormalities of the dopaminergic system within the striatum. These preliminary findings should be interpreted cautiously, however, given that the sample sizes were small and the subjects in these studies were not neuroleptic naive. Therefore, some of the observed abnormalities may be a consequence of past exposure to antidopaminergic medications or other differences between the groups that are unrelated to the TS diagnosis. Nonetheless, these data provide initial evidence supporting a dopaminergic hypothesis; specifically, TS appears to be associated with fundamental dopaminergic abnormalities within the striatum, and tic symptoms can be exacerbated by exposure to dopamimetic agents as well as attenuated by treatment with dopamine antagonist medications.

Glutamatergic Systems and the Pathogenesis of OCD and Related Disorders

Because CSTC circuits rely predominantly on glutamatergic transmission, investigators have posited that glutamatergic dysfunction may play a role in the pathophysiology of OCD. Newer neuroimaging modalities such as magnetic resonance spectroscopy allow for measurement of glutamate and related neurochemical concentrations in predetermined brain regions. Numerous studies have since implicated glutamate dysfunction in OCD in various brain regions (Gnanavel et al. 2014; Rosenberg et al. 2000, 2004; Yücel et al. 2007), whereas others have not identified glutamatergic dysfunction (Brennan et al. 2015). Additionally, some of the candidate genes associated with OCD, such as the solute carrier gene *SLCA1A*, are associated with glutamatergic function. In part as a result of these findings, investigators have conducted clinical trials in subjects with OCD using glutamatergic agents such as riluzole (Grant et al. 2014), memantine (Ghaleiha et al. 2013; Haghighi et al. 2013), ketamine (Rodriguez et al. 2013), and *N*-acetylcysteine (Costa et al. 2017) with mixed but generally positive results.

Neurochemistry Across the Obsessive-Compulsive Spectrum

Pathophysiological heterogeneity may explain why some subtypes of OCD are responsive to SRIs alone and some to SRIs plus dopamine antagonists, whereas others are wholly unresponsive to either of these interventions. For instance, tic-related OCD appears to be relatively SRI refractory and preferentially responsive to the combination of SRIs plus dopamine antagonists (McDougle et al. 1994a, 1994b). One possible explanation is that BDD and non-tic-related OCD involve primary orbitofrontal dysfunction or pathophysiology, whereas tic-related OCD and TS involve primary striatal pathology. Therefore, serotonergic modulation at the level of the orbitofrontal cortex might be sufficient for antiobsessional effects in BDD or non-tic-related OCD, whereas dopaminergic modulation within the striatum synergizes with orbitofrontal serotonergic modulation to relieve tic-related OCD, and pure TS responds to dopamine modulation at the level of the striatum but not to serotonergic modulation at the level of the orbitofrontal cortex.

Endocrine/HPA Axis Function

Because abnormalities of the hypothalamic-pituitary-adrenal (HPA) axis have been demonstrated in other anxiety disorders, some researchers have focused on HPA axis function in OCD. In multiple studies, investigators have examined peripheral measures of HPA axis function in patients with OCD. One study found increased levels of corticotropin-releasing hormone in the cerebrospinal fluid of patients with OCD (Altemus et al. 1992), whereas another study failed to find a difference in patients with OCD or TS versus healthy control subjects (Chappell et al. 1996). Another study (Gehris et al. 1990) found increased 24-hour urinary cortisol levels in subjects with OCD. Finally, three studies found increased serum concentrations of cortisol in OCD cohorts (Catapano et al. 1992; Kluge et al. 2007; Monteleone et al. 1994), whereas three other studies found no difference (Brambilla et al. 1997, 2000; Kawano et al. 2013). One study (Kluge et al. 2007) also found increased adrenocorticotropic hormone secretion in subjects with OCD.

HPA axis challenge studies have been performed in subjects with OCD as well. Dexamethasone suppression test studies in OCD cohorts have had inconsistent results, with some studies demonstrating nonsuppression (Catapano et al. 1990; Cottraux et al. 1984) and others failing to find abnormalities (Coryell et al. 1989; Jenike et al. 1987; Lieberman et al. 1985; Lucey et al. 1992; Vallejo et al. 1988). In one study, challenge with corticotropin-releasing hormone was associated with blunted adrenocorticotropic hormone secretion in subjects with OCD (Bailly et al. 1994). Two studies (Khanna et al. 2001; Zohar et al. 1987) found hyporesponsivity of the HPA axis following meta-chlorophenylpiperazine challenge, whereas two others failed to detect abnormalities (Charney et al. 1988; Hollander et al. 1992).

In summary, although HPA axis dysfunction is clearly present in other anxiety disorders, results of studies examining HPA axis function in OCRD have been inconsistent at best. These outcomes are likely to reflect the noncentrality of HPA axis function to the pathophysiology of OCD. Nevertheless, some abnormalities have been detected as epiphenomena due to the nonspecific anxiety symptoms associated with OCD. However, further studies of the role of the HPA axis in OCD need to be conducted.

Possible Autoimmune Etiology

Over the past few decades, a fascinating scientific story has emerged about the potential role of autoimmune mechanisms in the pathogenesis of OCRD. It had long been appreciated that Sydenham's chorea, one manifestation of acute rheumatic fever, is accompanied by neuropsychiatric symptoms reminiscent of OCD and TS. Unlike that of OCD or TS, however, much about the pathogenesis of Sydenham's chorea has been known since the mid-1970s. In particular, a study by Husby et al. (1976) suggested that the damage to the basal ganglia characteristic of Sydenham's chorea is mediated by antineuronal antibodies as part of an autoimmune response to group A β-hemolytic streptococcal (GABHS) infection. Hence, it was proposed that a similar process might cause OCD or TS in a subset of cases (Swedo et al. 1994). Critical clinical research initiated in the late 1980s demonstrated that OCD symptoms were common among children with Sydenham's chorea and that these symptoms often preceded motor manifestations of the disease (Swedo et al. 1989a, 1993). A series of studies involving children with OCD and TS showed that antineuronal antibodies were present in a subset of cases (Leonard et al. 1989; Rettew et al. 1992: Swedo et al. 1989b). Longitudinal study of several such cases indicated characteristic features of abrupt onset and discrete episodes of symptom exacerbation, which are often associated with demonstrable GABHS infection (Allen et al. 1995; Ayoub and Wannamaker 1966; Berrios et al. 1985; Swedo et al. 1998). Interestingly, a few longitudinal cases have been reported in which serial neuroimaging data demonstrated acute changes in striatal volume that paralleled the clinical course (Giedd et al. 1995). Taken together, these findings led to the designation of pediatric autoimmune neuropsychiatric disorders associated with streptococcal infections (PANDAS), as named by Swedo (2002), which was more recently changed to pediatric acute-onset neuropsychiatric syndrome (PANS). The autoimmune mechanisms of pathogenesis in this subtype of OCRD suggest new possibilities in terms of early diagnosis and treatment, including prophylaxis with antibiotics or plasmapheresis.

It is believed that a vulnerability to rheumatic fever, and hence to PANDAS, may be inherited as an autosomal recessive trait (Gibofsky et al. 1991). A monoclonal antibody against the B lymphocyte antigen D8/17 appears to serve as a genetic marker for susceptibility to rheumatic fever; preliminary studies have indicated significantly greater D8/17 binding in cases of OCD and TS (Murphy et al. 1997; Swedo et al. 1997). Given that PANDAS cases bear striking similarity early-onset and tic-related OCD as well as TS, it is tempting to consider that PANDAS may account for a substantial proportion of childhood-onset cases of OCRD. The relative frequency of OCD and TS attributable to PANDAS, in fact, remains unknown. However, it is interesting to note that family genetic data suggest a different inheritance pattern for PANDAS than has been observed in the large pedigrees of OCD and TS studied to date.

Other Biological Factors

Although most biological factors related to the pathophysiology of OCD are discussed in other sections of this chapter, it is worth noting that OCD may also develop following birth injury (Capstick and Seldrup 1977), temporal lobe epilepsy (Kettl and Marks 1986), head injury (McKeon et al. 1984), or cerebrovascular accident (Akaho et al. 2019). Specifically, damage to the basal ganglia is particularly associated with the development of OCD symptoms (Tonkonogy and Barreira 1989), as are diseases associated with degeneration of the basal ganglia (e.g., Huntington's disease, Parkinson's disease) (Cummings and Cunningham 1992; Müller et al. 1997).

Neuroanatomy and Pathophysiology

Relevant Normal Neuroanatomy

Contemporary neuroanatomical models of OCRD have emphasized the role of CSTC circuitry. In a series of classic articles, Alexander et al. (1986) introduced and reviewed the organization of multiple parallel, segregated CSTC circuits. Briefly, each CSTC circuit involves projections from various cortical zones to specific corresponding subterritories of striatum, which in turn send projections via other intermediate basal ganglia targets to ramify within the thalamus. These circuits are ultimately closed via reciprocal projections from the thalamus back to the very same prefrontal cortical regions from which the corticostriatal projections originated. Several levels of complexity must be considered with regard to the anatomy and function of these circuits in order to appreciate their role in the pathophysiology of OCD and related disorders. Therefore, we begin by describing the key elements of these circuits as well as their functional significance.

The *prefrontal cortex* mediates various cognitive functions, including response inhibition, planning, organizing, controlling, and verifying operations. Consequently, prefrontal dysfunction is associated with disinhibition, disorganization, inflexibility, perseveration, and stereotypy (Miller and Cohen 2001). The prefrontal cortex comprises several functional subterritories. The dorsolateral prefrontal cortex plays a role in learning and memory as well as planning and other complex cognitive (i.e., executive) functions. The ventral prefrontal cortex can be further subdivided into two functional domains: the posteromedial orbitofrontal cortex is a component of the paralimbic system and has a role in affective and motivational functions, as we discuss later, and the anterior and lateral orbitofrontal cortices represent the structural and functional intermediaries between the lateral prefrontal and paralimbic prefrontal zones. For instance, the anterior and lateral orbitofrontal cortices seem to have a role in response inhibition and regulation of behavior based on social context as well as in other affectively tinged cognitive operations (Rolls 2004).

The *paralimbic system* is the name given to a contiguous belt of cortex that forms the functional conduit between other cortical areas and the limbic system proper. The constituents of the paralimbic belt include the posteromedial orbitofrontal cortex as well as the cingulate, anterior temporal, parahippocampal, and insular cortices (Mesulam 1985). This system is believed to integrate abstracted representations of the outside world with inner emotional states, so that appropriate meaning and priority can be assigned to information as it is processed. Convergent data from human neuroimaging studies, together with previous animal and human research, suggest that the paralimbic system plays a critical role in mediating intense emotional states or arousal; in particular, this system has been implicated in anxiety (Rauch and Shin 1997; Rauch et al. 1994, 1995, 1996, 1997). Furthermore, it has long been appreciated that paralimbic elements serve to modulate the autonomic responses, including heart rate and blood pressure, that represent the somatic manifestations of intense affects or heightened arousal (Mesulam 1985).

The *striatum* comprises the caudate nucleus, putamen, and nucleus accumbens (also called the ventral striatum). Historically, the basal ganglia, including the striatum, were thought to play a circumscribed role limited to the modulation of motor functions. More recently, however, a much more complicated scheme has been adopted that recognizes the role of the striatum in cognitive and affective functions as well (Packard and Knowlton 2002).

Parallel, segregated CSTC circuits differ from one another on the basis of their distinct projection zones within the cortex, striatum, and thalamus and thus the particular functions each subserves. For the purposes of this review, we briefly describe four of these CSTC circuits: 1) the circuit involving projections from the sensorimotor cortex via the putamen subserves sensorimotor functions; 2) the corticostriatal circuit involving projections from the paralimbic cortex via the nucleus accumbens subserves affective or motivational functions; 3) projections from the anterior and lateral orbitofrontal cortices via the ventromedial caudate nucleus constitute the ventral cognitive circuit, which is thought to mediate context-related operations and response inhibition; and 4) projections from the dorsolateral prefrontal cortex via the dorsolateral caudate nucleus constitute the dorsal cognitive circuit, which is thought to mediate working memory and other executive functions.

Two major branches of the CSTC circuits exist. The corticothalamic branch provides a reciprocal excitatory monosynaptic communication between the cortex and the thalamus that purportedly mediates consciously initiated output (corticothalamic) and consciously accessible input (thalamocortical) streams. The cortico-striato-thalamic branch represents a collateral pathway that serves to modulate transmission at the level of the thalamus. Purportedly, the function of the striatum in this context is to process information automatically and without conscious representation. Thus, the healthy striatum, by exerting a balance of suppression or enhancement at the level of thalamus, serves to 1) filter out extraneous input, 2) ensure refined output, and 3) mediate stereotyped, rule-based processes without necessitating the allocation of conscious resources (Kravitz and Kreitzer 2012; Kravitz et al. 2010). In this way, the striatum regulates the content, and facilitates the quality, of information processing within the explicit (i.e., conscious) domain by fine-tuning input and output. In addition, it enhances the efficiency of the brain by carrying out some nonconscious functions, thereby reducing the computational load on conscious processing systems.

The *direct* and *indirect* cortico-striato-thalamic pathways represent a third level of complexity. Each cortico-striato-thalamic collateral consists of both a "direct" and an "indirect" pathway. These two systems operate in parallel, with opposing ultimate influences at the level of the thalamus. The direct system is so named because it involves direct projections from the striatum to the globus pallidus interna, with a net excitatory influence on the thalamus. Conversely, the indirect system involves indirect projections from the striatum via the globus pallidus externa to the globus pallidus interna and has a net inhibitory effect at the level of the thalamus. Thus, the direct and indirect pathways are generally believed to have opposite effects on CSTC circuits, although complexities in communication between the two pathways exist (Calabresi et al. 2014). Although these two systems share many features in common, they are characterized by important neurochemical differences. Specifically, whereas the direct system uses the neuropeptide substance P as a transmitter, the indirect system uses enkephalin instead.

Corticostriatal Hypothesis of OCD

Since the early 1990s, neurobiological models of OCD have emphasized the role of the frontal cortex and striatum (Graybiel and Rauch 2000; Pauls et al. 2014; Stein 2000). The scheme of corticostriatal circuitry fits well with emerging data implicating the elements of those circuits. Convergent results from neuroimaging studies indicate hyperactivity of the orbitofrontal cortex, anterior cingulate cortex, and (less consistently) caudate nucleus at rest, and attenuation of these abnormalities with effective treatment (Pauls et al. 2014). Neuropsychological studies were consistent with subtle deficits involving frontostriatal functions (Abramovitch et al. 2013). Neurosurgical procedures, including ablative limbic system procedures and deep brain stimulation, that interrupted this circuit appeared to reduce OCD symptoms (Greenberg et al. 2010). There is heuristic appeal to the hypothesis that positive feedback loops between the cortex and thalamus might mediate circular, repetitive thoughts, whereas the striatum might mediate fixed action patterns in the form of repetitive behaviors or compulsions (Pauls et al. 2014).

Although several early versions of this model were suggested, each posited an overdriven corticothalamic reverberating circuit. It has been proposed that a hyperactive caudate nucleus might be the cause of net excitation of the thalamus or that the apparent hyperactivity in the caudate represented insufficient compensation for intrinsic striatal dysfunction, such that inhibition of the thalamus through the cortico-striato-thalamic collateral was inadequate (Modell et al. 1989). As researchers came to appreciate the ramifications of the direct and indirect systems within the cortico-striato-thalamic collateral branch, the models evolved. A revised version suggested that in psychiatrically healthy individuals, an appropriate balance between the direct and indirect systems enables the collateral to optimally modulate activity at the thalamus, whereas in individuals with OCD, a shift toward dominance of the direct system could result in excitation or disinhibition at the thalamus, thereby overdriving the corticothalamic branch (Dougherty et al. 2018). Thus, the corticostriatal models of OCD accommodate much of the available data.

Striatal Topography Model of OCD and Related Disorders

Baxter et al. (1990) were the first to clearly articulate what has come to be known as the striatal topography model of OCRD (Leckman et al. 1992; Rauch and Baxter 1998; Rauch et al. 1998c). As the phenomenological, familial, and neurobiological relationships between OCD and TS became appreciated, it was hypothesized that the two disorders might share a fundamental pathophysiology whereby the clinical manifestations of each disease are governed by the precise topography of dysfunction within the striatum. The researchers suggested that different corticostriatal circuits might mediate different symptoms and might therefore define a spectrum of different disease entities. Originally, they proposed that ventromedial caudate/accumbens involvement might mediate obsessions, dorsolateral caudate dysfunction might mediate compulsions, and putamen involvement might mediate the tics of TS. Subsequently, inspired by results of symptom provocation studies, we proposed that the paralimbic system (including posteromedial orbitofrontal cortex) mediates affective manifestations, including the anxiety of OCD or BDD and the "urges" of TS or trichotillomania, whereas the ventral cognitive circuit, comprising the anterior and lateral orbitofrontal cortices and ventromedial caudate, mediates obsessional symptoms (Rauch and Baxter 1998; Rauch et al. 1998c). Further support for the striatal topography model comes from imaging studies that indicate structural abnormalities involving the caudate in OCD (Pauls et al. 2014) and the putamen in TS (Peterson et al. 1993; Singer et al. 1993) and trichotillomania (O'Sullivan et al. 1997).

Neuroanatomical Correlates of Factor-Analyzed Symptom Dimensions

Although PANS offers the potential for identifying a subtype of obsessive-compulsive spectrum conditions with a homogeneous etiology, optimal strategies for characterizing spectrum subtypes based on pathophysiology and phenomenology are yet to be established. Several strategies have been employed for subtyping OCRD based on symptomatology. The approach of factor analysis has been used to determine clusters of intercorrelated OCD symptoms that can be treated as orthogonal factors for describing clinical presentation (Katerberg et al. 2010). Because these factors are independent of one another, it is reasonable to hypothesize that each reflects a separate underlying aspect of pathophysiology. Rauch et al. (1998a) tested this modular approach to the characterization of OCD by seeking neuroanatomical correlates of symptom severity for each factor using PET. In this preliminary study, the symptom factors employed included 1) checking and religious, aggressive, and sexual obsessions; 2) symmetry and ordering; and 3) washing and cleaning (Baer 1994; Leckman et al. 1997). Notably, factors 1 and 2 had previously been associated with tic-related OCD. Interestingly, Rauch et al. (1998a) found that during a nominally neutral state, factor 1 was positively correlated with bilateral striatal activity, factor 2 was negatively correlated with right caudate activity, and factor 3 was positively correlated with orbitofrontal and anterior cingulate cortical activity. Mataix-Cols et al. (2004) examined subjects with OCD and control subjects using functional MRI and found that subjects with OCD had greater activation in the bilateral ventromedial prefrontal regions and right caudate nucleus associated with washing; greater activation of the putamen/globus pallidus, thalamus, and dorsal cortical areas associated with checking; greater activation of the left precentral gyrus and right orbitofrontal cortex associated with hoarding; and greater activation of the left occipitotemporal regions with aversive and symptom-unrelated factors. Although preliminary, these results suggest that different symptom dimensions are associated with activity within different modules of the CSTC circuits of interest (Rauch et al. 1998b).

Conclusion

Evolving brain imaging techniques represent the most powerful tools for characterizing in vivo human neuroanatomy, neurophysiology, and neurochemistry at modest temporal and spatial resolution. Categorical approaches will aim to identify discrete subtypes of patients, based on the measures reviewed in this chapter as well as on symptomatology and treatment response. Dimensional approaches will aim to consider these as continuous variables. Only time will tell which of these approaches is superior for describing the obsessive-compulsive spectrum. Concretely, prospective imaging studies can generate and test hypotheses regarding the elements of neuroimaging profiles that predict treatment response for medications, behavior therapy, or other therapies. Simultaneously, phenomenological characteristics can be correlated with both brain imaging indices and treatment outcomes. Thus, by triangulating across such multifaceted data sets, it should be possible to achieve a robust and valid clinical-neurobiological basis for diagnosis and subtyping across the OCRD.

As various pathophysiological entities are dissected, the hope is that each one will give way to specific treatments. Basic pharmacological research will continue to explore the receptor changes and, perhaps more importantly, the downstream molecular effects of currently available therapies. Such research will progressively illuminate the salient changes necessary to ameliorate symptoms in each of the subtypes of the obsessive-compulsive spectrum. Once these targets are established, it will be possible to rationally design new and, ideally, better treatments. Although this paragraph implies a focus on pharmacotherapy, an analogous process will, in fact, be necessary to advance nonpharmacological treatments, including behavior therapy as well as noninvasive neurostimulation and neurosurgical approaches.

These are exciting times in psychiatric neuroscience as the field moves closer to the promise of a diagnostic scheme that reflects pathophysiology. In this context, OCD is a model disorder. Even though technical advances in neuroimaging, genetics, and pharmacology have provided new tools with which to elucidate the pathogenesis of OCD, there should be renewed enthusiasm for the essential contribution of careful phenomenological characterization. It should already be clear that OCD, as defined in DSM-5 (American Psychiatric Association 2013), is not one disease, but several. Conversely, in some cases, OCD and TS may not be different diseases pathogenetically but, rather, different faces of the very same one.

Key Points

- The neurotransmitters most likely implicated in the pathophysiology of OCD include serotonin and dopamine and possibly glutamate.

- A specific cortico-striato-thalamo-cortical circuit that includes the orbitofrontal cortex, caudate nucleus, and thalamus is dysfunctional in subjects with OCD. This dysfunction has been repeatedly demonstrated in neuroimaging studies. Successful treatment attenuates this dysfunction.

- Studies of hypothalamic-pituitary-adrenal axis function in subjects with OCD have been inconsistent.

- Some cases of OCD may be associated with an autoimmune response (pediatric acute-onset neuropsychiatric syndrome), and these cases provide evidence of striatal pathology in OCD.

References

Abramovitch A, Abramowitz JS, Mittelman A: The neuropsychology of adult obsessive-compulsive disorder: a meta-analysis. Clin Psychol Rev 33(8):1163–1171, 2013 24128603

Akaho R, Deguchi I, Kigawa H, Nishimura K: Obsessive-compulsive disorder following cerebrovascular accident: a case report and literature review. J Stroke Cerebrovasc Dis 28(4):e17–e21, 2019 30638936

Alexander GE, DeLong MR, Strick PL: Parallel organization of functionally segregated circuits linking basal ganglia and cortex. Annu Rev Neurosci 9:357–381, 1986 3085570

Allen AJ, Leonard HL, Swedo SE: Case study: a new infection-triggered, automimmune subtype of pediatric OCD and Tourette's syndrome. J Am Acad Child Adolesc Psychiatry 34:307–311, 1995

Altemus M, Pigott T, Kalogeras KT, et al: Abnormalities in the regulation of vasopressin and corticotropin releasing factor secretion in obsessive-compulsive disorder. Arch Gen Psychiatry 49(1):9–20, 1992 1370198

American Psychiatric Association: Diagnostic and Statistical Manual of Mental Disorders, 5th Edition. Arlington, VA, American Psychiatric Association, 2013

Ayoub EM, Wannamaker LW: Streptococcal antibody titers in Sydenham's chorea. Pediatrics 38(6):946–956, 1966 5928726

Baer L: Factor analysis of symptom subtypes of obsessive compulsive disorder and their relation to personality and tic disorders. J Clin Psychiatry 55(suppl):18–23, 1994 8077163

Bailly D, Servant D, Dewailly D, et al: Corticotropin releasing factor stimulation test in obsessive compulsive disorder. Biol Psychiatry 35(2):143–146, 1994 8167212

Barr LC, Goodman WK, Price LH, et al: The serotonin hypothesis of obsessive compulsive disorder: implications of pharmacologic challenge studies. J Clin Psychiatry 53(suppl):17–28, 1992 1532961

Baxter LR, Schwartz JM, Guze BH, et al: Neuroimaging in obsessive-compulsive disorder: seeking the mediating neuroanatomy, in Obsessive-Compulsive Disorder: Theory and Management, 2nd Edition. Edited by Jenike MA, Minichiello WE, Chicago, IL, Year Book Medical Publishers, 1990, pp 167–188

Ben-Pazi A, Szechtman H, Eilam D: The morphogenesis of motor rituals in rats treated chronically with the dopamine agonist quinpirole. Behav Neurosci 115(6):1301–1317, 2001 11770061

Berrios X, Quesney F, Morales A, et al: Are all recurrences of "pure" Sydenham's chorea true recurrences of acute rheumatic fever? Pediatrics 10(6):867–872, 1985

Blier P, Bouchard C: Modulation of 5-HT release in the guinea-pig brain following long-term administration of antidepressant drugs. Br J Pharmacol 113(2):485–495, 1994 7834200

Blier P, de Montigny C: Current advances and trends in the treatment of depression. Trends Pharmacol Sci 15(7):220–226, 1994 7940983

Blier P, Chaput Y, de Montigny C: Long-term 5-HT reuptake blockade, but not monoamine oxidase inhibition, decreases the function of terminal 5-HT autoreceptors: an electrophysiological study in the rat brain. Naunyn Schmiedebergs Arch Pharmacol 337(3):246–254, 1988 3260661

Brambilla F, Bellodi L, Perna G, et al: Noradrenergic receptor sensitivity in obsessive compulsive disorder: II. Cortisol response to acute clonidine administration. Psychiatry Res 69(2–3):163–168, 1997 9109184

Brambilla F, Perna G, Bussi R, et al: Dopamine function in obsessive compulsive disorder: cortisol response to acute apomorphine stimulation. Psychoneuroendocrinology 25(3):301–310, 2000 10737700

Brennan BP, Tkachenko O, Schwab ZJ, et al: An examination of rostral anterior cingulate cortex function and neurochemistry in obsessive-compulsive disorder. Neuropsychopharmacology 40(8):1866–1876, 2015 25662837

Calabresi P, Picconi B, Tozzi A, et al: Direct and indirect pathways of basal ganglia: a critical reappraisal. Nat Neurosci 17(8):1022–1030, 2014 25065439

Campbell KM, de Lecea L, Severynse DM, et al: OCD-like behaviors caused by a neuropotentiating transgene targeted to cortical and limbic D1+ neurons. J Neurosci 19(12):5044–5053, 1999a 10366637

Campbell KM, McGrath MJ, Burton FH: Differential response of cortical-limbic neuropotentiated compulsive mice to dopamine D1 and D2 receptor antagonists. Eur J Pharmacol 371(2–3):103–111, 1999b 10357247

Campbell KM, Veldman MB, McGrath MJ, et al: TS+OCD-like neuropotentiated mice are supersensitive to seizure induction. Neuroreport 11(10):2335–2338, 2000 10923696

Capstick N, Seldrup J: Obsessional states: a study in the relationship between abnormalities occurring at the time of birth and the subsequent development of obsessional symptoms. Acta Psychiatr Scand 56(5):427–431, 1977 596233

Catapano F, Monteleone P, Maj M, et al: Dexamethasone suppression test in patients with primary obsessive-compulsive disorder and in healthy controls. Neuropsychobiology 23(2):53–56, 1990 2077433

Catapano F, Monteleone P, Fuschino A, et al: Melatonin and cortisol secretion in patients with primary obsessive-compulsive disorder. Psychiatry Res 44(3):217–225, 1992 1289919

Chappell P, Leckman J, Goodman W, et al: Elevated cerebrospinal fluid corticotropin-releasing factor in Tourette's syndrome: comparison to obsessive compulsive disorder and normal controls. Biol Psychiatry 39(9):776–783, 1996 8731518

Charney DS, Goodman WK, Price LH, et al: Serotonin function in obsessive-compulsive disorder: a comparison of the effects of tryptophan and m-chlorophenylpiperazine in patients and healthy subjects. Arch Gen Psychiatry 45(2):177–185, 1988 3337615

Corchs F, Nutt DJ, Hince DA, et al: Evidence for serotonin function as a neurochemical difference between fear and anxiety disorders in humans? J Psychopharmacol 29(10):1061–1069, 2015 26187054

Coryell WH, Black DW, Kelly MW, et al: HPA axis disturbance in obsessive-compulsive disorder. Psychiatry Res 30(3):243–251, 1989 2694203

Costa DLC, Diniz JB, Requena G, et al: Randomized, double-blind, placebo-controlled trial of N-acetylcysteine augmentation for treatment-resistant obsessive-compulsive disorder. J Clin Psychiatry 78(7):e766–e773, 2017 28617566

Cottraux JA, Bouvard M, Claustrat B, et al: Abnormal dexamethasone suppression test in primary obsessive-compulsive patients: a confirmatory report. Psychiatry Res 13(2):157–165, 1984 6596583

Cummings JL, Cunningham K: Obsessive-compulsive disorder in Huntington's disease. Biol Psychiatry 31(3):263–270, 1992 1532132

de Leeuw AS, Den Boer JA, Slaap BR, et al: Pentagastrin has panic-inducing properties in obsessive compulsive disorder. Psychopharmacology (Berl) 126(4):339–344, 1996 8878350

Denys D, van der Wee N, Janssen J, et al: Low level of dopaminergic D2 receptor binding in obsessive-compulsive disorder. Biol Psychiatry 55(10):1041–1045, 2004 15121489

Dougherty DD, Rauch SL, Jenike MA: Pharmacological treatments for obsessive-compulsive disorder, in A Guide to Treatments That Work, 3rd Edition. Edited by Nathan PE, Gorman JM. New York, Oxford University Press, 2007, pp 447–473

Dougherty DD, Brennan BP, Stewart SE, et al: Neuroscientifically informed formulation and treatment planning for patients with obsessive-compulsive disorder: a review. JAMA Psychiatry 75(10):1081–1087, 2018

Einat H, Szechtman H: Perseveration without hyperlocomotion in a spontaneous alternation task in rats sensitized to the dopamine agonist quinpirole. Physiol Behav 57(1):55–59, 1995 7878126

el Mansari M, Bouchard C, Blier P: Alteration of serotonin release in the guinea pig orbitofrontal cortex by selective serotonin reuptake inhibitors: relevance to treatment of obsessive-compulsive disorder. Neuropsychopharmacology 13(2):117–127, 1995 8597523

Figee M, de Koning P, Klaassen S, et al: Deep brain stimulation induces striatal dopamine release in obsessive-compulsive disorder. Biol Psychiatry 75(8):647–652, 2014 23938318

Fineberg NA, Bullock T, Montgomery DB, et al: Serotonin reuptake inhibitors are the treatment of choice in obsessive compulsive disorder. Int Clin Psychopharmacol 7(suppl 1):43–47, 1992 1517558

Frye PE, Arnold LE: Persistent amphetamine-induced compulsive rituals: response to pyridoxine (B6). Biol Psychiatry 16(6):583–587, 1981 7260219

Gehris TL, Kathol RG, Black DW, et al: Urinary free cortisol levels in obsessive-compulsive disorder. Psychiatry Res 32(2):151–158, 1990 2367600

Ghaleiha A, Entezari N, Modabbernia A, et al: Memantine add-on in moderate to severe obsessive-compulsive disorder: randomized double-blind placebo-controlled study. J Psychiatr Res 47(2):175–180, 2013 23063327

Gibofsky A, Khanna A, Suh E, et al: The genetics of rheumatic fever: relationship to streptococcal infection and autoimmune disease. J Rheumatol Suppl 30:1–5, 1991 1941846

Giedd JN, Rapoport JL, Kruesi MJ, et al: Sydenham's chorea: magnetic resonance imaging of the basal ganglia. Neurology 45(12):2199–2202, 1995 8848193

Gnanavel S, Sharan P, Khandelwal S, et al: Neurochemicals measured by (1)H-MR spectroscopy: putative vulnerability biomarkers for obsessive compulsive disorder. MAGMA 27(5):407–417, 2014 24338164

Goodman WK, McDougle CJ, Price LH, et al: m-Chlorophenylpiperazine in patients with obsessive-compulsive disorder: absence of symptom exacerbation. Biol Psychiatry 38(3):138–149, 1995 7578657

Gorman JM, Liebowitz MR, Fyer AJ, et al: Lactate infusions in obsessive-compulsive disorder. Am J Psychiatry 142(7):864–866, 1985 4014509

Grant PJ, Joseph LA, Farmer CA, et al: 12-week, placebo-controlled trial of add-on riluzole in the treatment of childhood-onset obsessive-compulsive disorder. Neuropsychopharmacology 39(6):1453–1459, 2014 24356715

Graybiel AM, Rauch SL: Toward a neurobiology of obsessive-compulsive disorder. Neuron 28(2):343–347, 2000 11144344

Greenberg BD, Rauch SL, Haber SN: Invasive circuitry-based neurotherapeutics: stereotactic ablation and deep brain stimulation for OCD. Neuropsychopharmacology 35(1):317–336, 2010 19759530

Haghighi M, Jahangard L, Mohammad-Beigi H, et al: In a double-blind, randomized and placebo-controlled trial, adjuvant memantine improved symptoms in inpatients suffering from refractory obsessive-compulsive disorders (OCD). Psychopharmacology (Berl) 228(4):633–640, 2013 23525525

Hesse S, Müller U, Lincke T, et al: Serotonin and dopamine transporter imaging in patients with obsessive-compulsive disorder. Psychiatry Res 140(1):63–72, 2005 16213689

Hienert M, Gryglewski G, Stamenkovic M, et al: Striatal dopaminergic alterations in Tourette's syndrome: a meta-analysis based on 16 PET and SPECT neuroimaging studies. Transl Psychiatry 8(1):143, 2018 30072700

Ho Pian KL, Westenberg HG, den Boer JA, et al: Effects of meta-chlorophenylpiperazine on cerebral blood flow in obsessive-compulsive disorder and controls. Biol Psychiatry 44(5):367–370, 1998 9755360

Hollander E, DeCaria CM, Nitescu A, et al: Serotonergic function in obsessive-compulsive disorder: behavioral and neuroendocrine responses to oral m-chlorophenylpiperazine and fenfluramine in patients and healthy volunteers. Arch Gen Psychiatry 49(1):21–28, 1992 1728249

Hoyer D, Clarke DE, Fozard JR, et al: International Union of Pharmacology classification of receptors for 5-hydroxytryptamine (serotonin). Pharmacol Rev 46(2):157–203, 1994 7938165

Husby G, van de Rijn I, Zabriskie JB, et al: Antibodies reacting with cytoplasm of subthalamic and caudate nuclei neurons in chorea and acute rheumatic fever. J Exp Med 144(4):1094–1110, 1976 789810

Jenike MA, Baer L, Brotman AW, et al: Obsessive-compulsive disorder, depression, and the dexamethasone suppression test. J Clin Psychopharmacol 7(3):182–184, 1987 3597805

Katerberg H, Delucchi KL, Stewart SE, et al: Symptom dimensions in OCD: item-level factor analysis and heritability estimates. Behav Genet 40(4):505–517, 2010 20361247

Kawano A, Tanaka Y, Ishitobi Y, et al: Salivary alpha-amylase and cortisol responsiveness following electrical stimulation stress in obsessive-compulsive disorder patients. Psychiatry Res 209(1):85–90, 2013 23266021

Kettl PA, Marks IM: Neurological factors in obsessive compulsive disorder: two case reports and a review of the literature. Br J Psychiatry 149:315–319, 1986 3779297

Khanna S, John JP, Reddy LP: Neuroendocrine and behavioral responses to mCPP in obsessive-compulsive disorder. Psychoneuroendocrinology 26(2):209–223, 2001 11087965

Kim CH, Koo MS, Cheon KA, et al: Dopamine transporter density of basal ganglia assessed with [123I]IPT SPET in obsessive-compulsive disorder. Eur J Nucl Med Mol Imaging 30(12):1637–1643, 2003 14513291

Kluge M, Schüssler P, Künzel HE, et al: Increased nocturnal secretion of ACTH and cortisol in obsessive compulsive disorder. J Psychiatr Res 41(11):928–933, 2007 17049559

Koizumi HM: Obsessive-compulsive symptoms following stimulants [letter]. Biol Psychiatry 20(12):1332–1333, 1985

Kravitz AV, Kreitzer AC: Striatal mechanisms underlying movement, reinforcement, and punishment. Physiology (Bethesda) 27(3):167–177, 2012 22689792

Kravitz AV, Freeze BS, Parker PR, et al: Regulation of parkinsonian motor behaviours by optogenetic control of basal ganglia circuitry. Nature 466(7306):622–626, 2010 20613723

Leckman JF, Pauls DL, Peterson BS, et al: Pathogenesis of Tourette syndrome: clues from the clinical phenotype and natural history. Adv Neurol 58:15–24, 1992 1414618

Leckman JF, Grice DE, Boardman J, et al: Symptoms of obsessive-compulsive disorder. Am J Psychiatry 154(7):911–917, 1997 9210740

Lee J, Kim BH, Kim E, et al: Higher serotonin transporter availability in early onset obsessive-compulsive disorder patients undergoing escitalopram treatment: a [11C]DASB PET study. Hum Psychopharmacol 33(1):e2642, 2018 29210107

Leonard HL, Lenane MC, Swedo SE, et al: Tics and Tourette's disorder: a 2- to 7-year follow-up of 54 obsessive-compulsive children. Am J Psychiatry 149:1244–1251, 1989

Lesch KP, Aulakh CS, Wolozin BL, et al: Regional brain expression of serotonin transporter mRNA and its regulation by reuptake inhibiting antidepressants. Brain Res Mol Brain Res 17(1–2):31–35, 1993 8381906

Lieberman JA, Kane JM, Sarantakos S, et al: Dexamethasone suppression tests in patients with obsessive-compulsive disorder. Am J Psychiatry 142(6):747–751, 1985 4003598

Lucey JV, Barry S, Webb MG, et al: The desipramine-induced growth hormone response and the dexamethasone suppression test in obsessive-compulsive disorder. Acta Psychiatr Scand 86(5):367–370, 1992 1336635

Marazziti D, Zohar J, Cassano G: Biological dissection of obsessive-compulsive disorder, in Current Insights in Obsessive-Compulsive Disorder. Edited by Berend B, Hollander E, Marazziti D, et al. Chichester, UK, Wiley and Sons, 1994, pp 137–148

Mataix-Cols D, Wooderson S, Lawrence N, et al: Distinct neural correlates of washing, checking, and hoarding symptom dimensions in obsessive-compulsive disorder. Arch Gen Psychiatry 61(6):564–576, 2004

McDougle CJ, Goodman WK, Leckman JF, et al: Haloperidol addition in fluvoxamine-refractory obsessive-compulsive disorder: a double-blind, placebo-controlled study in patients with and without tics. Arch Gen Psychiatry 51(4):302–308, 1994a 8161290

McDougle CJ, Goodman WK, Price LH: Dopamine antagonists in tic-related and psychotic spectrum obsessive compulsive disorder. J Clin Psychiatry 55(suppl):24–31, 1994b 7521326

McGrath MJ, Campbell KM, Parks CR 3rd, et al: Glutamatergic drugs exacerbate symptomatic behavior in a transgenic model of comorbid Tourette's syndrome and obsessive-compulsive disorder. Brain Res 877(1):23–30, 2000 10980239

McKeon J, McGuffin P, Robinson P: Obsessive-compulsive neurosis following head injury: a report of four cases. Br J Psychiatry 144:190–192, 1984 6704606

Mesulam M-M: Patterns in behavioral neuroanatomy: association areas, the limbic system, and hemispheric specialization, in Principles of Behavioral Neurology. Edited by Mesulam M-M. Philadelphia, PA, FA Davis, 1985, pp 1–70

Miller EK, Cohen JD: An integrative theory of prefrontal cortex function. Annu Rev Neurosci 24:167–202, 2001 11283309

Modell J, Mountz J, Curtis G, et al: Neurophysiologic dysfunction in basal ganglia/limbic striatal and thalamocortical circuits as a pathogenetic mechanism of obsessive compulsive disorder. J Neuropsychiatry Clin Neurosci 1:27–36, 1989

Monteleone P, Catapano F, Del Buono G, et al: Circadian rhythms of melatonin, cortisol and prolactin in patients with obsessive-compulsive disorder. Acta Psychiatr Scand 89(6):411–415, 1994 8085472

Müller N, Putz A, Kathmann N, et al: Characteristics of obsessive-compulsive symptoms in Tourette's syndrome, obsessive-compulsive disorder, and Parkinson's disease. Psychiatry Res 70(2):105–114, 1997 9194204

Murphy TK, Goodman WK, Fudge MW, et al: B lymphocyte antigen D8/17: a peripheral marker for childhood-onset obsessive-compulsive disorder and Tourette's syndrome? Am J Psychiatry 154(3):402–407, 1997 9054790

Novelli E, Nobile M, Diaferia G, et al: A molecular investigation suggests no relationship between obsessive-compulsive disorder and the dopamine D2 receptor. Neuropsychobiology 29(2):61–63, 1994 8170527

O'Sullivan R, Rauch SL, Breiter HC, et al: Reduced basal ganglia volumes in trichotillomania measured via morphometric magnetic resonance imaging. Biol Psychiatry 42(1):39–45, 1997 9193740

Packard MG, Knowlton BJ: Learning and memory functions of the basal ganglia. Annu Rev Neurosci 25:563–593, 2002 12052921

Pauls DL, Abramovitch A, Rauch SL, et al: Obsessive-compulsive disorder: an integrative genetic and neurobiological perspective. Nat Rev Neurosci 15(6):410–424, 2014 24840803

Perna G, Bertani A, Arancio C, et al: Laboratory response of patients with panic and obsessive-compulsive disorders to 35% CO_2 challenges. Am J Psychiatry 152(1):85–89, 1995 7802126

Peterson B, Riddle MA, Cohen DJ, et al: Reduced basal ganglia volumes in Tourette's syndrome using three-dimensional reconstruction techniques from magnetic resonance images. Neurology 43(5):941–949, 1993 8492950

Pigott TA, Zohar J, Hill JL, et al: Metergoline blocks the behavioral and neuroendocrine effects of orally administered m-chlorophenylpiperazine in patients with obsessive-compulsive disorder. Biol Psychiatry 29(5):418–426, 1991 2018816

Piñeyro G, Blier P, Dennis T, et al: Desensitization of the neuronal 5-HT carrier following its long-term blockade. J Neurosci 14(5 pt 2):3036–3047, 1994 8182457

Pogarell O, Hamann C, Pöpperl G, et al: Elevated brain serotonin transporter availability in patients with obsessive-compulsive disorder. Biol Psychiatry 54(12):1406–1413, 2003 14675805

Rasmussen SA, Goodman WK, Woods SW, et al: Effects of yohimbine in obsessive compulsive disorder. Psychopharmacology (Berl) 93(3):308–313, 1987 2829264

Rauch SL, Baxter LR: Neuroimaging models of obsessive-compulsive disorders, in Obsessive Compulsive Disorders: Theory and Management, 3rd Edition. Edited by Jenike MA, Baer L, Minichiello WE. St. Louis, MO, Mosby-Year Book, 1998, pp 289–317

Rauch SL, Shin LM: Functional neuroimaging studies in posttraumatic stress disorder. Ann NY Acad Sci 821:83–98, 1997 9238196

Rauch SL, Jenike MA, Alpert NM, et al: Regional cerebral blood flow measured during symptom provocation in obsessive-compulsive disorder using oxygen 15-labeled carbon dioxide and positron emission tomography. Arch Gen Psychiatry 51(1):62–70, 1994

Rauch SL, Savage CR, Alpert NM, et al: A positron emission tomographic study of simple phobic symptom provocation. Arch Gen Psychiatry 52(1):20–28, 1995 7811159

Rauch SL, van der Kolk BA, Fisler RE, et al: A symptom provocation study of posttraumatic stress disorder using positron emission tomography and script-driven imagery. Arch Gen Psychiatry 53(5):380–387, 1996 8624181

Rauch SL, Savage CR, Alpert NM, et al: The functional neuroanatomy of anxiety: a study of three disorders using positron emission tomography and symptom provocation. Biol Psychiatry 42(6):446–452, 1997 9285080

Rauch SL, Dougherty DD, Shin LM, et al: Neural correlates of factor-analyzed OCD symptom dimensions: a PET study. CNS Spectr 3(3):37–43, 1998a

Rauch SL, Whalen PJ, Curran T, et al: Thalamic deactivation during early implicit sequence learning: a functional MRI study. Neuroreport 9(5):865–870, 1998b 9579681

Rauch SL, Whalen PJ, Dougherty DD, et al: Neurobiological models of obsessive-compulsive disorders, in Obsessive Compulsive Disorders: Theory and Management, 3rd Edition. Edited by Jenike MA, Baer L, Minichiello WE. St. Louis, MO, Mosby-Year Book, 1998c, pp 222–253

Reimold M, Smolka MN, Zimmer A, et al: Reduced availability of serotonin transporters in obsessive-compulsive disorder correlates with symptom severity—a [11C]DASB PET study. J Neural Transm (Vienna) 114(12):1603–1609, 2007 17713719

Rettew DC, Swedo SE, Leonard HL, et al: Obsessions and compulsions across time in 79 children and adolescents with obsessive-compulsive disorder. J Am Acad Child Adolesc Psychiatry 31(6):1050–1056, 1992 1429404

Rodriguez CI, Kegeles LS, Levinson A, et al: Randomized controlled crossover trial of ketamine in obsessive-compulsive disorder: proof-of-concept. Neuropsychopharmacology 38(12):2475–2483, 2013 23783065

Rolls ET: The functions of the orbitofrontal cortex. Brain Cogn 55(1):11–29, 2004 15134840

Rosenberg DR, MacMaster FP, Keshavan MS, et al: Decrease in caudate glutamatergic concentrations in pediatric obsessive-compulsive disorder patients taking paroxetine. J Am Acad Child Adolesc Psychiatry 39(9):1096–1103, 2000 10986805

Rosenberg DR, Mirza Y, Russell A, et al: Reduced anterior cingulate glutamatergic concentrations in childhood OCD and major depression versus healthy controls. J Am Acad Child Adolesc Psychiatry 43(9):1146–1153, 2004 15322418

Simpson HB, Lombardo I, Slifstein M, et al: Serotonin transporters in obsessive-compulsive disorder: a positron emission tomography study with [(11)C]McN 5652. Biol Psychiatry 54(12):1414–1421, 2003 14675806

Singer HS, Hahn IH, Moran TH: Abnormal dopamine uptake sites in postmortem striatum from patients with Tourette's syndrome. Ann Neurol 30(4):558–562, 1991 1838678

Singer HS, Reiss AL, Brown JE, et al: Volumetric MRI changes in basal ganglia of children with Tourette's syndrome. Neurology 43(5):950–956, 1993 8492951

Stein DJ: Neurobiology of the obsessive-compulsive spectrum disorders. Biol Psychiatry 47(4):296–304, 2000 10686264

Swedo SE: Pediatric autoimmune neuropsychiatric disorders associated with streptococcal infections (PANDAS). Mol Psychiatry 7(suppl 2):S24–S25, 2002 12142939

Swedo SE, Rapoport JL, Cheslow DL, et al: High prevalence of obsessive-compulsive symptoms in patients with Sydenham's chorea. Am J Psychiatry 146(2):246–249, 1989a 2912267

Swedo SE, Rapoport JL, Leonard H, et al: Obsessive-compulsive disorder in children and adolescents: clinical phenomenology of 70 consecutive cases. Arch Gen Psychiatry 46(4):335–341, 1989b 2930330

Swedo SE, Leonard HL, Schapiro MB, et al: Sydenham's chorea: physical and psychological symptoms of St Vitus dance. Pediatrics 91(4):706–713, 1993 8464654

Swedo SE, Leonard HL, Kiessling LS: Speculations on antineuronal antibody-mediated neuropsychiatric disorders of childhood. Pediatrics 93(2):323–326, 1994 8121747

Swedo SE, Leonard HL, Mittleman BB, et al: Identification of children with pediatric autoimmune neuropsychiatric disorders associated with streptococcal infections by a marker associated with rheumatic fever. Am J Psychiatry 154(1):110–112, 1997 8988969

Swedo SE, Leonard HL, Garvey M, et al: Pediatric autoimmune neuropsychiatric disorders associated with streptococcal infections: clinical description of the first 50 cases. Am J Psychiatry 155:264–271, 1998

Szechtman H, Sulis W, Eilam D: Quinpirole induces compulsive checking behavior in rats: a potential animal model of obsessive-compulsive disorder (OCD). Behav Neurosci 112(6):1475–1485, 1998 9926830

Szechtman H, Eckert MJ, Tse WS, et al: Compulsive checking behavior of quinpirole-sensitized rats as an animal model of obsessive-compulsive disorder (OCD): form and control. BMC Neurosci 2:4, 2001 11316464

Thorén P, Asberg M, Cronholm B, et al: Clomipramine treatment of obsessive-compulsive disorder. I. A controlled clinical trial. Arch Gen Psychiatry 37(11):1281–1285, 1980 7436690

Tonkonogy J, Barreira P: Obsessive-compulsive disorder and caudate-frontal lesion. Neuropsychiatry Neuropsychol Behav Neurol 2:203–209, 1989

Vallejo J, Olivares J, Marcos T, et al: Dexamethasone suppression test and primary obsessional compulsive disorder. Compr Psychiatry 29(5):498–502, 1988 3180759

van der Wee NJ, Stevens H, Hardeman JA, et al: Enhanced dopamine transporter density in psychotropic-naive patients with obsessive-compulsive disorder shown by [123I]beta-CIT SPECT. Am J Psychiatry 161(12):2201–2206, 2004 15569890

Yücel M, Harrison BJ, Wood SJ, et al: Functional and biochemical alterations of the medial frontal cortex in obsessive-compulsive disorder. Arch Gen Psychiatry 64(8):946–955, 2007 17679639

Zitterl W, Aigner M, Stompe T, et al: [123I]-beta-CIT SPECT imaging shows reduced thalamus-hypothalamus serotonin transporter availability in 24 drug-free obsessive-compulsive checkers. Neuropsychopharmacology 32(8):1661–1668, 2007 17192774

Zohar J, Insel TR: Obsessive-compulsive disorder: psychobiological approaches to diagnosis, treatment, and pathophysiology. Biol Psychiatry 22(6):667–687, 1987 3036259

Zohar J, Mueller EA, Insel TR, et al: Serotonergic responsivity in obsessive-compulsive disorder: comparison of patients and healthy controls. Arch Gen Psychiatry 44(11):946–951, 1987 3675134

Recommended Readings

Hudak R, Dougherty DD (eds): Clinical Obsessive-Compulsive Disorder in Adults and Children. New York, Cambridge University Press, 2011

Pittenger C (eds): Obsessive-Compulsive Disorder: Phenomenology, Pathophysiology, and Treatment. New York, Oxford University Press, 2017

Steketee G (ed): The Oxford Handbook of Obsessive Compulsive and Spectrum Disorders. New York, Oxford University Press, 2011

CHAPTER 17

Pharmacotherapy for OCD

Benedetta Grancini, M.D.

Kevin J. Craig, M.B.B.Ch., M.Phil., MRCPsych

Eduardo Cinosi, M.B.B.S., MRCPsych

Ayotunde Shodunke, M.B.B.S., M.Sc., MRCPsych

Jemma Reid, M.B.B.S., MRCPsych

Zoya Marinova, M.D., Ph.D.

Naomi A. Fineberg, M.B.B.S., M.A., MRCPsych

OCD is a common, enduring, lifespan illness (Skoog and Skoog 1999). Prior to the 1960s, it was considered untreatable. Since then, a relatively narrow range of pharmacotherapies have been adopted: clomipramine in the 1960s, selective serotonin reuptake inhibitors (SSRIs) in the 1980s, and dopamine antagonist augmentation in the 1990s (for a review, see Fineberg and Gale 2005). Nowadays, with good care and optimal drug treatment, most patients with OCD can look forward to substantial symptomatic improvement. Recognition and accurate diagnosis are the first steps in the proper treatment of this condition. If the diagnosis of OCD is overlooked, then inappropriate treatment may be prescribed. For example, patients with OCD often present with symptoms of depression or anxiety, but not all antidepressants and few, if

This chapter was adapted from the chapter "Pharmacotherapy for Obsessive-Compulsive Disorder" by Naomi A. Fineberg and Kevin J. Craig from the previous edition of this volume and from "Benefits and Limitations of Pharmacological Interventions in Obsessive Compulsive Disorder," by the same authors, which appeared in *Clinical Neuropsychiatry* 3:345–363, 2006. We also gratefully acknowledge limited use of material from the chapter "Pharmacotherapy for Obsessive-Compulsive Disorder" by Wayne K. Goodman, M.D., that appeared in the first edition of this volume.

any, anxiolytic medications are effective in the presence of OCD. Moreover, OCD often goes untreated for approximately 10 years in adult patients (Poyraz et al. 2015) and 2–3 years in pediatric patients (Walitza et al. 2011). This delay negatively impacts a wide variety of clinical outcomes, such as poor treatment response and higher risk of general medical conditions (Aguglia et al. 2018).

The current standard of care in the United Kingdom is to offer either behavioral psychotherapy or medication as first-line treatment (National Institute for Health and Clinical Excellence 2005). The form of behavioral therapy that has been most effective in OCD is referred to as exposure and response prevention (ERP) (see Chapter 18, "Psychological Treatment for OCD," for a description of the use of behavioral therapy in OCD). At present, the principal pharmacotherapy for OCD involves a trial of a serotonin reuptake inhibitor (SRI), based on broad scientific evidence for the effectiveness of this class in long-term treatment and relapse prevention and their tolerability. Although we recognize the importance of all aspects of management, in this chapter we focus on pharmacological approaches to treatment.

First-Line Treatments

Modern pharmacotherapy for OCD began with the observation that clomipramine, which has potency for blocking serotonin reuptake compared with other tricyclic antidepressants (TCAs), relieved obsessive-compulsive symptoms (Fineberg and Gale 2005). The hypothesis that serotonin might be involved in the pathophysiology of OCD was supported by several studies favorably comparing SRIs to the noradrenergic TCA desipramine as well as monoamine oxidase inhibitors (Fineberg and Gale 2005). Although SRIs represent the cornerstone of pharmacological management for OCD, approximately 40% of patients fail to respond to first-line treatment (Pallanti et al. 2002a). A significant portion of this chapter is therefore devoted to biological approaches to SRI nonresponders.

Evaluation of Treatment Response

The 10-item Yale-Brown Obsessive Compulsive Scale (Y-BOCS; Goodman et al. 1989) and the Clinical Global Impression–Severity (CGI-S) and –Improvement (CGI-I) scales (Guy 1976) represent pivotal rating instruments for measuring OCD severity and treatment response. Although no universally accepted definition of treatment response exists, a CGI-I rating of improved or very much improved and a decrease in Y-BOCS scores of 25% or 35% are widely used criteria and appear to separate active from inactive treatments (Simpson et al. 2006). A mean 25% improvement in Y-BOCS score was associated with improved quality of life in a combined analysis of trial data (Hollander et al. 2010). Even using modest criteria, response rates in acute-phase OCD trials of SSRIs have rarely exceeded 65% (see Tables 17–1 and 17–2).

The concept of *remission* for OCD is also debated, and although no definition is universally accepted (Pallanti et al. 2002a), remission may be described as a brief period during which sufficient improvement has occurred that the individual has minimal symptoms of OCD. Study authors have chosen remission criteria ranging from Y-BOCS scores of less than 16 to scores of 7 or lower (Simpson et al. 2006).

TABLE 17–1. **OCD response rates in randomized placebo-controlled trials of SSRIs in the adult population**

Drug and daily dosage (duration in weeks)	CGI much or very much improved (A), %	25% or 35% improvement on baseline Y-BOCS (B), %	A+B, %	Study
Citalopram 20 mg (12)	57	—	—	Montgomery et al. 2001
Citalopram 40 mg (12)	52	—	—	Montgomery et al. 2001
Citalopram 60 mg (12)	65	—	—	Montgomery et al. 2001
Clomipramine (12)	55	—	—	Zohar and Judge 1996
Escitalopram 20 mg (24)	—	70[*]	—	Stein et al. 2007
Fluoxetine 20 mg (8)	—	—	36	Montgomery et al. 1993
Fluoxetine 40 mg (8)	—	—	48	Montgomery et al. 1993
Fluoxetine 60 mg (8)	—	—	47	Montgomery et al. 1993
Fluoxetine 20 mg (8)	—	32[**]	—	Tollefson et al. 1994
Fluoxetine 40 mg (8)	—	34[**]	—	Tollefson et al. 1994
Fluoxetine 60 mg (8)	—	35[**]	—	Tollefson et al. 1994
Fluvoxamine (8)	43	—	—	Goodman et al. 1989
Fluvoxamine (10)	33	—	—	Goodman et al. 1996
Fluvoxamine CR (12)	34	63[*]	—	Hollander et al. 2003d
Fluvoxamine CR (12)	—	45[**]	—	Hollander et al. 2003d
Paroxetine (12)	55	—	—	Zohar and Judge 1996
Paroxetine (24)	—	67[*]	—	Stein et al. 2007
Sertraline (12)	39	—	—	Greist et al. 1995a
Sertraline (12)	41	—	—	Kronig et al. 1999

Note. For a review, see Skapinakis et al. 2016a.
—=data not reported; CGI=Clinical Global Impression (Guy 1976); CR=controlled release; SSRI=selective serotonin reuptake inhibitor; Y-BOCS=Yale-Brown Obsessive Compulsive Scale (Goodman et al. 1989).
[*]25% improvement on baseline Y-BOCS; [**]35% improvement on baseline Y-BOCS.

Recovery involves the achievement of a higher goal (Burchi et al. 2018), including a combination of symptomatic, durational, and functional (objective and subjective) criteria, such as a Y-BOCS score of 12 or lower plus self-reported measures of functional improvement lasting at least 2 years.

Serotonin Reuptake Inhibitors

Clomipramine in Acute-Phase OCD Treatment Trials

Clomipramine was conclusively established as an effective treatment for OCD in double-blind, placebo-controlled trials, including large-scale multicenter studies with reasonably heterogeneous patients. The studies demonstrated a decrease in Y-BOCS scores and improved social and emotional well-being. Clomipramine was also effective in patients with OCD and comorbid depression, a state experienced by roughly two-thirds of patients with OCD (Fineberg and Gale 2005).

TABLE 17–2.   **Response rates in randomized placebo-controlled trials of SSRIs in pediatric OCD**

Drug and daily dosage *(duration)*	CGI much or very much improved, %	25% improvement on baseline CY-BOCS, %	Other outcome measure	Study
Fluoxetine 20 mg (8 weeks)	—	—	Mean decrease of CY-BOCS (44%) and CGI (33%)	Riddle et al. 1992
Fluoxetine 20–60 mg (13 weeks)	55	—	Rate of clinical response (CY-BOCS improved by 40%) 49%	Geller et al. 2001
Fluoxetine 60–80 mg (8 weeks)	57	—		Liebowitz et al. 2002
Fluvoxamine 50–200 mg (10 weeks)	42	30		Riddle et al. 2001
Paroxetine 10–50 mg (10 weeks)	47	65		Geller et al. 2004
Sertraline (8 weeks)	42	53		March et al. 1998
Sertraline (12 weeks)	—	—	Rate of clinical remission (CY-BOCS <10) 21%	Pediatric OCD Treatment Study Team 2004

Note.   For reviews, see Skapinakis et al. 2016a and Geller et al. 2004.
—=data not reported; CGI=Clinical Global Impression (Guy 1976); CY-BOCS=Children's Yale-Brown Obsessive Compulsive Scale (Scahill et al. 1997); SSRI=selective serotonin reuptake inhibitor.

Selective Serotonin Reuptake Inhibitors in Acute-Phase OCD Treatment Trials

All SSRIs (citalopram, escitalopram, fluoxetine, fluvoxamine, paroxetine, sertraline) were effective for obsessive-compulsive symptoms in a series of placebo-controlled trials (see Fineberg and Craig 2010); trial length usually ranged from 8–12 weeks, with response rates varying from 32% to 70% (see Tables 17–1 and 17–2). Focusing on depression comorbidity in OCD, Hoehn-Saric et al. (2000) reported superiority for sertraline over the primarily norepinephrine reuptake inhibitor desipramine for both obsessive and depressive symptoms, highlighting the importance of treating OCD comorbid with depression with an SSRI.

Although some improvements may emerge within the first weeks of SRI treatment, several weeks are needed for a full effect. Sometimes progress seems remarkably slow. Side effects such as nausea and agitation tend to emerge early but usually abate over time. Because gains accrue for at least 6 months (Stein et al. 2007), with open-label follow-up data suggesting at least 2 years (Rasmussen et al. 1997), patients should not discontinue or change the drug prematurely. A trial of at least 12 weeks at the maximum tolerated dosage and regular interim quantitative assessments are usually advisable for judging effectiveness. Even though individuals experiencing very little clinical improvement in the first few weeks are unlikely to improve with continued treatment (da Conceição Costa et al. 2013) and the chance of improvement after switching from an ineffective SRI to another SRI is low (see "Switching Between Serotonin Reuptake Inhibitors" later in this chapter), as long as the original treatment is tolerated and at least some signs of benefit are seen, administration should continue for sufficient time to allow improvements to develop.

Although the response to treatment with SRIs is characteristically partial, between 30% and 60% of patients with OCD reach a clinically relevant level of improvement during acute treatment studies. This figure increased to around 70% by 24 weeks in an extended double-blind study by Stein et al. (2007) (see Table 17–1). An important consideration is that the patients studied in randomized controlled trials (RCTs) are often drawn from centers specializing in OCD, which can result in lower response rates because more patients with treatment-resistant illness are seen at such sites. Open-label studies, which more closely reflect typical clinical practice, usually find higher rates of SRI response than do RCTs. In a multicenter escitalopram relapse prevention trial, 320 of 468 (68%) patients receiving open-label escitalopram (10 or 20 mg/day) achieved clinical response status by the 16-week endpoint (Fineberg et al. 2007b).

Remission rates represent a more exacting marker of treatment success and have been estimated to be around 40%–45%, with trial lengths ranging from 16 to 24 weeks. In clinical trials, first-line treatment with an SSRI led to remission or clinically meaningful improvement in around 45% and 75% of cases, respectively (Fineberg et al. 2007a; Stein et al. 2007).

Selective Serotonin Reuptake Inhibitor Versus Clomipramine as First-Line Treatment

The clinical effectiveness of a medication depends on a balance among efficacy, safety, and tolerability. The best way to determine the comparative effectiveness of treatments is through a randomized, head-to-head, double-blind comparison. Several published studies compared clomipramine with SSRIs (Table 17–3). To date, these studies failed to find evidence of superior efficacy for any SRI tested; however, SSRIs were generally better tolerated with fewer serious side effects than clomipramine.

SSRIs are generally safe and well tolerated, with RCTs (as listed in Table 17–1) reporting adverse event–related withdrawal rates of around 5%–15%. SSRIs are associated with initially increased nausea, nervousness, insomnia, somnolence, dizziness, and diarrhea. Sexual side effects, including reduced libido and delayed orgasm, affected up to 30% of individuals (Monteiro et al. 1987). Three controlled studies have compared the clinical effectiveness of different SSRIs in OCD, and the results were not strong enough to support the superior efficacy of any one compound (reviewed in Fineberg and Gale 2005). Pharmacokinetic variation is relevant in determining which SSRI to use in order to avoid unwanted drug–drug interactions. Fluoxetine, paroxetine, and to a lesser extent fluvoxamine and sertraline inhibit the cytochrome P450 isoenzyme CYP2D6, which metabolizes TCAs, including clomipramine, dopamine antagonists/antipsychotics, antiarrhythmics, and β-blockers. Fluvoxamine also inhibits both CYP1A2 and CYP3A4, which eliminate warfarin, TCAs, benzodiazepines, and some antiarrhythmics. Citalopram and escitalopram are relatively free from hepatic interactions; however, dose-dependent prolongation of the electrocardiogram (ECG) QT interval associated with citalopram (and to a lesser extent escitalopram; U.S. Food and Drug Administration 2011) argues for caution in using these agents in

TABLE 17–3.   **Controlled studies comparing SSRIs with clomipramine in OCD treatment**

Drug and study	N	Design (daily dosage, *mg*)	Outcome	
			Tolerability	Efficacy
Citalopram				
Pidrman and Tuma 1998	24	CMI vs. CIT	CIT=CMI	CIT=CMI
Fluoxetine				
Pigott et al. 1990	11	CMI (50–250) vs. FLX (20–80)	FLX>CMI	CMI=FLX
Lopez-Ibor et al. 1996	30 vs. 24	CMI (150) vs. FLX (40)	FLX=CMI	CMI=FLX on primary criterion CMI>FLX on other criteria
Fluvoxamine				
Smeraldi et al. 1992	10	CMI (200) vs. FLV (200)	FLV=CMI	CMI=FLV
Freeman et al. 1994	30 vs. 34	CMI (150–250) vs. FLV (150–250)	FLV>CMI (on severe effects)	CMI=FLV
Koran et al. 1996	42 vs. 37	CMI (100–250) vs. FLV (100–250)	FLV=CMI	CMI=FLV
Milanfranchi et al. 1997	13 vs.13	CMI (50–300) vs. FLV (50–300)	FLV=CMI	CMI=FLV
Rouillon 1998	105 vs. 112	CMI (150–300) vs. FLV (150–300)	FLV>CMI	CMI=FLV
Paroxetine				
Zohar and Judge 1996	99 vs. 201 vs. 99	CMI (50–250) vs. PAR (20–60) vs. placebo	PAR>CMI	CMI>placebo PAR>placebo
Sertraline				
Bisserbe et al. 1997	82 vs. 86	CMI (50–200) vs. SER (50–200)	SER>CMI	SER=CMI

Note.   For a review, see Fineberg and Gale 2005.
CIT=citalopram; CMI=clomipramine; FLV=fluvoxamine; FLX=fluoxetine; PAR=paroxetine; SER=sertraline; SSRI=selective serotonin reuptake inhibitor.
Source.   Adapted from Fineberg and Gale 2005.

elderly individuals with OCD and in patients at elevated cardiac risk. Fluoxetine has a long half-life, resulting in fewer discontinuation effects, and therefore can be beneficial for patients whose adherence to medication is poor.

The SSRIs fluoxetine and paroxetine are also largely metabolized by CYP2D6, whereas citalopram and escitalopram are metabolized by CYP2C19. Genetic variants of CYP2D6 and CYP2C19 produce different metabolic profiles (i.e., poor, extensive, and ultrarapid metabolizers), which could theoretically affect the tolerability and, as seen in emerging evidence, clinical response to these medications in patients with OCD (Zai et al. 2014).

Most side effects of clomipramine can be predicted from its receptor binding profile: anticholinergic blockade (e.g., dry mouth and constipation), antihistaminic (H_1) binding (e.g., sedation and weight gain; Maina et al. 2004), and α-adrenergic blockade (e.g., orthostatic hypotension). Nausea, tremor, and impaired sexual performance also are common with clomipramine, as with other SRIs. Compared with the SSRIs, clomipramine is associated with a greater risk of potentially dangerous side effects, including prolongation of the ECG QT interval and seizures, especially at dosages greater than 250 mg/day. Keep in mind that intentional overdoses with clomipramine can be lethal. For patients with comorbid OCD and bipolar disorder, SSRIs are considered less likely than clomipramine to precipitate mania, but mood-stabilizing medication is still advised (Kaplan and Hollander 2003).

Combined Therapy Versus Monotherapy

Although combination of an SRI with cognitive-behavioral therapy (CBT), especially ERP, is generally considered superior to either treatment alone for the treatment of OCD (Fineberg et al. 2018), few controlled studies have addressed this. Those that did either had methodological shortcomings or produced negative findings (Skapinakis et al. 2016b).

Evidence for an enhancing effect of clomipramine added to exposure therapy remains inconsistent (Foa et al. 2005; Marks et al. 1988), but fluvoxamine has been shown to enhance the efficacy of exposure therapy (Cottraux et al. 1993) and multimodal CBT (Hohagen et al. 1998). Similar results were reported in a recent randomized controlled feasibility study by Fineberg et al. (2018); although the combined arm appeared to be the most clinically effective treatment acutely, in the long term (weeks 16–52), several analyses suggested advantages for sertraline compared to CBT. Conversely, an RCT of adults by O'Connor et al. (2006) did not show enhanced clinical outcomes for CBT plus fluvoxamine compared with CBT monotherapy. Another 12-week RCT of OCD in children (N=112) conducted by the Pediatric OCD Treatment Study Team (2004) reported some additional benefit for combined treatment compared to CBT alone or sertraline alone, although all three active arms showed significant clinical improvement. A secondary analysis of these data showed that young people with a positive family history of OCD and those with more severe symptoms responded less well to CBT (Garcia et al. 2010).

Meta-Analyses of Serotonin Reuptake Inhibitors

Meta-analyses cannot substitute for high-quality head-to-head comparator trials. By combining data from separate studies using specific rules, meta-analyses can provide more objective and quantifiable measures of treatment effect size than can narrative reviews. However, because they are subject to potential imbalances in populations studied and differing methodologies, combined analyses of OCD trials spanning several decades must be viewed with caution (Pigott and Seay 1999). For example, Skapinakis et al. (2016a), in a meta-analysis, found that the majority of randomized studies investigating psychological therapies did not restrict the use of medication in the interventional arm. In contrast, randomized studies of pharmacotherapy usually restricted the use of CBT in the drug treatment arm. Also, a significant difference reported in a large meta-analysis may reflect only a small difference in efficacy between the treatments that may not reach clinical relevance. For these reasons, the evidence from meta-analyses may be considered weaker than evidence from well-powered head-to-head studies.

Several meta-analyses have supported the efficacy of SSRIs in the treatment of OCD, reporting onset of significant benefit within the first 2 weeks of treatment (Issari et al. 2016; Soomro et al. 2008). The meta-analysis by Skapinakis et al. (2016a) confirmed the effectiveness of psychological interventions, clomipramine, SSRIs, or combined treatment (SRI plus CBT) in adult patients with OCD.

Whereas most meta-analyses demonstrated similar significant advantages for all SRIs over placebo, some showed superiority for clomipramine over SSRIs (reviewed in Fineberg and Gale 2005). However, strong heterogeneity across individual studies may have biased the results in favor of clomipramine.

The United Kingdom's National Institute for Health and Clinical Excellence (2005) systematically accessed both unpublished and published randomized studies, which were included in the meta-analysis only if they met stringent methodological criteria, in order to develop an evidence-based treatment guideline. Clomipramine and SSRIs were indistinguishable in terms of efficacy, but clomipramine was associated with higher rates of premature and adverse events. Thus, in the guideline, SSRIs were recommended over clomipramine as first-line agents.

Geller et al. (2003a) performed a meta-analysis of pharmacotherapy for childhood OCD and recommended, in the absence of head-to-head studies, that clomipramine generally should not be used before the SSRIs in children because of its more problematic side effect profile. Fineberg et al. (2004) reported similar treatment response for adults and children with OCD, with the greatest incremental treatment gains within the first 2 weeks of SSRI treatment. Three recent meta-analyses evaluated all available treatments for pediatric OCD (i.e., CBT, clomipramine, SSRIs, and combined treatment; Ivarsson et al. 2015; McGuire et al. 2015; Skapinakis et al. 2016a) and found them all to be effective, with some advantage for psychological interventions over medication. However, the poorer methodological rigor that occurs in studies of psychological interventions has resulted in inflated effect size (McGuire et al. 2015; Skapinakis et al. 2016a).

Dosage Selection and Titration

Clomipramine and fluvoxamine have not been investigated using fixed-dosage comparator groups, and most studies using flexible dosages titrated toward the upper end of the range showed efficacy and tolerability for dosages as high as 300 mg/day of clomipramine and 150–300 mg/day of fluvoxamine (Fineberg and Gale 2005). Because clomipramine lowers the seizure threshold and is associated with clinically relevant cardiotoxicity, it should usually be prescribed within recommended dosage limits (Fineberg et al. 2015).

Studies using fixed-dosage comparator groups showed a clear positive dose-response relationship for paroxetine and fluoxetine, but the evidence for superiority of high dosages for sertraline and citalopram was less clear-cut (Fineberg and Gale 2005). A fixed-dosage escitalopram study (Stein et al. 2007) found a clear superiority for 20 mg/day. A dose-dependent effect of citalopram and escitalopram on extending the ECG QT interval was reported (U.S. Food and Drug Administration 2011), and therefore the maximum licensed dosage was reduced, although a recent study did not show evidence of elevated cardiac risk with higher dosages of citalopram (Zivin et al. 2013). Notwithstanding, dosages of citalopram and escitalopram exceeding the FDA's approved limit should be used with caution, and in "at-risk" individuals it is advisable to provide additional ECG monitoring for adverse effects on cardiac conduction (Fineberg et al. 2015). A meta-analysis by Bloch et al. (2010) confirmed that higher dosages of SSRIs were associated with improved treatment efficacy as well as greater side effects. These results argue for a moderate dose-response relationship and further controlled exploration of higher SSRI dosages for OCD.

Although rapid upward titration of medications may produce earlier responses in patients with OCD, long-term benefits of this approach have not been established (Fineberg and Gale 2005). Slow upward titration could ameliorate SRI-related adverse effects, particularly for children, elderly patients, and patients with comorbidities. Longer-term side effects, such as sleep disturbance, headache, and sexual dysfunction, may be dosage related and are common causes of drug discontinuation. Expert consensus currently favors beginning with moderate dosages, with upward dosage titrations to maximum should symptoms persist (National Institute for Health and Clinical Excellence 2005).

Other Antidepressants

For first-line treatment of OCD, few rational alternatives to SRIs exist. Venlafaxine has generated some interest due to its predominantly serotonergic action at low dosages. Venlafaxine was not significantly better than placebo in an 8-week double-blind trial of 30 patients with OCD (Yaryura-Tobias and Neziroglu 1996). In a subsequent non-placebo-controlled study by Denys et al. (2003), no significant differences were found between patients assigned to receive venlafaxine 300 mg/day (n=75) and those who received paroxetine 60 mg/day (n=75); the response rate was 40% in both groups. However, in a study of nonresponders in the same group of patients, a more favorable response was found for venlafaxine-treated individuals switched to paroxetine than vice versa (Denys et al. 2004). Pallanti et al. (2004) compared two groups receiving citalopram with and without open-label mirtazapine; the addition of mirtazapine produced only short-lived additional benefit.

Combinations

Combinations of SRIs have been found useful in some studies of OCD (Pallanti et al. 1999) but not others (Diniz et al. 2010). Caution is required if clomipramine is combined with SSRIs, especially those that potentially cross-react at the hepatic microsomes. For example, ECG changes have been reported in cases involving the combination of clomipramine with fluvoxamine (Szegedi et al. 1996). Combining SSRIs with clomipramine therefore is not usually recommended unless adequate safety provisions are in place, such as ECG monitoring and regular assay of clomipramine plus norclomipramine plasma levels (which generally should not exceed 450 ng/mL)—because a relationship exists between TCA plasma concentration, adverse effects, and toxicity (Baumann et al. 2005). As discussed, prolongation of the QT interval with higher dosages of citalopram (and to a lesser extent escitalopram; U.S. Food and Drug Administration 2011) also argues for caution combining citalopram and clomipramine (Fineberg et al. 2015).

Long-Term Efficacy Data

Maintenance Serotonin Reuptake Inhibitors and Long-Term Trials

Because OCD is a chronic illness, treatment needs to remain effective for the long term. Double-blind studies lasting up to 12 months have shown that patients who responded to acute treatment benefited from continuing with medication, with no evidence of tolerance developing (Greist et al. 1995b; Tollefson et al. 1994). Additional improvements in OCD symptoms and a reduced incidence of side effects have been found in a 2-year follow-up with open-label sertraline (Rasmussen et al. 1997). These results suggest that treatment continues to be effective in the longer term, especially if higher dosages are maintained (Tollefson et al. 1994), and that further benefits accrue with ongoing treatment. The findings do not support dosage reduction.

Relapse Prevention

Relapse prevention is an essential therapeutic goal, not only to protect against the suffering and distress related to acute illness but also because relapse significantly impairs functional disability and quality of life (Hollander et al. 2010). A naturalistic study found that approximately 60% of patients who responded to treatment at a U.S. specialist center relapsed over a 5-year follow-up period, with a higher relapse rate for patients with comorbid obsessive-compulsive personality disorder (Eisen et al. 2013).

Conventional relapse prevention trials randomly assign responders taking open-label drugs to either continuation or a gradual switch to placebo and then measure subsequent relapse rates (Fineberg et al. 2007a). To date, the results of relapse prevention studies in OCD have been mixed, largely owing to methodological differences. Table 17–4 shows the results of a meta-analysis of the published relapse prevention studies of adults with OCD (Fineberg et al. 2007a). Studies examining the short-term effects of discontinuing clomipramine or SSRIs under double-blind, placebo-controlled conditions showed a rapid and incremental worsening of symptoms in most patients with OCD who were switched to placebo (reviewed in Fineberg and Gale 2005), implying that treatment needs to be continued to remain effective. Fluoxetine, escitalopram, and paroxetine showed significantly lower relapse rates than placebo, whereas sertraline was unable to demonstrate a significant advantage compared to placebo on the a priori criterion of preventing relapse, almost certainly because the study's criterion for relapse was too strictly defined. Another relapse-prevention study in a child and adolescent cohort found a numerically increased rate of relapse for placebo compared to paroxetine (43.9% vs. 34.7%), but the difference did not reach statistical significance, possibly because the follow-up phase was too short (16 weeks). Interestingly, in this study, comorbidity was associated with a significantly increased rate of relapse after drug discontinuation (Geller et al. 2004).

Koran et al. (2005b) investigated relapse rates following double-blind, placebo-controlled discontinuation of open-label mirtazapine—an agent without evidence of acute OCD efficacy. Y-BOCS scores continued to improve for patients given mirtazapine but worsened for those given placebo, hinting that mirtazapine may have long-term efficacy in preventing relapse in OCD.

TABLE 17–4.   **Double-blind, placebo-controlled studies of relapse prevention in adult OCD**

Drug (study)	Duration of prior drug treatment, *weeks*	*N* in DP	Follow-up after DP, *weeks*	Outcome
Escitalopram (Fineberg et al. 2007b)	16	158	24	*Time to relapse on placebo< escitalopram* *Relapse rate on placebo > escitalopram*
Fluoxetine (Romano et al. 2001)	20	71	52	Relapse rate on placebo= pooled fluoxetine *Relapse rate on placebo> fluoxetine 60 mg*
Paroxetine (Hollander et al. 2003a)	12	105	24	*Relapse rate on placebo> paroxetine*
Sertraline (Koran et al. 2002)	52	223	28	Relapse rate on placebo= sertraline Acute exacerbation of OCD on placebo> sertraline Dropout due to relapse on placebo>sertraline

Note.   Text in *italic* indicates positive outcomes on the a priori criterion for relapse.
DP=discontinuation phase.
Source.   Adapted from Fineberg et al. 2007a.

Taken together, these results support relapse prevention as a realistic treatment target and suggest that continuation of an SSRI at an effective dosage level protects patients against relapse. Existing data do not support any time period after which drug discontinuation appears safe. However, even if medication is continued, protection is not complete: roughly one-quarter of adult patients relapse despite treatment adherence. The possibility that some patients may retain response at a lower dosage or after drug discontinuation must be weighed against the possibility that reinstatement of treatment after relapse may be associated with a poorer response (Maina et al. 2001).

Treatment-Refractory Populations

Serotonin Reuptake Inhibitor Resistance

Research into SRI resistance has been hindered by lack of consensus on a definition of resistant OCD (Pallanti et al. 2002a; Simpson et al. 2006). Fineberg et al. (2006a) suggested that failure to improve baseline Y-BOCS scores by 25% after treatment with at least two SRIs given at maximally tolerated standard dosages for at least 12 weeks constitutes clinically meaningful SRI resistance.

Different factors may account for patient nonresponse to an adequate trial of an SRI. Obsessive-compulsive symptoms may interfere with adherence. Compulsive hoarding responds particularly poorly compared to other symptom dimensions in

SSRI studies (Carey et al. 2008). According to meta-analysis, other factors linked with poor SRI response in adults with OCD include early onset, longer duration, more severe illness, and poor response to previous therapy. For childhood OCD, comorbidity (e.g., depression, tics, conduct disorder, ADHD) has been linked to treatment resistance (Geller et al. 2003b).

Dosing in Treatment-Resistant OCD

Few studies have addressed higher-dosage SSRIs as treatments for resistant OCD. A controlled study of sertraline 250–400 mg/day showed an improved response compared with sertraline 200 mg/day on some symptom severity measures (Ninan et al. 2006). An open 12-week trial (Rabinowitz et al. 2008) of escitalopram (30–50 mg/day) found significant within-group improvement in Y-BOCS scores and overall good tolerability. Double-blind studies are required to confirm the efficacy and tolerability of high-dosage SSRIs in treatment-resistant OCD.

Risks are greater for increasing dosages of clomipramine because of its inherent toxicity, and other strategies are usually preferable. In addition, recent FDA warnings of a dosage-dependent increase in the ECG QTc interval associated with citalopram and escitalopram suggest that caution is required when escalating dosages. In such cases, regular ECG monitoring is advisable.

Intravenous Administration

Altering the mode of drug delivery may be another way to gain control of intractable OCD. Two double-blind trials (Fallon et al. 1998; Koran et al. 1997) supported the short-term efficacy of intravenous clomipramine in patients with treatment-refractory OCD. Disadvantages include availability at only a few research settings and limited evidence of long-term benefits. Similar findings reported by Pallanti et al. (2002b), in a short open-label trial of intravenous citalopram, require substantiation under double-blind conditions.

Switching Between Serotonin Reuptake Inhibitors

According to the Expert Consensus Guidelines (March et al. 1997), clinicians should usually delay switching medication until after an adequate trial (8–12 weeks at maximally tolerated dosage). Limited evidence supports switching from one SSRI to another rather than continuing treatment with the same drug. In one review, 11%–33% of patients whose illness did not respond to the first SRI showed clinically meaningful response to a second SRI, with decreasing likelihood of responding to subsequent changes to other agents (Fineberg et al. 2006b). A small open-label study (Koran and Saxena 2002) found that response rates for switching from one SSRI to another (0%–20%) were lower compared with switching to clomipramine (33%–40%). Two additional small open-label studies suggested that patients whose OCD did not respond to one or more SRIs might benefit from a change to venlafaxine (Hollander et al. 2002, 2003c).

Combined Treatments

Serotonin Reuptake Inhibitor Plus Dopamine Antagonists

No positive trials of dopamine antagonists as monotherapy for OCD have been published that meet contemporary clinical trial standards. Clozapine and aripiprazole monotherapy were not beneficial in open-label trials (Connor et al. 2005; McDougle et al. 1995). However, growing evidence supports the use of adjunctive dopamine antagonists with SRIs in treatment-resistant OCD. The balance of evidence from a growing number of small RCTs suggests that augmentation with haloperidol, risperidone, olanzapine, aripiprazole, or quetiapine is beneficial (reviewed in Reid et al. 2017). An RCT of paliperidone augmentation did not find a statistically significant benefit, probably due to its small sample size (Storch et al. 2013). Meta-analyses of trials of adjunctive dopamine antagonists also suggest efficacy based on Y-BOCS score reductions and remission rates (Bloch et al. 2006; Dold et al. 2013, 2015; Komossa et al. 2010; Skapinakis et al. 2007; Veale et al. 2014). Of the adjunctive dopamine antagonists considered, efficacy was convincingly reported for risperidone (0.5–6 mg/day), aripiprazole (10–15 mg/day), and haloperidol (mean 6 mg/day); quetiapine (50–600 mg/day) was less consistent, possibly because some of the quetiapine studies included more refractory cases. An analysis by Bloch et al. (2006) found that patients with comorbid tic disorders were particularly responsive to adjunctive dopamine antagonists. A single positive open-label study of the more selective dopamine antagonist amisulpride (200–600 mg/day) used as an adjunct to SRIs (Metin et al. 2003) merits replication under controlled conditions. Table 17–5 illustrates responder rates in double-blind studies of adjunctive dopamine antagonists, which varied from 27% to 64% depending on the chosen criterion.

Dose-ranging studies are required to establish the optimal dosage, and head-to-head studies are needed to test the relative efficacy and tolerability across second- and first-generation agents. Long-term studies are also required to test for sustained efficacy, tolerability, and relapse prevention. One small study has reported a high level of relapse following open-label discontinuation (Maina et al. 2003).

Serotonin Reuptake Inhibitor Plus Behavior Therapy

Few clinical trials have addressed the role of adjunctive CBT for patients presenting a partial response to SRI monotherapy. Simpson et al. (2008) found a significant between-group advantage for ERP compared to stress management training in an 8-week randomized controlled study of 111 patients who had partially responded to an SRI; this continued over a 6-month open follow-up period in a subgroup of responders with stable SRI dosages and maintenance sessions (Foa et al. 2013).

In another 8-week RCT of 100 SSRI partial responders (Simpson et al. 2013), those in the adjunctive ERP arm showed a significantly greater improvement in Y-BOCS scores and higher response rates compared with those in either the adjunctive risperidone or pill placebo arms.

Focusing on pediatric OCD, Franklin et al. (2011) found that CBT and medication management showed a significantly greater effect than medication management only or medication management plus instructions in CBT.

Other Treatments

Novel and Experimental Drug Treatments

Several novel treatments have been proposed and tested in resistant OCD, but very few show promise. Table 17–6 lists some of those that have *not* been shown effective to date in available studies. Some useful results are discussed in the following sections.

TABLE 17–5.   Responder rates in double-blind randomized controlled trials of adjunctive dopamine antagonists in SRI-resistant OCD

Drug and study	≥25% improvement (Y-BOCS)	≥35% improvement (Y-BOCS)	≥25% improvement (Y-BOCS+ CGI-I≤2)	≥35% improvement (Y-BOCS+ CGI-I≤2)
Haloperidol				
McDougle et al. 1994				64%+Y-BOCS <16
Olanzapine				
Bystritsky et al. 2004	46%			
Shapira et al. 2004	41%			
Quetiapine				
Denys et al. 2004				40%
Carey et al. 2005			40%	
Fineberg et al. 2005	27%			
Kordon et al. 2008		33%		
Risperidone				
McDougle et al. 2000				50%
Hollander et al. 2003b			40%	
Erzegovesi et al. 2005		50%		
Simpson et al. 2013	23%			
Aripiprazole				
Sayyah et al. 2012	53%			
Muscatello et al. 2011	69%	25%		
Paliperidone				
Storch et al. 2013		35%		

Note. For a review, see Veale et al. 2014.
CGI-I=Clinical Global Impression Severity Improvement scale (Guy 1976); SRI=serotonin reuptake inhibitor; Y-BOCS=Yale-Brown Obsessive Compulsive Scale (Goodman et al. 1989).

Glutamatergic Modulation

Several lines of research, from neuroimaging to genetics, are converging to suggest that abnormal glutamatergic transmission may be important in OCD (for a review, see Marinova et al. 2017), leading to small RCTs involving drugs modulating glutamate, both in adult (Table 17–7) and pediatric (Table 17–8) patients with OCD. Adjunctive memantine arguably showed consistent evidence of efficacy (Kishi et al. 2018). Lamotrigine also showed evidence of efficacy in two small RCTs, whereas topiramate and riluzole showed a therapeutic effect in some but not all studies, and topiramate showed a possible preferential effect on compulsions. Further evidence is needed for ketamine (still experimental, with a potentially rapid onset of action), *N*-acetylcysteine (contradictory results to date), glycine (positive trend for efficacy in one RCT), minocycline (efficacy in one RCT), and L-carnosine (efficacy in one RCT) (Marinova et al. 2017).

TABLE 17–6. **Double-blind, placebo-controlled trials of agents with no proven effect in OCD**

Drug	Clinical group	Study
Buspirone	Augmentation in refractory OCD	Grady et al. 1993
Buspirone	Augmentation in refractory OCD	McDougle et al. 1993
Buspirone	Augmentation in refractory OCD	Pigott et al. 1992
Clonazepam	Augmentation in refractory OCD	Crockett et al. 2004
Desipramine	Augmentation in refractory OCD	Barr et al. 1997
Lithium	Augmentation in refractory OCD	McDougle et al. 1991
Lithium	Augmentation in refractory OCD	Pigott et al. 1991
Naloxone	Monotherapy	Keuler et al. 1996
Oxytocin	Monotherapy	Epperson et al. 1996
Pindolol	Augmentation in refractory OCD	Dannon et al. 2000
St. John's wort	Augmentation in refractory OCD	Kobak et al. 2005

Opiate Agonists and Antagonists

Oral morphine augmentation was shown to be effective in a double-blind crossover study of 23 patients with treatment-resistant OCD (Koran et al. 2005a). The analysis showed a significant decrease in Y-BOCS scores for morphine versus placebo but not for lorazepam versus placebo. In contrast, two randomized trials of opiate antagonists, one of naloxone and the other naltrexone, found no significant effect (Amiaz et al. 2008; Keuler et al. 1996).

Other Agents

Two placebo-controlled pharmacological challenge studies demonstrated improvement in OCD symptoms following single-dose administration of the dopamine releaser D-amphetamine (Insel et al. 1983; Joffe et al. 1991). Two serotonin 5-HT$_3$ receptor antagonists have been investigated, ondansetron in five studies and granisetron in one study; overall, the evidence for 5-HT$_3$ antagonists is inconclusive (Serata et al. 2015). A few studies have shown promise for inositol, a key metabolic precursor in G protein–coupled receptors; small open-label studies have shown contradictory results for inositol in OCD and putative obsessive-compulsive spectrum disorders (Harvey et al. 2002; Levine 1997; Nemets et al. 2001).

Immune Modulation

Some cases of childhood-onset OCD may be related to an infection-triggered autoimmune process similar to that of Sydenham's chorea. Although pediatric autoimmune neuropsychiatric disorders associated with streptococcal infections (PANDAS) and

TABLE 17–7. Double-blind randomized controlled trials of glutamate-modulating drugs in adult patients with OCD

Compound	Duration and dosage	Patients, N	Outcome	Study
Monotherapy				
Ketamine	Ketamine and saline intravenously infused at least 1 week apart in random order; dosage: 0.5 mg/kg	15	Ketamine>placebo at 7 days	Rodriguez et al. 2013
Augmentation of psychotropic regimen				
Riluzole	12 weeks + 2 weeks lead-on placebo; final dosage: 100 mg/day	38	Riluzole=placebo	Pittenger 2015
	10 weeks; final dosage: 100 mg/day	50	Riluzole>placebo	Emamzadehfard et al. 2016
Memantine	8 weeks; final dosage: 20 mg/day	42	Memantine>placebo	Ghaleiha et al. 2013
	12 weeks; dosage: 5–10 mg/day	40	Memantine>placebo	Haghighi et al. 2013
	12 weeks; dosage: 20 mg/day	32	Memantine>placebo	Modarresi et al. 2018
Glycine	12 weeks; final dosage: 60 g/day	24	Trend ($P=0.053$); glycine>placebo	Greenberg et al. 2009
Topiramate	12 weeks; dosage: 100–200 mg/day	49	Topiramate>placebo	Mowla et al. 2010
	12 weeks; dosage: 50–400 mg/day	36	Topiramate = placebo (topiramate>placebo for compulsions only)	Berlin et al. 2011
	12 weeks; dosage range: 100–200 mg/day	38	Topiramate=placebo	Afshar et al. 2014
Lamotrigine	16 weeks; final dosage: 100 mg/day	40	Lamotrigine>placebo	Bruno et al. 2012
	12 weeks; final dosage: 100 mg/day	53	Lamotrigine>placebo	Khalkhali et al. 2016
N-acetylcysteine (NAC)	12 weeks; dosage: up to 2.4 g/day	48	NAC>placebo	Afshar et al. 2012
	16 weeks; dosage: 3 g/day	44	NAC=placebo	Sarris et al. 2015
	10 weeks; dosage: 2 g/day	44	NAC>placebo	Paydary et al. 2016
	16 weeks; dosage: 3 g/day	40	NAC=placebo	Costa et al. 2017
	10 weeks; dosage: up to 2.4 g/day	34	NAC>placebo	Ghanizadeh et al. 2017

TABLE 17–7. Double-blind randomized controlled trials of glutamate-modulating drugs in adult patients with OCD *(continued)*

Compound	Duration and dosage	Patients, N	Outcome	Study
Minocycline	10 weeks; dosage: 200 mg/day	102	Minocycline>placebo	Esalatmanesh et al. 2016
L-Carnosine	10 weeks; dosage: 500 mg bid	44	L-Carnosine>placebo	Arabzadeh et al. 2017
Augmentation of psychotherapy				
D-Cycloserine (DCS)	12 CBT sessions with DCS 4 hours before each; dosage: 250 mg/CBT session	24	DCS=placebo	Storch et al. 2007
	10 CBT sessions with DCS 2 hours before each; dosage: 125 mg/CBT session	25	DCS=placebo	Kushner et al. 2007
	10 CBT sessions with DCS 1 hour before each; dosage: 100 mg/CBT session	23	DCS=placebo	Wilhelm et al. 2008
	DCS 1 hour before five CBT tasks during a 12-week internet-based CBT; dosage: 50 mg/CBT task	128	DCS=placebo	Andersson et al. 2015
	Six guided exposure sessions with DCS 1 hour before each; dosage: 125 mg/session	39	DCS=placebo	de Leeuw et al. 2017

Note.   CBT=cognitive-behavioral therapy.
Source.   Adapted from Marinova et al. 2017.

TABLE 17–8.   **Double-blind RCTs of glutamate-modulating drugs in pediatric patients with OCD**

Compound	Duration and dosage	Study sample, N	Outcome	Study
Augmentation of psychotropic regimen				
Riluzole	12 weeks; final dosage: 100 mg/day	60	Riluzole=placebo	Grant et al. 2014
Augmentation of psychotherapy				
D-Cycloserine (DCS)	10 CBT sessions with DCS 1 hour before each of 7 sessions; dosage: weight adjusted	30	DCS=placebo	Storch et al. 2010
	9 CBT sessions with DCS 1 hour before each of 5 sessions; dosage: weight adjusted	17	DCS=placebo	Farrell et al. 2013
	14 CBT sessions with DCS immediately after each of 10 sessions; dosage: 50 mg	27	DCS=placebo	Mataix-Cols et al. 2014
	10 CBT sessions with DCS 1 hour prior to each of 7 sessions; dosage: weight adjusted	142	DCS=placebo	Storch et al. 2016

Note.   CBT=cognitive-behavioral therapy.
Source.   Adapted from Marinova et al. 2017.

pediatric acute-onset neuropsychiatric syndrome (PANS) remain controversial diagnostic concepts, they have stimulated new research into possible links among bacterial pathogens, autoimmune reactions, and neuropsychiatric symptoms. Inconclusive trials with immunomodulatory treatments or antimicrobial prophylaxis have been performed (reviewed in Murphy et al. 2006). Additional recent evidence has hinted at a potential therapeutic role for anti-inflammatory agents (Spartz et al. 2017). To date, however, the use of immune-modulating treatments for patients with early and acute-onset OCD remains controversial (Burchi and Pallanti 2018).

Conclusion

Figure 17–1 shows a suggested treatment pathway for patients with OCD. SRIs produce a rapid onset and a broad spectrum of actions and can be used to treat a wide range of conditions, including depression and anxiety, that occur comorbid with OCD. SSRIs offer advantages over clomipramine in terms of safety and tolerability and usually constitute first-line treatments. They appear to be cost-effective compared with other treatment options (National Institute for Health and Clinical Excellence 2005). Higher dosages usually offer greater benefits, and gains continue to

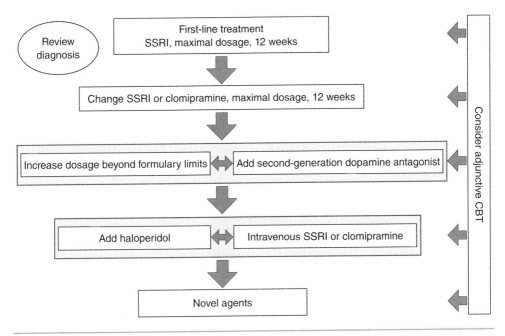

FIGURE 17–1. OCD: a pharmacological pathway.

CBT=cognitive-behavioral therapy; SSRI=selective serotonin reuptake inhibitor.

accrue gradually over weeks and months. For approximately 70% of patients, SSRIs effect a clinically meaningful response, and around 40% of patients enter remission after sustained treatment. Ongoing treatment protects against relapse for most cases.

For SRI-resistant cases, the strongest evidence supports the use of adjunctive dopamine antagonists, shown to be clinically effective in up to two-thirds of cases, with a particularly beneficial effect in those with comorbid tic disorders. Their long-term effects remain unclear, however, and trials in other diagnostic groups suggest significant adverse effects. Rational alternatives include increasing the dosage of the SSRI or switching SRIs.

Improving the diagnosis and delivery of health care to patients with OCD must continue to be a high priority. Further research should target new therapeutic approaches and standardized methods to measure treatment response so that treatment choices can be guided by sound evidence. Novel techniques such as analysis of large data sets (big data) and transcriptomics may signal new candidate drugs with different and varied methods of action for future systematic exploration.

Key Points

- Serotonin reuptake inhibitors (SRIs) remain the cornerstone of pharmacological treatment and lead to substantial clinical improvement, if continued for long enough, in the majority of patients with OCD.

- Selective serotonin reuptake inhibitors (SSRIs) are the preferred first-line treatment for OCD. Clomipramine is preferred for those whose illness fails to respond to or who cannot tolerate SSRIs.

- Gradual dosage titration upward within licensed limits, while clinical response and side effects are measured, is usually appropriate.

- An initial treatment period of at least 12 weeks at maximally tolerated dosage levels is advisable to properly judge effectiveness.

- Rating scales (e.g., Yale-Brown Obsessive Compulsive Scale, Clinical Global Impression–Severity scale, Clinical Global Impression–Improvement scale) are helpful to standardize assessment of clinical response.

- For most patients with OCD, symptoms respond only partially to SRIs, and in about one-third, the response is poor.

- Maintenance treatment appears to protect against relapse.

- In patients with treatment-resistant OCD, combining pharmacotherapy with cognitive-behavioral therapy, increasing dosages, or switching between SRIs are practical next steps.

- Growing evidence supports the efficacy of adding dopamine antagonists at the lower end of their dosing range to SRI medication, but long-term data are lacking, and for many patients, the response remains unsatisfactory.

- Novel agents under investigation for OCD include compounds modulating glutamatergic activity, immune modulators, neuropeptides, and opioid modulators. The use of these compounds is still at an experimental stage, and long-term data are lacking.

References

Afshar H, Roohafza H, Mohammad-Beigi H, et al: N-acetylcysteine add-on treatment in refractory obsessive-compulsive disorder: a randomized, double-blind, placebo-controlled trial. J Clin Psychopharmacol 32(6):797–803, 2012

Afshar H, Akuchekian S, Mahaky B, et al: Topiramate augmentation in refractory obsessive-compulsive disorder: a randomized, double-blind, placebo-controlled trial. J Res Med Sci 19(10):976–981, 2014

Aguglia A, Signorelli MS, Albert U, et al: The impact of general medical conditions in obsessive-compulsive disorder. Psychiatry Investig 15(3):246–253, 2018 29475243

Amiaz R, Fostick L, Gershon A, et al: Naltrexone augmentation in OCD: a double-blind placebo-controlled cross-over study. Eur Neuropsychopharmacol 18(6):455–461, 2008 18353618

Andersson E, Hedman E, Enander J, et al: d-Cycloserine vs placebo as adjunct to cognitive behavioural therapy for obsessive-compulsive disorder and interaction with antidepressants: a randomized clinical trial. JAMA Psychiatry 72(7):659–667, 2015

Arabzadeh S, Shahhossenie M, Mesgarpour B, et al: L-carnosine as an adjuvant to fluvoxamine in treatment of obsessive compulsive disorder: a randomized double-blind study. Hum Psychopharmacol 32(4), 2017 28485008

Barr LC, Goodman WK, Anand A, et al: Addition of desipramine to serotonin reuptake inhibitors in treatment-resistant obsessive-compulsive disorder. Am J Psychiatry 154(9):1293–1295, 1997 9286191

Baumann P, Ulrich S, Eckermann G, et al: The AGNP-TDM Expert Group Consensus Guidelines: focus on therapeutic monitoring of antidepressants. Dialogues Clin Neurosci 7(3):231–247, 2005 16156382

Berlin HA, Koran LM, Jenike MA, et al: Double-blind, placebo-controlled trial of topiramate augmentation in treatment-resistant obsessive-compulsive disorder. J Clin Psychiatry 72(5):716–721, 2011

Bisserbe JC, Lane RM, Flament MF: A double-blind comparison of sertraline and clomipramine in outpatients with obsessive-compulsive disorder. Eur Psychiatry 12:82–93, 1997

Bloch MH, Landeros-Weisenberger A, Kelmendi B, et al: A systematic review: antipsychotic augmentation with treatment refractory obsessive-compulsive disorder. Mol Psychiatry 11(7):622–632, 2006 16585942

Bloch MH, McGuire J, Landeros-Weisenberger A, et al: Meta-analysis of the dose-response relationship of SSRI in obsessive-compulsive disorder. Mol Psychiatry 15(8):850–855, 2010 19468281

Bruno A, Micò U, Pandolfo G, et al: Lamotrigine augmentation of serotonin reuptake inhibitors in treatment-resistant obsessive-compulsive disorder: a double-blind, placebo-controlled study. J Psychopharmacol (Oxf) 26(11):1456–1462, 2012

Burchi E, Pallanti S: Antibiotics for PANDAS? Limited evidence: review and putative mechanisms of action. Prim Care Companion CNS Disord 20(3), 2018 29722936

Burchi E, Hollander E, Pallanti S: From treatment response to recovery: a realistic goal in OCD. Int J Neuropsychopharmacol 21(11):1007–1013, 2018 30184141

Bystritsky A, Ackerman DL, Rosen RM, et al: Augmentation of serotonin reuptake inhibitors in refractory obsessive-compulsive disorder using adjunctive olanzapine: a placebo-controlled trial. J Clin Psychiatry 20(11):565–568, 2004 29722936

Carey PD, Vythilingum B, Seedat S, et al: Quetiapine augmentation of SRIs in treatment refractory obsessive-compulsive disorder: a double-blind, randomised, placebo-controlled study. BMC Psychiatry 5:5, 2005 15667657

Carey PD, Fineberg N, Lochner C, et al: Escitalopram in obsessive-compulsive disorder (OCD): response of symptom dimensions to pharmacotherapy. Poster presented at International Anxiety Disorders Symposium, Cape Town, South Africa, March 2008

Connor KM, Payne VM, Gadde KM, et al: The use of aripiprazole in obsessive-compulsive disorder: preliminary observations in 8 patients. J Clin Psychiatry 66(1):49–51, 2005

Costa DL, Diniz JB, Requena G, et al: Randomized, double-blind, placebo-controlled trial of N-acetylcysteine augmentation for treatment-resistant obsessive-compulsive disorder. J Clin Psychiatry 78(7):e766–e773, 2017 28617566

Cottraux J, Mollard E, Bouvard M, et al: Exposure therapy, fluvoxamine, or combination treatment in obsessive-compulsive disorder: one-year followup. Psychiatry Res 49(1):63–75, 1993 8140182

Crockett BA, Churchill E, Davidson JR: A double-blind combination study of clonazepam with sertraline in obsessive-compulsive disorder. Ann Clin Psychiatry 16(3):127–132, 2004 15517844

da Conceição Costa DL, Shavitt RG, Castro Cesar RC, et al: Can early improvement be an indicator of treatment response in obsessive-compulsive disorder? Implications for early treatment decision-making. J Psychiatr Res 47(11):1700–1707, 2013 23948637

Dannon PN, Sasson Y, Hirschmann S, et al: Pindolol augmentation in treatment-resistant obsessive compulsive disorder: a double-blind placebo controlled trial. Eur Neuropsychopharmacol 10(3):165–169, 2000 10793318

de Leeuw AS, van Megen HJ, Kahn RS, et al: d-Cycloserine addition to exposure sessions in the treatment of patients with obsessive-compulsive disorder. Eur Psychiatry 40:38–44, 2017

Denys D, van der Wee N, van Megen HJ, et al: A double blind comparison of venlafaxine and paroxetine in obsessive-compulsive disorder. J Clin Psychopharmacol 23(6):568–575, 2003 14624187

Denys D, van Megen HJ, van der Wee N, et al: A double-blind switch study of paroxetine and venlafaxine in obsessive-compulsive disorder. J Clin Psychiatry 65(1):37–43, 2004 14744166

Diniz JB, Shavitt RG, Pereira CA, et al: Quetiapine versus clomipramine in the augmentation of selective serotonin reuptake inhibitors for the treatment of obsessive-compulsive disorder: a randomized, open-label trial. J Psychopharmacol 24(3):297–307, 2010 19164490

Dold M, Aigner M, Lanzenberger R, et al: Antipsychotic augmentation of serotonin reuptake inhibitors in treatment-resistant obsessive-compulsive disorder: a meta-analysis of double-blind, randomized, placebo-controlled trials. Int J Neuropsychopharmacol 16(3):557–574, 2013 22932229

Dold M, Aigner M, Lanzenberger R, et al: Antipsychotic augmentation of serotonin reuptake inhibitors in treatment-resistant obsessive-compulsive disorder: an update meta-analysis of double-blind, randomized, placebo-controlled trials. Int J Neuropsychopharmacol 18(9), 2015 25939614

Eisen JL, Sibrava NJ, Boisseau CL, et al: Five-year course of obsessive-compulsive disorder: predictors of remission and relapse. J Clin Psychiatry 74(3):233–239, 2013 23561228

Emamzadehfard S, Kamaloo A, Paydary K, et al: Riluzole in augmentation of fluvoxamine for moderate to severe obsessive-compulsive disorder: randomized, double-blind, placebo-controlled study. Psychiatry Clin Neurosci 70(8):332–341, 2016

Epperson CN, McDougle CJ, Price LH: Intranasal oxytocin in obsessive-compulsive disorder. Biol Psychiatry 40(6):547–549, 1996 8879477

Erzegovesi S, Guglielmo E, Siliprandi F, et al: Low-dose risperidone augmentation of fluvoxamine treatment in obsessive-compulsive disorder: a double-blind, placebo-controlled study. Eur Neuropsychopharmacol 15(1):69–74, 2005 15572275

Esalatmanesh S, Abrishami Z, Zeinoddini A, et al: Minocycline combination therapy with fluvoxamine in moderate-to-severe obsessive-compulsive disorder: a placebo-controlled, double-blind, randomized trial. Psychiatry Clin Neurosci 70(11):517–526, 2016

Fallon BA, Liebowitz MR, Campeas R, et al: Intravenous clomipramine for obsessive-compulsive disorder refractory to oral clomipramine: a placebo-controlled study. Arch Gen Psychiatry 55(10):918–924, 1998 9783563

Farrell LJ, Waters AM, Boschen MJ, et al: Difficult-to-treat pediatric obsessive-compulsive disorder: feasibility and preliminary results of a randomized pilot trial of d-cycloserine-augmented behavior therapy. Depress Anxiety 30(8):723–731, 2013

Fineberg N, Craig KJ: Pharmacotherapy for obsessive-compulsive disorder, in Textbook of Anxiety Disorders, 2nd Edition. Edited by Stein DJ, Hollander E, Rothbaum BO. Washington, DC, American Psychiatric Publishing, 2010, pp 311–338

Fineberg NA, Gale TM: Evidence-based pharmacotherapy of obsessive-compulsive disorder. Int J Neuropsychopharmacol 8(1):107–129, 2005 15450126

Fineberg N, Heyman I, Jenkins R, et al: Does childhood and adult obsessive compulsive disorder (OCD) respond the same way to treatment with serotonin reuptake inhibitors (SRIs)? Eur Neuropsychopharmacol 14(suppl 3):S191, 2004

Fineberg NA, Sivakumaran T, Roberts A, et al: Adding quetiapine to SRI in treatment-resistant obsessive-compulsive disorder: a randomized controlled treatment study. Int Clin Psychopharmacol 20(4):223–226, 2005 15933483

Fineberg NA, Gale TM, Sivakumaran T: A review of antipsychotics in the treatment of obsessive compulsive disorder. J Psychopharmacol 20(1):97–103, 2006a 16204331

Fineberg NA, Nigam N, Sivakumaran T: Pharmacological strategies for treatment-resistant obsessive compulsive disorder. Psychiatr Ann 36:464–474, 2006b

Fineberg NA, Pampaloni I, Pallanti S, et al: Sustained response versus relapse: the pharmacotherapeutic goal for obsessive-compulsive disorder. Int Clin Psychopharmacol 22(6):313–322, 2007a 17917549

Fineberg NA, Tonnoir B, Lemming O, et al: Escitalopram prevents relapse of obsessive-compulsive disorder. Eur Neuropsychopharmacol 17(6–7):430–439, 2007b 17240120

Fineberg NA, Reghunandanan S, Simpson HB, et al: Obsessive-compulsive disorder (OCD): practical strategies for pharmacological and somatic treatment in adults. Psychiatry Res 227(1):114–125, 2015 25681005

Fineberg NA, Baldwin DS, Drummond LM, et al: Optimal treatment for obsessive compulsive disorder: a randomized controlled feasibility study of the clinical-effectiveness and cost-effectiveness of cognitive-behavioural therapy, selective serotonin reuptake inhibitors and their combination in the management of obsessive compulsive disorder. Int Clin Psychopharmacol 33(6):334–348, 2018 30113928

Foa EB, Liebowitz MR, Kozak MJ, et al: Randomized, placebo-controlled trial of exposure and ritual prevention, clomipramine, and their combination in the treatment of obsessive-compulsive disorder. Am J Psychiatry 162(1):151–161, 2005 15625214

Foa EB, Simpson HB, Liebowitz MR, et al: Six-month follow-up of a randomized controlled trial augmenting serotonin reuptake inhibitor treatment with exposure and ritual prevention for obsessive-compulsive disorder. J Clin Psychiatry 74(5):464–469, 2013 23759449

Franklin ME, Sapyta J, Freeman JB, et al: Cognitive behavior therapy augmentation of pharmacotherapy in pediatric obsessive-compulsive disorder: the Pediatric OCD Treatment Study II (POTS II) randomized controlled trial. JAMA 306(11):1224–1232, 2011 21934055

Freeman CPC, Trimble MR, Deakin JFW, et al: Fluvoxamine versus clomipramine in the treatment of obsessive-compulsive disorder: a multicenter, randomized, double-blind parallel group comparison. J Clin Psychiatry 55:301–305, 1994

Garcia AM, Sapyta JJ, Moore PS, et al: Predictors and moderators of treatment outcome in the Pediatric Obsessive Compulsive Treatment Study (POTS I). J Am Acad Child Adolesc Psychiatry 49(10):1024–1033; quiz 1086, 2010 20855047

Geller DA, Hoog SL, Heiligenstein JH, et al: Fluoxetine treatment for obsessive-compulsive disorder in children and adolescents: a placebo-controlled clinical trial. J Am Acad Child Adolesc Psychiatry 40(7):773–779, 2001 11437015

Geller DA, Biederman J, Stewart SE, et al: Which SSRI? A meta-analysis of pharmacotherapy trials in pediatric obsessive-compulsive disorder. Am J Psychiatry 160(11):1919–1928, 2003a 14594734

Geller DA, Coffey B, Faraone S, et al: Does comorbid attention-deficit/hyperactivity disorder impact the clinical expression of pediatric obsessive-compulsive disorder? CNS Spectr 8(4):259–264, 2003b 12679741

Geller DA, Wagner KD, Emslie G, et al: Paroxetine treatment in children and adolescents with obsessive-compulsive disorder: a randomized, multicenter, double-blind, placebo-controlled trial. J Am Acad Child Adolesc Psychiatry 43(11):1387–1396, 2004 15502598

Ghaleiha A, Entezari N, Modabbernia A, et al: Memantine add-on in moderate to severe obsessive-compulsive disorder: randomized double-blind placebo-controlled study. J Psychiatr Res 47(2):175–180, 2013

Ghanizadeh A, Mohammadi MR, Bahraini S, et al: Efficacy of N-acetylcysteine augmentation on obsessive compulsive disorder: a multicenter randomized double blind placebo controlled clinical trial. Iran J Psychiatry 12(2):134–141, 2017 28659986

Goodman WK, Price LH, Rasmussen SA, et al: The Yale-Brown Obsessive Compulsive Scale. II. Validity. Arch Gen Psychiatry 46(11):1012–1016, 1989 2510699

Goodman WK, Kozak MJ, Liebowitz M, et al: Treatment of obsessive-compulsive disorder with fluvoxamine: a multicentre, double-blind, placebo-controlled trial. Int Clin Psychopharmacol 11(1):21–29, 1996 8732310

Grady TA, Pigott TA, L'Heureux F, et al: Double-blind study of adjuvant buspirone for fluoxetine-treated patients with obsessive-compulsive disorder. Am J Psychiatry 150(5):819–821, 1993 8480832

Grant PJ, Joseph LA, Farmer CA, et al: 12-week, placebo-controlled trial of add-on riluzole in the treatment of childhood-onset obsessive-compulsive disorder. Neuropsychopharmacology 39(6):1453–1459, 2014

Greenberg WM, Benedict MM, Doerfer J, et al: Adjunctive glycine in the treatment of obsessive-compulsive disorder in adults. J Psychiatr Res 43(6):664–670, 2009

Greist J, Chouinard G, DuBoff E, et al: Double-blind parallel comparison of three dosages of sertraline and placebo in outpatients with obsessive-compulsive disorder. Arch Gen Psychiatry 52(4):289–295, 1995a 7702445

Greist JH, Jefferson JW, Kobak KA, et al: A 1 year double-blind placebo-controlled fixed dose study of sertraline in the treatment of obsessive-compulsive disorder. Int Clin Psychopharmacol 10(2):57–65, 1995b 7673657

Guy W: ECDEU Assessment Manual for Psychopharmacology, Revised. Bethesda, MD, U.S. Department of Health, Education and Welfare, 1976

Haghighi M, Jahangard L, Mohammad-Beigi H, et al: In a double-blind, randomized and placebo-controlled trial, adjuvant memantine improved symptoms in inpatients suffering from refractory obsessive-compulsive disorders (OCD). Psychopharmacology (Berl) 228(4):633–640, 2013

Harvey BH, Brink CB, Seedat S, et al: Defining the neuromolecular action of myo-inositol: application to obsessive-compulsive disorder. Prog Neuropsychopharmacol Biol Psychiatry 26(1):21–32, 2002 11853115

Hoehn-Saric R, Ninan P, Black DW, et al: Multicenter double-blind comparison of sertraline and desipramine for concurrent obsessive-compulsive and major depressive disorders. Arch Gen Psychiatry 57(1):76–82, 2000 10632236

Hohagen F, Winkelmann G, Rasche-Rüchle H, et al: Combination of behaviour therapy with fluvoxamine in comparison with behaviour therapy and placebo. Results of a multicentre study. Br J Psychiatry Suppl (35):71–78, 1998 9829029

Hollander E, Bienstock CA, Koran LM, et al: Refractory obsessive-compulsive disorder: state-of-the-art treatment. J Clin Psychiatry 63(suppl 6):20–29, 2002 12027116

Hollander E, Allen A, Steiner M, et al: Acute and long-term treatment and prevention of relapse of obsessive-compulsive disorder with paroxetine. J Clin Psychiatry 64(9):1113–1121, 2003a 14628989

Hollander E, Baldini Rossi N, Sood E, et al: Risperidone augmentation in treatment-resistant obsessive-compulsive disorder: a double-blind, placebo-controlled study. Int J Neuropsychopharmacol 6(4):397–401, 2003b 14604454

Hollander E, Friedberg J, Wasserman S, et al: Venlafaxine in treatment-resistant obsessive-compulsive disorder. J Clin Psychiatry 64(5):546–550, 2003c 12755657

Hollander E, Koran LM, Goodman WK, et al: A double-blind, placebo-controlled study of the efficacy and safety of controlled-release fluvoxamine in patients with obsessive-compulsive disorder. J Clin Psychiatry 64(6):640–647, 2003d 12823077

Hollander E, Stein DJ, Fineberg NA, et al: Quality of life outcomes in patients with obsessive-compulsive disorder: relationship to treatment response and symptom relapse. J Clin Psychiatry 71(6):784–792, 2010 20492845

Insel TR, Hamilton JA, Guttmacher LB, et al: d-Amphetamine in obsessive-compulsive disorder. Psychopharmacology (Berl) 80(3):231–235, 1983 6412267

Issari Y, Jakubovski E, Bartley CA, et al: Early onset of response with selective serotonin reuptake inhibitors in obsessive-compulsive disorder: a meta-analysis. J Clin Psychiatry 77(5):e605–e611, 2016 27249090

Ivarsson T, Skarphedinsson G, Kornør H, et al: The place of and evidence for serotonin reuptake inhibitors (SRIs) for obsessive compulsive disorder (OCD) in children and adolescents: views based on a systematic review and meta-analysis. Psychiatry Res 227(1):93–103, 2015 25769521

Joffe RT, Swinson RP, Levitt AJ: Acute psychostimulant challenge in primary obsessive-compulsive disorder. J Clin Psychopharmacol 11(4):237–241, 1991 1680885

Kaplan A, Hollander E: A review of pharmacologic treatments for obsessive-compulsive disorder. Psychiatr Serv 54(8):1111–1118, 2003 12883138

Keuler DJ, Altemus M, Michelson D, et al: Behavioral effects of naloxone infusion in obsessive-compulsive disorder. Biol Psychiatry 40(2):154–156, 1996 8793049

Khalkhali M, Aram S, Zarrabi H, et al: Lamotrigine augmentation versus placebo in serotonin reuptake inhibitors-resistant obsessive-compulsive disorder: a randomized controlled trial. Iran J Psychiatry 11(2):104–114, 2016

Kishi T, Matsuda Y, Iwata N: Combination therapy of serotonin reuptake inhibitors and memantine for obsessive-compulsive disorder: a meta-analysis of double-blind, randomized, placebo-controlled trials. J Alzheimers Dis 64(1):43–48, 2018 29865079

Kobak KA, Taylor LV, Bystritsky A, et al: St John's wort versus placebo in obsessive-compulsive disorder: results from a double-blind study. Int Clin Psychopharmacol 20(6):299–304, 2005 16192837

Komossa K, Depping AM, Meyer M, et al: Second-generation antipsychotics for obsessive compulsive disorder. Cochrane Database Syst Rev (12):CD008141, 2010 21154394

Koran LM, Saxena S: Issues and strategies in treating refractory obsessive-compulsive disorder. CNS Spectr 5:24–31, 2002

Koran LM, McElroy SL, Davidson JR, et al: Fluvoxamine versus clomipramine for obsessive-compulsive disorder: a double-blind comparison. J Clin Psychopharmacol 16(12):121–129, 1996 8690827

Koran LM, Sallee FR, Pallanti S: Rapid benefit of intravenous pulse loading of clomipramine in obsessive-compulsive disorder. Am J Psychiatry 154(3):396–401, 1997 9054789

Koran LM, Hackett E, Rubin A, et al: Efficacy of sertraline in the long-term treatment of obsessive-compulsive disorder. Am J Psychiatry 159(1):88–95, 2002 11772695

Koran LM, Aboujaoude E, Bullock KD, et al: Double-blind treatment with oral morphine in treatment-resistant obsessive-compulsive disorder. J Clin Psychiatry 66(3):353–359, 2005a 15766302

Koran LM, Gamel NN, Choung HW, et al: Mirtazapine for obsessive-compulsive disorder: an open trial followed by double-blind discontinuation. J Clin Psychiatry 66(4):515–520, 2005b 15816795

Kordon A, Wahl K, Koch N, et al: Quetiapine addition to serotonin reuptake inhibitors in patients with severe obsessive-compulsive disorder: a double-blind, randomized, placebo-controlled study. J Clin Psychopharmacol 28(5):550–554, 2008

Kronig MH, Apter J, Asnis G, et al: Placebo-controlled, multicenter study of sertraline treatment for obsessive-compulsive disorder. J Clin Psychopharmacol 19(2):172–176, 1999 10211919

Kushner MG, Kim SW, Donahue C, et al: d-Cycloserine augmented exposure therapy for obsessive-compulsive disorder. Biol Psychiatry 62(8):835–838, 2007

Levine J: Controlled trials of inositol in psychiatry. Eur Neuropsychopharmacol 7(2):147–155, 1997 9169302

Liebowitz MR, Turner SM, Piacentini J, et al: Fluoxetine in children and adolescents with OCD: a placebo-controlled trial. J Am Acad Child Adolesc Psychiatry 41(12):1431–1438, 2002 12447029

Lopez-Ibor J Jr, Saiz J, Cottraux J, et al: Double-blind comparison of fluoxetine versus clomipramine in the treatment of obsessive compulsive disorder. Eur Neuropsychopharmacol 6:111–118, 1996

Maina G, Albert U, Bogetto F: Relapses after discontinuation of drug associated with increased resistance to treatment in obsessive-compulsive disorder. Int Clin Psychopharmacol 16(1):33–38, 2001 11195258

Maina G, Albert U, Ziero S, et al: Antipsychotic augmentation for treatment resistant obsessive-compulsive disorder: what if antipsychotic is discontinued? Int Clin Psychopharmacol 18(1):23–28, 2003 12490771

Maina G, Albert U, Salvi V, et al: Weight gain during long-term treatment of obsessive-compulsive disorder: a prospective comparison between serotonin reuptake inhibitors. J Clin Psychiatry 65(10):1365–1371, 2004 15491240

March JS, Frances A, Kahn DA, et al: The Expert Consensus Guideline Series: treatment of obsessive compulsive disorder. J Clin Psychiatry 58(suppl):1–72, 1997

March JS, Biederman J, Wolkow R, et al: Sertraline in children and adolescents with obsessive-compulsive disorder: a multicenter randomized controlled trial. JAMA 280(10):1752–1756, 1998 9842950

Marinova Z, Chuang DM, Fineberg N: Glutamate-modulating drugs as a potential therapeutic strategy in obsessive-compulsive disorder. Curr Neuropharmacol 15(7):977–995, 2017 28322166

Marks IM, Lelliott P, Basoglu M, et al: Clomipramine, self-exposure and therapist-aided exposure for obsessive-compulsive rituals. Br J Psychiatry 152:522–534, 1988 3167404

Mataix-Cols D, Turner C, Monzani B, et al: Cognitive-behavioural therapy with post-session d-cycloserine augmentation for paediatric obsessive-compulsive disorder: pilot randomised controlled trial. Br J Psychiatry 204(1):77–78, 2014

McDougle CJ, Price LH, Goodman WK, et al: A controlled trial of lithium augmentation in fluvoxamine-refractory obsessive-compulsive disorder: lack of efficacy. J Clin Psychopharmacol 11(3):175–184, 1991 1820757

McDougle CJ, Goodman WK, Leckman JF, et al: Limited therapeutic effect of addition of buspirone in fluvoxamine-refractory obsessive-compulsive disorder. Am J Psychiatry 150(4):647–649, 1993 8465885

McDougle CJ, Goodman WK, Leckman JF, et al: Haloperidol addition in fluvoxamine-refractory obsessive-compulsive disorder: a double-blind, placebo-controlled study in patients with and without tics. Arch Gen Psychiatry 51(4):302–308, 1994 8161290

McDougle CJ, Barr LC, Goodman WK, et al: Lack of efficacy of clozapine monotherapy in refractory obsessive-compulsive disorder. Am J Psychiatry 152(12):1812–1814, 1995 8526253

McDougle CJ, Epperson CN, Pelton GH, et al: A double-blind, placebo-controlled study of risperidone addition in serotonin reuptake inhibitor–refractory obsessive-compulsive disorder. Arch Gen Psychiatry 57(8):794–801, 2000 10920469

McGuire JF, Piacentini J, Lewin AB, et al: A meta-analysis of cognitive behavior therapy and medication for child obsessive compulsive disorder: moderators of treatment efficacy, response, and remission. Depress Anxiety 32(8):580–593, 2015 26130211

Metin O, Yazici K, Tot S, et al: Amisulpiride augmentation in treatment resistant obsessive-compulsive disorder: an open trial. Hum Psychopharmacol 18(6):463–467, 2003 12923825

Milanfranchi A, Ravagli S, Lensi P, et al: A double-blind study of fluvoxamine and clomipramine in the treatment of obsessive compulsive disorder. Int Clin Psychopharmacol 12:131–136, 1997

Modarresi A, Sayyah M, Razooghi S, et al: Memantine augmentation improves symptoms in serotonin reuptake inhibitor-refractory obsessive-compulsive disorder: a randomized controlled trial. Pharmacopsychiatry 51(6):263–269, 2018 29100251

Monteiro WO, Noshirvani HF, Marks IM, Lelliott PT: Anorgasmia from clomipramine in obsessive-compulsive disorder. A controlled trial. Br J Psychiatry 151:107–112, 1987 3315086

Montgomery SA, McIntyre A, Osterheider M, et al: A double-blind, placebo-controlled study of fluoxetine in patients with DSM-III-R obsessive-compulsive disorder. The Lilly European OCD Study Group. Eur Neuropsychopharmacol 3(2):143–152, 1993 8364350

Montgomery SA, Kasper S, Stein DJ, et al: Citalopram 20 mg, 40 mg and 60 mg are all effective and well tolerated compared with placebo in obsessive-compulsive disorder. Int Clin Psychopharmacol 16(2):75–86, 2001 11236072

Mowla A, Khajeian AM, Sahraian A, et al: Topiramate augmentation in resistant OCD: a double-blind placebo-controlled clinical trial. CNS Spectr 15(11):613–617, 2010

Murphy TK, Sajid MW, Goodman WK: Immunology of obsessive-compulsive disorder. Psychiatr Clin North Am 29(2):445–469, 2006 16650717

Muscatello MR, Bruno A, Pandolfo G, et al: Effect of aripiprazole augmentation of serotonin reuptake inhibitors or clomipramine in treatment-resistant obsessive-compulsive disorder: a double-blind, placebo-controlled study. J Clin Psychopharmacol 31(2):174–179, 2011

National Institute for Health and Clinical Excellence: Obsessive-Compulsive Disorder and Body Dysmorphic Disorder: Treatment. London, NICE, 2005. Available at: http://www.nice.org.uk /Guidance/CG31. Accessed June 22, 2019.

Nemets B, Fux M, Levine J, et al: Combination of antidepressant drugs: the case of inositol. Hum Psychopharmacol 16(1):37–43, 2001 12404596

Ninan PT, Koran LM, Kiev A, et al: High-dose sertraline strategy for nonresponders to acute treatment for obsessive-compulsive disorder: a multicenter double-blind trial. J Clin Psychiatry 67(1):15–22, 2006 16426083

O'Connor KP, Aardema F, Robillard S, et al: Cognitive behaviour therapy and medication in the treatment of obsessive-compulsive disorder. Acta Psychiatr Scand 113(5):408–419, 2006 16603032

Pallanti S, Quercioli L, Paiva RS, et al: Citalopram for treatment-resistant obsessive-compulsive disorder. Eur Psychiatry 14(2):101–106, 1999 10572334

Pallanti S, Hollander E, Bienstock C, et al: Treatment non-response in OCD: methodological issues and operational definitions. Int J Neuropsychopharmacol 5(2):181–191, 2002a 12135542

Pallanti S, Quercioli L, Koran LM: Citalopram intravenous infusion in resistant obsessive-compulsive disorder: an open trial. J Clin Psychiatry 63(9):796–801, 2002b 12363120

Pallanti S, Quercioli L, Bruscoli M: Response acceleration with mirtazapine augmentation of citalopram in obsessive-compulsive disorder patients without comorbid depression: a pilot study. J Clin Psychiatry 65(10):1394–1399, 2004 15491244

Paydary K, Akamaloo A, Ahmadipour A, et al: N-acetylcysteine augmentation therapy for moderate-to-severe obsessive-compulsive disorder: randomized, double-blind, placebo-controlled trial. J Clin Pharmacol Ther 41(2):214–219, 2016

Pediatric OCD Treatment Study Team: Cognitive-behavior therapy, sertraline, and their combination for children and adolescents with obsessive-compulsive disorder: the Pediatric OCD Treatment Study (POTS) randomized controlled trial. JAMA 292(16):1969–1976, 2004 15507582

Pidrman V, Tuma I: Citalopram versus clomipramine in double-blind therapy of obsessive compulsive disorder, in Abstracts From 11th Congress of the European College of Neuropsychopharmacology Paris, France, October 31–November 4, 1998

Pigott TA, Seay SM: A review of the efficacy of selective serotonin reuptake inhibitors in obsessive-compulsive disorder. J Clin Psychiatry 60(2):101–106, 1999 10084636

Pigott TA, Pato MT, Bernstein SE, et al: Controlled comparisons of clomipramine and fluoxetine in the treatment of obsessive compulsive disorder. Behavioral and biological results. Arch Gen Psychiatry 47:926–932, 1990

Pigott TA, Pato MT, L'Heureux F, et al: A controlled comparison of adjuvant lithium carbonate or thyroid hormone in clomipramine-treated patients with obsessive-compulsive disorder. J Clin Psychopharmacol 11(4):242–248, 1991 1918422

Pigott TA, L'Heureux F, Hill JL, et al: A double-blind study of adjuvant buspirone hydrochloride in clomipramine-treated patients with obsessive-compulsive disorder. J Clin Psychopharmacol 12(1):11–18, 1992 1552034

Pittenger C: Glutamatergic agents for OCD and related disorders. Curr Treat Options Psychiatry 2(3):271–283, 2015

Poyraz CA, Turan S, Saglam NG, et al: Factors associated with the duration of untreated illness among patients with obsessive compulsive disorder. Compr Psychiatry 58:88–93, 2015 25596625

Rabinowitz I, Baruch Y, Barak Y: High-dose escitalopram for the treatment of obsessive-compulsive disorder. Int Clin Psychopharmacol 23(1):49–53, 2008 18090508

Rasmussen S, Hackett E, DuBoff E, et al: A 2-year study of sertraline in the treatment of obsessive-compulsive disorder. Int Clin Psychopharmacol 12(6):309–316, 1997 9547132

Reid JE, Reghunandanan S, Roberts A, Fineberg NA: Obsessive-compulsive disorder: standard evidence-based pharmacological treatment, in Obsessive-Compulsive Disorder, Phenomenology, Pathophysiology and Treatment, Edited by Pittenger C. New York, Oxford University Press, 2017, pp 443–462

Riddle MA, Scahill L, King RA, et al: Double-blind, crossover trial of fluoxetine and placebo in children and adolescents with obsessive-compulsive disorder. J Am Acad Child Adolesc Psychiatry 31(6):1062–1069, 1992 1429406

Riddle MA, Reeve EA, Yaryura-Tobias JA, et al: Fluvoxamine for children and adolescents with obsessive-compulsive disorder: a randomized, controlled, multicenter trial. J Am Acad Child Adolesc Psychiatry 40(2):222–229, 2001 11211371

Rodriguez CI, Kegeles LS, Levinson A, et al: Randomized controlled crossover trial of ketamine in obsessive-compulsive disorder: proof-of-concept. Neuropsychopharmacology 38(12):2475–2483, 2013

Romano S, Goodman W, Tamura R, et al: Long-term treatment of obsessive-compulsive disorder after an acute response: a comparison of fluoxetine versus placebo. J Clin Psychopharmacol 21:46–52, 2001 11199947

Rouillon F: A double-blind comparison of fluvoxamine and clomipramine in OCD. Eur Neuropsychopharmacol 8(suppl):260–261, 1998

Sarris J, Oliver G, Camfield DA, et al: N-acetyl cysteine (NAC) in the treatment of obsessive-compulsive disorder: a 16-week, double-blind, randomised, placebo-controlled study. CNS Drugs 29(9):801–809, 2015

Sayyah M, Sayyah M, Boostani H, et al: Effects of aripiprazole augmentation in treatment-resistant obsessive-compulsive disorder (a double blind clinical trial). Depress Anxiety 29(10):850–854, 2012

Scahill L, Riddle MA, McSwiggin-Hardin M, et al: Children's Yale-Brown Obsessive Compulsive Scale: reliability and validity. J Am Acad Child Adolesc Psychiatry 36(6):844–852, 1997 9183141

Serata D, Kotzalidis GD, Rapinesi C, et al: Are 5-HT3 antagonists effective in obsessive-compulsive disorder? A systematic review of literature. Hum Psychopharmacol 30(2):70–84, 2015 25676060

Shapira NA, Ward HE, Mandoki M, et al: A double-blind, placebo-controlled trial of olanzapine addition in fluoxetine-refractory obsessive-compulsive disorder. Biol Psychiatry 55(5):553–555, 2004 15023585

Simpson HB, Huppert JD, Petkova E, et al: Response versus remission in obsessive-compulsive disorder. J Clin Psychiatry 67(2):269–276, 2006 16566623

Simpson HB, Foa EB, Liebowitz MR, et al: A randomized, controlled trial of cognitive-behavioral therapy for augmenting pharmacotherapy in obsessive-compulsive disorder. Am J Psychiatry 165(5):621–630, 2008 18316422

Simpson HB, Foa EB, Liebowitz MR, et al: Cognitive-behavioral therapy vs risperidone for augmenting serotonin reuptake inhibitors in obsessive-compulsive disorder: a randomized clinical trial. JAMA Psychiatry 70(11):1190–1199, 2013 24026523

Skapinakis P, Papatheodorou T, Mavreas V: Antipsychotic augmentation of serotonergic antidepressants in treatment-resistant obsessive-compulsive disorder: a meta-analysis of the randomized controlled trials. Eur Neuropsychopharmacol 17(2):79–93, 2007 16904298

Skapinakis P, Caldwell D, Hollingworth W, et al: A systematic review of the clinical effectiveness and cost-effectiveness of pharmacological and psychological interventions for the management of obsessive-compulsive disorder in children/adolescents and adults. Health Technol Assess 20(43):1–392, 2016a 27306503

Skapinakis P, Caldwell D, Hollingworth W, et al: Pharmacological and psychotherapeutic interventions for management of obsessive-compulsive disorder in adults: a systematic review and network meta-analysis. Lancet Psychiatry 3(8):730–739, 2016b 27318812

Skoog G, Skoog I: A 40-year follow-up of patients with obsessive-compulsive disorder [see comments]. Arch Gen Psychiatry 56(2):121–127, 1999 10025435

Smeraldi E, Ergovesi S, Bianchi I: Fluvoxamine versus clomipramine treatment in obsessive-compulsive disorder: a preliminary study. New Trends in Experimental and Clinical Psychiatry 8:63–65, 1992

Soomro GM, Altman D, Rajagopal S, et al: Selective serotonin re-uptake inhibitors (SSRIs) versus placebo for obsessive compulsive disorder (OCD). Cochrane Database Syst Rev (1):CD001765, 2008 18253995

Spartz EJ, Freeman GM Jr, Brown K, et al: Course of neuropsychiatric symptoms after introduction and removal of nonsteroidal anti-inflammatory drugs: a pediatric observational study. J Child Adolesc Psychopharmacol 27(7):652–659, 2017 28696783

Stein DJ, Andersen EW, Tonnoir B, et al: Escitalopram in obsessive-compulsive disorder: a randomized, placebo-controlled, paroxetine-referenced, fixed-dose, 24-week study. Curr Med Res Opin 23(4):701–711, 2007 17407626

Storch EA, Merlo LJ, Bengtson M, et al: d-Cycloserine does not enhance exposure-response prevention therapy in obsessive-compulsive disorder. Int Clin Psychopharmacol 22:230–237, 2007

Storch EA, Murphy TK, Goodman WK, et al: A preliminary study of d-cycloserine augmentation of cognitive-behavioral therapy in pediatric obsessive-compulsive disorder. Biol Psychiatry 68(11):1073–1076, 2010

Storch EA, Goddard AW, Grant JE, et al: Double-blind, placebo-controlled, pilot trial of paliperidone augmentation in serotonin reuptake inhibitor-resistant obsessive-compulsive disorder. J Clin Psychiatry 74(6):e527–e532, 2013 23842022

Storch EA, Wilhelm S, Sprich S, et al: Efficacy of augmentation of cognitive behavior therapy with weight-adjusted d-cycloserine vs placebo in pediatric obsessive-compulsive disorder: a randomized clinical trial. JAMA Psychiatry 73(8):779–788, 2016

Szegedi A, Wetzel H, Leal M, et al: Combination treatment with clomipramine and fluvoxamine: drug monitoring, safety, and tolerability data. J Clin Psychiatry 57(6):257–264, 1996 8666584

Tollefson GD, Rampey AH Jr, Potvin JH, et al: A multicenter investigation of fixed-dose fluoxetine in the treatment of obsessive-compulsive disorder. Arch Gen Psychiatry 51(7):559–567, 1994 8031229

U.S. Food and Drug Administration: FDA Drug Safety Communication: revised recommendations for Celexa (citalopram hydrobromide) related to a potential risk of abnormal heart rhythms with high doses. MedWatch, August 2011. Available at: www.fda.gov/Drugs/DrugSafety/ucm297391.htm. Accessed June 21, 2019.

Veale D, Miles S, Smallcombe N, et al: Atypical antipsychotic augmentation in SSRI treatment refractory obsessive-compulsive disorder: a systematic review and meta-analysis. BMC Psychiatry 14:317, 2014 25432131

Walitza S, Melfsen S, Jans T, et al: Obsessive-compulsive disorder in children and adolescents. Dtsch Arztebl Int 108(11):173–179, 2011 21475565

Wilhelm S, Buhlmann U, Tolin DF, et al: Augmentation of behavior therapy with d-cycloserine for obsessive-compulsive disorder. Am J Psychiatry 165(3):335–341, 2008

Yaryura-Tobias JA, Neziroglu FA: Venlafaxine in obsessive-compulsive disorder. Arch Gen Psychiatry 53(7):653–654, 1996 8660133

Zai G, Brandl EJ, Müller DJ, et al: Pharmacogenetics of antidepressant treatment in obsessive-compulsive disorder: an update and implications for clinicians. Pharmacogenomics 15(8):1147–57, 2014 25084207

Zivin K, Pfeiffer PN, Bohnert AS, et al: Evaluation of the FDA warning against prescribing citalopram at doses exceeding 40 mg. Am J Psychiatry 170(6):642–650, 2013 23640689

Zohar J, Judge R: Paroxetine versus clomipramine in the treatment of obsessive-compulsive disorder. OCD Paroxetine Study Investigators. Br J Psychiatry 169(4):468–474, 1996 8894198

Recommended Readings

Baldwin DS, Anderson IM, Nutt DJ, et al: Evidence-based pharmacological treatment of anxiety disorders, post-traumatic stress disorder and obsessive-compulsive disorder: a revision of the 2005 guidelines from the British Association for Psychopharmacology. J Psychopharmacol 28(5):403, 2014

Fineberg NA, Reghunandanan S, Simpson HB, et al: Obsessive-compulsive disorder (OCD): practical strategies for pharmacological and somatic treatment in adults. Psychiatry Res 227(1):114–125, 2015 25681005

Fineberg NA, Apergis-Schoute AM, Vaghi MM, et al: Mapping compulsivity in the DSM-5 obsessive compulsive and related disorders: cognitive domains, neural circuitry, and treatment. Int J Neuropsychopharmacol 21(1):42–58, 2018

Marinova Z, Chuang DM, Fineberg N: Glutamate-modulating drugs as a potential therapeutic strategy in obsessive-compulsive disorder. Curr Neuropharmacol 15(7):977–995, 2017 28322166

National Institute for Health and Clinical Excellence: Obsessive-Compulsive Disorder and Body Dysmorphic Disorder: Treatment. London, National Institute for Health and Clinical Excellence, 2005

Reid JE, Reghunandanan S, Roberts A, et al: Obsessive-compulsive disorder: standard evidence-based pharmacological treatment, in Obsessive-Compulsive Disorder, Phenomenology, Pathophysiology and Treatment. Edited by Pittenger C. New York, Oxford University Press, 2017, pp 443–462

Reghunandanan S, Fineberg NA, Stein DS (eds): Obsessive Compulsive Disorder, 2nd Edition. Oxford, UK, Oxford Psychiatry Library, Oxford University Press, 2015

Sachdev RA, Ruparelia R, Reid JE, et al: Pharmacological treatments for obsessive-compulsive and related disorders: a transdiagnostic perspective, in Transdiagnostic Approach to Obsessions, Compulsions and Related Phenomena. Edited by Fontenelle L, Yucel M. Cambridge, UK, Cambridge University Press, 2019, pp 183–207

Skapinakis P, Caldwell D, Hollingworth W, et al: Pharmacological and psychotherapeutic interventions for management of obsessive-compulsive disorder in adults: a systematic review and network meta-analysis. Lancet Psychiatry 3(8):730–739, 2016 27318812

CHAPTER 18

Psychological Treatment for OCD

Jonathan S. Abramowitz, Ph.D.

Jennifer L. Buchholz, M.A.

OCD is a condition characterized by persistent anxiety and involving recurrent, unwanted, and seemingly bizarre thoughts, images, impulses, or doubts that evoke distress (*obsessions*; e.g., persistent violent and morally repugnant ideas, such as "Jesus is dead") and repetitive behavioral or mental rituals performed to reduce this distress (*compulsions*; e.g., excessive praying, confessing, and asking for assurances to prevent a feared consequence, such as going to hell). Obsessional fears tend to involve issues related to uncertainty about personal safety or the safety of others. Compulsions are deliberately performed to reduce this uncertainty and control anxiety. Although not a diagnostic criterion, phobic-like avoidance is a cardinal feature of OCD. Most people with OCD attempt to avoid situations and stimuli that trigger obsessional fear and urges to ritualize. For example, someone with obsessions about germs might avoid public washrooms, and someone with obsessions about causing fires might avoid using the oven.

Research consistently reveals that certain types of obsessions and compulsions co-occur within patients (Abramowitz et al. 2010). These include 1) obsessions about contamination, with decontamination (e.g., washing) rituals; 2) obsessions regarding responsibility for harm, with checking and reassurance-seeking rituals; 3) obsessions about order or symmetry, with arranging rituals; and 4) obsessions with violent, sexual, moral, or blasphemous themes, with covert rituals such as mental neutralizing (e.g., praying, compulsive thought suppression). Some individuals also have excessive concerns about numbers causing bad luck or about their health.

Although many people with OCD recognize that their obsessional fears and rituals are senseless and excessive, others strongly believe their rituals serve to prevent the occurrence of disastrous consequences (i.e., they have "poor insight" [Foa et al. 1995]). Such insight occurs on a continuum of severity and might vary over time and across different types of obsessions. For some patients, feared consequences include an identifiable disaster (e.g., "I will get AIDS if I touch a toilet"), whereas others fear that if rituals are not performed, feelings of anxiety, uncertainty, disgust, or incompleteness will persist indefinitely or rise to unmanageable levels.

In this chapter, we begin with a historical overview of the development of effective psychological treatment techniques for OCD—most notably, exposure and response prevention (ERP)—with an emphasis on translational research that has bridged the gap from the animal behavior laboratory to the psychotherapy clinic. Next, we discuss the practical application and mechanisms of ERP, before reviewing the empirical literature that establishes its efficacy and predictors of outcome. We turn then to other psychosocial approaches, including cognitive therapy (CT) and acceptance and commitment therapy (ACT), a relatively new development in the treatment of OCD, and discuss their use in psychological treatment as guided by empirical research. Various formats for psychological treatment are reviewed, followed by a focus on treatment-refractory groups. We conclude with a discussion of some additional recent advances in the treatment of OCD.

Historical Overview

Development of Behavioral Treatment for OCD: A Translational Perspective

Prior to the 1970s and 1980s, treatment for OCD consisted largely of psychodynamic psychotherapy approaches derived from psychoanalytic ideas of unconscious motivation. Although anecdotal reports exist (Freud 1909/1955), virtually no scientific studies assessing the efficacy of these approaches have been published. Nonetheless, the general consensus of clinicians was that OCD was an unmanageable condition with a poor prognosis. This admission speaks to how little confidence clinicians placed in such approaches. Indeed, available reports suggest that the effects of psychodynamically oriented therapies are neither robust nor durable for OCD.

By the last quarter of the twentieth century, however, the prognostic picture for OCD had improved dramatically. This was due in large part to the work of Victor Meyer (1966) and other behaviorally oriented clinicians and researchers (e.g., Jack Rachman, Isaac Marks), who relied on behavioral models of obsessive-compulsive behavior established in the 1950s to guide the synthesis of behaviorally based therapies for humans. These historical developments provide us with some of the clearest and most compelling examples of translational research in the mental health field. Thus, we begin by placing contemporary psychological treatment for OCD in its historical context.

Early Laboratory Research

The early work of Richard Solomon et al. (1953) provides an elegant, yet often overlooked, animal behavior model of OCD. Solomon and colleagues studied dogs in shuttle boxes (small rooms divided in two by a hurdle, over which the animals could jump). Each half of the box was separately furnished with a metal grate that could be independently electrified to give the dogs an electric shock through their paws. In addition, a flickering light served as a conditioned stimulus. The researchers produced a compulsive ritual-like behavior in the dogs by pairing the flickering light with an electric shock (the shock occurred 10 seconds after the light was turned on). The dogs soon learned to terminate exposure to the shock by jumping into the other compartment of the shuttle box, which was not electrified. After several trials, the dogs learned to altogether *avoid* the shock by jumping to the nonelectrified compartment in response to the flickering light (i.e., within 10 seconds). In other words, the experimenter had produced a conditioned "escape" response to the light—that is, jumping from one compartment of the box to the other.

Once this conditioned response was established, the electricity was disconnected, and the dogs never received another shock. Nevertheless, the animals continued to jump across the hurdle each time the conditioned stimulus (the light) was turned on. This continued for hundreds (and in some cases, thousands) of trials despite no actual risk of shock. Apparently, the dogs had acquired an obsessive-compulsive behavior—jumping across the hurdle—that reduced their fear of shock and thus was maintained by negative reinforcement (the removal of an aversive stimulus such as emotional distress). This serves as an animal analogue to human OCD, in which, as described earlier, compulsive behavior is triggered by fear associated with situations or stimuli such as toilets, unlucky numbers, or obsessional thoughts (conditioned stimuli) that pose no more than acceptable risk of harm. This fear is then reduced by compulsive rituals (e.g., washing) and avoidance behaviors, which serve as an escape from distress and thereby are negatively reinforced and become habitual.

Solomon et al. (1953) also studied the *reduction* of the compulsive jumping behavior of their "obsessive-compulsive" dogs using various techniques, the most effective of which involved a combination of procedures now known as *exposure and response prevention*. Specifically, the experimenter turned on the flickering light (analogous to in vivo *exposure*, as described in the next subsection) and increased the height of the hurdle in the shuttle box so that the dogs were unable to jump (analogous to *response prevention*). When this was done, the dogs immediately showed signs of a strong fear response—yelping, running around the chamber, defecating and urinating—because they expected to receive a shock. Gradually, however, this emotional reaction subsided—because the shock was never given—until the dogs finally displayed calmness without the slightest hint of distress. In behavioral terms, this experimental paradigm produced *extinction* of the fear. After several "extinction trials," the entire emotional and behavioral response was extinguished, so that even when the light was turned on and the height of the hurdle was lowered, the dogs did not jump.

During the 1960s and 1970s, OCD researchers adapted similar research paradigms to human beings with OCD (Rachman and Hodgson 1980). Of course, no electric shocks were used, but the adaptation was as follows: patients with handwashing rituals, after providing informed consent, were seated at a table with a container of dirt and miscellaneous garbage. The experimenter asked the patients to place their hands in the mixture and explained that no washing would be permitted for some length of time. When the patients began the procedure, an increase in anxiety, fear, and urges to wash were observed. This increase in distress was akin to the dogs' response once the light was turned on and the hurdle had been increased in height, making jumping (i.e., escape) impossible. Like Solomon's dogs, the patients with OCD also evidenced a gradual reduction in distress and in urges to wash. This procedure was repeated on subsequent days, the study revealing that, after some time, extinction was complete and the OCD symptoms were reduced.

From the Laboratory to the Clinic

Victor Meyer (1966) first reported the application of ERP to OCD. He helped inpatients deliberately confront, for 2 hours each day, situations and stimuli they usually avoided (e.g., floors, bathrooms). The purpose of the repeated and prolonged confrontation was to induce obsessional fears of contamination and illness as well as urges to ritualize; however, the patients also were helped to refrain from performing compulsive rituals after exposure. Of Meyer's 15 patients, 10 responded extremely well to this therapy, and the remainder evidenced partial improvement. Follow-up studies conducted several years later found that only two of those who had been successfully treated had relapsed (Meyer et al. 1974).

As in this original work, contemporary ERP entails therapist-guided, systematic, repeated, and prolonged exposure to situations that provoke obsessional fear, along with abstinence from compulsive behaviors. This exposure might occur in the form of actual confrontation with feared low-risk situations (i.e., in vivo exposure), imaginal confrontation with the feared disastrous consequences of confronting the low-risk situations (i.e., imaginal exposure), or confrontation with physiological sensations associated with anxiety (i.e., interoceptive exposure). For example, an individual who fears causing bad luck if she steps on the cracks in the sidewalk could practice stepping on them, imagining being held responsible for harming others because she had stepped on the cracks and inducing the physiological experiences associated with anxiety (e.g., elevated heart rate, hyperventilation).

Refraining from compulsive rituals (response prevention) is a vital component of treatment because the performance of compulsive rituals would prematurely discontinue exposure and prevent the patient from learning 1) that the obsessional stimulus is not truly dangerous and 2) that anxiety is safe and tolerable and subsides on its own, even if the ritual is not performed. Thus, ERP requires that patients remain in the exposure situation until they learn that feared situations and obsessional thoughts are safe, that anxiety itself is safe, and that compulsive rituals and avoidance are therefore not necessary to escape from obsessional distress.

Exposure and Response Prevention

In this section, we discuss the procedure involved in ERP. Table 18–1 summarizes the components of this intervention for patients with OCD.

Assessment

A course of ERP begins with a thorough assessment of the patient's particular obsessional thoughts, stimuli that trigger these obsessions, rituals and avoidance behaviors, and the anticipated harmful consequences of confronting feared situations without performing rituals. Comorbid conditions that may complicate treatment are identified, and plans for their management are established. Although the behavioral

TABLE 18–1.   **Components of exposure and response prevention (ERP) treatment for OCD**

Assessment	Therapist uses a semistructured interview and self-report instruments to gather information about the patient's obsessional thoughts, triggering stimuli, avoidance behaviors, and compulsive rituals.
Education and treatment planning	Therapist socializes the patient to the cognitive-behavioral model of OCD and explains the rationale for ERP. Together they develop a list of exposure items to be confronted and compulsive rituals to be resisted.
In vivo exposure	Patient engages repeatedly and for prolonged periods with environmental cues that provoke obsessional fear.
Imaginal exposure	Patient engages repeatedly and for prolonged periods with obsessional thoughts, images, and doubts that provoke anxiety and uncertainty.
Response prevention	Patient resists urges to complete compulsive rituals to learn that such rituals are not necessary to manage obsessional thoughts and anxiety.
Reducing family accommodation	Therapist helps those close to the person with OCD to reduce their involvement in avoidance patterns or rituals.

assessment focuses on obsessive-compulsive psychopathology, the patient learns a great deal about the context in which OCD occurs, the complications it causes, factors that precipitate symptomatic episodes (e.g., life stress), and situations associated with fewer symptoms (e.g., vacations).

Some patients with OCD may be reluctant to disclose their obsessions and compulsions because they are embarrassed or ashamed, because they believe that admitting them aloud will produce a negative outcome, or perhaps because they have experienced their obsessions and carried out their rituals so often and for so long that they no longer recognize them as abnormal. The use of a checklist of common obsessions and compulsions, such as the symptom checklist that accompanies the Yale-Brown Obsessive Compulsive Scale (Y-BOCS; Goodman et al. 1989a, 1989b), often helps elicit this information more completely.

In addition, identifying all of the circumstances, both external (situations and stimuli) and internal (intrusive thoughts), that trigger obsessional distress and compulsive urges is crucial to designing an effective ERP program. This *functional assessment* should elicit information about the involvement of family, friends, and coworkers in the patient's rituals, because such involvement is quite common. It should also involve an assessment of the functional interference associated with OCD symptoms.

Education and Treatment Planning

Before actual treatment commences, the therapist socializes patients to a psychological model of OCD based on the behavioral model discussed earlier (see "Historical Overview"). Patients are given a clear rationale for how ERP is expected to be helpful in reducing OCD. This educational component is an important step in therapy because it helps motivate patients to tolerate the distress that typically accompanies exposure practice. A helpful rationale includes information about how ERP involves the provocation of temporary distress during prolonged exposure to foster learning that obsessional fears are unfounded and that anxiety is safe and manageable. Informa-

TABLE 18–2.   **Example of an exposure list**

Exposure item	SUDS score
Touching door handles and handrails	45
Images of "herpes germs"	55
Shaking hands with others	65
Using public telephones	70
Touching garbage cans	75
Touching sweat from another person	80
Using public bathrooms	85
Touching drops of own urine	90
Touching paper towel with small smudge of feces	95

Note.   SUDS=Subjective Units of Distress Scale. Scores range from 0 (no distress) to 100 (maximum distress).

tion gathered during the assessment sessions is then used to plan, collaboratively with patients, the specific exposure exercises that will be pursued.

In planning for ERP, the therapist and the patient must engineer experiences in which the patient confronts stimuli that evoke obsessional anxiety but in which feared outcomes do not materialize and the only explanation is that the obsessional stimuli are not as dangerous as the patient thought. The exposure treatment plan, or *exposure list*, is a list of specific situations, stimuli, and thoughts that the patient will confront during therapy. The situations may be arranged hierarchically according to the degree of *subjective units of distress* that exposure would provoke, but this is not essential. Prolonged confrontation with each exposure list item, one at a time, is conducted repeatedly (without rituals) until the patient's expectations of feared outcomes (including fears of not being able to manage obsessions and anxiety) have been disconfirmed. It is critical that items on the exposure list match patients' specific obsessional fears. For example, an individual with obsessional fears of germs must be exposed to the sources of feared germs. If the patient believes public bathrooms and public telephones are "contaminated," exposure must include confrontation with these things. An example of an exposure list for such a patient appears in Table 18–2.

In addition to explaining and planning the exposure list during the educational stage of ERP, the therapist must acquaint patients with *response prevention* procedures. Importantly, "response prevention" does not imply that the therapist actively prevents patients from performing rituals. Instead, the therapist encourages patients to resist urges to perform rituals on their own.

Exposure Therapy Sessions

Although a gradual approach is not essential, exposure exercises typically begin with moderately distressing situations, stimuli, and images and progress to the most distressing situations that must be confronted during treatment. Beginning with less anxiety-evoking exposure tasks increases the likelihood that patients will learn to manage the distress and complete the exposure exercises successfully. Moreover, having success with initial exposures increases confidence in the treatment and helps motivate patients to persevere during later, more difficult, exercises. Each exposure session lasts from 60 to 90 minutes and usually includes in vivo exposure to an actual situation or stimulus and imaginal exposure to the obsessional thoughts and doubts provoked by the fear stimulus. At the end of each treatment session, the therapist assigns homework, instructing patients to continue exposure for several hours and in different contexts without the therapist. Exposure to the most anxiety-evoking situations is not left to the end of the treatment but rather is practiced about midway through the schedule of exposure tasks. This tactic allows patients ample opportunity to repeat exposure to the most difficult situations in different contexts to allow generalization of treatment effects. During the later treatment sessions, the therapist emphasizes how important it is for patients to continue to apply the ERP procedures learned during treatment. Depending on the patients' particular obsessions and compulsions, and on the practicality of confronting actual feared situations, treatment sessions might involve varying amounts of situational and imaginal exposure practice, sometimes necessitating that a patient and therapist leave the office or clinic to perform the exercises (Abramowitz 2006).

Compulsive rituals evolve to control discomfort after exposure to triggers, and response prevention removes this source of relief. At the beginning of therapy, therefore, short-term increases in obsessions and discomfort often occur as ritualistic urges are resisted. Strategies can be used to enable patients to continue exposure without resorting to ritual behaviors. For example, patients can remind themselves that distress is uncomfortable but not unbearable and that the aim of treatment is to learn how to live life even when obsessional thoughts and anxiety are present. A gradual approach to stopping rituals might be considered if patients have difficulty completely refraining, although complete abstinence from rituals should be upheld as a goal for therapy.

Some clinicians teach patients relaxation techniques to help manage anxiety that accompanies ERP, but this practice is counterproductive and should not be used. If exposure-induced anxiety is reduced or terminated via relaxation, this prevents patients from learning that anxiety is safe, manageable, and temporary. Such learning is crucial in overcoming OCD. Thus, relaxation techniques become as maladaptive as compulsive rituals. Moreover, the use of relaxation teaches patients that feelings of anxiety are something to be resisted, fought off, or escaped from. This is contrary to the idea of exposure therapy, which teaches patients to *endure* anxiety—a universal and adaptive experience that does not have serious consequences—regardless of intensity. In short, despite the intuitive appeal of techniques for directly reducing anxiety, relaxation training has no place in the treatment of OCD. (In fact, as reviewed in later sections of this chapter, it is used as a placebo intervention in controlled treatment studies.) Durable improvement in OCD requires that patients repeatedly experience the evocation of obsessional fear and subsequently observe that even when no rituals, escape, or avoidance behaviors are performed, feared disasters do not occur and the subjective distress is safe and manageable.

Managing Symptom Accommodation by Others

Individuals with OCD try to structure their environment so as to minimize their obsessional anxiety. Thus, patients may involve significant others in their OCD symptoms, such as by asking a partner to carry out checking rituals or provide reassurance to decrease obsessive doubts or by demanding that family members take off their "contaminated" clothes when they enter the house. In many instances, such symptom accommodation becomes a way of life for the family or couple because it provides short-term relief for the patient. Over the long term, however, this behavior inadvertently maintains OCD symptoms, because it has the same effect as if the patient were personally performing the ritual or avoidance behavior. Because symptom accommodation is counterproductive to ERP, significant others must be educated about the nature and treatment of OCD and taught more productive ways of managing patients' obsessional distress and requests for help with rituals. Specifically, family members can be taught to respond to requests for rituals by saying things like, "I know you feel very anxious right now, but I'm not supposed to do that ritual for you anymore. How can I help you get through this without reinforcing your OCD symptoms?" (Abramowitz 2006).

Mechanisms of Action

Traditional explanations for the effects of ERP emphasize *emotional processing*—the notion that 1) repeated and prolonged exposure corrects fear-based associations, which then leads to fear extinction (the type of learning that occurs during exposure), and 2) habituation of fear within and between exposure sessions is an index of such learning (e.g., Foa and Kozak 1986). More recent research on learning and memory has led to an updated *inhibitory learning framework* for understanding the effects of ERP. This model proposes that ERP does not result in "unlearning" fear-based associations but rather that it facilitates new safety-based associations that exist in memory alongside older fear-based associations. Thus, ERP is effective to the extent that it leads to the development of new safety learning that is strong enough to inhibit the older fear-based learning (Craske et al. 2008; Jacoby and Abramowitz 2016). Although not altogether incompatible with emotional processing accounts, the inhibitory learning model is distinct in that it proposes that learning fear *tolerance* leads to more durable inhibition of fear-based associations than does fear *reduction* (habituation) during exposure (Craske et al. 2008).

Efficacy and Effectiveness of Exposure and Response Prevention

Expert consensus treatment guidelines state that ERP is the first-line psychosocial intervention for OCD (Koran and Simpson 2013). In this section, we review empirical research on the outcome of ERP. Before turning to a review of individual treatment trials, let us first consider results from meta-analytic studies.

Meta-Analytic Findings

Data from a large number of controlled and uncontrolled outcome trials consistently indicate that ERP is extremely helpful in reducing OCD symptoms. A comprehensive meta-analysis of the controlled studies across various cognitive-behavioral interventions for OCD indicated that ERP was the most effective approach, with average symptom improvement rates of 50%–70% (Olatunji et al. 2013). This meta-analysis revealed a very large treatment effect size of 1.39 relative to control treatments (e.g., anxiety management training, relaxation) at posttreatment and a medium effect size of 0.43 at follow-up. These findings suggest that most patients with OCD who undergo treatment with ERP experience substantial short- and long-term benefit. Moreover, a meta-analysis of 13 randomized controlled trials (RCTs) directly comparing ERP to serotonin reuptake inhibitor (SRI) medications for OCD revealed small to medium effect sizes (0.37, 0.22) favoring ERP over selective serotonin reuptake inhibitors (SSRIs; Romanelli et al. 2014).

Randomized Controlled Trials

The Y-BOCS (Goodman et al. 1989a, 1989b), a 10-item semistructured clinical interview, is considered the gold standard as a measure of OCD severity. Because of its respectable psychometric properties (Taylor 1995), the Y-BOCS is widely used in OCD treatment outcome research and provides a measuring stick by which to compare results across studies. When administering the Y-BOCS, the interviewer rates the following five parameters for obsessions (items 1–5) and compulsions (items 6–10) on a scale from 0 (no symptoms) to 4 (extreme): time, interference with functioning, distress, resistance, and control. The total score is the sum of the 10 items and therefore ranges from 0 to 40. Y-BOCS scores of 0–7 tend to indicate subclinical OCD symptoms; scores of 8–15, mild symptoms; 16–25, moderate symptoms; 26–35, severe symptoms; and 36–40, extreme severity.

The efficacy of ERP for OCD was established via a handful of RCTs conducted in the 1990s and 2000s. Table 18–3 summarizes the results of the five most rigorous studies that used the Y-BOCS as an outcome measure. Two studies compared ERP with a credible psychotherapy control condition. Fals-Stewart et al. (1993) randomly assigned patients to individual ERP, group ERP, or a progressive relaxation control treatment. All treatments included 24 sessions delivered on a twice-weekly basis over 12 weeks. Although both ERP regimens were found to be superior to relaxation, no differences were found between group and individual ERP. Average improvement in the ERP groups was 41% on the Y-BOCS (vs. 9% for relaxation), and posttreatment scores fell within the mild range of severity.

In the second study, Lindsay et al. (1997) compared ERP to anxiety management training (AMT), a credible placebo treatment consisting of breathing retraining, relaxation, and problem-solving therapy. Both treatments were intensive: 15 daily sessions conducted over a 3-week period. On average, patients receiving ERP improved almost 62% from pretreatment to posttreatment on the Y-BOCS, with endpoint scores again in the mild range. In contrast, the AMT group showed a 6% *increase* in symptoms following treatment. The clear superiority of ERP over credible placebo therapies such as relaxation and AMT indicates that improvement in OCD symptoms can be attributed to the ERP procedures themselves, over and above any nonspecific factors such as time, attention, or expectancy of positive outcome.

van Balkom et al. (1998) examined the relative efficacy of five treatment conditions: 1) ERP, 2) CT, 3) ERP plus fluvoxamine, 4) CT plus fluvoxamine, and 5) waitlist control. As Table 18–3 indicates, ERP fared somewhat less well in this study than in other RCTs. A likely explanation for the 32% symptom reduction is that the ERP protocol was less than optimal. All exposure was conducted as homework assignments rather than in session under therapist supervision. Moreover, therapists did not discuss expectations of disastrous consequences with patients during the first 8 weeks of ERP

TABLE 18–3.   **Effects of exposure and response prevention (ERP) in randomized controlled trials**

		Y-BOCS total score, *mean (SD)*					
		ERP group			Control group		
Study	Control condition	*n*	Pre	Post	*n*	Pre	Post
Fals-Stewart et al. 1993*	Relaxation	31	20.2	12.1	32	19.9	18.1
Lindsay et al. 1997	Anxiety management	9	28.7 (4.6)	11.0 (3.8)	9	24.4 (7.0)	25.9 (5.8)
van Balkom et al. 1998	Waiting list	19	25.0 (7.9)	17.1 (8.4)	18	26.8 (6.4)	26.4 (6.8)
Foa et al. 2005	Pill placebo	29	24.6 (4.8)	11.0 (7.9)	26	25.0 (4.0)	22.2 (6.4)
Nakatani et al. 2005	Pill placebo	10	29.9 (3.1)	12.9 (4.9)	8	30.5 (3.7)	28.4 (5.5)

Note.   Y-BOCS=Yale-Brown Obsessive Compulsive Scale.
*Standard deviation not reported in the study.

because this would have overlapped substantially with CT. The waiting list was associated with a 2% reduction in OCD symptoms.

Foa et al. (2005) examined the relative efficacy of four treatment conditions: 1) intensive ERP (15 daily sessions including in-session exposure), 2) clomipramine, 3) combined treatment (ERP plus clomipramine), and 4) pill placebo. ERP produced a 50% Y-BOCS score reduction, which was far superior to the effects of pill placebo (11%). Moreover, endpoint Y-BOCS scores fell to within the mild range of OCD severity. In a similar study, Nakatani et al. (2005) randomly assigned patients to receive either weekly ERP sessions, fluvoxamine, or pill placebo. The ERP group evinced a mean Y-BOCS score reduction of 58%, which was superior to that reported for the placebo group (7%). Moreover, at posttest, the ERP group's Y-BOCS scores were again within the mild range of symptoms. Overall, then, the findings from RCTs suggest that ERP produces substantial and clinically meaningful improvement in OCD symptoms and that symptom reduction is attributable to the specific effects of these treatment procedures and not to nonspecific or "common" factors of psychotherapy.

Comparisons With Medication

Numerous randomized, double-blind, placebo-controlled trials have established the efficacy of pharmacotherapy with SRIs (e.g., fluvoxamine) for OCD (Montgomery et al. 1993; see Chapter 17, "Pharmacotherapy for Obsessive-Compulsive Disorder"). Given that both ERP and SRIs are effective treatments, researchers have attempted to examine their relative efficacy. For example, the study by Foa et al. (2005) included comparisons among 12 weeks of ERP, of clomipramine, and of the combination of ERP plus clomipramine. Immediately following treatment, all active therapies showed superiority to placebo, yet ERP (mean 50% Y-BOCS reduction) was superior to clomipramine (mean 35% Y-BOCS reduction). It is important to note that patients in this study received intensive ERP, meaning daily treatment sessions. Thus, this treatment regimen is not necessarily representative of typical clinical practice.

The study by Nakatani et al. (2005) also included a relevant comparison between ERP and fluvoxamine. The ERP program consisted of 12 weekly treatment sessions in which exposure exercises were planned for practice between sessions. Thus, most of the ERP work was conducted by the patient alone rather than supervised by a therapist. Still, the 58% Y-BOCS reduction with ERP was significantly greater than the 29% reduction observed in the fluvoxamine group. These two studies indicate that ERP, even in patient-directed format, is a more effective treatment than pharmacotherapy with SRIs such as fluvoxamine. No recent studies have compared ERP to other forms of medication.

Combining Exposure and Response Prevention With Medication

Benzodiazepines are contraindicated during ERP (Deacon 2006) because their use serves as a safety signal and prevents the patient from learning that obsessional fear declines naturally even if the medication is not used. With regard to simultaneous treatment with ERP and SRIs, available studies generally indicate superior outcome compared with SRI monotherapy but not with ERP alone (Cottraux et al. 1990; Foa et al. 2005; Hohagen et al. 1998; O'Connor et al. 1999; van Balkom et al. 1998). Importantly, many of the available studies have limitations, such as the exclusion of patients with comorbidity—perhaps the very patients who would show the greatest benefit from combined treatment. Some investigators have examined pairing ERP with pharmacological cognitive enhancers such as D-cycloserine (DCS), yohimbine hydrochloride, and methylene blue (Williams et al. 2014). These agents are thought to facilitate ERP by acting on brain regions implicated in fear learning and extinction (Singewald et al. 2015). The most well studied of these agents is DCS, a partial agonist of the glutamatergic NMDA receptor in the amygdala (which is involved in fear conditioning and extinction). Placebo-controlled studies with OCD samples, however, yield inconsistent findings, with effect sizes ranging from 0.89 (in favor of DCS; Kushner et al. 2007) to −0.19 (in favor of placebo; Storch et al. 2007). Finally, a few studies have found that adding ERP improves outcome following one or more adequate trials of SRIs (Kampman et al. 2002; Simpson et al. 1999; Tenneij et al. 2005; Tolin et al. 2004). Results found by Tenneij et al. (2005) suggest that even medication *responders* can benefit further from adjunctive ERP. These data have substantial clinical implications, given that medication is the most widely available and most widely used form of treatment for OCD, yet it typically produces modest improvement.

Effectiveness of Exposure and Response Prevention in Non-Research Settings

Although RCTs substantiate the efficacy of ERP, such studies are conducted under highly controlled research conditions. Thus, an important question concerns whether the beneficial effects of this treatment extend beyond the "ivory tower" to typical service delivery settings that serve less rarefied patient populations and where therapists do not receive supervision from top experts on ERP. Several studies have addressed this issue, reporting on outcomes in naturalistic settings (Franklin et al. 2000; Rothbaum and Shahar 2000; Warren and Thomas 2001). In the largest study, Franklin et al. (2000) examined outcomes for 110 consecutively referred individuals with OCD who received 15 sessions of intensive ERP on an outpatient fee-for-service basis. Half of this sample had comorbid Axis I or Axis II diagnoses, and patients were denied ERP only if they were actively psychotic, abusing substances, or suicidal. Patients treated with ERP showed improvement as reflected by mean Y-BOCS scores that decreased from 26.8 to 11.8 (60% reduction in OCD symptoms). Moreover, only 10 patients dropped out of treatment prematurely.

In a multicultural naturalistic study, Friedman et al. (2003) found that although treatment was effective in reducing OCD and depressive symptoms, many patients reported significant residual symptoms after therapy. Mean Y-BOCS scores for African American patients decreased from 23.5 pretreatment to 17.2 posttreatment (27% reduction), and those for white patients decreased from 26.03 pretreatment to 17.65 posttreatment (32% reduction). No between-group differences in treatment outcomes were found. Taken together, the findings from these naturalistic studies indicate that the effects of ERP for OCD can be transportable from highly controlled research settings to typical clinical settings that serve more heterogeneous patient populations.

Predictors of Outcome With Exposure and Response Prevention

Although ERP is a highly effective intervention, not all patients show a satisfactory response. Therefore, it would be desirable to be able to predict whether a given patient is likely to respond. Although a multitude of studies have provided relatively inconsistent findings, a number of variables appear to be associated reliably with outcome. In one systematic review, Knopp et al. (2013) found that hoarding symptoms, increased anxiety and OCD symptom severity, unemployment, and being single/not married were associated with poorer treatment outcomes, whereas medication use, age of OCD onset, strength of OCD-related cognitions, and educational level failed to show an association with outcomes. Although some studies have found that the severity of depressive symptoms predicts poorer response to ERP (Abramowitz et al. 2000), a meta-analytic review did not detect consistency in this finding across numerous controlled studies (Olatunji et al. 2013).

Results also have been conflicting as to whether the patient's level of marital satisfaction affects the efficacy of ERP for OCD (Emmelkamp et al. 1990; Hafner 1982; Riggs et al. 1992). What is clearer is that hostility toward the patient from relatives is associated with poor response and premature dropout from ERP (Chambless and Steketee 1999). In contrast, when relatives express dissatisfaction with the patient's symptoms, but not personal rejection, such constructive criticism may have motivational properties that enhance treatment response (Chambless and Steketee 1999).

Other Psychosocial Approaches

Cognitive Therapy

Whereas behavioral approaches to understanding OCD date back to the 1960s, the application of cognitive principles to understanding and treating OCD is more recent, having occurred during the 1980s and 1990s. The basis of *cognitive therapy* is the rational and evidence-based challenging and correction of the irrational thoughts and beliefs that underlie obsessional fear (Clark 2004). Compared with ERP, cognitive approaches incorporate fewer prolonged exposures to fear cues. However, some authors champion *cognitive-behavioral therapy* (CBT), which entails CT combined with "behavioral experiments"—essentially mini-exposure exercises used to demonstrate erroneous beliefs and assumptions (e.g., using knives around a loved one to test beliefs about acting on unwanted urges to stab).

Cognitive interventions for OCD were derived from 1) cognitive formulations of OCD, which posit that particular sorts of dysfunctional beliefs play an important role in the psychopathology of this disorder, and 2) the assertion that modifying faulty thinking patterns could reduce OCD symptoms. Over the past 30 years, various cognitive models have been proposed, most of which represent variations of Salkovskis's (1996) formulation. These models begin with the well-established finding that unwanted intrusive thoughts (e.g., those regarding sex, aggression, and harm) are universal experiences (Rachman and de Silva 1978). Clinical obsessions arise, however, when these intrusions are misinterpreted as having serious implications for which the person having the thoughts would be personally responsible (e.g., "Thinking about harming the baby means I'm a dangerous person who must take extra care to ensure that I don't lose control"). Such an appraisal evokes distress and motivates the person to try to suppress or remove the unwanted intrusion (e.g., by replacing it with a "good" thought) and to attempt to prevent harmful events associated with the thought (e.g., by avoiding the baby).

Compulsions and avoidance behaviors are conceptualized as instrumental for averting or undoing harm or for reducing the perceived responsibility for aversive outcomes. However, compulsions prevent the correction of mistaken beliefs by robbing the person of the opportunity to see that obsessional fears are unfounded. That is, when a compulsive ritual is performed and the feared event does not take place, the individual mistakenly attributes this to the ritual rather than to the low probability of danger (e.g., "If I had not avoided bathing the infant, I would have drowned her").

Based on these models, CT for OCD focuses on modifying pathological interpretations of intrusive thoughts and correcting the associated dysfunctional beliefs (Clark 2004; Wilhelm and Steketee 2006). Treatment begins by educating patients about the cognitive model and the rationale for CT. For example, patients are taught that their intrusive thoughts are not indicative of anything important but that a problem arises if such thoughts are perceived as unacceptable or threatening. Patients are helped to understand that *the way that* they interpret the intrusive thoughts is the source of the problem, leading to distress and to maladaptive behaviors such as compulsions. Once the unwanted intrusions are correctly perceived as nonthreatening, then the obsessions and the associated compulsions can be eliminated.

How effective are cognitive treatments, compared with ERP? A meta-analysis by Abramowitz et al. (2002) that included five studies directly comparing ERP and CT/CBT suggested no difference in the effectiveness of these treatment modalities. Closer examination, however, revealed that effect sizes for the cognitive treatments were larger when behavioral experiments were included in the cognitive protocols. In other words, ERP and CBT have similar treatment efficacy, yet CT that does not include exposure in any form appears to be less effective than ERP or CBT. Moreover, the efficacy of ERP was most likely to be greater than that of both CT and CBT when

ERP involved therapist-assisted exposure rather than only homework-based exposure. Properly implemented ERP involves both types of exposure.

Acceptance and Commitment Therapy

An even more recent development in the psychological treatment of OCD is the application of ACT, which is grounded in functional contextualism and relational frame theory (Hayes et al. 2011). ACT is an experiential approach that suggests that the context (e.g., historical, situational) in which behavior evolves is useful for predicting and changing psychological events. Events with a similar form may serve different functions; for example, counting is only conceptualized as a compulsion in OCD when considered in relation to the presence of obsessions, the client's history, and the function of the counting. ACT sessions involve metaphorical discussions of these concepts, with "homework" suggestions to supplement what has been discussed. ACT's effectiveness is gauged by the degree to which patients experience improvement in valued living (individually defined) as opposed to reduction in psychological symptoms.

Specifically, ACT aims to foster *psychological flexibility*—that is, being present in the moment without becoming entangled in private experiences such as thoughts and emotions—and a willingness to experience unwanted private events (e.g., obsessional thoughts, anxiety). Accordingly, the goal of ACT for OCD is to help patients strive toward what is important and meaningful to them despite the presence of unwanted thoughts, anxiety, and urges to perform rituals. This is accomplished through acceptance (embracing private experiences without trying to change them), cognitive defusion (seeing obsessions as *words* rather than as *rules*), awareness of the present moment (nonjudgmentally attending to the present), self-as-context (developing perspective as someone who *experiences* fears versus *being* one's fears), values (motivating one's therapeutic work toward meaningful areas of life), and committed action (moving in the direction of one's values).

Although ACT does not include explicit ERP techniques, it does aim to broaden patients' engagement with feared stimuli and to improve their quality of life. Accordingly, we have developed an ACT-based ERP program (see Twohig et al. 2015 for a full description) that aims to 1) foster patients' willingness to experience obsessions, anxiety, and uncertainty and respond flexibly in their presence; 2) help patients recognize thoughts and feelings as neither right nor wrong (i.e., "cognitive defusion"); and 3) help patients move toward what they value in their lives. This program makes use of numerous ACT metaphors that are discussed in the context of OCD and its treatment. *Willingness*, in this context, refers to being open to "experiencing one's own experience" without trying to change, avoid, or escape it. Patients are helped to understand the goal of treatment as developing a healthier and more welcoming (e.g., more peaceful) relationship with OCD-related thoughts and anxiety (rather than trying to reduce these experiences).

Patients are also helped to shift away from rigidly evaluating obsessional thoughts and other OCD-related private experiences as facts (e.g., "dangerous," "immoral") and instead to simply observe these experiences and decide for themselves how much weight to give them. An exemplary metaphor is a game of chess with its two opposing teams. One team's pieces represent obsessional thoughts and anxiety, whereas the other team's pieces represent feelings of safety and being in control. The therapist can point out that the two opposing teams are actually both within the patient; in other words, as soon as the patient chooses a team, he or she is fighting him- or herself and therefore cannot win the game. The therapist and patient can discuss how things would be different if the patient assumed the role of *chess board* instead of one of the teams. As the board, the patient is in contact with the pieces (noticing them and remaining aware of what they are doing), but the outcome of the game is not important. ERP presents opportunities to practice "being the board."

In an RCT for OCD, Twohig et al. (2010) compared the effectiveness of eight sessions of ACT to progressive relaxation training (with no in-session exposure). ACT involved no explicit ERP instructions, although patients engaged between sessions in values-based "behavioral commitments" (e.g., pursuing a meaningful activity without engaging in compulsions) without reference to explicit goals of anxiety reduction. ACT produced superior OCD symptom reduction relative to relaxation at posttreatment (47% vs. 27%) and at follow-up (51% vs. 36%). In a direct comparison between ACT-informed ERP and traditional ERP, no differences were found in outcome, in quality of life, or in dropout rate or compliance with exposure (Twohig et al. 2018).

Interpersonal Aspects of OCD and Treatment

Given that many individuals with OCD are involved in close relationships (e.g., marriages), more and more consideration has been given to understanding this condition from an interpersonal perspective. Importantly, a bidirectional association exists in which OCD symptoms often lead to a strain on close relationships, and aspects of the relationship contribute to the maintenance of OCD. For example, nonaffected spouses or partners might (albeit inadvertently) maintain their loved ones' OCD symptoms by "helping" with avoidance and rituals (e.g., checking or providing reassurance for the patient) (Calvocoressi et al. 1999). Such *symptom accommodation* can occur among relationally distressed as well as nondistressed couples and might be performed to prevent the person with OCD from becoming overly anxious (or hostile) or simply as a way of expressing care and concern within the relationship. Interpersonal factors impact OCD symptoms when avoidance and rituals give rise to relationship conflict, which elevates stress and exacerbates OCD symptoms. Finally, couples might struggle with chronic relationship discord unrelated to OCD (e.g., financial or childcare concerns) that increases stress and worsens obsessions and compulsions (Abramowitz et al. 2013b).

This bidirectional association suggests that for patients in intimate relationships, ERP could be enhanced by involving the partner in treatment and addressing the ways in which relationship factors maintain OCD. A handful of older studies that examined "partner-assisted" ERP for OCD reported mixed results. Mehta (1990), for example, found that including a partner as a coach during ERP was more effective than when ERP did not involve such a coach. Emmelkamp et al. (1990), however, found no between-group differences in a similarly designed comparison. Earlier still, Emmelkamp and de Lange (1983) had reported that partner-assisted ERP was more effective than unassisted ERP at posttest but not at 1-month follow-up.

We (Abramowitz et al. 2013b) recently developed a comprehensive couples-based ERP program focusing on communication training, partner-assisted exposure, and accommodation reduction. This program begins with an assessment of OCD symptoms as well as ways the couple has structured their environment so as to accommodate OCD. Next, the conceptual model of OCD and rationale for ERP are presented to both partners to increase patience and hopefulness and to reduce misunderstanding and criticism. The patient's partner is then taught how to assist with exposure therapy by serving as a coach and helping the patient "get through" the obsessional anxiety as opposed to trying to alleviate this distress. The patient and partner are taught two types of communication skills to help them complete exposure practices as a team: 1) *emotional expressiveness*, in which the partners are taught how to discuss with one another how they feel (as opposed to offering solutions), and 2) *decision making* as a team regarding implementing ERP. When symptom accommodation is present, treatment focuses on changing such interaction patterns. Finally, for couples who experience relationship distress outside the context of OCD (e.g., over finances or childcare), general couple or family interventions (e.g., communication training) are used to optimize family and relationship functioning more broadly.

In a trial of 16 couples who received this treatment (Abramowitz et al. 2013a), we found a large within-group effect size on OCD symptoms at posttreatment (55% symptom reduction; effect size 2.68) that was maintained at 12-month follow-up (56% symptom reduction; effect size 2.42). Moreover, these effect sizes were notably larger than for comparable individual ERP-based treatment (e.g., Vogel et al. [2004] reported within-group effect sizes of 2.06 at 12-month follow-up). Partners also evidenced medium to large reductions in their level of accommodation of OCD symptoms and showed improvement in their own levels of distress and relationship satisfaction and functioning (e.g., better communication, less criticism) (Belus et al. 2014).

Special Populations

Mental Ritualizers

It was long thought that some individuals with OCD had obsessions without compulsive rituals (referred to as "pure obsessions"). Moreover, such patients were considered highly resistant to ERP (Baer 1994). More recently, however, clearer recognition of the frequency of mental rituals (often mistaken for obsessions because they are not visibly apparent behaviors) and covert neutralizing responses ("mini-rituals") has led to a reconceptualization of pure obsessions as "obsessions with covert rituals" (Abramowitz et al. 2003; Clark and Guyitt 2008; Rachman 1993). This conceptualization led to the development of effective treatment for such patients. Specifically, Freeston et al. (1997) obtained excellent results with a treatment package that contained the following elements: 1) education about cognitive and behavioral models of OCD; 2) ERP, consisting of in-session and homework exposure in which the patient repeatedly writes out the obsession, says it aloud, or records it on a continuous-loop recording and then plays it back repeatedly on a portable device (Salkovskis and Westbrook 1989) while refraining from covert rituals and mental compulsions; and 3) CT, targeting exaggerated responsibility, inappropriate interpretations of intrusive thoughts, and inflated estimates of the probability and severity of negative outcomes. Compared with patients in a waitlist control group, treated patients achieved substantial improvement: among all treated patients ($n=28$), Y-BOCS scores improved from 23.9 to 9.8 (62%) after an average of 25.7 sessions over 19.2 weeks. Moreover, treated patients retained their gains at 6-month follow-up (mean Y-BOCS score 10.8; 55% symptom reduction from baseline). This study demonstrated that ERP and CT can be successfully combined in the management of a presentation of OCD that had previously been considered resistant to psychological treatment.

Patients With Treatment-Refractory OCD

Patients with poor insight about their OCD symptoms improve less with ERP than do those who have greater insight (Foa et al. 1999). Perhaps patients with poor insight have difficulty making changes as a result of exposure exercises. Alternatively, those with poor insight may be more reluctant to confront obsessional situations during therapy because of their fears. Although ERP is recommended even for patients with poor insight, those who struggle with this approach may benefit from the addition of cognitive techniques. A second augmentative approach in such cases is pharmacotherapy with SSRIs, and some psychiatrists will even prescribe antipsychotic medication for such patients.

Some comorbid Axis I conditions can impede the effects of CBT for OCD. Major depressive disorder (Abramowitz and Foa 2000) and generalized anxiety disorder (Steketee et al. 2001) are particularly associated with poorer response to ERP. Perhaps seriously depressed patients become demoralized and experience difficulties in complying with CBT instructions. Strong negative affect also may exacerbate OCD symptoms and limit treatment gains. For patients with generalized anxiety disorder, pervasive worry concerning other life issues is liable to detract from the time and emotional resources available for learning skills from ERP treatment (Steketee et al. 2001). Other Axis I conditions likely to interfere with ERP are those involving psychotic and manic symptoms that produce alterations in perception, cognition, and judgment. Active substance abuse or dependence also rules out the use of CBT. These problems presumably impede patients' ability to follow treatment instructions on their own or to attend to the cognitive changes that CBT aims to facilitate. It is therefore important for patients to receive treatment for these comorbid conditions before attempting ERP for OCD.

Practical Techniques

Cognitive and behavioral (i.e., ERP) treatments are time-limited, skills-based therapies in which the therapist takes a role akin to that of a coach or teacher, and the patient takes the role of student. Treatment is typically provided on an individual basis and generally lasts from 12 to 20 sessions. Although each session has a more or less specific agenda, session time is generally spent helping patients develop skills for reducing obsessions and compulsions. Homework practice is assigned for patients to complete between sessions to gain mastery of these skills. As suggested in the previous literature review, treatment can take place on various schedules, including weekly or twice-weekly sessions. A few specialty clinics offer treatment for OCD on an intensive basis, meaning 15 daily outpatient treatment sessions over a period of approximately 3 weeks. A practical advantage of the intensive approach over less intensive schedules is that massed sessions allow for regular therapist supervision, permitting rapid correction of subtle avoidance, rituals, or suboptimal exposure practice that might otherwise compromise outcome. Therefore, intensive therapy is recommended in cases of severe OCD and when patients encounter extreme difficulty resisting compulsive urges. The primary disadvantage of intensive therapy is that such a course entails frequent meetings, which can present scheduling issues for both the clinician and the patient.

Group Cognitive-Behavioral Therapy

Group CBT programs that emphasize ERP and cognitive techniques have been found to be effective in reducing OCD symptoms (Anderson and Rees 2007; McLean et al. 2001; Volpato Cordioli et al. 2003). In one study, a 12-week program of group therapy emphasizing ERP was more effective than group therapy emphasizing CT techniques, although both programs were more effective than a waitlist control condition (McLean et al. 2001). In another investigation, group CBT resulted in significant improvement relative to results for the waitlist group, and patients continued to improve at 3-month follow-up (Volpato Cordioli et al. 2003). In the only study directly comparing individual and group CBT (involving CT and ERP techniques) for OCD, Anderson and Rees (2007) found that receiving 10 weeks of either treatment was more effective than being on the waitlist but that no differences were found between group and individual treatments. Average posttest and follow-up Y-BOCS scores were in the 16–18 range (indicating mild symptom severity). Strengths of a group approach to the treatment of OCD include the support and cohesion that are nonspecific effects of group therapy. Potential disadvantages, however, include the relative lack of attention to each individual's particular symptom presentation, particularly given the heterogeneity of OCD.

Residential and Hospital-Based Treatment

Although most psychiatric hospitals are equipped to provide standard care for patients with OCD, programming in such facilities is often limited by the short duration of stay and lack of expertise in implementing ERP. Therefore, the initial focus in most hospitals is on stabilizing patients via medication and nonspecific psychotherapy (e.g., supportive counseling, stress management training). Now, however, a handful of residential facilities in the United States have specialized programs offering long-term inpatient treatment for severe OCD. The programs typically include individual and group ERP and cognitive interventions, medication management, and supportive therapy for comorbid psychiatric conditions. Lengths of stay may vary from a few weeks to a month or longer. Two facilities that offer such services as of this writing are the Obsessive-Compulsive Disorders Institute at McLean Hospital (Belmont, Massachusetts) and the Obsessive-Compulsive Disorder Center at Rogers Memorial Hospital (Oconomowoc, Wisconsin).

One advantage of specialized residential OCD programs is that they provide constant supervision for patients requiring help with implementing treatment (i.e., conducting self-directed ERP). Moreover, such programs are ideal for individuals who lack family or friends to assist with treatment or who have severe impairment in functioning, suicidal risk, or comorbid medical complications. A disadvantage, however, is that such programs often are costly. In addition, patients with obsessions and compulsions regarding specific places or stimuli (e.g., bathrooms at home) may have difficulty reproducing these feared situations within the hospital setting for the purposes of exposure. Thus, generalization of treatment effects must be considered. The only study to directly compare inpatient and outpatient ERP for OCD found no differences in outcome between 20 sessions of outpatient and 5.4 months of inpatient treatment (van den Hout et al. 1988).

Internet, Telehealth, and Smartphone Applications

Innovative delivery formats that increase accessibility to ERP are gaining popularity. Internet, telehealth, and smartphone application (app) platforms show promise for improving treatment dissemination by enabling low-cost and efficient alternatives to traditional face-to-face therapy. In this section, we review several such approaches.

Andersson et al. (2012) conducted an RCT investigating the efficacy of an internet-based CBT (iCBT) program for OCD that gave patients access to self-help modules *and* an online therapist. They found that participants in the iCBT group had larger improvements (40% Y-BOCS score reduction) than those assigned to an attention control group (10% reduction). CBT delivery methods that use telephone and webcam communication have also demonstrated efficacy. In a systematic literature review, Tumur et al. (2007) reported that BTSteps, a software program and touch-tone telephone system that provided automated guidance, consistently led to symptom reduction (effect size 0.84), and demonstrated acceptability and feasibility. Storch et al. (2011) found that children and adolescents with OCD who were assigned to family-based CBT delivered via web camera had 56% greater improvement in OCD symptoms, whereas those assigned to a waitlist control group had only 13% improvement.

A number of smartphone apps have been designed to walk individuals through assessment, education, and ERP. One app, the Mayo Clinic Anxiety Coach, is designed to deliver ERP for OCD (and other anxiety-related problems). Case examples suggest that this app enhances treatment of pediatric OCD (Whiteside et al. 2014). Additional apps have been developed for OCD assessment and treatment, but empirical support has not yet been established (Van Ameringen et al. 2017). For example, Apple's iTunes offers a mobile Y-BOCS assessment app and an OCD treatment app based on ERP principles. Although neither has been formally validated, the latter is currently being studied.

Mataix-Cols and Marks (2006) proposed a stepped-care model for the treatment of OCD in which individuals with less severe symptoms receive immediate access to self-guided treatment, freeing up time for therapists to work face-to-face with patients who have more complex symptoms. Reducing the time clinicians spend with each patient means that more people can receive effective treatment without increasing cost or therapist burden. More research is needed, however, to identify patient characteristics associated with adherence and outcome. Wootton et al. (2011) found that only 22% of patients believed that online therapy would improve their symptoms substantially; thus, many individuals are unwilling to incorporate technology into treatment. Despite the various challenges involved, the integration of technology and behavioral health is an exciting step toward improving access and adherence to evidence-based treatments for OCD.

Conclusion

Few psychological disorders result in as much distress and functional impairment as OCD (Barlow 2002). Despite the lack of a definitive theory of the etiology of obsessions and compulsions, research has led to a very clear understanding of the processes that *maintain* these symptoms. ERP and CT, which are derived from this understanding, have received consistent empirical support, leading to a good prognosis for most patients. By far the most studied psychological intervention for OCD is ERP, which often produces substantial, immediate, and durable reductions in OCD symptoms. Evidence from effectiveness studies suggests that ERP is transportable to nonresearch settings and therefore should be a first-line treatment modality for patients with OCD in general clinical settings (March et al. 1997). Moreover, ERP is quite helpful in alleviating OCD symptoms that do not respond satisfactorily to pharmacotherapy. Even though these results are encouraging, full remission with psychological treatment is not the standard (Abramowitz 1998); response is, in fact, highly variable. Researchers are beginning to uncover factors that reliably predict poor response to ERP, including severe depression and lack of insight into the senselessness of obsessional fears.

Given the significant advances in OCD research and treatment over the past century, it is heartening to look back at how far we have come. We can also look forward with hope that researchers will address critical areas that warrant further study. For example, patient motivation to begin treatment, especially given the anxiety-provoking nature of ERP, is a problem. Readiness programs, in which patients read case histories or discuss treatment with former patients, might decrease refusal rates and increase treatment compliance. From the clinician's perspective, engineering and executing successful exposure-based therapy can often be a challenge. Indeed, the greatest barrier to successful treatment of OCD is that relatively few clinicians receive the kind of training needed to become proficient in these procedures. Therefore, research and development of programs for teaching service providers how to implement psychological treatments for OCD will have a major impact on improving access to these effective interventions.

Key Points

- Exposure and response prevention (ERP) involves helping patients engage with feared stimuli and obsessional thoughts while resisting the urge to perform compulsive rituals.

- ERP is the most effective treatment for OCD, as demonstrated in controlled comparisons with other forms of psychological treatment as well as with selective serotonin reuptake inhibitors (SSRIs).

- Although adding SSRIs or clomipramine does not enhance the efficacy of ERP, the effects of these medications can be augmented by adding ERP.

- ERP is also known to be effective in nonresearch clinical settings.

- Severe comorbid depression, generalized anxiety disorder, and poor insight into the senselessness of the obsessions and compulsions of OCD are predictors of poor outcome with ERP.

- Cognitive therapy is an efficacious treatment for OCD, but it is not as effective as ERP.

References

Abramowitz JS: Does cognitive-behavioral therapy cure obsessive-compulsive disorder? A meta-analytic evaluation of clinical significance. Behav Ther 29:339–355, 1998

Abramowitz JS: Understanding and Treating Obsessive-Compulsive Disorder: A Cognitive-Behavioral Approach. Mahwah, NJ, Erlbaum, 2006

Abramowitz JS, Foa EB: Does comorbid major depressive disorder influence outcome of exposure and response prevention for OCD? Behav Ther 31:795–800, 2000

Abramowitz JS, Franklin ME, Street GP, et al: Effects of comorbid depression on response to treatment for obsessive-compulsive disorder. Behav Ther 31:517–528, 2000

Abramowitz JS, Franklin ME, Foa EB: Empirical status of cognitive-behavioral therapy for obsessive-compulsive disorder: a meta-analytic review. Rom J Cogn Behav Psychother 2:89–104, 2002

Abramowitz JS, Franklin ME, Schwartz SA, et al: Symptom presentation and outcome of cognitive-behavioral therapy for obsessive-compulsive disorder. J Consult Clin Psychol 71(6):1049–1057, 2003 14622080

Abramowitz JS, Deacon BJ, Olatunji BO, et al: Assessment of obsessive-compulsive symptom dimensions: development and evaluation of the Dimensional Obsessive-Compulsive Scale. Psychol Assess 22(1):180–198, 2010 20230164

Abramowitz JS, Baucom DH, Boeding S, et al: Treating obsessive-compulsive disorder in intimate relationships: a pilot study of couple-based cognitive-behavior therapy. Behav Ther 44(3):395–407, 2013a 23768667

Abramowitz JS, Baucom DH, Wheaton MG, et al: Enhancing exposure and response prevention for OCD: a couple-based approach. Behav Modif 37(2):189–210, 2013b 22619395

Anderson RA, Rees CS: Group versus individual cognitive-behavioural treatment for obsessive-compulsive disorder: a controlled trial. Behav Res Ther 45(1):123–137, 2007 16540080

Andersson E, Enander J, Andrén P, et al: Internet-based cognitive behaviour therapy for obsessive-compulsive disorder: a randomized controlled trial. Psychol Med 42:2193–2203, 2012 22348650

Baer L: Factor analysis of symptom subtypes of obsessive compulsive disorder and their relation to personality and tic disorders. J Clin Psychiatry 55(suppl):18–23, 1994 8077163

Barlow DH: Anxiety and Its Disorders. New York, Guilford, 2002

Belus JM, Baucom DH, Abramowitz JS: The effect of a couple-based treatment for OCD on intimate partners. J Behav Ther Exp Psychiatry 45(4):484–488, 2014 25086352

Calvocoressi L, Mazure CM, Kasl SV, et al: Family accommodation of obsessive-compulsive symptoms: instrument development and assessment of family behavior. J Nerv Ment Dis 187(10):636–642, 1999 10535658

Chambless DL, Steketee G: Expressed emotion and behavior therapy outcome: a prospective study with obsessive-compulsive and agoraphobic outpatients. J Consult Clin Psychol 67(5):658–665, 1999 10535232

Clark DA: Cognitive-Behavioral Therapy for OCD. New York, Guilford, 2004

Clark DA, Guyitt B: Pure obsessions: conceptual misnomer or clinical anomaly?, in Obsessive Compulsive Disorder: Subtypes and Spectrum Conditions. Edited by Abramowitz JS, McKay D, Taylor S. Amsterdam, Netherlands, Elsevier, 2008, pp 53–75

Cottraux J, Mollard E, Bouvard M, et al: A controlled study of fluvoxamine and exposure in obsessive-compulsive disorder. Int Clin Psychopharmacol 5(1):17–30, 1990 2110206

Craske MG, Kircanski K, Zelikowsky M, et al: Optimizing inhibitory learning during exposure therapy. Behav Res Ther 46(1):5–27, 2008 18005936

Deacon BJ: The effect of pharmacotherapy on the effect of exposure therapy, in Handbook of Exposure Therapies. Edited by Richard D, Lauterbach D. Amsterdam, Netherlands, Elsevier, 2006, pp 311–333

Emmelkamp PM, de Lange I: Spouse involvement in the treatment of obsessive-compulsive patients. Behav Res Ther 21(4):341–346, 1983

Emmelkamp PMG, de Haan E, Hoogduin CAL: Marital adjustment and obsessive-compulsive disorder. Br J Psychiatry 156:55–60, 1990 1967545

Fals-Stewart W, Marks AP, Schafer J: A comparison of behavioral group therapy and individual behavior therapy in treating obsessive-compulsive disorder. J Nerv Ment Dis 181(3):189–193, 1993 8445378

Foa EB, Kozak MJ: Emotional processing of fear: exposure to corrective information. Psychol Bull 99(1):20–35, 1986 2871574

Foa EB, Kozak MJ, Goodman WK, et al: DSM-IV field trial: obsessive-compulsive disorder. Am J Psychiatry 152(1):90–96, 1995 7802127

Foa EB, Abramowitz JS, Franklin ME, et al: Feared consequences, fixity of belief, and treatment outcome in patients with obsessive-compulsive disorder. Behav Ther 30:717–724, 1999

Foa EB, Liebowitz MR, Kozak MJ, et al: Randomized, placebo-controlled trial of exposure and ritual prevention, clomipramine, and their combination in the treatment of obsessive-compulsive disorder. Am J Psychiatry 162:151–161, 2005 15625214

Franklin ME, Abramowitz JS, Kozak MJ, et al: Effectiveness of exposure and ritual prevention for obsessive-compulsive disorder: randomized compared with nonrandomized samples. J Consult Clin Psychol 68(4):594–602, 2000 10965635

Freeston MH, Ladouceur R, Gagnon F, et al: Cognitive-behavioral treatment of obsessive thoughts: a controlled study. J Consult Clin Psychol 65(3):405–413, 1997 9170763

Freud S: Notes upon a case of obsessional neurosis (1909), in Standard Edition of the Complete Psychological Works of Sigmund Freud, Vol 10. Translated and edited by Strachey J. London, Hogarth, 1955, pp 151–318

Friedman S, Smith LC, Halpern B, et al: Obsessive-compulsive disorder in a multi-ethnic urban outpatient clinic: initial presentation and treatment outcome with exposure and ritual prevention. Behav Ther 34:397–410, 2003

Emmelkamp PM, de Haan E, Hoogduin CA: Marital adjustment and obsessive-compulsive disorder. Br J Psychiatry 156:55–60, 1990 1967545

Goodman WK, Price LH, Rasmussen SA, et al: The Yale-Brown Obsessive Compulsive Scale. I. Development, use, and reliability. Arch Gen Psychiatry 46(11):1006–1011, 1989a 2684084

Goodman WK, Price LH, Rasmussen SA, et al: The Yale-Brown Obsessive Compulsive Scale. II. Validity. Arch Gen Psychiatry 46(11):1012–1016, 1989b 2510699

Hafner RJ: Marital interaction in persisting obsessive-compulsive disorders. Aust N Z J Psychiatry 16(3):171–178, 1982 6960888

Hayes SC, Strosahl KD, Wilson KG: Acceptance and Commitment Therapy: The Process and Practice of Mindful Change. New York, Guilford, 2011

Hohagen F, Winkelmann G, Rasche-Rüchle H, et al: Combination of behaviour therapy with fluvoxamine in comparison with behaviour therapy and placebo. Results of a multicentre study. Br J Psychiatry Suppl 173(35):71–78, 1998 9829029

Jacoby RJ, Abramowitz JS: Inhibitory learning approaches to exposure therapy: a critical review and translation to obsessive-compulsive disorder. Clin Psychol Rev 49:28–40, 2016 27521505

Kampman M, Keijsers GPJ, Hoogduin CAL, et al: Addition of cognitive-behaviour therapy for obsessive-compulsive disorder patients non-responding to fluoxetine. Acta Psychiatr Scand 106(4):314–319, 2002 12225499

Knopp J, Knowles S, Bee P, et al: A systematic review of predictors and moderators of response to psychological therapies in OCD: do we have enough empirical evidence to target treatment? Clin Psychol Rev 33(8):1067–1081, 2013 24077387

Koran LM, Simpson HB: Guideline Watch (March 2013): Practice Guideline for the Treatment of Patients With Obsessive-Compulsive Disorder. Arlington, VA, American Psychiatric Association, March 2013. Available at: https://psychiatryonline.org/pb/assets/raw/sitewide/practice_guidelines/guidelines/ocd-watch.pdf. Accessed June 24, 2019.

Kushner MG, Kim SW, Donahue C, et al: d-Cycloserine augmented exposure therapy for obsessive-compulsive disorder. Biol Psychiatry 62(8):835–838, 2007 17588545

Lindsay M, Crino R, Andrews G: Controlled trial of exposure and response prevention in obsessive-compulsive disorder. Br J Psychiatry 171:135–139, 1997 9337948

March JS, Frances A, Carpenter D, et al: The Expert Consensus Guidelines series: treatment of obsessive-compulsive disorder. J Clin Psychiatry 58(suppl 4):1–71, 1997

Mataix-Cols D, Marks IM: Self-help with minimal therapist contact for obsessive-compulsive disorder: a review. Eur Psychiatry 21(2):75–80, 2006

McLean PD, Whittal ML, Thordarson DS, et al: Cognitive versus behavior therapy in the group treatment of obsessive-compulsive disorder. J Consult Clin Psychol 69(2):205–214, 2001 11393598

Mehta M: A comparative study of family-based and patient-based behavioural management in obsessive-compulsive disorder. Br J Psychiatry 157:133–135, 1990

Meyer V: Modification of expectations in cases with obsessional rituals. Behav Res Ther 4(4):273–280, 1966 5978682

Meyer V, Levy R, Schnurer A: The behavioral treatment of obsessive-compulsive disorders, in Obsessional States. Edited by Beech H. London, Methuen, 1974, pp 233–258

Montgomery SA, McIntyre A, Osterheider M, et al: A double-blind, placebo-controlled study of fluoxetine in patients with DSM-III-R obsessive-compulsive disorder. Eur Neuropsychopharmacol 3(2):143–152, 1993 8364350

Nakatani E, Nakagawa A, Nakao T, et al: A randomized controlled trial of Japanese patients with obsessive-compulsive disorder—effectiveness of behavior therapy and fluvoxamine. Psychother Psychosom 74(5):269–276, 2005 16088264

O'Connor K, Todorov C, Robillard S, et al: Cognitive-behaviour therapy and medication in the treatment of obsessive-compulsive disorder: a controlled study. Can J Psychiatry 44(1):64–71, 1999 10076743

Olatunji BO, Davis ML, Powers MB, et al: Cognitive-behavioral therapy for obsessive-compulsive disorder: a meta-analysis of treatment outcome and moderators. J Psychiatr Res 47(1):33–41, 2013 22999486

Rachman S: Obsessions, responsibility, and guilt. Behav Res Ther 31(2):149–154, 1993 8442740

Rachman S, de Silva P: Abnormal and normal obsessions. Behav Res Ther 16(4):233–248, 1978

Rachman S, Hodgson R: Obsessions and Compulsions. Englewood Cliffs, NJ, Prentice Hall, 1980

Riggs DS, Hiss H, Foa EB: Marital distress and the treatment of obsessive compulsive disorder. Behav Ther 23:585–597, 1992

Romanelli RJ, Wu FM, Gamba R, et al: Behavioral therapy and serotonin reuptake inhibitor pharmacotherapy in the treatment of obsessive-compulsive disorder: a systematic review and meta-analysis of head-to-head randomized controlled trials. Depress Anxiety 31(8):641–652, 2014 24390912

Rothbaum BO, Shahar F: Behavioral treatment of obsessive-compulsive disorder in a naturalistic setting. Cognit Behav Pract 7:262–270, 2000

Salkovskis PM: Cognitive-behavioral approaches to the understanding of obsessional problems, in Current Controversies in the Anxiety Disorders. Edited by Rapee R. New York, Guilford, 1996, pp 103–133

Salkovskis PM, Westbrook D: Behaviour therapy and obsessional ruminations: can failure be turned into success? Behav Res Ther 27(2):149–160, 1989 2930440

Simpson HB, Gorfinkle KS, Liebowitz MR: Cognitive-behavioral therapy as an adjunct to serotonin reuptake inhibitors in obsessive-compulsive disorder: an open trial. J Clin Psychiatry 60(9):584–590, 1999 10520976

Singewald N, Schmuckermair C, Whittle N, et al: Pharmacology of cognitive enhancers for exposure-based therapy of fear, anxiety and trauma-related disorders. Pharmacol Ther 149:150–190, 2015 25550231

Solomon RL, Kamin LJ, Wynne LC: Traumatic avoidance learning: the outcomes of several ex-
    tinction procedures with dogs. J Abnorm Psychol 48(2):291–302, 1953 13052353

Steketee G, Chambless DL, Tran GQ: Effects of Axis I and II comorbidity on behavior therapy
    outcome for obsessive-compulsive disorder and agoraphobia. Compr Psychiatry 42(1):76–
    86, 2001 11154720

Storch EA, Merlo LJ, Bengtson M, et al: D-Cycloserine does not enhance exposure-response
    prevention therapy in obsessive-compulsive disorder. Int Clin Psychopharmacol
    22(4):230–237, 2007 17519647

Storch EA, Caporino NE, Morgan JR, et al: Preliminary investigation of web-camera delivered
    cognitive-behavioral therapy for youth with obsessive-compulsive disorder. Psychiatry
    Res 189:407–412, 2011 21684018

Taylor S: Assessment of obsessions and compulsions: reliability, validity, and sensitivity to
    treatment effects. Clin Psychol Rev 15:261–296, 1995

Tenneij NH, van Megen HJ, Denys DA, et al: Behavior therapy augments response of patients
    with obsessive-compulsive disorder responding to drug treatment. J Clin Psychiatry
    66(9):1169–1175, 2005 16187776

Tolin DF, Maltby N, Diefenbach GJ, et al: Cognitive-behavioral therapy for medication nonre-
    sponders with obsessive-compulsive disorder: a wait-list-controlled open trial. J Clin Psy-
    chiatry 65(7):922–931, 2004 15291681

Tumur I, Kaltenthaler E, Ferriter M, et al: Computerised cognitive behaviour therapy for obses-
    sive-compulsive disorder: a systematic review. Psychother Psychosom 76(4):196–202, 2007
    17570957

Twohig MP, Hayes SC, Plumb JC, et al: A randomized clinical trial of acceptance and commit-
    ment therapy versus progressive relaxation training for obsessive-compulsive disorder.
    J Consult Clin Psychol 78(5):705–716, 2010 20873905

Twohig MP, Abramowitz JS, Bluett EJ, et al: Exposure therapy for OCD from an acceptance and
    commitment therapy (ACT) framework. J Obsessive Compuls Relat Disord 6:167–173, 2015

Twohig MP, Abramowitz JS, Smith BM, et al: Adding acceptance and commitment therapy to
    exposure and response prevention for obsessive-compulsive disorder: a randomized con-
    trolled trial. Behav Res Ther 108:1–9, 2018 29966992

Van Ameringen M, Turna J, Khalesi Z, et al: There is an app for that! The current state of mobile
    applications (apps) for DSM-5 obsessive-compulsive disorder, posttraumatic stress disor-
    der, anxiety and mood disorders. Depress Anxiety 34(6):526–539, 2017 28569409

van Balkom AJ, de Haan E, van Oppen P, et al: Cognitive and behavioral therapies alone versus
    in combination with fluvoxamine in the treatment of obsessive compulsive disorder.
    J Nerv Ment Dis 186(8):492–499, 1998 9717867

van den Hout M, Emmelkamp P, Kraaykamp H, et al: Behavioral treatment of obsessive-
    compulsives: inpatient vs outpatient. Behav Res Ther 26(4):331–332, 1988 3214397

Vogel PA, Stiles TC, Götestam KG: Adding cognitive therapy elements to exposure therapy for
    obsessive compulsive disorder: a controlled study. Behav Cogn Psychother 32:275–290, 2004

Volpato Cordioli A, Heldt E, Braga Bochi D, et al: Cognitive-behavioral group therapy in obses-
    sive-compulsive disorder: a randomized clinical trial. Psychother Psychosom 72(4):211–
    216, 2003 12792126

Warren R, Thomas JC: Cognitive-behavior therapy of obsessive-compulsive disorder in private
    practice: an effectiveness study. J Anxiety Disord 15(4):277–285, 2001 11474814

Whiteside SP, Ale CM, Vickers Douglas K, et al: Case examples of enhancing pediatric OCD
    treatment with a smartphone application. Clin Case Stud 13:80–94, 2014

Wilhelm S, Steketee G: Cognitive Therapy for Obsessive-Compulsive Disorder: A Guide for
    Practitioners. Oakland, CA, New Harbinger, 2006

Williams MT, Davis DM, Powers M, et al: Current trends in prescribing medications for obsessive-
    compulsive disorder: best practices and new research. Dir Psychiatry 34:247–261, 2014

Wootton BM, Titov N, Dear BF, et al: The acceptability of Internet-based treatment and charac-
    teristics of an adult sample with obsessive compulsive disorder: an internet survey. PLoS
    One 6(6):e20548, 2011 21673987

Recommended Readings

Abramowitz JS: Obsessive-Compulsive Disorder: Advances in Psychotherapy—Evidence-Based Practice. Cambridge, MA, Hogrefe and Huber, 2006

Abramowitz JS: Understanding and Treating Obsessive-Compulsive Disorder: A Cognitive-Behavioral Approach. Mahwah, NJ, Erlbaum, 2006

Abramowitz JS, Taylor S, McKay D (eds): Clinical Handbook of Obsessive-Compulsive Disorder and Related Problems. Baltimore, MD, Johns Hopkins University Press, 2008

Antony MM, Purdon C, Summerfeldt L (eds): Psychological Treatment of Obsessive-Compulsive Disorder: Fundamentals and Beyond. Washington, DC, American Psychological Association Press, 2008

Kozak MJ, Foa EB: Mastery of Obsessive Compulsive Disorder: Therapist's Guide. San Antonio, TX, Psychological Corporation, 1997

Wilhelm S, Steketee G: Cognitive Therapy for Obsessive-Compulsive Disorder: A Guide for Practitioners. Oakland, CA, New Harbinger, 2006

Websites of Interest

Anxiety and Depression Association of America: www.adaa.org
Association for Behavioral and Cognitive Therapies: www.abct.org
International OCD Foundation: www.iocdf.org

CHAPTER 19

The Obsessive-Compulsive Spectrum of Disorders

Elisabetta Burchi, M.D.

Michael Diamond, M.D.

Erin Shanahan, B.S.

Dan J. Stein, M.D.

Eric Hollander, M.D.

Since the nineteenth century, OCD has been thought to share underlying features with a range of other psychiatric conditions. Interest in a spectrum of obsessive-compulsive-related disorders has increased since the 1990s (Hollander 1993), and converging evidence supports an overlap of obsessive-compulsive phenomenology, comorbidity, family history, underlying neurocircuitry, and treatment response across various conditions. In DSM-5 (American Psychiatric Association 2013), OCD was moved out of the "Anxiety Disorders" chapter and a new chapter, "Obsessive-Compulsive and Related Disorders" (OCRD), was created. ICD-11 will similarly have a new chapter on these disorders. Although the current classification in DSM-5 is still categorical and based on symptoms, the new nosological grouping in part reflects advancement in pathophysiological knowledge. The disorders classified alongside OCD in this DSM-5 chapter, which are grouped based on similarities on a number of diagnostic validators as well as on considerations regarding clinical utility, include body dysmorphic disorder (BDD), hoarding disorder (HD), trichotillomania (hair-pulling disorder), excoriation (skin-picking) disorder (ED), substance/medication-induced OCRD, and OCRD due to another medical condition. This group does not cover all the conditions that may be characterized by obsessive-compulsive features and, resorting to a dimensional approach, constructs such as compulsivity may be used transdiagnostically to characterize conditions that go beyond the boundaries of the OCRD chapter, pointing to a compulsive-impulsive spectrum (Stein and Hollander 1993). Furthermore, studies informed by the Research Domain Criteria framework are now dissecting traditional diagnoses and proposing putative biological validators of such a spectrum (Brooks et al. 2017).

The organization of this chapter mirrors that of the DSM-5 chapter on OCRD. For each condition, updated data on assessment, pathophysiology, and treatment are provided, with particular attention to comparisons with OCD (Table 19–1). The discussion of OCD has been earmarked to a separate chapter.

Body Dysmorphic Disorder

BDD is defined by a distressing preoccupation with a subjectively perceived defect in one's appearance and by the performance of repetitive behaviors or mental acts in response to this preoccupation (American Psychiatric Association 2013). Previously classified as a somatoform disorder, BDD is now classified in the OCRD chapter in DSM-5.

BDD affects around 2% of the population (Buhlmann et al. 2010), and prevalence may be higher in college students (Bohne et al. 2002). Notably, more than 10% of patients looking for dermatological care may be affected by BDD (Veale et al. 2016). Preoccupations experienced by patients with BDD regarding perceived and mostly subjective physical flaws often are described as obsessional, persistent, and time consuming (DSM-5 Criteria A and B). These preoccupations are associated with feelings of shame, anxiety, guilt, and significant distress (Criterion C). Many patients with BDD believe that their concerns are appropriate and also demonstrate delusions of reference (Phillips et al. 2014). In response to their physical concerns, patients with BDD may report repetitive behaviors such as mirror-checking, camouflaging, requests for reassurance, and skin picking.

The current conceptualization of BDD within an obsessive-compulsive spectrum is based on some overlap with OCD in areas of clinical characteristics and treatment (Malcolm et al. 2018). However, such overlaps may reflect similarities across a large cluster of conditions, and few studies to date have directly compared BDD and OCD on biological and dimensional parameters. Areas of overlap between BDD and OCD include onset in adolescence or young adulthood, chronic course, and global functional impairment. Also, patients with either disorder present with fear of negative evaluation and disgust propensity.

In contrast, significantly poorer insight and more delusionality have been found in patients with BDD than in patients with OCD (Toh et al. 2017). Whereas in BDD the focus of concern is restricted to appearance and imagined ugliness, in OCD a broad range of preoccupations may be present, only some of which are somatic in nature. Importantly, subjects with BDD exhibit extraordinarily higher levels of suicidal thoughts and behaviors compared to other psychiatric groups that have been established as begin at high risk for suicidal thoughts, including patients with OCD, eating disorders, or bipolar disorder (Angelakis et al. 2016). Among the hypothesized moderators underlying this characteristic are specific symptoms of BDD such as body image concerns and psychiatric comorbidities. Compared with patients with OCD,

TABLE 19–1. Four key obsessive-compulsive spectrum disorders: clinical features, neurobiology, and treatments

Disorder	Clinical features	Neurobiology	Treatments	Clinical points
Body dysmorphic disorder	Distressful preoccupation with a subjectively perceived defect in one's appearance Performance of repetitive behaviors or mental acts in response to this preoccupation, such as mirror checking, camouflaging, requests for reassurance, and skin picking	Enhanced activity of the amygdala, insula, and orbitofrontal cortex in relation to fear, disgust, and happiness	First line: SSRIs in high doses and CBT Possible augmentation: buspirone, venlafaxine, and dopamine D_2 antagonists	Complementary assessment of suicidal risk and comorbid depression Screening regarding cosmetic surgery
Hoarding disorder	Persistent difficulty discarding or parting with possessions regardless of value, usually due to distress or perceived need to possess given items Accumulation of possessions compromises intended use of living spaces	Enhanced activity of the anterior cingulate cortex and insula when patients are tasked to discard their own objects Increased precentral gyrus activation during successful response inhibition	Pharmacotherapy: SSRIs Tailored CBT such as ERP Motivational interviewing in individuals with poor insight	Explore comorbidity with anxiety and mood disorders Symptoms usually ego-syntonic
Trichotillomania	Automatic or focused pulling out of one's own hair, leading to hair loss and marked functional impairment	Focal involvement of frontostriatal circuits Difficulty inhibiting motor behavior and spatial working memory Symptom severity has been correlated with reduced cerebellar volume	First line: CBT (combination of stimulus control, HRT, and acceptance-based therapy) SSRIs most used, but no strong evidence of efficacy; preliminary evidence of NAC efficacy	Obsessive component may be absent Associations with other body-focused compulsive behaviors Investigate trichophagia

TABLE 19–1. **Four key obsessive-compulsive spectrum disorders: clinical features, neurobiology, and treatments** *(continued)*

Disorder	Clinical features	Neurobiology	Treatments	Clinical points
Excoriation disorder	Damaging one's own skin to the point of creating lesions Feelings of loss of control, embarrassment, and shame related to the index behavior	Abnormalities in activation of right dorsal striatum, bilateral anterior cingulate, and right medial frontal regions involved in habit formation underpinning grooming behavior Enhanced activation of amygdala, insula, and orbitofrontal cortex associated with emotional reactivity (fear, disgust, and happiness)	CBT and DBT Reversal behavioral therapy; SSRIs; preliminary evidence for NAC	Comorbidity with trichotillomania

Note. CBT=cognitive-behavioral therapy; DBT=dialectical behavior therapy; ERP=exposure and response prevention; HRT=habit reversal therapy; NAC=*N*-acetylcysteine; SSRI=selective serotonin reuptake inhibitor.

patients with BDD show a higher prevalence of major depressive disorder, social anxiety disorder, and substance use disorders (Malcolm et al. 2018). Interestingly, lifetime comorbidity rates of BDD and OCD are almost three times higher in samples with a primary diagnosis of BDD than in those with primary OCD (27.5% vs. 10.4%) (Frías et al. 2015).

Although the development of BDD has been associated with past experiences of trauma, the underlying neurobiology of BDD is not yet established. Some studies have shown increased total white matter volume and caudate volume asymmetry, aligning BDD with the striatal topography model of OCRD (Tasios and Michopoulos 2017). However, indirect comparisons with studies conducted in OCD suggest that BDD pathophysiology may involve more widespread white matter changes and greater abnormalities within the limbic system (specifically the amygdala), the visual processing areas, and the orbitofrontal cortex rather than the corticostriatal regions (Bohon et al. 2012; Feusner et al. 2010a, 2010b). The severity of BDD symptoms has been associated with greater volume of the right amygdala. Changes in the volume of the amygdala are not typically observed in OCD overall but have been more discretely associated with harm and checking symptoms. Despite the fact that BDD and OCD appear to share similar mild impairments in broad neurocognitive functioning (Toh et al. 2017), patients with BDD, compared with patients with OCD, seem to present with greater hyperactivity of detail-oriented visual systems (Beilharz et al. 2017) and worse facial affect recognition, particularly in relation to disgust and anger (Toh et al. 2017). These findings align with clinical observations of detail-oriented bias in people with BDD. On the other hand, in OCD more attention has been devoted to executive dysfunction related to fronto-cortico-striatal activity.

Functional MRI (fMRI) studies have found that patients with BDD interpret visual information that is holistic in nature via neural pathways meant for detailed information (Feusner et al. 2011). An fMRI study comparing visual processing networks in patients with BDD and patients with anorexia nervosa found similar patterns of connectivity, suggesting reduced introspection in both disorders as well as a tendency to assign inappropriate importance to visual information (Moody et al. 2015). Disturbances in visual processing may underpin the disordered beliefs in BDD that appear circumscribed to appearance-based concerns, which is different from the "magical thinking style"—that is, the more cognitive bias—that underpins OCD obsessions.

Current evidence suggests that BDD often goes undiagnosed. This may be due to patients' shame about their symptoms or to poor insight and a desire for non–mental health treatment, such as cosmetic surgery. Thus, therapists often must ask explicitly about BDD symptoms during the psychiatric interview. Accurate diagnosis of BDD can be aided by use of brief screening instruments such as the Yale-Brown Obsessive-Compulsive Scale Modified for Body Dysmorphic Disorder (BDD-YBOCS; Phillips et al. 1997), a 12-item semistructured clinician-administered interview that is considered the gold standard. As a convention in the field, a pre- to posttreatment score reduction of at least 30% on the BDD-YBOCS denotes "treatment response."

Considering the relatively high risk of suicide in this population, a specific assessment of suicide risk should also be performed. In addition, given the associations between cosmetic treatments and negative outcomes in terms of BDD symptom severity (Bowyer et al. 2016), patients should be encouraged toward evidence-based treatment for BDD as opposed to cosmetic interventions.

The mainstay of treatment in BDD consists of a combination of pharmacotherapy and cognitive-behavioral therapy (CBT), with response rates across studies varying from about 50% to 80% (Phillips 2017). As is the case in treatment of OCD, first-line pharmacological treatment of BDD is centered around the use of high-dose selective serotonin reuptake inhibitors (SSRIs) (Hong et al. 2019).

CBT is effective both alone and in combination with pharmacotherapy for long-term maintenance therapy and relapse prevention in patients with BDD (Krebs et al. 2017). Particular attention may be devoted to the component of self-disgust in BDD, which, as in OCD, may be resistant to extinction during therapy, highlighting its potential importance to treatment outcomes (Wilver et al. 2018). Interestingly, the presence and severity of delusional beliefs do not affect the probability of recovery in BDD (Phillips et al. 2013).

Buspirone, venlafaxine, and second-generation antipsychotics may prove to be viable options for augmentation (Hong et al. 2019). Among other treatment options, oxytocin may be promising, given the overlapping symptom domains and frequent comorbidity with autism spectrum disorder and the association with excessive grooming behaviors (Vasudeva and Hollander 2017). Neuromodulation techniques, specifically repetitive transcranial magnetic stimulation and bilateral deep brain stimulation, have shown promise in complex, treatment-resistant BDD (Mahato et al. 2016; Park et al. 2017).

Hoarding Disorder

HD is now included as a distinct disorder in DSM-5. HD is characterized by persistent difficulty in parting with possessions, regardless of their value (Criterion A); this difficulty is due to distress associated with discarding (Criterion B) and results in accumulation of possessions that clutter living spaces (Criterion C). HD was formerly classified as a subtype of OCD and a symptom of obsessive-compulsive personality disorder. HD is now recognized as its own disorder due to differences with OCD that lie in symptoms, underlying brain activity, clinical course, and response to treatment.

Prevalence of HD is estimated to be 2%–6% in the adult population and 2% in adolescents (Pertusa et al. 2010). Age of impairment is usually later in HD than in OCD, and the course of the disease is often chronic rather than remittent, with progressive worsening over each decade of life (Ayers et al. 2010). Individuals who engage in hoarding often do not engage in other OCD-like behaviors, such as checking. Additionally, behaviors in HD are usually ego-syntonic rather than ego-dystonic, as in OCD (Albert et al. 2015).

Phenotypic similarities may be observed in individuals with HD and OCD. This is the case when a patient with OCD may not discard an object due to fear of consequences associated with discarding. However, the diagnosis of OCD would be given only if the clutter and consumption of living space is a direct result of typical obsessions and compulsions.

Hoarding may be seen in individuals with degenerative and neurodevelopmental disorders such as dementia and Prader-Willi syndrome, as well as in those with anxiety and mood disorders. In fact, although hoarding was commonly seen as a component of OCD, its comorbidity lies more with anxiety and mood disorders, such as generalized anxiety disorder (31%–37%) and major depressive disorder (26%–31%), with only 15%–20% of those with HD fitting a diagnosis of OCD (Mataix-Cols et al. 2013; Tolin et al. 2011).

Patients do not typically self-report hoarding because they do not find it distressing, and it is the existence of another comorbid condition that often brings patients with HD to a clinician's attention. For example, symptoms associated with generalized anxiety disorder may be distressing enough to cause a patient to seek treatment, which then allows a clinician to tease out a comorbid HD diagnosis (Tolin et al. 2011). Although hoarding behavior does not always cause distress to the individual due to lack of insight, it may cause significant distress to family members and others living in the home, prompting these significant others to bring a patient with HD to a physician. When the issue is brought to a clinician's attention, the diagnosis of HD can be confirmed using DSM-5 criteria or the Structured Interview for Hoarding Disorder (Nordsletten et al. 2013). In addition, other tools and assessments can be used to determine severity, changes over time, and response to treatment, including the Saving Inventory–Revised (Frost et al. 2004), Hoarding Rating Scale (Tolin et al. 2010), and Clutter Image Rating Scale (Frost et al. 2008; Tolin et al. 2007).

HD may run in families, with 50% of those meeting the diagnosis of HD having a first-degree family member who also hoards (American Psychiatric Association 2013). Specific genes contributing to HD may, in part, overlap with OCD and other OCRD such as BDD (Monzani et al. 2014).

Patients with HD have shown impairments in spatial planning, visuospatial learning, working memory, and cognitive control (Grisham et al. 2007). Recent neurofunctional studies have further elucidated the difference between HD and OCD, showing distinct patterns of brain activation during executive performance (Suñol et al. 2019; Tolin et al. 2012). Specifically, alterations in HD resemble an impulsive-like pattern of response, with associated hyperactivation of the right lateral orbitofrontal cortex and abnormal deactivation of the frontal regions during error processing (Suñol et al. 2019). In addition, patients with HD exhibit a biphasic abnormality in the anterior cingulate cortex and insula function that is stimulus dependent and related to problems in identifying the emotional significance of a stimulus, generating an appropriate emotional response, or regulating their affective state during decision making (Tolin et al. 2012).

The predominant psychosocial theories of pathogenesis have postulated that traumatic events and early material deprivation of items can later lead to the development of HD. However, these theories have not been supported by research to date (Landau et al. 2010).

Although no gold standard intervention has been established, patients with HD are treated with a similar approach to that used for patients with OCD, with tailored CBT and pharmacotherapy (Steketee 2018). To date, research on pharmacological treatment for patients with HD is limited, and only one-third of individuals with HD respond to psychotherapeutic or pharmacological therapies, with poor response to serotonergic medication (Bloch et al. 2014). Recent studies with paroxetine (Saxena et al. 2007), however, showed similar outcomes in patients with HD and OCD. Research on venlafaxine has shown some promising results, although true efficacy has yet to be established (Saxena and Sumner 2014). CBT has proven benefits, specifically tailored exposure and response prevention, typically involving home visits and at-home homework sessions. Motivational interviewing is useful in patients with poor insight. Other therapies include group therapy, individual therapy via webcam, family support groups, and skills training in discarding and acquisition (Steketee 2018).

Trichotillomania (Hair-Pulling Disorder)

Trichotillomania is a condition characterized by recurrent pulling of one's own hair leading to hair loss and marked functional impairment (American Psychiatric Association 2013). Previously defined as an impulse-control disorder, given the association between trichotillomania and other body-focused compulsive behavior disorders such as ED (Lochner et al. 2005), trichotillomania is now included in the DSM-5 chapter on OCRD. Although hair pulling, as a behavior, appears to be quite common, trichotillomania prevalence ranges from 0.5% to 2.0%, with typical onset during adolescence. When untreated, trichotillomania is commonly chronic, with fluctuations in intensity over time (Grant and Chamberlain 2016).

In trichotillomania, pulling can be undertaken at any bodily region that has hair, but the scalp is the most common site (Woods et al. 2006). Pulling behavior may be "automatic" or "focused," generally when the patient sees or feels a hair that is "not right" (Christenson and Mackenzie 1995). Triggers to pull hair may be sensory (e.g., physical sensations), emotional (e.g., feeling anxious, bored, tense), or cognitive (e.g., thoughts about appearance) (Woods and Houghton 2014). In contrast to compulsive behaviors in OCD, hair pulling is seldom driven by cognitive intrusions, and therefore obsessional thoughts are not included in the diagnostic criteria. Moreover, unlike the often-upsetting experience of performing rituals reported by patients with OCD, the experience of pulling hair is often described by patients with trichotillomania as pleasurable (White et al. 2013).

The small number of studies in which the pathophysiology of trichotillomania has been researched yielded results indicating a genetic component and potential neurostructural and neurofunctional alterations (Grant and Chamberlain 2016). The Hoxb8 knockout mouse (Greer and Capecchi 2002), the Sapap3 knockout mouse (Welch et al. 2007), and the Slitrk5 knockout mouse (Shmelkov et al. 2010) have been proposed as promising models, because these are characterized by elevated grooming. These three genes are all involved in the wiring of corticostriatal circuits, and *SAPAP3* variants have been associated with pathological grooming in humans (Bienvenu et al. 2009). In trichotillomania, as in OCD, some evidence indicates involvement of the basal ganglia, amygdala, bilateral cingulate cortex, right frontal cortex, and presupplementary motor area (Chamberlain et al. 2009, 2010). Consistent with their similarities in underlying neurocircuitry, OCD and trichotillomania seem to share overlapping difficulty in inhibiting motor behavior (Chamberlain et al. 2006) and in spatial working memory (Chamberlain et al. 2007). However, a more restricted profile of cognitive dysfunction has been found in patients with trichotillomania than in patients with OCD, suggesting a more focal involvement of elements of frontostriatal circuitry (Chamberlain et al. 2007). In addition, symptom severity has specifically been correlated to reduced cerebellar volume in trichotillomania (Keuthen et al. 2007). Finally, a dampening of nucleus accumbens responses to reward anticipation (but relative hypersensitivity to gain and loss outcomes) as compared to control subjects has been reported, suggesting that a disordered reward process may play a role in the pathophysiology of trichotillomania (White et al. 2013) and OCD (Figee et al. 2011).

Given that hair pulling may have numerous etiologies, a comprehensive, multimodal assessment is suggested. Use of trichoscopy, a dermoscopy method of hair and scalp evaluation, may help distinguish trichotillomania from other types of hair loss. The Structured Clinical Interview for DSM-5 Disorders (First et al. 2016) currently includes a section to address trichotillomania diagnosis. The diagnostic assessment can be augmented by a functional behavioral assessment to evaluate the antecedents that influence how and when a person pulls, which may ultimately guide treatment planning. Clinician and self-report scales such as the National Institute of Mental Health Trichotillomania Symptoms Severity Scale (Swedo et al. 1998), the Y-BOCS Trichotillomania (Stanley et al. 1999), and the Massachusetts General Hospital Hairpulling Scale (Keuthen et al. 1995) have demonstrated good psychometric proprieties.

Although the diagnosis of trichotillomania is fairly straightforward, a thorough assessment should routinely determine the presence of comorbidities and possible severe sequelae. In fact, trichotillomania often presents together with other comorbid psychiatric conditions, such as other OCRD, mood disorders, anxiety disorders, and neurodevelopmental disorders (Woods and Houghton 2014). Moreover, post-pulling behavior may be clinically relevant, such as in those patients (more than 20%) who eat the hair after pulling it out. This behavior, called *trichophagia*, may result in undigested masses of hair called *trichobezoars*, which can potentially lead to gastrointestinal obstruction (Grant and Odlaug 2008).

Despite the relatively few treatment studies conducted in the trichotillomania population, CBT seems to be the most empirically validated treatment and may include stimulus control, habit reversal therapy, and acceptance-based therapy (Woods and Houghton 2014). Evidence supporting pharmacological options is scarce (Cison et al. 2018). In fact, despite the fact that SSRIs are the most commonly prescribed treatment option, a Cochrane Review concluded that no strong evidence has been found of a treatment effect for SSRIs in trichotillomania (Rothbart et al. 2013). Based on preliminary evidence regarding the efficacy of *N*-acetylcysteine (NAC), olanzapine, and clomipramine, further studies on glutamate modulators, dopamine antagonists, and serotonergic tricyclic antidepressants are needed. Other therapies tested in trichotillomania include opioid antagonists (naltrexone; Grant et al. 2014) and cannabinoid agonists (dronabinol; Grant et al. 2011).

Excoriation (Skin-Picking) Disorder

ED is characterized by picking at one's own skin to the point of creating lesions (DSM-5 Criterion A). DSM-5 mentions that in addition to skin picking, skin rubbing, squeezing, lancing, and biting may occur. Individuals most commonly pick at the face, arms, or hands, with a specific focus on areas of minor skin irritations such as scabs, calluses, or pimples. Fingernails are commonly used, but pins, tweezers, or other objects are also used (Grant and Odlaug 2008; Tucker et al. 2011). Despite their repeated attempts to decrease this behavior, people with ED often have a difficult time stopping (Criterion B). Excoriation may cause clinically significant distress, such as feelings of loss of control, embarrassment, and shame. In addition, it causes significant impairments in social, occupational, or other areas of functioning (Criterion C).

Research suggests that ED has a strong genetic load. Interestingly, a multivariate twin modeling study found that OCRD may be influenced by two distinct liability factors; one of these is common to all OCRD, whereas the other may be exclusive to trichotillomania and ED. These and other findings suggest a close etiological relationship between trichotillomania and ED (Lochner et al. 2002; Monzani et al. 2014; Odlaug and Grant 2008; Snorrason et al. 2012). Currently, gene-searching efforts in trichotillomania and ED are still in their infancy; however, some promising susceptibility genes have been identified, such as *SAPAP3* (Bienvenu et al. 2009; Welch et al. 2007; Züchner et al. 2009).

Despite small sample sizes, neuroanatomical research has suggested that patients with ED have abnormalities in white matter distribution involved in motor generation and suppression that are similar to those found in patients with trichotillomania. These findings provide additional support to the hypothesis that ED and trichotillomania share underlying mechanisms (Grant et al. 2013).

Functional studies have found abnormalities in activation of the right dorsal striatum, bilateral cingulate cortex, and medial prefrontal regions involved in habit formation, action monitoring, and inhibition in individuals with ED (Odlaug et al. 2016). A recent fMRI study conducted in women with ED found that participants who scored higher on self-rated trait anxiety/depression measures reported higher intensities of fear, disgust, and happiness during picture viewings, with enhanced activation of the amygdala, insula, and orbitofrontal cortex, areas that mediate affective responses and affective awareness (Wabnegger et al. 2018).

Instruments have been developed to assess variables such as the frequency of picking behaviors and the psychosocial impairment related to picking. The Skin Picking Scale–Revised (Snorrason et al. 2012), an eight-item scale that assesses both symptom severity and impairment, has demonstrated good psychometric properties in both adults and adolescents (Gallinat et al. 2017). Other instruments address the specific etiological mechanisms that have been proposed in ED. For example, the Skin Picking Reward Scale measures how strongly skin picking is "liked" (i.e., the degree of pleasurable feelings).

Available psychotherapies for ED include CBT, dialectical behavior therapy, habit reversal training, acceptance-enhanced behavior therapy, and acceptance and commitment therapy, as well as differential reinforcement of other behavior, incompatible behavior, and alternative behavior (Roos et al. 2015). Habit reversal training is the treatment for ED with the greatest empirical support. This treatment first focuses on the nuances of the patients' unique pulling behaviors and then targets their specific symptoms. Treatment may include awareness training and self-monitoring, stimulus control, and competing response procedures. A key goal of the therapy is to help patients learn to recognize their pulling urges. Once this is accomplished, they can avoid situations in which pulling is more likely or adopt behaviors that can be used instead of pulling (Sarah et al. 2013).

A 2016 meta-analysis concluded that behavioral treatments demonstrated significant benefits compared to SSRIs, lamotrigine, and inactive controls (Schumer et al. 2016). However, SSRIs have been a mainstay of pharmacotherapy, with fluoxetine, citalopram, and escitalopram demonstrating improvement on measures of skin-picking behavior (Lochner et al. 2017), and evidence from a randomized controlled trial has indicated that NAC should also be considered as a potential intervention (Grant et al. 2016). Given the overlapping underpinnings between ED and trichotillomania, opioid antagonists and glutamatergic agents should be further studied as treatments for ED.

Substance/Medication-Induced Obsessive-Compulsive and Related Disorder

As stated in DSM-5, substances such as cocaine, amphetamines and other stimulants, heavy metals, toxins, and some prescription medications may induce symptoms such as obsessions, compulsions, skin picking, hair-pulling, or other body-focused repetitive behaviors (DSM-5 Criterion A). The diagnosis of substance/medication-induced OCRD is given only when symptoms develop during the use of a substance or medication or soon thereafter (Criterion B). In the case of prescription medications, symptoms usually develop during the treatment period and typically subside once treatment has ended. This diagnosis should not be given when the symptoms are present only during the course of delirium or when symptoms can be explained by another medical condition.

Obsessive-Compulsive and Related Disorder Due to Another Medical Condition

Sometimes, clinically significant obsessive-compulsive symptoms are proven to be the direct pathophysiological consequence of a diagnosed medical condition. Infections, degenerative disorders, traumatic brain injury, and cerebrovascular lesions directly involving the frontal lobes and basal ganglia may lead to onset of OCD. Other medical conditions that may indirectly cause compulsive behaviors include anemia, kidney failure, liver diseases, or skin conditions in which pruritus may precipitate skin picking. The presence of features that are atypical of most OCRD, such as late and abrupt age of onset, may suggest this diagnosis and consequently the appropriate treatment.

Some controversy exists about whether to include pediatric autoimmune neuropsychiatric disorder associated with streptococcal infections (PANDAS) in this DSM-5 category. The difficulty in operationalizing the association between Group A streptococcal disease infection and abrupt onset and exacerbations of OCD and tic symptoms led to the definition of a new umbrella category called pediatric acute-onset neuropsychiatric syndrome (PANS). This new category highlights the fact that several agents other than *Streptococcus* may be involved in the onset of obsessive-compulsive symptoms (Chang et al. 2015). Use of immunotherapy and antibiotic therapy for PANDAS/PANS has been researched, but studies that improve the quality of evidence to guide interventions are still needed (Burchi and Pallanti 2018). Although PANS is not included in DSM-5 as a distinct syndrome, patients with acute-onset OCRD should be evaluated for inflammatory, infective, and immunological abnormalities.

Other Specified Obsessive-Compulsive and Related Disorder

According to DSM-5, when a patient's presenting symptoms are characteristic of OCRD but do not meet the full criteria for any of the disorders in the spectrum, a diagnosis of "other specified obsessive-compulsive and related disorder" is provided. This diagnosis can be given, for example, to patients with obsessive thoughts about body odor (also termed *olfactory reference syndrome*).

Conclusion

Recent advances, particularly in neurogenetics and neuroimaging, have contributed to understanding OCRD as a group characterized by overlapping phenomenological characteristics and pathophysiological underpinnings. The recognition of this new nosological grouping is clinically valuable because it encourages appropriate assessment and treatment of several conditions that are often overlooked. The concept of an obsessive-compulsive spectrum that extends beyond the DSM-5 OCRD chapter is currently guiding a number of research efforts and may also be used by clinicians to complement current categorical diagnoses with a dimensional approach.

Key Points

- Controversy exists about the extent to which different disorders are related to OCD, but certain obsessive-compulsive spectrum disorders have clear overlaps in phenomenology and psychobiology.

- The construct of an OCD spectrum has heuristic value insofar as it encourages diagnosis and treatment of a range of disorders that are often overlooked by clinicians and researchers.

- Some putative obsessive-compulsive spectrum disorders respond selectively to selective serotonin reuptake inhibitors and to cognitive-behavioral therapy.

References

Albert U, Cori DD, Barbaro F, et al: Hoarding disorder: a new obsessive-compulsive related disorder in the DSM. Journal of Psychopathology 21:354–364, 2015

American Psychiatric Association: Diagnostic and Statistical Manual of Mental Disorders, 5th Edition. Arlington, VA, American Psychiatric Association, 2013

Angelakis I, Gooding PA, Panagioti M: Suicidality in body dysmorphic disorder (BDD): a systematic review with meta-analysis. Clin Psychol Rev 49:55–66, 2016 27607741

Ayers CR, Saxena S, Golshan S, et al: Age at onset and clinical features of late life compulsive hoarding. Int J Geriatr Psychiatry 25(2):142–149, 2010

Beilharz F, Castle DJ, Grace S, et al: A systematic review of visual processing and associated treatments in body dysmorphic disorder. Acta Psychiatr Scand 136(1):16–36, 2017 28190269

Bienvenu OJ, Wang Y, Shugart YY, et al: Sapap3 and pathological grooming in humans: results from the OCD collaborative genetics study. Am J Med Genet B Neuropsychiatr Genet 150B(5):710–720, 2009 19051237

Bloch MH, Bartley CA, Zipperer L, et al: Meta-analysis: hoarding symptoms associated with poor treatment outcome in obsessive-compulsive disorder. Mol Psychiatry 19(9):1025–1030, 2014 24912494

Bohne A, Wilhelm S, Keuthen NJ, et al: Prevalence of body dysmorphic disorder in a German college student sample. Psychiatry Res 109(1):101–104, 2002 11850057

Bohon C, Hembacher E, Moller H, et al: Nonlinear relationships between anxiety and visual processing of own and others' faces in body dysmorphic disorder. Psychiatry Res 204(2–3):132–139, 2012 23137801

Bowyer L, Krebs G, Mataix-Cols D, et al: A critical review of cosmetic treatment outcomes in body dysmorphic disorder. Body Image 19:1–8, 2016

Brooks SJ, Lochner C, Shoptaw S, et al: Using the Research Domain Criteria (RDoC) to conceptualize impulsivity and compulsivity in relation to addiction. Prog Brain Res 235:177–218, 2017 29054288

Buhlmann U, Glaesmer H, Mewes R, et al: Updates on the prevalence of body dysmorphic disorder: a population-based survey. Psychiatry Res 178(1):171–175, 2010 20452057

Burchi E, Pallanti S: Antibiotics for PANDAS? Limited evidence: review and putative mechanisms of action. Prim Care Companion CNS Disord 20(3):17r02232, 2018 29722936

Chamberlain SR, Fineberg NA, Blackwell AD, et al: Motor inhibition and cognitive flexibility in obsessive-compulsive disorder and trichotillomania. Am J Psychiatry 163(7):1282–1284, 2006 16816237

Chamberlain SR, Fineberg NA, Blackwell AD, et al: A neuropsychological comparison of obsessive-compulsive disorder and trichotillomania. Neuropsychologia 45(4):654–662, 2007 17005210

Chamberlain SR, Odlaug BL, Boulougouris V, et al: Trichotillomania: neurobiology and treatment. Neurosci Biobehav Rev 33(6):831–842, 2009 19428495

Chamberlain SR, Hampshire A, Menzies LA, et al: Reduced brain white matter integrity in trichotillomania: a diffusion tensor imaging study. Arch Gen Psychiatry 67(9):965–971, 2010 20819990

Chang K, Frankovich J, Cooperstock M, et al: Clinical evaluation of youth with pediatric acute-onset neuropsychiatric syndrome (PANS): recommendations from the 2013 PANS Consensus Conference. J Child Adolesc Psychopharmacol 25(1):3–13, 2015 25325534

Christenson GA, Mackenzie TB: Trichotillomania, body dysmorphic disorder, and obsessive-compulsive disorder. J Clin Psychiatry 56(5):211–212, 1995 7737961

Cison H, Kus A, Popowicz E, et al: Trichotillomania and trichophagia: modern diagnostic and therapeutic methods. Dermatol Ther (Heidelb) 8(3):389–398, 2018 30099694

Feusner JD, Bystritsky A, Hellemann G, et al: Impaired identity recognition of faces with emotional expressions in body dysmorphic disorder. Psychiatry Res 179(3):318–323, 2010a 20493560

Feusner JD, Moody T, Hembacher E, et al: Abnormalities of visual processing and frontostriatal systems in body dysmorphic disorder. Arch Gen Psychiatry 67(2):197–205, 2010b 20124119

Feusner JD, Hembacher E, Moller H, et al: Abnormalities of object visual processing in body dysmorphic disorder. Psychol Med 41(11):2385–2397, 2011

Figee M, Vink M, de Geus F, et al: Dysfunctional reward circuitry in obsessive-compulsive disorder. Biol Psychiatry 69(9):867–874, 2011 21272861

First MB, Williams JBW, Karg RS, et al: Structured Clinical Interview for DSM-5 Disorders, Clinician Version (SCID-5-CV). Arlington, VA, American Psychiatric Association, 2016

Frías Á, Palma C, Farriols N, et al: Comorbidity between obsessive-compulsive disorder and body dysmorphic disorder: prevalence, explanatory theories, and clinical characterization. Neuropsychiatr Dis Treat 11:2233–2244, 2015 26345330

Frost RO, Steketee G, Grisham J: Measurement of compulsive hoarding: Saving Inventory–Revised. Behav Res Ther 42(10):1163–1182, 2004 15350856

Frost RO, Steketee G, Tolin DF, et al: Development and validation of the clutter image rating. J Psychopathol Behav 30:193–203, 2008

Gallinat C, Keuthen NJ, Stefini A, et al: The assessment of skin picking in adolescence: psycho-metric properties of the Skin Picking Scale–Revised (German version). Nord J Psychiatry 71(2):145–150, 2017

Grant JE, Chamberlain SR: Trichotillomania. Am J Psychiatry 173(9):868–874, 2016 27581696

Grant JE, Odlaug BL: Clinical characteristics of trichotillomania with trichophagia. Compr Psychiatry 49(6):579–584, 2008

Grant JE, Odlaug BL, Chamberlain SR, et al: Dronabinol, a cannabinoid agonist, reduces hair pulling in trichotillomania: a pilot study. Psychopharmacology (Berl) 218(3):493–502, 2011 21590520

Grant JE, Odlaug BL, Hampshire A, et al: White matter abnormalities in skin picking disorder: a diffusion tensor imaging study. Neuropsychopharmacology 38(5):763–769, 2013 23303052

Grant JE, Odlaug BL, Schreiber LR, et al: The opiate antagonist, naltrexone, in the treatment of trichotillomania: results of a double-blind, placebo-controlled study. J Clin Psychopharmacol 34(1):134–138, 2014 24145220

Grant JE, Chamberlain SR, Redden SA, et al: N-acetylcysteine in the treatment of excoriation disorder: a randomized clinical trial. JAMA Psychiatry 73(5):490–496, 2016 27007062

Greer JM, Capecchi MR: Hoxb8 is required for normal grooming behavior in mice. Neuron 33(1):23–34, 2002 11779477

Grisham JR, Brown TA, Savage CR, et al: Neuropsychological impairment associated with compulsive hoarding. Behav Res Ther 45(7):1471–1483, 2007 17341416

Hollander E (ed): Obsessive-Compulsive Related Disorders. Washington, DC, American Psychiatric Press, 1993

Hong K, Nezgovorova V, Uzunova G, et al: Pharmacological treatment of body dysmorphic disorder. Curr Neuropharmacol 17(8):697–702, 2019 29701157

Keuthen NJ, O'Sullivan RL, Ricciardi JN, et al: The Massachusetts General Hospital (MGH) Hairpulling Scale: 1. development and factor analyses. Psychother Psychosom 64(3–4):141–145, 1995

Keuthen NJ, Makris N, Schlerf JE, et al: Evidence for reduced cerebellar volumes in trichotillomania. Biol Psychiatry 61(3):374–381, 2007 16945351

Krebs G, de la Cruz LF, Monzani B, et al: Long-term outcomes of cognitive-behavioral therapy for adolescent body dysmorphic disorder. Behav Ther 48(4):462–473, 2017

Landau D, Iervolino AC, Pertusa A, et al: Stressful life events and material deprivation in hoarding disorder. J Anxiety Disord 25(2):192–202, 2011

Lochner C, du Toit PL, Zungu-Dirwayi N, et al: Childhood trauma in obsessive-compulsive disorder, trichotillomania, and controls. Depress Anxiety 15(2):66–68, 2002

Lochner C, Seedat S, du Toit PL, et al: Obsessive-compulsive disorder and trichotillomania: a phenomenological comparison. BMC Psychiatry 5:2, 2005 15649315

Lochner C, Roos A, Stein DJ: Excoriation (skin-picking) disorder: a systematic review of treatment options. Neuropsychiatr Dis Treat 13:1867–1872, 2017 28761349

Mahato RS, San Gabriel MC, Longshore CT, et al: A case of treatment-resistant depression and body dysmorphic disorder: the role of electroconvulsive therapy revisited. Innov Clin Neurosci 13(7-8):37–40, 2016 27672487

Malcolm A, Labuschagne I, Castle D, et al: The relationship between body dysmorphic disorder and obsessive-compulsive disorder: a systematic review of direct comparative studies. Aust N Z J Psychiatry 52(11):1030–1049, 2018 30238784

Mataix-Cols D, Billotti D, Fernández de la Cruz L, et al: The London field trial for hoarding disorder. Psychol Med 43(4):837–847, 2013 22883395

Monzani B, Rijsdijk F, Harris J, et al: The structure of genetic and environmental risk factors for dimensional representations of DSM-5 obsessive-compulsive spectrum disorders. JAMA Psychiatry 71(2):182–189, 2014 24369376

Moody TD, Sasaki MA, Bohon C, et al: Functional connectivity for face processing in individuals with body dysmorphic disorder and anorexia nervosa. Psychol Med 45(16):3491–3503, 2015 26219399

Nordsletten AE, de la Cruz LF, Pertusa A, et al: The Structured Interview for Hoarding Disorder (SIHD): development, usage and further validation. J Obsessive Compuls Relat Disord 2(3):346–350, 2013

Odlaug BL, Grant JE: Trichotillomania and pathologic skin picking: clinical comparison with an examination of comorbidity. Ann Clin Psychiatry 20(2):57–63, 2008 18568576

Odlaug BL, Hampshire A, Chamberlain SR, et al: Abnormal brain activation in excoriation (skin-picking) disorder: evidence from an executive planning fMRI study. Br J Psychiatry 208(2):168–174, 2016 26159604

Park HR, Kim IH, Kang H, et al: Nucleus accumbens deep brain stimulation for a patient with self-injurious behavior and autism spectrum disorder: functional and structural changes of the brain: report of a case and review of literature. Acta Neurochir (Wien) 159(1):137–143, 2017 27807672

Pertusa A, Frost RO, Fullana MA, et al: Refining the diagnostic boundaries of compulsive hoarding: a critical review. Clin Psychol Rev 30(4):371–386, 2010 20189280

Phillips KA (ed): Pharmacotherapy and other somatic treatments for body dysmorphic disorder, in Body Dysmorphic Disorder: Advances in Research and Clinical Practice. New York, Oxford University Press, 2017

Phillips KA, Hollander E, Rasmussen SA, et al: A severity rating scale for body dysmorphic disorder: development, reliability, and validity of a modified version of the Yale-Brown Obsessive Compulsive Scale. Psychopharmacol Bull 33(1):17–22, 1997

Phillips KA, Menard W, Quinn E, et al: A 4-year prospective observational follow-up study of course and predictors of course in body dysmorphic disorder. Psychol Med 43(5):1109–1117, 2013 23171833

Phillips KA, Hart AS, Simpson HB, et al: Delusional versus nondelusional body dysmorphic disorder: recommendations for DSM-5. CNS Spectr 19(1):10–20, 2014 23659348

Roos A, Grant JE, Fouche JP, et al: A comparison of brain volume and cortical thickness in excoriation (skin picking) disorder and trichotillomania (hair pulling disorder) in women. Behav Brain Res 279:255–258, 2015 25435313

Rothbart R, Amos T, Siegfried N, et al: Pharmacotherapy for trichotillomania. Cochrane Database Syst Rev (11):CD007662, 2013 24214100

Sarah HM, Hana FZ, Hilary ED, et al: Habit reversal training in trichotillomania: guide for the clinician. Expert Rev Neurother 13(9):1069–1077, 2013

Saxena S, Brody AL, Maidment KM, et al: Paroxetine treatment of compulsive hoarding. J Psychiatr Res 41(6):481–487, 2007

Saxena S, Sumner J: Venlafaxine extended-release treatment of hoarding disorder. Int Clin Psychopharmacol 29(5):266–273, 2014 24722633

Schumer MC, Bartley CA, Bloch MH: Systematic review of pharmacological and behavioral treatments for skin picking disorder. J Clin Psychopharmacol 36(2):147–152, 2016 26872117

Shmelkov SV, Hormigo A, Jing D, et al: Slitrk5 deficiency impairs corticostriatal circuitry and leads to obsessive-compulsive-like behaviors in mice. Nat Med 16(5):598–602, 2010 20418887

Snorrason I, Belleau EL, Woods DW: How related are hair pulling disorder (trichotillomania) and skin picking disorder? A review of evidence for comorbidity, similarities and shared etiology. Clin Psychol Rev 32(7):618–629, 2012

Stanley MA, Breckenridge JK, Snyder AG, et al: Clinician-rated measures of hair pulling: a preliminary psychometric evaluation. Journal of Psychopathology and Behavioral Assessment 21(2):157–170, 1999

Stein DJ, Hollander E: The spectrum of obsessive-compulsive related disorders, in Obsessive-Compulsive Related Disorders. Edited by Hollander E. Washington, DC, American Psychiatric Press, 1993, pp 241–271

Steketee G: Presidential address: team science across disciplines: advancing CBT research and practice on hoarding. Behav Ther 49(5):643–652, 2018

Suñol M, Martínez-Zalacaín I, Picó-Pérez M, et al: Differential patterns of brain activation between hoarding disorder and obsessive-compulsive disorder during executive performance. Psychol Med 25:1–8, 2019 30907337

Swedo SE, Leonard HL, Garvey M, et al: Pediatric autoimmune neuropsychiatric disorders associated with streptococcal infections: clinical description of the first 50 cases. Am J Psychiatry 155(2):264–271, 1998 9464208

Tasios K, Michopoulos I: Body dysmorphic disorder: latest neuroanatomical and neuropsychological findings. Psychiatriki 28(3):242–250, 2017 29072188

Toh WL, Castle DJ, Mountjoy RL, et al: Insight in body dysmorphic disorder (BDD) relative to obsessive-compulsive disorder (OCD) and psychotic disorders: revisiting this issue in light of DSM-5. Compr Psychiatry 77:100–108, 2017 28651226

Tolin DF, Frost RO, Steketee G: An open trial of cognitive-behavioral therapy for compulsive hoarding. Behav Res Ther 45(7):1461–1470, 2007

Tolin DF, Villavicencio A: Inattention, but not OCD, predicts the core features of hoarding disorder. Behav Res Ther 49(2):120–125, 2011 21193171

Tolin DF, Frost RO, Steketee G: A brief interview for assessing compulsive hoarding: the Hoarding Rating Scale–Interview. Psychiatry Res 178(1):147–152, 2010 20452042

Tolin DF, Stevens MC, Villavicencio AL, et al: Neural mechanisms of decision making in hoarding disorder. Arch Gen Psychiatry 69(8):832–841, 2012 22868937

Tucker BT, Woods DW, Flessner CA, et al: The Skin Picking Impact Project: phenomenology, interference, and treatment utilization of pathological skin picking in a population-based sample. J Anxiety Disord 25(1):88–95, 2011

Vasudeva SB, Hollander E: Body dysmorphic disorder in patients with autism spectrum disorder: a reflection of increased local processing and self-focus. Am J Psychiatry 174(4):313–316, 2017 28366095

Veale D, Gledhill LJ, Christodoulou P, et al: Body dysmorphic disorder in different settings: a systematic review and estimated weighted prevalence. Body Image 18:168–186, 2016 27498379

Wabnegger A, Übel S, Suchar G, et al: Increased emotional reactivity to affective pictures in patients with skin-picking disorder: evidence from functional magnetic resonance imaging. Behav Brain Res 336:151–155, 2018 28866131

Welch JM, Lu J, Rodriguiz RM, et al: Cortico-striatal synaptic defects and OCD-like behaviours in Sapap3-mutant mice. Nature 448(7156):894–900, 2007 17713528

White MP, Shirer WR, Molfino MJ, et al: Disordered reward processing and functional connectivity in trichotillomania: a pilot study. J Psychiatr Res 47(9):1264–1272, 2013 23777938

Wilver NL, Summers BJ, Garratt GH, et al: An initial investigation of the unique relationship between disgust propensity and body dysmorphic disorder. Psychiatry Res 269:237–243, 2018

Woods DW, Houghton DC: Diagnosis, evaluation, and management of trichotillomania. Psychiatr Clin North Am 37(3):301–317, 2014 25150564

Woods DW, Flessner CA, Franklin ME, et al: The Trichotillomania Impact Project (TIP): exploring phenomenology, functional impairment, and treatment utilization. J Clin Psychiatry 67(12):1877–1888, 2006 25150564

Züchner S, Wendland JR, Ashley-Koch AE, et al: Multiple rare SAPAP3 missense variants in trichotillomania and OCD. Mol Psychiatry 14(1):6, 2009

Recommended Readings

Fineberg NA, Apergis-Schoute AM, Vaghi MM, et al: Mapping compulsivity in the DSM-5 obsessive compulsive and related disorders: cognitive domains, neural circuitry, and treatment. Int J Neuropsychopharmacol 21(1):42–58, 2018 29036632

Grant JE, Fineberg N, van Ameringen M, et al: New treatment models for compulsive disorders. Eur Neuropsychopharmacol 26(5):877–884, 2016

Hollander E, Braun A, Simeon D: Should OCD leave the anxiety disorders in DSM-V? The case for obsessive compulsive-related disorders. Depress Anxiety 25(4):317–329, 2008 18412058

Marras A, Fineberg N, Pallanti S: Obsessive compulsive and related disorders: comparing DSM-5 and ICD-11. CNS Spectr 21(4):324–333, 2016

Stein DJ: Neurobiology of the obsessive–compulsive spectrum disorders. Biol Psychiatry 47(4):296–304, 2000

Weingarden H, Renshaw KD: Shame in the obsessive compulsive related disorders: a conceptual review. J Affect Disord 171:74–84, 2015

PART V

Panic Disorder and Agoraphobia

CHAPTER 20

Phenomenology of Panic Disorder

Amanda Waters Baker, Ph.D.

Olivia Losiewicz, B.A.

Mark H. Pollack, M.D.

Jordan W. Smoller, M.D., Sc.D.

Michael W. Otto, Ph.D.

Elizabeth Hoge, M.D.

Naomi Simon, M.D., M.Sc.

Panic disorder (PD) is characterized by recurrent unexpected panic attacks, followed by at least 1 month of anxiety about future attacks or the implications of the attacks or at least 1 month of significant behavior change because of attacks. PD was not defined as a discrete disorder until DSM-III (American Psychiatric Association 1980), although investigations into the phenomenology and treatment of panic-like symptoms began in the mid-twentieth century. Until DSM-5 (American Psychiatric Association 2013), agoraphobia (fear of situations in which escape may be difficult) was considered part of PD, but now it is defined as a separate disorder. This chapter reviews PD epidemiology, clinical features, associated impairment, and psychiatric comorbidity.

Epidemiology

The lifetime prevalence rates of panic attacks and PD have been estimated through several epidemiological studies, including the National Comorbidity Survey Replication (NCS-R) and National Epidemiologic Survey on Alcohol and Related Conditions (NESARC). Both surveys included individuals ages 18 years and older (Grant et al. 2006; Kessler et al. 2012). The NCS-R, conducted from 2001 to 2003, used the DSM-IV criteria as diagnosed by the Composite International Diagnostic Interview (CIDI; American Psychiatric Association 1994; Kessler and Üstün 2004; Wittchen et al. 1991). This nationwide survey was based on a probability sample of the continental United States (N=9,282) and was designed to study prevalence and correlates of DSM-IV (Kessler et al. 2012). These data were also included in a cross-national epidemiological study from the World Mental Health Survey Initiative (de Jonge et al. 2016). The NESARC also used DSM-IV criteria as well as face-to-face interviews with a representative sample of 43,093 Americans from 2001 to 2002.

Findings from the World Mental Health Survey suggest a 13.2% lifetime prevalence of DSM-5 panic attacks. This study found that the lifetime prevalence of PD was 1.7% across 25 different countries, and 3.0% in the United States specifically. In the NCS-R, the lifetime prevalence of panic attacks (without PD) was 22%, although the lifetime prevalence of PD (with and without agoraphobia) was 4.7% (Kessler et al. 2006). Kessler et al. (2012) found the proportion of people who will eventually develop PD at some time in their life to be 6.8% and the 12-month prevalence rate of PD to be 2.4%.

PD is more common in women; the female-to-male ratio is approximately 2:1, and the lifetime prevalence is approximately 5% in women and 2% in men (Roy-Byrne et al. 2018). Although the median age at onset for PD is 24 years, approximately half of adult patients with PD report experiencing significant difficulties with anxiety during childhood (Pollack et al. 1996). The onset of PD has been reported to occur spontaneously (Biederman et al. 1997), but most individuals with PD identify a life stressor occurring within the year prior to panic onset, which may be associated with its onset (Manfro et al. 1996; Roy-Byrne et al. 1986). It is unclear whether patients with PD experience more life stressors than other individuals or whether they are more sensitive to the aversive effects of life events because of differences in neurobiology, genetic endowment, temperamental predisposition, or conditioning.

PD is found across racial and ethnic backgrounds, although it is more frequently diagnosed in white Americans than in Asian, Latinx, or African Americans (Asnaani et al. 2009). Notably, different racial groups experience specific panic symptoms at different rates. For example, white Americans experience more trembling and shaking than African Americans and Hispanic Americans, whereas Hispanic Americans experience more choking sensations than white Americans and African Americans (Asnaani et al. 2009). Theories explaining these variations include cultural differences and health differences between the groups (see Chapter 4, "Cultural and Social Aspects of Anxiety Disorders"). Cultural factors should be considered in the assessment of individuals presenting with panic and somatic symptoms.

Other risk factors for PD include being younger than age 60 years; being unemployed; being divorced, separated, or widowed; having a lower level of education; having a lower household income; having more stressful life events; and being foreign born (Asnaani et al. 2009; de Jonge et al. 2016).

Clinical Features

PD is a common, distressing, and often disabling condition in which patients experience recurrent unexpected panic attacks followed by at least 1 month of persistent concerns about having additional attacks (i.e., anticipatory anxiety), worry about the implications of the attack, or a significant change in behavior (e.g., avoidance) related to the attacks (Box 20–1). The panic attacks cannot be due to the physiological effects of a substance or a medical condition or be better accounted for by anxiety episodes occurring in conjunction with other psychiatric disorders (see "Differential Diagnosis" at end of this section).

Box 20–1. DSM-5 diagnostic criteria for panic disorder

A. Recurrent unexpected panic attacks. A panic attack is an abrupt surge of intense fear or intense discomfort that reaches a peak within minutes, and during which time four (or more) of the following symptoms occur:

Note: The abrupt surge can occur from a calm state or an anxious state.

1. Palpitations, pounding heart, or accelerated heart rate.
2. Sweating.
3. Trembling or shaking.
4. Sensations of shortness of breath or smothering.
5. Feelings of choking.
6. Chest pain or discomfort.
7. Nausea or abdominal distress.
8. Feeling dizzy, unsteady, light-headed, or faint.
9. Chills or heat sensations.
10. Paresthesias (numbness or tingling sensations).
11. Derealization (feelings of unreality) or depersonalization (being detached from oneself).
12. Fear of losing control or "going crazy."
13. Fear of dying.

Note: Culture-specific symptoms (e.g., tinnitus, neck soreness, headache, uncontrollable screaming or crying) may be seen. Such symptoms should not count as one of the four required symptoms.

B. At least one of the attacks has been followed by 1 month (or more) of one or both of the following:

1. Persistent concern or worry about additional panic attacks or their consequences (e.g., losing control, having a heart attack, "going crazy").
2. A significant maladaptive change in behavior related to the attacks (e.g., behaviors designed to avoid having panic attacks, such as avoidance of exercise or unfamiliar situations).

C. The disturbance is not attributable to the physiological effects of a substance (e.g., a drug of abuse, a medication) or another medical condition (e.g., hyperthyroidism, cardiopulmonary disorders).

D. The disturbance is not better explained by another mental disorder (e.g., the panic attacks do not occur only in response to feared social situations, as in social anxiety disorder; in response to circumscribed phobic objects or situations, as in specific phobia; in response to obsessions, as in obsessive-compulsive disorder; in response to reminders of traumatic events, as in posttraumatic stress disorder; or in response to separation from attachment figures, as in separation anxiety disorder).

Box 20–2.   DSM-5 specifier for panic attack

Note: Symptoms are presented for the purpose of identifying a panic attack; however, panic attack is not a mental disorder and cannot be coded. Panic attacks can occur in the context of any anxiety disorder as well as other mental disorders (e.g., depressive disorders, posttraumatic stress disorder, substance use disorders) and some medical conditions (e.g., cardiac, respiratory, vestibular, gastrointestinal). When the presence of a panic attack is identified, it should be noted as a specifier (e.g., "posttraumatic stress disorder with panic attacks"). For panic disorder, the presence of panic attack is contained within the criteria for the disorder and panic attack is not used as a specifier.

An abrupt surge of intense fear or intense discomfort that reaches a peak within minutes, and during which time four (or more) of the following symptoms occur:

Note: The abrupt surge can occur from a calm state or an anxious state.

1. Palpitations, pounding heart, or accelerated heart rate
2. Sweating
3. Trembling or shaking
4. Sensations of shortness of breath or smothering
5. Feelings of choking
6. Chest pain or discomfort
7. Nausea or abdominal distress
8. Feeling dizzy, unsteady, light-headed, or faint
9. Chills or heat sensations
10. Paresthesias (numbness or tingling sensations)
11. Derealization (feelings of unreality) or depersonalization (being detached from oneself)
12. Fear of losing control or "going crazy"
13. Fear of dying

Note: Culture-specific symptoms (e.g., tinnitus, neck soreness, headache, uncontrollable screaming or crying) may be seen. Such symptoms should not count as one of the four required symptoms.

Panic attacks are periods of intense fear, apprehension, or discomfort that develop suddenly and reach a peak of intensity within 10 minutes of the initiation of symptoms. The DSM-5 panic attack specifier requires that 4 of 13 symptoms be present to diagnose a panic attack (Box 20–2). Notably, most of the symptoms (i.e., 11 of 13) of a panic attack are physical rather than emotional; this fact may contribute to the frequent presentation of PD in general medical settings and increased rates of medical services use among affected patients (Simon and VonKorff 1991). The sudden onset of panic attacks and their episodic nature distinguish them from the more diffuse symptoms characterizing anticipatory or generalized anxiety. Panic attacks are not unique to PD and may occur on exposure to feared events in any of the anxiety disorders as well as in mood, psychotic, and substance use disorders (Asmundson et al. 2014). DSM-5 recognizes the importance of panic attacks in other disorders and denotes them as specifiers (e.g., someone may be diagnosed with "PTSD with panic attacks"). Panic attacks also are reported, albeit infrequently, in individuals without anxiety disorders. Compared with panic attacks occurring in PD, these panic episodes are less likely to involve fears of dying, having a heart attack, and losing control and tend to occur in stressful situations such as public speaking or interpersonal conflicts and before tests and examinations (Norton et al. 1992). Panic attacks are notably associated with increased symptom severity of various disorders, suicidal ideation and behavior, and diminished treatment response among those with other anxiety and mental disorders (Asmundson et al. 2014).

The diagnostic criteria for PD emphasize anxiety about panic attacks as a core feature, including concerns about additional attacks, worry about the implications of the attacks, and significant changes in behavior (e.g., avoidance) associated with the attacks. This places central attention on a patient's phobic responses to the panic attacks themselves and their perceived consequences (e.g., "I'm having a heart attack"; "I may faint"). In contrast, other disorders may be characterized by panic responses that accompany feared responses to other phobic events, such as exposure to a social situation in social anxiety disorder, to a trauma cue in PTSD, or to an obsessional concern (e.g., contamination) in OCD.

Panic attacks that occur with fewer than 4 of the 13 panic symptoms specified by DSM-5 are *limited-symptom attacks*. Many patients with PD have a combination of full- and limited-symptom attacks. For some individuals, the early phases of treatment may be characterized by a decrease in full-symptom attacks with a transient increase in limited-symptom attacks as treatment begins to become effective. Although limited-symptom attacks incorporate fewer symptoms, they still may be quite distressing and associated with significant impairment and treatment-seeking behavior (Klerman et al. 1991).

The severity and frequency of panic attacks vary; some patients experience episodes once or twice a week, whereas others experience multiple attacks on a daily basis. The frequency of panic attacks may be a misleading indicator of the true severity of the condition because some patients may reduce the frequency of attacks by avoiding situations that trigger them (e.g., agoraphobic avoidance).

Course and Relationship With Agoraphobia

Agoraphobia refers to a patient's fear or avoidance of situations from which escape might be difficult or embarrassing or in which help may not be readily available in the event of a panic attack or other embarrassing or debilitating problems. Agoraphobic situations may include being away from home alone; traveling on public transportation; being in open spaces such as parking lots and bridges; being in enclosed spaces such as elevators, tunnels, or grocery stores; and standing in long lines. Agoraphobia also may occur in any situation in which the patient previously experienced a panic attack. Despite their fear, some patients may push themselves through the agoraphobic situation, whereas others avoid the situations or can face them only with a trusted companion. Some patients become homebound for fear of losing control outside the perceived relative safety of their home. For some, the avoidance behavior may be cued by interoceptive or internal stimuli, such as rapid heart rate, which may occur in the context of physical exercise or sexual arousal. Through conditioning, these stimuli may trigger a cognitive cascade of alarm and result in avoidance of physical exertion or other situations that cause autonomic arousal.

Box 20-3.   DSM-5 diagnostic criteria for agoraphobia

A. Marked fear or anxiety about two (or more) of the following five situations:

  1. Using public transportation (e.g., automobiles, buses, trains, ships, planes)
  2. Being in open spaces (e.g., parking lots, marketplaces, bridges)
  3. Being in enclosed places (e.g., shops, theaters, cinemas)
  4. Standing in line or being in a crowd
  5. Being outside of the home alone

B. The individual fears or avoids these situations because of thoughts that escape might be difficult or help might not be available in the event of developing panic-like symptoms or other incapacitating or embarrassing symptoms (e.g., fear of falling in the elderly; fear of incontinence).

C. The agoraphobic situations almost always provoke fear or anxiety.

D. The agoraphobic situations are actively avoided, require the presence of a companion, or are endured with intense fear or anxiety.

E. The fear or anxiety is out of proportion to the actual danger posed by the agoraphobic situations and to the sociocultural context.

F. The fear, anxiety, or avoidance is persistent, typically lasting for 6 months or more.

G. The fear, anxiety, or avoidance causes clinically significant distress or impairment in social, occupational, or other important areas of functioning.

H. If another medical condition (e.g., inflammatory bowel disease, Parkinson's disease) is present, the fear, anxiety, or avoidance is clearly excessive.

I. The fear, anxiety, or avoidance is not better explained by the symptoms of another mental disorder—for example, the symptoms are not confined to specific phobia, situational type; do not involve only social situations (as in social anxiety disorder); and are not related exclusively to obsessions (as in obsessive-compulsive disorder), perceived defects or flaws in physical appearance (as in body dysmorphic disorder), reminders of traumatic events (as in posttraumatic stress disorder), or fear of separation (as in separation anxiety disorder).

Note: Agoraphobia is diagnosed irrespective of the presence of panic disorder. If an individual's presentation meets criteria for panic disorder and agoraphobia, both diagnoses should be assigned.

Source. Reprinted from American Psychiatric Association: *Diagnostic and Statistical Manual of Mental Disorders,* 5th Edition. Arlington, VA, American Psychiatric Association, 2013. Copyright © 2013 American Psychiatric Association. Used with permission.

DSM-5 includes agoraphobia as its own disorder, but DSM-IV-TR (American Psychiatric Association 2000) included agoraphobia as part of two conditions: PD with agoraphobia and agoraphobia without a history of PD. DSM-5 separated the two conditions because of evidence that agoraphobia without panic attacks has different incidence rates, gender distributions, and treatment strategies (Box 20–3) (Wittchen et al. 2008). Studies framing agoraphobia as its own disorder have had high reliability (Asmundson et al. 2014).

Core Features

A wealth of studies support fears of anxiety-related sensations as a core feature predisposing to and helping maintain PD. These fears—often assessed with the Anxiety

Sensitivity Index (Reiss et al. 1986)—predict the onset or maintenance of PD, mediate improvement during cognitive-behavioral treatment of PD, and predict relapse following medication discontinuation for PD (Gallagher et al. 2013; Smits et al. 2018). Accordingly, continued attention to these fears in preventive and intervention models is warranted.

Impairment Associated With Panic Disorder

Examination of the health and social consequences of PD has demonstrated significant associated impairment and disability. For example, individuals with PD experience greater impairment of quality of life and well-being than nonanxious individuals (Barrera and Norton 2009) and impairment equal to that of people with medical illness such as diabetes (Davidoff et al. 2012). Although Cramer et al. (2005) found that the impairment associated with PD is equal to that of major depression, Carta et al. (2015) found that the impairment associated with depression is greater than that with PD. Regardless, studies agree that PD worsens well-being. Also, although many patients with PD achieve improvements in quality of life with effective treatment, many patients with panic continue to be below community levels of quality of life, suggesting that PD should be directly targeted in treatment (Davidoff et al. 2012). Individuals with PD, like those with many other psychiatric disorders, experience frequent, severe impairment in their home, work, and social functioning (Alonso et al. 2018). Panic has been associated with high rates of vocational dysfunction (including less productivity) and financial dependence as well as excessive use of medical services (Klerman et al. 1991; Roy-Byrne et al. 1999). A European study examining the economic costs of PD, including medical and nonmedical costs such as lost productivity, found an annual per-capita cost of 10,269 euros (Batelaan et al. 2007).

PD is common in the general medical setting (range 2%–13%; median prevalence 4%–6% [Roy-Byrne et al. 1999]) and is associated with increased health care use. Recent studies have found that anxiety is one of the most commonly cited psychiatric complaints in primary care (McCombe et al. 2018), with up to 9.7% of primary care patients having PD (Roca et al. 2009). Like other psychiatric conditions, PD is often unrecognized and untreated in primary care settings; the World Health Organization documented that the diagnosis of panic was overlooked in half the affected patients in primary care (Lecrubier and Üstün 1998). Furthermore, suicidal ideation is underreported by people with PD (Teismann et al. 2018).

Underrecognition of PD may be attributable in part to the typical presentation of panic patients with predominantly somatic symptoms (e.g., chest pain) rather than psychological symptoms (Bridges and Goldberg 1985). One study indicated that patients with PD were five to eight times more likely than nonaffected individuals to be high users of medical services (Simon and VonKorff 1991). Even the presence of panic attacks not meeting full criteria for PD may be associated with significant impairment in functioning and treatment seeking (Klerman et al. 1991). Recognition and treatment of PD in general medical settings is critical, given the association of the disorder with adverse effects across multiple domains of functioning and the demonstration that treatment results in symptomatic relief, improvement in role functioning, decreased use of medical resources, and reduction in overall costs (Batelaan et al. 2012; Hofmann et al. 2012).

Comorbidity

PD may be complicated by the presence of comorbid conditions, including other anxiety disorders as well as depression and alcohol use disorder. One study (Tilli et al. 2012) found that 98% of participants with PD had at least one lifetime comorbid diagnosis. The NCS-R found that co-occurring anxiety disorders were most common, with 66% of individuals with PD meeting criteria for another anxiety disorder and 94% of individuals with PD with agoraphobia meeting criteria for another anxiety disorder (Calkins et al. 2016). The specific comorbidity rates for PD with and without agoraphobia were as follows: specific phobias (34% and 67%, respectively), social anxiety disorder (31% and 67%, respectively), generalized anxiety disorder (21% and 15%, respectively), and PTSD (22% and 40%, respectively).

Major depressive disorder is among the most common conditions comorbid with PD, with a lifetime prevalence of 38% in epidemiological samples (Kessler et al. 2006) and possibly higher in clinical samples (Kessler et al. 1998). Depression may either predate or emerge after onset of PD and may reflect a reactive demoralization or frustration with the negative effects of panic or the emergence of an independent condition.

PD comorbidity with bipolar disorder has been examined in several studies. Data from a treatment-seeking population of individuals with bipolar disorder suggest lifetime rates of panic with or without agoraphobia of approximately 18% in bipolar I and 14% in bipolar II disorder (Simon et al. 2004b). Moreover, panic has been associated with earlier age at onset of bipolar disorder, shorter euthymic periods, poorer quality of life, greater substance abuse comorbidity, higher levels of suicidality, and poorer response to treatment, both prospectively and retrospectively (Otto et al. 2006; Simon et al. 2004b). Unfortunately, there remains a paucity of data to guide treatment of patients with panic and bipolar comorbidity, although the presence of bipolar disorder has important implications for treatment selection for PD, such as avoiding monotherapy with antidepressants and prioritizing mood stabilization (Simon et al. 2004a).

Alcohol use disorders may also be present in a significant subset of individuals with PD. One study suggested that approximately 34% of adults with PD with agoraphobia meet criteria for at least one lifetime substance use disorder (Conway et al. 2006). Some individuals report that their abuse of alcohol developed in the context of an attempt to self-medicate their anxiety. However, the temporal relation between alcohol abuse and PD tends to follow diagnostic patterns, with mean age at onset in the late teens and early 20s for alcohol abuse and the late 20s for PD (Otto et al. 1992). One study found that approximately one-half of individuals with panic and substance use disorders had an earlier onset of the substance use disorder (Sareen et al. 2006). It is of note that individuals with anxiety disorders who attempt to self-medicate do appear to be at increased risk for substance use comorbidity as well as mood disorders and suicidality (Bolton et al. 2006). Clinically, the presence of alcohol and other substance use disorders may be associated with poor outcome and should be considered in all individuals presenting with panic and other anxiety disorders. Patients abusing alcohol or drugs require focused substance abuse treatment, in addition to the treatment directed at the PD, to facilitate comprehensive recovery.

The presence of comorbidity in PD bodes poorly for a variety of psychological, functional, and treatment outcomes. For instance, increased rates of suicide and suicide attempts have been associated with PD, with some research suggesting that inflated rates of lifetime suicide attempts are the result of co-occurring psychiatric conditions (e.g., depression or alcohol abuse). Evidence suggests that the presence of PD is associated with increased rates of suicide attempts, even when comorbidity and a history of childhood abuse are accounted for (Goodwin and Roy-Byrne 2006; Nam et al. 2016). Similarly, the lifetime risk of suicide attempts by patients with PD and major depressive disorder is more than double that of patients with only one of the two disorders (Cox et al. 1994; Fawcett et al. 1990). High anxiety-sensitivity-related cognitive concerns about the potential threat of physical symptoms has emerged as a potential risk factor of death from suicide (Rappaport et al. 2014).

Medical disorders also occur more commonly and are associated with increased impairment in individuals with PD (Kessler et al. 2003; Sareen et al. 2005). In particular, panic is associated with respiratory conditions, including asthma (Goodwin et al. 2003) and chronic obstructive pulmonary disease (Karajgi et al. 1990). The overlap of anxiety sensitivity with the experience of panic symptoms and greater dyspnea in patients with chronic obstructive pulmonary disease, as well as the relationship between respiratory and anxiety neurocircuitry, remains under active investigation (Livermore et al. 2012). PD also occurs commonly with migraines, particularly migraines with aura; the odds of PD are 3.76 times greater among individuals with migraines than those without migraines (Smitherman et al. 2013). Another report combining prior panic studies that examined both thyroid history and test results also supports significantly elevated rates of thyroid dysfunction (6.5%), suggesting that patients with PD should be screened at least once for thyroid disease (Simon et al. 2002). Comorbidity of PD with vertigo due to vestibular dysfunction also may occur, with some symptom overlap and the development of agoraphobic avoidance, including avoidance of environmental factors that may heighten dizziness (Staab et al. 2004). Cardiac symptoms and disease are another important area of medical overlap with PD (Smoller et al. 2007). Many somatic symptoms such as heart palpitations or chest pain that occur during panic attacks may not be easily differentiated from those due to a primary cardiac disorder; many patients with PD seek care initially complaining of cardiac symptoms. Although the precise etiology of these associations is unknown, PD may have implications for cardiac health and mortality, with several studies supporting increased risk for fatal coronary heart disease, changes in QT and heart rate variability, and sudden death (Albert et al. 2005). Treatment of PD with selective serotonin reuptake inhibitors, in contrast to tricyclic antidepressants, has been associated with a significant improvement in heart rate variability, which theoretically may decrease risk for mortality due to sudden cardiac death potentially due to alterations in autonomic activity (Pohl et al. 2000; Yeragani et al. 2000).

Differential Diagnosis

Although PD is commonly comorbid with other anxiety disorders, the nature of the panic attacks differentiates the disorders. To distinguish between social anxiety and PD, focusing on the patient's core fears may help with diagnosis. In PD, the patient's central fear is of having a panic attack and may manifest in situations outside of social ones. Patients with social anxiety disorder focus primarily on the possibility of humiliation or embarrassment in social situations and may panic upon exposure to social scrutiny. For many patients, both types of fears may be present, and the diagnosis of both conditions is warranted.

Generalized anxiety disorder (GAD) is also frequently comorbid with PD (Kessler et al. 2006). In GAD, patients are excessively worried about life activities or stressors, with the anxiety not solely focused on anticipation of recurrent panic attacks. The episodic and crescendo nature of panic attacks as compared with the more persistent, but often less intense, anxiety associated with GAD is another distinguishing feature.

Patients with specific phobias, PTSD, and OCD may also experience panic attacks, but these are typically cued by exposure to or anticipation of specific phobic situations (e.g., heights or other phobic situations in the case of specific phobias, situations evocative of events associated with trauma in the case of PTSD, and contamination in patients with OCD). For these conditions, panic attacks are cued by specific situations and do not occur spontaneously unless PD is also present.

Evaluation

A semistructured interview with a clinician is the first step when diagnosing PD. For example, clinical researchers frequently use the Structured Clinical Interview for DSM-5 (First et al. 2016) to diagnose PD and to distinguish it from other overlapping disorders. Another gold standard instrument in clinical practice for PD assessment and severity monitoring with treatment is the seven-item Panic Disorder Severity Scale (PDSS), which is available in clinician-administered and self-report versions (Houck et al. 2002; Shear et al. 1997). The PDSS assesses panic symptom severity, anticipatory anxiety, avoidance due to the fear of having a panic attack, and associated work and social impairment due to PD. Screening tools such as the PD module of the Patient Health Questionnaire can be used in primary care or community settings (Wittkampf et al. 2011).

A medical evaluation is often recommended to rule out medical conditions, such as thyroid conditions or arrhythmias that can mimic the symptoms of PD, prior to giving a PD diagnosis. PD may be diagnosed in addition to a medical condition and can often worsen the physical symptoms of that medical condition, making it difficult to distinguish without careful clinical assessment.

Conclusion

PD is a common, distressing, and disabling condition. It is frequently complicated by comorbid agoraphobia and other psychiatric disorders. It often presents in the general medical setting and is associated with increased use of medical services, underscoring the need for timely recognition and treatment as well as careful differential diagnosis.

Key Points

- Recent epidemiological data suggest a lifetime prevalence of 2%–5% for panic disorder (PD) with and without associated agoraphobia.

- PD is two to three times more commonly diagnosed in women than men, with a typical age at onset in the third decade, although many patients report a history of anxiety beginning in childhood.

- Although panic attacks are often the most dramatic feature of PD, comprehensive evaluation of affected individuals should include not only panic attack frequency and severity but also anticipatory anxiety, avoidance, and functioning.

- PD is associated with significant distress and dysfunction as well as increased use of medical resources, greater risk for adverse cardiovascular events, and overall reduced quality of life.

- PD is often complicated by the presence of comorbid conditions, including other anxiety disorders, mood disorders, substance abuse, and medical disorders.

References

Albert CM, Chae CU, Rexrode KM, et al: Phobic anxiety and risk of coronary heart disease and sudden cardiac death among women. Circulation 111(4):480–487, 2005 15687137

Alonso J, Mortier P, Auerbach RP, et al: Severe role impairment associated with mental disorders: results of the WHO World Mental Health Surveys International College Student Project. Depress Anxiety 35(9):802–814, 2018 29847006

American Psychiatric Association: Diagnostic and Statistical Manual of Mental Disorders, 3rd Edition. Washington, DC, American Psychiatric Association, 1980

American Psychiatric Association: Diagnostic and Statistical Manual of Mental Disorders, 4th Edition. Washington, DC, American Psychiatric Association, 1994

American Psychiatric Association: Diagnostic and Statistical Manual of Mental Disorders, 4th Edition, Text Revision. Washington, DC, American Psychiatric Association, 2000

American Psychiatric Association: Diagnostic and Statistical Manual of Mental Disorders, 5th Edition. Arlington, VA, American Psychiatric Association, 2013

Asmundson GJ, Taylor S, Smits JAJ: Panic disorder and agoraphobia: an overview and commentary on DSM-5 changes. Depress Anxiety 31(6):480–486, 2014 24865357

Asnaani A, Gutner CA, Hinton DE, et al: Panic disorder, panic attacks and panic attack symptoms across race-ethnic groups: results of the collaborative psychiatric epidemiology studies. CNS Neurosci Ther 15(3):249–254, 2009 19691544

Barrera TL, Norton PJ: Quality of life impairment in generalized anxiety disorder, social phobia, and panic disorder. J Anxiety Disord 23(8):1086–1090, 2009 19640675

Batelaan N, Smit F, de Graaf R, et al: Economic costs of full-blown and subthreshold panic disorder. J Affect Disord 104(1–3):127–136, 2007 17466380

Batelaan NM, Rhebergen D, de Graaf R, et al: Panic attacks as a dimension of psychopathology: evidence for associations with onset and course of mental disorders and level of functioning. J Clin Psychiatry 73(9):1195–1202, 2012 23059148

Biederman J, Faraone SV, Marrs A, et al: Panic disorder and agoraphobia in consecutively referred children and adolescents. J Am Acad Child Adolesc Psychiatry 36(2):214–223, 1997 9031574

Bolton J, Cox B, Clara I, et al: Use of alcohol and drugs to self-medicate anxiety disorders in a nationally representative sample. J Nerv Ment Dis 194(11):818–825, 2006 17102705

Bridges KW, Goldberg DP: Somatic presentation of DSM III psychiatric disorders in primary care. J Psychosom Res 29(6):563–569, 1985 4087223

Calkins AW, Bui E, Taylor CT, et al: Anxiety disorders, in Massachusetts General Hospital: Comprehensive Clinical Psychiatry, 2nd Edition. Edited by Stern TA, Fava M, Willens T, et al. Philadelphia, PA, Mosby Elsevier, 2016, pp 353–367

Carta MG, Moro MF, Aguglia E, et al: The attributable burden of panic disorder in the impairment of quality of life in a national survey in Italy. Int J Soc Psychiatry 61(7):693–699, 2015 25770204

Conway KP, Compton W, Stinson FS, et al: Lifetime comorbidity of DSM-IV mood and anxiety disorders and specific drug use disorders: results from the National Epidemiologic Survey on Alcohol and Related Conditions. J Clin Psychiatry 67(2):247–257, 2006 16566620

Cox BJ, Direnfeld DM, Swinson RP, et al: Suicidal ideation and suicide attempts in panic disorder and social phobia. Am J Psychiatry 151:882–887, 1994

Cramer V, Torgersen S, Kringlen E: Quality of life and anxiety disorders: a population study. J Nerv Ment Dis 193(3):196–202, 2005 15729110

Davidoff J, Christensen S, Khalili DN, et al: Quality of life in panic disorder: looking beyond symptom remission. Qual Life Res 21(6):945–959, 2012 21935739

de Jonge P, Roest AM, Lim CC, et al: Cross-national epidemiology of panic disorder and panic attacks in the World Mental Health surveys. Depress Anxiety 33:1155–1177, 2016 27775828

Fawcett J, Scheftner WA, Fogg L, et al: Time-related predictors of suicide in major affective disorder. Am J Psychiatry 147:1189–1194, 1990

First MB, Williams JBW, Karg RS, et al: Structured Clinical Interview for DSM-5 Disorders, Clinician Version (SCID-5-CV). Arlington, VA, American Psychiatric Association, 2016

Gallagher MW, Payne LA, White KS, et al: Mechanisms of change in cognitive behavioral therapy for panic disorder: the unique effects of self-efficacy and anxiety sensitivity. Behav Res Ther 51(11):767–777, 2013 24095901

Goodwin RD, Roy-Byrne P: Panic and suicidal ideation and suicide attempts: results from the National Comorbidity Survey. Depress Anxiety 23(3):124–132, 2006 16502406

Goodwin RD, Jacobi F, Thefeld W: Mental disorders and asthma in the community. Arch Gen Psychiatry 60(11):1125–1130, 2003 14609888

Grant BF, Hasin DS, Stinson FS, et al: The epidemiology of DSM-IV panic disorder and agoraphobia in the United States: results from the National Epidemiologic Survey on Alcohol and Related Conditions. J Clin Psychiatry 67(3):363–374, 2006 16649821

Hofmann SG, Asnaani A, Vonk IJJ, et al: The efficacy of cognitive behavioral therapy: a review of meta-analyses. Cognit Ther Res 36(5):427–440, 2012 23459093

Houck PR, Spiegel DA, Shear MK, et al: Reliability of the self-report version of the Panic Disorder Severity Scale. Depress Anxiety 15(4):183–185, 2002 12112724

Karajgi B, Rifkin A, Doddi S, et al: The prevalence of anxiety disorders in patients with chronic obstructive pulmonary disease. Am J Psychiatry 147(2):200–201, 1990 2301659

Kessler RC, Ustün TB: The World Mental Health (WMH) Survey Initiative version of the World Health Organization (WHO) Composite International Diagnostic Interview (CIDI). Int J Methods Psychiatr Res 13(2):93–121, 2004 15297906

Kessler RC, Stang PE, Wittchen HU, et al: Lifetime panic-depression comorbidity in the National Comorbidity Survey. Arch Gen Psychiatry 55(9):801–808, 1998 9736006

Kessler RC, Ormel J, Demler O, et al: Comorbid mental disorders account for the role impairment of commonly occurring chronic physical disorders: results from the National Comorbidity Survey. J Occup Environ Med 45(12):1257–1266, 2003 14665811

Kessler RC, Chiu WT, Jin R, et al: The epidemiology of panic attacks, panic disorder, and agoraphobia in the National Comorbidity Survey Replication. Arch Gen Psychiatry 63(4):415–424, 2006 16585471

Kessler RC, Petukhova M, Sampson NA, et al: Twelve-month and lifetime prevalence and lifetime morbid risk of anxiety and mood disorders in the United States. Int J Methods Psychiatr Res 21(3):169–184, 2012 22865617

Klerman GL, Weissman MM, Ouellette R, et al: Panic attacks in the community. Social morbidity and health care utilization. JAMA 265(6):742–746, 1991 1990190

Lecrubier Y, Ustün TB: Panic and depression: a worldwide primary care perspective. Int Clin Psychopharmacol 13(suppl 4):S7–S11, 1998 9690959

Livermore N, Sharpe L, McKenzie D: Catastrophic interpretations and anxiety sensitivity as predictors of panic-spectrum psychopathology in chronic obstructive pulmonary disease. J Psychosom Res 72(5):388–392, 2012 22469282

Manfro GG, Otto MW, McArdle ET, et al: Relationship of antecedent stressful life events to childhood and family history of anxiety and the course of panic disorder. J Affect Disord 41(2):135–139, 1996 8961041

McCombe G, Fogarty F, Swan D, et al: Identified mental disorders in older adults in primary care: a cross-sectional database study. Eur J Gen Pract 24(1):84–91, 2018 29353511

Nam YY, Kim CH, Roh D: Comorbid panic disorder as an independent risk factor for suicide attempts in depressed outpatients. Compr Psychiatry 67:13–18, 2016 27095329

Norton GR, Cox BJ, Malan J: Nonclinical panickers: a critical review. Clin Psychol Rev 12:121–139, 1992

Otto MW, Pollack MH, Sachs GS, et al: Alcohol dependence in panic disorder patients. J Psychiatr Res 26(1):29–38, 1992 1560407

Otto MW, Simon NM, Wisniewski SR, et al: Prospective 12-month course of bipolar disorder in out-patients with and without comorbid anxiety disorders. Br J Psychiatry 189:20–25, 2006 16816301

Pohl R, Jampala V, Balon R, et al: Effects of nortriptyline and paroxetine on QT variability in patients with panic disorder. Depress Anxiety 11:126–130, 2000

Pollack MH, Otto MW, Sabatino S, et al: Relationship of childhood anxiety to adult panic disorder: correlates and influence on course. Am J Psychiatry 153(3):376–381, 1996 8610825

Rappaport LM, Moskowitz DS, Galynker I, et al: Panic symptom clusters differentially predict suicide ideation and attempt. Compr Psychiatry 55(4):762–769, 2014 24439632

Reiss S, Peterson RA, Gursky DM, et al: Anxiety sensitivity, anxiety frequency and the prediction of fearfulness. Behav Res Ther 24:1–8, 1986

Roca M, Gili M, Garcia-Garcia M, et al: Prevalence and comorbidity of common mental disorders in primary care. J Affect Disord 119(1–3):52–58, 2009 19361865

Roy-Byrne PP, Geraci M, Uhde TW: Life events and course of illness in patients with panic disorder. Am J Psychiatry 143(8):1033–1035, 1986 3728719

Roy-Byrne PP, Stein MB, Russo J, et al: Panic disorder in the primary care setting: comorbidity, disability, service utilization, and treatment. J Clin Psychiatry 60(7):492–499, quiz 500, 1999 10453807

Roy-Byrne PP, Stein MB, Hermann R: Panic disorder in adults: epidemiology, pathogenesis, clinical manifestations, course, assessment, and diagnosis. UpToDate, June 2018. Available at: https://www.uptodate.com/contents/panic-disorder-in-adults-epidemiology-pathogenesis-clinical-manifestations-course-assessment-and-diagnosis. Accessed June 25, 2019.

Sareen J, Cox BJ, Clara I, et al: The relationship between anxiety disorders and physical disorders in the U.S. National Comorbidity Survey. Depress Anxiety 21(4):193–202, 2005 16075453

Sareen J, Chartier M, Paulus MP, et al: Illicit drug use and anxiety disorders: findings from two community surveys. Psychiatry Res 142(1):11–17, 2006 16712953

Shear MK, Brown TA, Barlow DH, et al: Multicenter collaborative Panic Disorder Severity Scale. Am J Psychiatry 154(11):1571–1575, 1997 9356566

Simon GE, VonKorff M: Somatization and psychiatric disorder in the NIMH Epidemiologic Catchment Area study. Am J Psychiatry 148(11):1494–1500, 1991 1928462

Simon NM, Blacker D, Korbly NB, et al: Hypothyroidism and hyperthyroidism in anxiety disorders revisited: new data and literature review. J Affect Disord 69(1–3):209–217, 2002 12103468

Simon NM, Otto MW, Weiss RD, et al: Pharmacotherapy for bipolar disorder and comorbid conditions: baseline data from STEP-BD. J Clin Psychopharmacol 24(5):512–520, 2004a 15349007

Simon NM, Otto MW, Wisniewski SR, et al: Anxiety disorder comorbidity in bipolar disorder patients: data from the first 500 participants in the Systematic Treatment Enhancement Program for Bipolar Disorder (STEP-BD). Am J Psychiatry 161(12):2222–2229, 2004b 15569893

Smitherman TA, Kolivas ED, Bailey JR: Panic disorder and migraine: comorbidity, mechanisms, and clinical implications. Headache 53(1):23–45, 2013 23278473

Smits JAJ, Otto MW, Powers MB, et al (eds): Anxiety Sensitivity: A Clinical Guide to Assessment and Treatment. San Diego, CA, Academic Press, 2018

Smoller JW, Pollack MH, Wassertheil-Smoller S, et al: Panic attacks and risk of incident cardiovascular events among postmenopausal women in the Women's Health Initiative Observational Study. Arch Gen Psychiatry 64(10):1153–1160, 2007 17909127

Staab JP, Ruckenstein MJ, Amsterdam JD: A prospective trial of sertraline for chronic subjective dizziness. Laryngoscope 114(9):1637–1641, 2004 15475796

Teismann T, Lukaschek K, Hiller TS, et al: Suicidal ideation in primary care patients suffering from panic disorder with or without agoraphobia. BMC Psychiatry 18(1):305, 2018 30249220

Tilli V, Suominen K, Karlsson H: Panic disorder in primary care: comorbid psychiatric disorders and their persistence. Scand J Prim Health Care 30(4):247–253, 2012 23113695

Wittchen HU, Robins LN, Cottler LB, et al: Cross-cultural feasibility, reliability and sources of variance of the Composite International Diagnostic Interview (CIDI). The Multicentre WHO/ADAMHA Field Trials. Br J Psychiatry 159:645–653, 658, 1991 1756340

Wittchen H-U, Nocon A, Beesdo K, et al: Agoraphobia and panic: prospective-longitudinal relations suggest a rethinking of diagnostic concepts. Psychother Psychosom 77(3):147–157, 2008 18277061

Wittkampf KA, Baas KD, van Weert HC, et al: The psychometric properties of the panic disorder module of the Patient Health Questionnaire (PHQ-PD) in high-risk groups in primary care. J Affect Disord 130(1–2):260–267, 2011 21075451

Yeragani VK, Pohl R, Jampala VC, et al: Effects of nortriptyline and paroxetine on QT variability in patients with panic disorder. Depress Anxiety 11(3):126–130, 2000 10875054

Recommended Readings

Craske MG, Waters AM: Panic disorder, phobias, and generalized anxiety disorder. Annu Rev Clin Psychol 1:197–225, 2005

Katon WJ: Panic disorder. N Engl J Med 354:2360–2367, 2006

Pollack MH, Otto MW (eds): Longitudinal Perspectives on Anxiety Disorders. Psychiatric Clinics of North America, Vol 18. Philadelphia, PA, WB Saunders, 1995

Rosenbaum JF, Pollack MH (eds): Panic Disorder and Its Treatment. New York, Marcel Dekker, 1998

Smoller JW, Sheidley BR, Tsuang MT (eds): Psychiatric Genetics: Applications in Clinical Practice. Washington, DC, American Psychiatric Publishing, 2008

Websites of Interest

Anxiety and Depression Association of America: www.adaa.org

Center for Anxiety and Traumatic Stress Disorders (Massachusetts General Hospital): www.mghanxiety.org

National Institute of Mental Health: Panic Disorder: www.nimh.nih.gov/health/topics/panic-disorder/index.shtml

CHAPTER 21

Pathogenesis of Panic Disorder

Ryan D. Webler, B.A.

Jeremy D. Coplan, M.D.

A panic attack is a sudden, simultaneous combination of intense physiological changes, somatic sensations, and conscious fear (American Psychiatric Association 2013). Although panic attacks may take several forms, a prototypical panic attack is triggered by the perception of a somatic change that prompts increased interoceptive awareness and a corresponding fear that something is physically wrong, often to a catastrophic degree. Physiological changes and conscious interpretations of these changes may spur a vicious circle; increased fear may, for example, provoke increased heart rate, which may spiral into the catastrophic interpretation that one is on the verge of death. Many panic attack victims experience additional attacks accompanied by worry about past or possible future attacks, as well as behavioral changes such as avoidance. These individuals are said to have panic disorder (American Psychiatric Association 2013).

In this chapter, we review the pathogenesis of panic disorder. We examine empirical evidence supportive of its current biological and psychological conceptions and review a range of pertinent neurochemical, pharmacological, neuroimaging, and psychological findings. Finally, we propose a revised neurobiological conception of panic disorder.

Biological Bases of Panic

Initial evidence for a biological basis of panic disorder came from the observation that a range of psychotropic medications, in addition to the tricyclic antidepressant (TCA) imipramine, eliminated or at least significantly ameliorated panic disorder symptoms. The acute pharmacological effects of psychotropic medications prompted speculation that specific neurotransmitter systems may be directly implicated in the onset, maintenance, or progression of panic disorder. Traditional biological theories therefore include noradrenergic (a component of acute TCA effects), serotonergic (selective serotonin reuptake inhibitor [SSRI] and TCA mechanism of action), and GABAergic/glutamatergic (high-potency benzodiazepine and D-cycloserine mechanism of action) systems.

The development of neural network theory has begun to expand our understanding of the pathogenesis of panic disorder beyond the neurochemical level. The triple network model (Menon 2011) implicates three main networks in the development and maintenance of psychopathology: the executive control network, salience network, and default mode network. Although functional connectivity data for panic disorder are currently lacking, a structural and functional neuroimaging literature is rapidly developing that bears on panic disorder–related dysfunction in major nodes implicated in the triple network model.

The contribution of the noradrenergic, serotonergic, and GABAergic/glutamatergic systems to the development of panic disorder is detailed in the following discussion. The pathogenesis of panic disorder is then expanded to include recent findings related to abnormalities within nodes of the central executive network, salience network, and default mode network.

Noradrenergic Theory

Several groups of investigators conducted important studies of the noradrenergic system in panic disorder. In keeping with the notion that noradrenergic stimulation would increase anxiety, they showed that yohimbine administration produced panic attacks in patients with panic disorder (Uhde et al. 1992). Studies that used clonidine, which stimulates release of growth hormone–releasing factor through α_2 agonism in the hypothalamus, indicated that the growth hormone response to clonidine was blunted in patients with panic disorder. In cognitively healthy subjects, under both baseline and stressful conditions, the noradrenergic system and the hypothalamic-pituitary-adrenal axis appear to work in synchrony. Elevations or reductions of activity within one system are accompanied by parallel changes in the other system. The coordinated interaction between these two systems has been cited by Chrousos and Gold (1992) as crucial for the mammalian organism's stress response.

Serotonergic Theory

The serotonergic system has long been a major area of focus not only for panic disorder but also for psychiatry as a whole. Although approximately 15 serotonin receptor subtypes have now been discovered (Palacios 2016), neurotransmission through serotonin type 1A (5-HT_{1A}) receptors located on pyramidal neurons of the hippocampus has been viewed as crucial in engendering a sense of resilience to the organism (Paul et al. 2014). If neurotransmission at this site is inadequate, anxiety and avoidant behavior may ensue. Serotonergic neurotransmission via the 5-HT_{1A} receptor is also an important stimulus for expression of brain-derived neurotrophic factor in the hippocampus. Brain-derived neurotrophic factor is a potent promoter of dentate gyrus neurogenesis, which has been associated with antidepressant and anxiolytic response (Quesseveur et al. 2013).

Hyperventilation is one of the cardinal physiological correlates of panic anxiety. Some researchers have suggested a link between the serotonergic system and hyperventilation derived from the clinical observation that serotonin exerts clinical benefit through enhancement of serotonin neurotransmission and that a normalization of ventilatory overdrive accompanies clinical improvement of panic disorder. Kent et al. (1996) depleted serotonin using a tryptophan-free highly concentrated amino acid mixture, which resulted in a reduction in serotonin neurotransmission along with an increase in minute ventilation in patients with panic disorder. However, control subjects' ventilatory function remained unaltered despite depletion. Evidence therefore indicates that serotonin does play a role in human ventilation and that patients with panic disorder are particularly sensitive to serotonin depletion. Enhancement of serotonin neurotransmission by an SSRI thus may exert therapeutic effects in part by normalizing aberrant ventilatory patterns.

GABAergic and Glutamatergic Theory

Various regions of the brain known to be associated with panic symptoms, including the orbitofrontal complex, amygdala, and insular cortex, have been identified neuroradiologically to have abnormalities in the binding of benzodiazepine-$GABA_A$ receptor complexes (Cameron et al. 2007; Malizia et al. 1998; Nuss 2015). Other studies have also shown decreases in benzodiazepine receptor complexes, particularly in the temporal cortex, hippocampus, and precuneus (Bremner et al. 2000; Kaschka et al. 1995).

The role that glutamate plays in anxiety disorders has received increased attention of late. A recent investigation linked optogenetic activation of glutamatergic terminals in the perifornical hypothalamus projecting to the basolateral amygdala with increased fear acquisition, delayed extinction, and increased long-term fear persistence (Molosh et al. 2018). Interestingly, the augmentation of cognitive-behavioral therapy (CBT) with the partial NMDA agonist D-cycloserine has been found to improve anxiolytic response in panic disorder (Otto et al. 2010). However, meta-analyses are less sanguine regarding D-cycloserine's clinical utility (Bürkner et al. 2017).

Neural Network Theory

Central Executive Network

The central executive network mediates processes such as selective attention, working memory, and decision making (Menon 2011) and has major nodes in the dorsolateral prefrontal cortex (PFC) and lateral posterior parietal cortex. Panic disorder–related volume reductions in these and other central executive network nodes have been identified (Lai and Wu 2012; Sobanski et al. 2010).

Several studies have shown central executive network aberrancies in patients with panic disorder that bear on treatment outcome and relate to disorder-specific emotional regulation. For example, aberrant dorsolateral PFC activation to threat stimuli has been found in panic disorder (Maddock et al. 2003), and the degree of dorsolateral PFC activation to threat has been linked to CBT response (Reinecke et al. 2014).

CBT fosters the development of emotional regulation strategies; a greater degree of pretreatment dorsolateral PFC dysfunction may prevent patients with panic disorder from recruiting the cognitive control resources necessary to benefit from CBT. The dorsolateral PFC plays a particularly important role in explicit emotional regulation. Decreased dorsolateral PFC activation during emotional regulation has been found in panic disorder (Ball et al. 2013) and has been negatively linked to self-reported anxiety during a carbon dioxide challenge (Balderston et al. 2017).

Salience Network

Increased attention and sensitivity to interoceptive and external threat cues is a hallmark of panic disorder. The salience network, which detects relevant interoceptive and external changes, may play a critical role in disorder-specific exaggerated response patterns to benign internal and external stimuli. Several studies have reported panic disorder–related volume decreases in two integral salience network nodes: the anterior cingulate cortex (ACC) and insular cortex (Asami et al. 2008; Lai and Wu 2012; Uchida et al. 2008). Interestingly, more recent evidence suggests that individuals with extensive bilateral lesions in another salience network node, the amygdala, may still experience panic attacks (Feinstein et al. 2013; Khalsa et al. 2016). The implications of this finding are discussed in "Updated Neuroanatomical Hypothesis of Panic Disorder" later in the chapter.

Hyperactivation to external threat has been consistently found across the salience network, including in the dorsomedial PFC, dorsal ACC, and insula (Brinkmann et al. 2017; Engel et al. 2016; Feldker et al. 2016). Several studies have found aberrant threat-induced amygdala activation in panic disorder (Feldker et al. 2017; Fonzo et al. 2015).

Connectivity differences between salience network nodes have also been identified. Demenescu et al. (2013) found a positive relationship between anxiety symptom severity and connectivity of the amygdala–ACC and dorsomedial PFC during fearful face processing (Demenescu et al. 2013). Another study linked nonresponse to CBT with a lack of inhibitory functional dorsal ACC–amygdala coupling (Lueken et al. 2013).

A link between insular activation and symptoms such as fear of cardiovascular symptoms and subjective breathing discomfort during the carbon dioxide challenge has been established (Feldker et al. 2018). Interestingly, reported fear of somatic symptoms in a study of interoceptive threat response to hyperventilation has been strongly linked to rostral dorsal ACC/dorsomedial PFC activity (Holtz et al. 2012). Activity in these regions has also been linked to conscious threat appraisal symptoms such as worry and catastrophizing (Kalisch and Gerlicher 2014).

Default Mode Network

The default mode network has nodes in the anterior medial PFC, posterior cingulate cortex, angular gyrus, and medial temporal lobe (Menon 2011) and plays an integral role in processes that may contribute to the development and maintenance of panic disorder, including fear extinction and emotional regulation. Dysfunction in default mode network regions critically implicated in both fear extinction and emotional regulation have been found in panic disorder.

Specific to the default mode network, the hippocampus and ventromedial PFC play crucial roles in important extinction and emotional regulation processes. The hippocampus encodes and distinguishes among contextually specific memories (Leutgeb et al. 2007) and may drive fear extinction and emotional regulation through downstream connections to medial prefrontal regions such as the ventromedial PFC,

TABLE 21–1.	Triple network model: panic disorder–related volume, activation, and connectivity differences		
	Central executive network	Salience network	Default mode network
Volume	↓	↓	↓
Activation	↓↑	↑	↓↑
Within-network connectivity	↔	↑	↓

which regulates threat/emotional processing activity in salience network regions such as the amygdala (Milad and Quirk 2012).

Increased panic disorder–related activations have been found in key default mode network regions, including the hippocampus and posterior ACC (Engel et al. 2016; Maddock et al. 2003). Increased hippocampal and subgenual ACC activations to safety conditions (Lueken et al. 2013) have also been identified and may be linked to increased panic disorder–related fear generalization, wherein related but distinct safety stimuli evoke increased activation (Lissek 2012).

Decreased ventromedial PFC activation to masked affective faces has been noted in patients with panic disorder relative to control subjects (Killgore et al. 2014; Tuescher et al. 2011). Reinforcing this finding, Marin et al. (2017) found lower ventromedial PFC activation to extinction recall in a transdiagnostic anxiety disorder group that included patients with panic disorder. Additionally, connectivity between two default mode network nodes, the ventromedial PFC and subgenual ACC, was increased in control subjects relative to patients with anxiety disorder; patients instead showed increased connectivity between the ventromedial PFC and salience network nodes such as the amygdala and insular cortex.

Table 21–1 depicts volume, activation, and within-network connectivity differences between patients with panic disorder and control subjects in the three major networks implicated in the triple network model. Downward-pointing arrows denote decreases; upward-pointing arrows denote increases; side arrows denote no difference. The literature summarized in this table is fledgling and developing. Conflicting findings (denoted by upward- and downward-pointing arrows) may relate to differences in methodology or the function of specific nodes within each network. No study to our knowledge has demonstrated a significant difference in central executive network connectivity between patients with panic disorder and control subjects.

Psychological Bases of Panic

Conditioning, Extinction, and Generalization

Conditioning, extinction, and generalization are foundational psychological concepts that refer to various aspects of fear learning. *Conditioning* refers to the process by which a benign (conditioned) stimulus temporally linked with an innately threatening (unconditioned) stimulus comes to elicit a defensive response. *Extinction* is an updating process by which a conditioned response is extinguished when a conditioned stimulus is repeatedly unpaired with an unconditioned stimulus. *Generalization* is the process by which stimuli sharing characteristics with a conditioned stimulus elicit similar responses despite having never been directly paired with an unconditioned stimulus.

The theoretical relevance of fear learning to panic disorder is intuitively clear. A panic attack may be associated with myriad interoceptive (e.g., tachycardia) and exteroceptive (e.g., context) cues. The panic attack may be considered the unconditioned stimulus, and the temporally associated interoceptive and exteroceptive cues may be considered conditioned stimuli. These conditioned stimuli may become capable of provoking defensive responses (autonomic or behavioral changes) and conscious fear. Stimuli perceptually similar or conceptually related to conditioned stimuli may also provoke defensive responses and conscious fear through generalization. CBT may promote extinction of these threat and fear responses by identifying and challenging fear-related cognitive distortions (e.g., catastrophic misinterpretations) and directly unpairing interoceptive or exteroceptive conditioned stimuli from the unconditioned panic attack through exposure.

Research on Pavlovian Fear Learning

Although decades of animal threat learning research have shed light on the behavioral features and neural substrates of conditioning, extinction, and generalization, researchers have only recently begun to investigate Pavlovian fear learning in humans. In an investigation of unpredictable and predictable fear learning, Grillon et al. (2008) found increased fear-potentiated startle to unpredictable threat but not predictable threat in patients with panic disorder compared to control subjects. The authors speculated that increased response to unpredictable threat may be an acquired trait spurred by frequent, uncued panic attacks or a premorbid, threat-sensitizing trait that increases vulnerability to panic disorder.

Additional work by Lissek et al. (2009) identified increased fear-potentiated startle to safety cues in patients with panic disorder, suggestive of a disorder-related deficit in fear-learning discrimination linked to increased fear generalization. The relationship between a putative discrimination deficit and fear generalization in panic disorder was subsequently reinforced by a perceptual gradient study that demonstrated increased fear generalization in panic disorder (Lissek et al. 2010).

Studies investigating fear extinction in panic disorder found increased physiological responses to conditioned stimuli during extinction (Michael et al. 2007; Otto et al. 2014). As described earlier, decreases in extinction-related activation in default mode network nodes such as the ventromedial PFC concurrent with increased salience network node activation have been shown in panic disorder (Marin et al. 2017).

Updated Neuroanatomical Hypothesis of Panic Disorder

In this section, we discuss research findings that support and further integrate Gorman's seminal neuroanatomical panic disorder model with other contemporary theories, including the triple network model (Gorman et al. 2000). It is important to note that much of the updated model remains provisional given the current lack of panic disorder–related functional connectivity data. It will be important to test this model against future findings that directly bear on functional connectivity between and within the larger networks containing these nodes.

Both animal models and clinical findings highlight the centrality of the amygdala in panic disorder. The amygdala is part of the salience network and plays a prominent role in identifying emotionally salient stimuli and linking these stimuli to innate, unconditioned stimuli (threat conditioning). The amygdala projects to several subcortical regions responsible for behavioral and physiological adjustments, including the parabrachial nucleus, the lateral nucleus of the hypothalamus, the locus coeruleus, the paraventricular nucleus of the hypothalamus, and periaqueductal gray matter. In addition, the amygdala projects to cortical regions of the salience network, including the dorsal ACC, which amplifies brief threat signals sent from the amygdala and projects these signals back to the amygdala, sustaining threat-related attention and arousal (Milad and Quirk 2012). Amygdala–dorsal ACC hyperconnectivity has been found in panic disorder and may contribute to disorder-related threat sensitivity and hyperarousal (Demenescu et al. 2013).

The amygdala's role in the conscious perception of panic is questionable in light of evidence that panic may emerge in the context of extensive bilateral amygdala lesions (Feinstein et al. 2013; Khalsa et al. 2016). Thus, the amygdala may play a crucial role in the propagation of an initial threat signal that is only later converted into a conscious threat percept by cortical nodes (LeDoux and Pine 2016). Indeed, specific panic symptoms such as fear of cardiovascular symptoms, subjective breathing discomfort, and fear of somatic symptoms have been correlated with downstream cortical salience network nodes such as the anterior insular cortex, dorsal ACC, and dorsomedial PFC (Holtz et al. 2012; Kalisch and Gerlicher 2014).

The salience network switches between the default mode network and the central executive network, activating the central executive network during the perception of salient cues (Goulden et al. 2014). Increased connectivity between the left inferior frontal gyrus, an executive control network node, and salience network nodes such as the amygdala, insula, and ACC has been found in panic disorder (Kircher et al. 2013). Functional connectivity between the salience network and central executive network may putatively facilitate the conscious feeling of fear in part by ushering salient threat cues into working memory, although this has not been directly studied.

In contrast to salience network nodes such as the dorsal ACC and insula, which differentially activate to threatening stimuli during fear conditioning, default mode network nodes such as the hippocampus and ventromedial PFC differentially activate to safety stimuli (Fullana et al. 2016). The hippocampus is particularly central to pattern separation; disorder-related hippocampal dysfunction may fuel fear generalization wherein benign and threatening stimuli are not properly distinguished (Lissek et al. 2014). Indeed, aberrantly increased hippocampal activation to safety stimuli has been evidenced in panic disorder (Lueken et al. 2013) and is suggestive of fear generalization (Lissek et al. 2014). Disorder-specific dysfunction in the ventromedial PFC may also contribute to increased generalization by compromising fear extinction (Marin et al. 2017).

An updated neurobiological hypothesis of panic disorder predicts that activation of the amygdala and its efferents leads to physiological adjustments such as increased blood pressure, heart rate, respiration, and arousal. Activation in functionally connected upstream salience network nodes such as the dorsal ACC, insular cortex, and dorsomedial PFC amplifies the original threat signal and may, in concert with cortical executive control network and default mode network nodes, represent the threat signal as a conscious fear percept. Dysfunctional default mode network nodes may be unable to extinguish the fear signal or appropriately identify the original interoceptive or exteroceptive stimulus as benign. Aberrant cortical processing in salience network, central executive network, and default mode network nodes may subsequently lead to a cognitive misinterpretation of the amygdala-orchestrated defensive physiological adjustments, leading to intensified physiological adjustments and catastrophizing.

Although aberrant activation in and between nodes of the three discussed networks has been noted in panic disorder, few studies have examined how these activation patterns change following treatment and how these changes relate to treatment-related improvement. Similarly, few studies have examined which neural network changes precede the development of panic disorder and which merely correlate with its onset.

It also remains unclear whether aberrant function in more than one of the discussed networks is necessary to cause panic disorder, whether dysfunction in one is sufficient, or whether dysfunction in one necessitates dysfunction in others (i.e., a cascading effect). Longitudinal studies using improved neuroimaging and computational techniques will likely shed light on which neural network changes underlie panic disorder symptoms.

Conclusion

The pathogenesis of panic disorder will likely advance as new findings from animal models and clinical sciences emerge. Psychological accounts of panic disorder grounded in fear-learning models (conditioning, extinction, generalization) provide a framework for identifying the brain–behavior relationships underlying panic disorder. Longitudinal studies may shed light on the precise neural network changes driving panic disorder.

Key Points

- A range of drugs are now widely accepted to be effective in panic disorder, which provides support for the biological basis of panic disorder, specifically implicating the noradrenergic, serotonergic, and GABAergic/glutamatergic systems.

- Selective serotonin reuptake inhibitors may act in panic disorder by diminishing arousal and defense escape behavior, decreasing levels of corticotropin-releasing factor, and correcting ventilatory patterns that are associated with panic disorder.

- The GABA/glutamate imbalance plays a pivotal role in the pathogenesis of panic disorder. Patients with panic disorder have been found to have deficient

GABA-benzodiazepine receptors in key sites of the fear network, including the prefrontal cortex, insula, and amygdala.

- Aberrant fear conditioning may drive panic disorder symptoms by linking panic attacks with conditioned interoceptive or exteroceptive cues that subsequently prompt future attacks. Generalization to perceptually similar or conceptually related benign stimuli may ensue.

- Disorder-specific findings related to the triple network model suggest that dysfunctional salience network, central executive network, and default mode network activity/connectivity may play a key role in the pathogenesis of panic disorder.

References

American Psychiatric Association: Diagnostic and Statistical Manual of Mental Disorders, 5th Edition. Arlington, VA, American Psychiatric Association, 2013

Asami T, Hayano F, Nakamura M, et al: Anterior cingulate cortex volume reduction in patients with panic disorder. Psychiatry Clin Neurosci 62(3):322–330, 2008 18588593

Balderston NL, Liu J, Roberson-Nay R, et al: The relationship between dlPFC activity during unpredictable threat and CO_2-induced panic symptoms. Transl Psychiatry 7(12):1266, 2017 29213110

Ball TM, Ramsawh HJ, Campbell-Sills L, et al: Prefrontal dysfunction during emotion regulation in generalized anxiety and panic disorders. Psychol Med 43(7):1475–1486, 2013 23111120

Bremner JD, Innis RB, White T, et al: SPECT [I-123]iomazenil measurement of the benzodiazepine receptor in panic disorder. Biol Psychiatry 47(2):96–106, 2000 10664825

Brinkmann L, Buff C, Feldker K, et al: Distinct phasic and sustained brain responses and connectivity of amygdala and bed nucleus of the stria terminalis during threat anticipation in panic disorder. Psychol Med 47(15):2675–2688, 2017 28485259

Bürkner PC, Bittner N, Holling H, et al: D-cycloserine augmentation of behavior therapy for anxiety and obsessive-compulsive disorders: a meta-analysis. PLoS One 12(3):e0173660, 2017 28282427

Cameron OG, Huang GC, Nichols T, et al: Reduced gamma-aminobutyric acid(A)-benzodiazepine binding sites in insular cortex of individuals with panic disorder. Arch Gen Psychiatry 64(7):793–800, 2007 17606813

Chrousos GP, Gold PW: The concepts of stress and stress system disorders: overview of physical and behavioral homeostasis. JAMA 267(9):1244–1252, 1992 1538563

Demenescu LR, Kortekaas R, Cremers HR, et al: Amygdala activation and its functional connectivity during perception of emotional faces in social phobia and panic disorder. J Psychiatr Res 47(8):1024–1031, 2013 23643103

Engel KR, Obst K, Bandelow B, et al: Functional MRI activation in response to panic-specific, non-panic aversive, and neutral pictures in patients with panic disorder and healthy controls. Eur Arch Psychiatry Clin Neurosci 266(6):557–566, 2016 26585457

Feinstein JS, Buzza C, Hurlemann R, et al: Fear and panic in humans with bilateral amygdala damage. Nat Neurosci 16(3):270–272, 2013 23377128

Feldker K, Heitmann CY, Neumeister P, et al: Brain responses to disorder-related visual threat in panic disorder. Hum Brain Mapp 37(12):4439–4453, 2016 27436308

Feldker K, Heitmann CY, Neumeister P, et al: Transdiagnostic brain responses to disorder-related threat across four psychiatric disorders. Psychol Med 47(4):730–743, 2017 27869064

Feldker K, Heitmann CY, Neumeister P, et al: Cardiorespiratory concerns shape brain responses during automatic panic-related scene processing in patients with panic disorder. J Psychiatry Neurosci 43(1):26–36, 2018 29252163

Fonzo GA, Ramsawh HJ, Flagan TM, et al: Common and disorder-specific neural responses to emotional faces in generalised anxiety, social anxiety and panic disorders. Br J Psychiatry 206(3):206–215, 2015 25573399

Fullana MA, Harrison BJ, Soriano-Mas C, et al: Neural signatures of human fear conditioning: an updated and extended meta-analysis of fMRI studies. Mol Psychiatry 21(4):500–508, 2016 26122585

Gorman JM, Kent JM, Sullivan GM, et al: Neuroanatomical hypothesis of panic disorder, revised. Am J Psychiatry 157(4):493–505, 2000

Goulden N, Khusnulina A, Davis NJ, et al: The salience network is responsible for switching between the default mode network and the central executive network: replication from DCM. Neuroimage 99:180–190, 2014 24862074

Grillon C, Lissek S, Rabin S, et al: Increased anxiety during anticipation of unpredictable but not predictable aversive stimuli as a psychophysiologic marker of panic disorder. Am J Psychiatry 165(7):898–904, 2008 18347001

Holtz K, Pané-Farré CA, Wendt J, et al: Brain activation during anticipation of interoceptive threat. Neuroimage 61(4):857–865, 2012 22440646

Kalisch R, Gerlicher AM: Making a mountain out of a molehill: on the role of the rostral dorsal anterior cingulate and dorsomedial prefrontal cortex in conscious threat appraisal, catastrophizing, and worrying. Neurosci Biobehav Rev 42:1–8, 2014 24525267

Kaschka W, Feistel H, Ebert D: Reduced benzodiazepine receptor binding in panic disorders measured by iomazenil SPECT. J Psychiatr Res 29(5):427–434, 1995 8748067

Kent JM, Coplan JD, Martinez J, et al: Ventilatory effects of tryptophan depletion in panic disorder: a preliminary report. Psychiatry Res 64(2):83–90, 1996 8912949

Khalsa SS, Feinstein JS, Li W, et al: Panic anxiety in humans with bilateral amygdala lesions: pharmacological induction via cardiorespiratory interoceptive pathways. J Neurosci 36(12):3559–3566, 2016 27013684

Killgore WD, Britton JC, Schwab ZJ, et al: Cortico-limbic responses to masked affective faces across PTSD, panic disorder, and specific phobia. Depress Anxiety 31(2):150–159, 2014 23861215

Kircher T, Arolt V, Jansen A, et al: Effect of cognitive-behavioral therapy on neural correlates of fear conditioning in panic disorder. Biol Psychiatry 73(1):93–101, 2013 22921454

Lai C-H, Wu Y-T: Fronto-temporo-insula gray matter alterations of first-episode, drug-naïve and very late-onset panic disorder patients. J Affect Disord 140(3):285–291, 2012 22386047

LeDoux JE, Pine DS: Using neuroscience to help understand fear and anxiety: a two-system framework. Am J Psychiatry 173(11):1083–1093, 2016 27609244

Leutgeb JK, Leutgeb S, Moser MB, et al: Pattern separation in the dentate gyrus and CA3 of the hippocampus. Science 315(5814):961–966, 2007 17303747

Lissek S: Toward an account of clinical anxiety predicated on basic, neurally mapped mechanisms of Pavlovian fear-learning: the case for conditioned overgeneralization. Depress Anxiety 29(4):257–263, 2012 22447565

Lissek S, Rabin SJ, McDowell DJ, et al: Impaired discriminative fear-conditioning resulting from elevated fear responding to learned safety cues among individuals with panic disorder. Behav Res Ther 47(2):111–118, 2009 19027893

Lissek S, Rabin S, Heller RE, et al: Overgeneralization of conditioned fear as a pathogenic marker of panic disorder. Am J Psychiatry 167(1):47–55, 2010 19917595

Lissek S, Bradford DE, Alvarez RP, et al: Neural substrates of classically conditioned fear-generalization in humans: a parametric fMRI study. Soc Cogn Affect Neurosci 9(8):1134–1142, 2014 23748500

Lueken U, Straube B, Konrad C, et al: Neural substrates of treatment response to cognitive-behavioral therapy in panic disorder with agoraphobia. Am J Psychiatry 170(11):1345–1355, 2013 23982225

Maddock RJ, Buonocore MH, Kile SJ, et al: Brain regions showing increased activation by threat-related words in panic disorder. Neuroreport 14(3):325–328, 2003 12634477

Malizia AL, Cunningham VJ, Bell CJ, et al: Decreased brain GABA(A)-benzodiazepine receptor binding in panic disorder: preliminary results from a quantitative PET study. Arch Gen Psychiatry 55(8):715–720, 1998 9707382

Marin MF, Zsido RG, Song H, et al: Skin conductance responses and neural activations during fear conditioning and extinction recall across anxiety disorders. JAMA Psychiatry 74(6):622–631, 2017 28403387

Menon V: Large-scale brain networks and psychopathology: a unifying triple network model. Trends Cogn Sci 15(10):483–506, 2011 21908230

Michael T, Blechert J, Vriends N, et al: Fear conditioning in panic disorder: enhanced resistance to extinction. J Abnorm Psychol 116(3):612–617, 2007 17696717

Milad MR, Quirk GJ: Fear extinction as a model for translational neuroscience: ten years of progress. Annu Rev Psychol 63:129–151, 2012 22129456

Molosh AI, Dustrude ET, Lukkes JL, et al: Panic results in unique molecular and network changes in the amygdala that facilitate fear responses. Mol Psychiatry August 14, 2018 30108314 Epub ahead of print

Nuss P: Anxiety disorders and GABA neurotransmission: a disturbance of modulation. Neuropsychiatr Dis Treat 11:165–175, 2015 25653526

Otto MW, Tolin DF, Simon NM, et al: Efficacy of d-cycloserine for enhancing response to cognitive-behavior therapy for panic disorder. Biol Psychiatry 67(4):365–370, 2010 19811776

Otto MW, Moshier SJ, Kinner DG, et al: De novo fear conditioning across diagnostic groups in the affective disorders: evidence for learning impairments. Behav Ther 45(5):619–629, 2014 25022773

Palacios JM: Serotonin receptors in brain revisited. Brain Res 1645:46–49, 2016 26740406

Paul ED, Johnson PL, Shekhar A, et al: The Deakin/Graeff hypothesis: focus on serotonergic inhibition of panic. Neurosci Biobehav Rev 46(Pt 3):379–396, 2014 24661986

Quesseveur G, David DJ, Gaillard MC, et al: BDNF overexpression in mouse hippocampal astrocytes promotes local neurogenesis and elicits anxiolytic-like activities. Transl Psychiatry 3:e253, 2013 23632457

Reinecke A, Thilo K, Filippini N, et al: Predicting rapid response to cognitive-behavioural treatment for panic disorder: the role of hippocampus, insula, and dorsolateral prefrontal cortex. Behav Res Ther 62:120–128, 2014 25156399

Sobanski T, Wagner G, Peikert G, et al: Temporal and right frontal lobe alterations in panic disorder: a quantitative volumetric and voxel-based morphometric MRI study. Psychol Med 40(11):1879–1886, 2010 20056020

Tuescher O, Protopopescu X, Pan H, et al: Differential activity of subgenual cingulate and brainstem in panic disorder and PTSD. J Anxiety Disord 25(2):251–257, 2011 21075593

Uchida RR, Del-Ben CM, Busatto GF, et al: Regional gray matter abnormalities in panic disorder: a voxel-based morphometry study. Psychiatry Res 163(1):21–29, 2008 18417322

Uhde TW, Tancer ME, Rubinow DR, et al: Evidence for hypothalamo-growth hormone dysfunction in panic disorder: profile of growth hormone (GH) responses to clonidine, yohimbine, caffeine, glucose, GRF and TRH in panic disorder patients versus healthy volunteers. Neuropsychopharmacology 6(2):101–118, 1992 1610485

Recommended Readings

Bouton ME, Mineka S, Barlow DH: A modern learning theory perspective on the etiology of panic disorder. Psychol Rev 108:4–32, 2001

Busch FN, Milrod BL, Singer MB: Theory and technique in psychodynamic treatment of panic disorder. J Psychother Pract Res 8:234–242, 1999

Caspi A, Moffitt TE: Gene-environment interactions in psychiatry: joining forces with neuroscience. Nat Rev Neurosci 7:583–590, 2006

Coplan JD, Andrews MW, Rosenblum LA, et al: Persistent elevations of cerebrospinal fluid concentrations of corticotropin-releasing factor in adult nonhuman primates exposed to early life stressors: implications for the pathophysiology of mood and anxiety disorders. Proc Natl Acad Sci USA 93:1619–1623, 1996

Goddard AW, Mason GF, Almai A, et al: Reductions in occipital cortex GABA levels in panic disorder detected with 1h-magnetic resonance spectroscopy. Arch Gen Psychiatry 58(6):556–561, 2001 11386984

Goossens L, Leibold N, Peeters R, et al: Brainstem response to hypercapnia: a symptom provocation study into the pathophysiology of panic disorder. J Psychopharmacol 28(5):449–456, 2014 24646808

Gorman JM, Kent JM, Sullivan GM, et al: Neuroanatomical hypothesis of panic disorder, revised. Am J Psychiatry 157:493–505, 2000

Graeff FG, Zangrossi H Jr: The dual role of serotonin in defense and the mode of action of antidepressants on generalized anxiety and panic disorders. Cent Nerv Syst Agents Med Chem 10(3):207–217, 2010 20528764

Hettema JM, Neale MC, Kendler KS: A review and meta-analysis of the genetic epidemiology of anxiety disorders. Am J Psychiatry 158:1568–1578, 2001

Howe AS, Buttenschøn HN, Bani-Fatemi A, et al: Candidate genes in panic disorder: meta-analyses of 23 common vari-ants in major anxiogenic pathways. Mol Psychiatry 21(5):665–679, 2016 26390831

Johnson PL, Truitt WA, Fitz SD, et al: Neural pathways underlying lactate induced panic. Neuropsychopharmacology 33:2093–2107, 2007

Klein DF: False suffocation alarms, spontaneous panics, and related conditions: an integrative hypothesis. Arch Gen Psychiatry 50:306–317, 1993

Lai CH, Wu YT: Changes in gray matter volume of remitted first-episode, drug-naïve, panic disorder patients after 6-week antidepressant therapy. J Psychiatr Res 47(1):122–127, 2013 23079534

LeDoux J: The Emotional Brain: The Mysterious Underpinning of Emotional Life. New York, Simon and Schuster, 1996

LeDoux JE, Brown R: A higher-order theory of emotional consciousness. Proc Natl Acad Sci USA 114(10):E2016–E2025, 2017 28202735

Yoon S, Jun CS, Jeong HS, et al: Altered cortical gyrification patterns in panic disorder: deficits and potential compensation. J Psychiatr Res 47(10):1446–1454, 2013 23871448

CHAPTER 22

Pharmacotherapy for Panic Disorder

Borwin Bandelow, M.D., Ph.D.

David S. Baldwin, M.A., D.M., FRCPsych

Phenomenology

Panic disorder with or without agoraphobia is a severe and often disabling condition, with lifetime prevalence rates of 1.6%–5.2% (panic disorder) and 0.8%–2.6% (agoraphobia) according to various epidemiological surveys (Bandelow and Michaelis 2015). Patients included in clinical studies have a mean age of 37.2 years, probably because the disorder seems to peak in terms of severity at this age (Bandelow and Schüller 2019). New-onset panic disorder is rarely found in late life. Hypotheses about the etiology of anxiety disorders are currently based on a combination of genetic or neurobiological and environmental factors, such as early childhood adversity or stressful exposure later in life (e.g., occupational stress and traumatic experiences) (Bandelow et al. 2016, 2017).

Pharmacological treatment of panic disorder emerged in 1959, when Donald F. Klein established the efficacy of the tricyclic antidepressant (TCA) imipramine (Klein and Fink 1962). In 1960, the first benzodiazepine, chlordiazepoxide, was introduced. Since the 1980s, selective serotonin reuptake inhibitors (SSRIs) have been given to patients with panic disorder (Den Boer and Westenberg 1988). In 2005, the serotonin-norepinephrine reuptake inhibitor (SNRI) venlafaxine was introduced. Since then, no new clinically available pharmacological treatments for panic disorder have emerged.

Psychological treatments play an important role in the treatment of panic disorder (see Chapter 23, "Psychotherapy for Panic Disorder"). However, in this chapter, we focus on psychopharmacological treatment and the relationship between medication and psychological treatment.

Psychopharmacological Treatment

The overview of pharmacotherapy of panic disorder in this chapter is based on comprehensive guidelines and meta-analyses (Baldwin et al. 2014; Bandelow et al. 2008, 2015a, 2015b) according to the principles of evidence-based medicine. Only randomized controlled studies that have undergone strict quality control have been included in these analyses. For first-line evidence, drugs were required to be superior to placebo in at least two double-blind, placebo-controlled studies and shown to be as effective as a reference drug. In the following subsections, assignment as first-line, second-line, or third-line drugs is based on the documented efficacy and tolerability of the medications. Drugs available for the treatment of panic disorder are listed in Table 22–1.

First-Line Treatment

Selective Serotonin Reuptake Inhibitors

The efficacy of the SSRIs in panic disorder has been proven in many controlled studies, and they are considered to be first-line drugs for this disorder because of their well-established efficacy and their relatively benign adverse effect profile. Efficacy has been shown for all currently available SSRIs (i.e., citalopram, escitalopram, fluvoxamine, fluoxetine, paroxetine, sertraline).

Usually, treatment with SSRIs is well tolerated. Restlessness, jitteriness, an increase in anxiety symptoms, and insomnia in the first days or weeks of treatment may hamper adherence. Lowering the starting dosage may reduce this "overstimulation." Other side effects include fatigue, dizziness, nausea, and anorexia or weight gain. Sexual dysfunction (decreased libido, impotence, or ejaculatory disturbances) may be a problem in long-term treatment (Baldwin 2004), and discontinuation syndromes have been observed. Anxiolytic effects typically start after 2–4 weeks, but in some patients beneficial effects emerge after 6–8 weeks. Doses are typically given in the morning or midday except in patients reporting daytime sedation, for whom nighttime administration may be preferable.

Serotonin-Norepinephrine Reuptake Inhibitor Venlafaxine

The side effect profile of venlafaxine is broadly similar to that of the SSRIs, although excessive perspiration may be more frequent. When higher dosages are prescribed (i.e., ≥300 mg/day), blood pressure should be monitored regularly.

Second-Line Treatment: Tricyclic Antidepressants

Treatment with TCAs has been shown to improve panic disorder. Treatment adherence with tricyclic drugs may be affected by adverse effects such as an initial increase in "jitteriness," dry mouth, postural hypotension, tachycardia, sedation, sexual dysfunction, and impaired psychomotor function that can impact safely driving a car. Weight gain may be a problem in long-term treatment. In general, the frequency of adverse events is somewhat higher for TCAs than for second-generation antidepressants, such as the SSRIs (Lecrubier and Judge 1997). Thus, the latter drugs should be tried first before TCAs are used. The dosage of TCAs should be titrated up slowly un-

TABLE 22–1. **Recommendations for drug treatment of panic disorder**

Treatment	Examples	Recommended daily dosage for adults, *mg*
Treatment of acute panic attacks		
Benzodiazepines	Alprazolam	0.5–2
	Lorazepam melting tablets	1–2.5
First-line treatment		
Selective serotonin reuptake inhibitors	Citalopram	20–60
	Escitalopram	10–20
	Fluoxetine	20–40
	Fluvoxamine	100–300
	Paroxetine	20–60
	Sertraline	50–200
Serotonin-norepinephrine reuptake inhibitor	Venlafaxine	75–225
Tricyclic antidepressant	Imipramine	75–250
Second-line treatment		
Tricyclic antidepressant	Clomipramine	75–250
Third-line treatment		
Benzodiazepines	Alprazolam	1.5–8
	Clonazepam	1–4
Monoamine oxidase inhibitor	Phenelzine	45–90
Reversible inhibitor of monoamine oxidase	Moclobemide	300–600

Note. These recommendations are based on randomized double-blind clinical studies published in peer-reviewed journals. Not all of the recommended drugs are licensed for these indications in every country.

til dosage levels as high as those used in the treatment of depression are reached. Patients should be informed that the onset of the anxiolytic effect of the drug may have a latency of 2–4 weeks (in some cases up to 6–8 weeks).

Third-Line Treatment: Benzodiazepines

The efficacy of benzodiazepines in panic disorder has been shown in many controlled clinical studies. The advantage of these drugs is that the anxiolytic effects often start swiftly after oral or parenteral application. In contrast to antidepressants, benzodiazepines do not cause initially increased nervousness. In general, they have a good record of safety, but because of CNS depression, benzodiazepine treatment may be associated with sedation, dizziness, prolonged reaction time, and other side effects. Cognitive function and driving skills may be affected adversely.

Tolerance seems to be rare (Rickels 1982), but dependency may develop after long-term treatment with benzodiazepines (e.g., over 4–8 months), especially in predisposed patients, such as those with a history of substance use disorders (Schweizer et al. 1998). Withdrawal reactions typically have their peak severity at 2 days for short-half-life and 4–7 days for long-half-life benzodiazepines. Prolonged withdrawal reactions have occasionally been reported. Thus, choosing treatment with benzodiaze-pines requires a careful weighing of risks and benefits.

Some controversy exists in the field as to whether benzodiazepines can be used as first-line agents in anxiety disorders. According to guidelines, routine use of these drugs is not recommended (Andrews et al. 2018; Bandelow et al. 2008, 2015a; National Institute for Health and Clinical Excellence 2011). In patients for whom other treatment modalities were not effective or were not tolerated because of side effects, year-long treatment with benzodiazepines may be justified. However, patients with a history of benzodiazepine abuse should be excluded from this treatment. Cognitive-behavioral interventions may facilitate benzodiazepine discontinuation (Spiegel 1999). Benzodiazepines may also be used in combination with antidepressants during the first weeks before the onset of effect of the antidepressants (Goddard et al. 2001), although overall efficacy of combination treatment does not appear to be superior to antidepressant alone. When treating comorbid panic disorder, one should be aware that benzodiazepines, in contrast to antidepressants, do not treat comorbid conditions, such as depression or OCD.

Other Medications

Some other available drugs have shown preliminary evidence or mixed results. These drugs may be used off-label in patients after nonresponse to standard treatments. One study showed the efficacy of the monoamine oxidase inhibitor phenelzine in panic disorder (Sheehan et al. 1980). In this study, phenelzine was superior to placebo and as effective as imipramine. However, because of the possibility of severe side effects and interactions with other drugs or food components, phenelzine is not considered a first-line drug and should be used only by experienced psychiatrists when other treatment modalities have been unsuccessful or have not been tolerated. To avoid overstimula-tion and insomnia, doses should be given in the morning and midday.

Moclobemide, a reversible inhibitor of monoamine oxidase A, may be a treatment option for otherwise unresponsive patients. However, findings with the drug were in-consistent, and some studies did not show superiority to placebo. Moclobemide is available in Canada and many other countries but not in the United States. Side effects include restlessness, insomnia, dry mouth, and headache. To avoid overstimulation and insomnia, doses should be given in the morning and midday.

Long-Term Treatment

Panic disorder tends to run a waxing and waning course, and as such, treatment usu-ally should continue for many months after symptomatic remission in order to reduce the risk of relapse. Some patients maintain their avoidance behavior even when panic attacks are resolved after successful treatment. This should be addressed in psycho-therapy sessions.

Several studies have investigated the long-term value of SSRI and TCA treatment. Some of these trials are long-term studies comparing a drug and placebo for a longer period (e.g., 26–60 weeks); others are relapse prevention studies, in which patients usu-ally receive open-label treatment with the study drug for a shorter period, after which responders are randomly assigned to either ongoing active drug treatment or placebo.

SSRIs, venlafaxine, TCAs, and moclobemide showed long-term efficacy in these studies. On the basis of these studies and clinical experience, expert consensus conferences generally recommend a duration of pharmacotherapy of 6 months (Baldwin et al. 2014) to 12 months (Andrews et al. 2018; Bandelow et al. 2008). Discontinuation should be gradual over approximately 2–4 weeks to minimize withdrawal symptoms.

Regarding SSRIs, the same dosages are usually prescribed in the maintenance treatment of panic disorder as in the acute treatment phase. To our knowledge, no studies have examined reduced dosages of SSRIs in maintenance treatment.

Comparisons of Antipanic Drugs

Few head-to-head comparisons of antipanic drugs have been published. In studies comparing the efficacy of TCAs and SSRIs, no differences in efficacy could be found between the two classes (Lecrubier and Judge 1997). Also, in patients with comorbid panic disorder and major depressive disorder, sertraline and imipramine were equally effective, but sertraline showed significantly greater tolerability and compliance than imipramine (Lepola et al. 2003). However, in most of these studies, the SSRIs were better tolerated than the TCAs. Comparisons among the SSRIs did not reveal differences in efficacy (Bandelow et al. 2004), although escitalopram showed evidence of superiority over citalopram on some outcome measures in one study (Bandelow et al. 2007b).

No direct comparisons have been made between the SSRIs and benzodiazepines in the treatment of panic disorder. In several studies alprazolam was compared with the TCA imipramine (Taylor et al. 1990). No differences could be found between the two drugs in terms of global improvement.

The relative efficacy of drugs was examined in a meta-analysis (Bandelow et al. 2015b), which was based on the pre/post effect sizes and showed substantial differences between the various medications. High effect sizes were found for the SNRI venlafaxine (pre/post effect size 2.43) and for the SSRIs fluoxetine (2.27) and paroxetine (2.16). The benzodiazepine clonazepam has also shown a high effect size in panic disorder (2.61). The advantages and disadvantages of antipanic drugs are summarized in Table 22–2.

Practical Guidelines for Treatment

Recommended dosages are indicated in Table 22–1. SSRIs have a rather "flat" response curve. However, for paroxetine, a dosage of 40 mg/day was more effective than 20 mg/day. Evidence of a dose-response relationship is inconsistent for most antidepressants, possibly due to the statistical difficulties associated with dosage-finding studies. However, according to clinical experience, some patients who have not responded to the lowest recommended dosage may respond to higher dosages within the therapeutic range.

Initiate TCAs at a low dosage and increase the dosage every 3–5 days. To increase compliance, it may be feasible to give all the antidepressant medication in a single dose, depending on the patient's tolerance. Benzodiazepine dosages should be as low as possible but as high as necessary to achieve an optimal treatment result. A treat-

TABLE 22–2.   **Advantages and disadvantages of antianxiety drugs**

Medication class	Advantages	Disadvantages
Selective serotonin reuptake inhibitors	No dependency Sufficient evidence from clinical studies Favorable side effect profile Relatively safe in overdose	Latency of effect 2–6 weeks Initial jitteriness, nausea, restlessness, sexual dysfunctions, and other side effects Withdrawal symptoms possible
Serotonin-norepinephrine reuptake inhibitor (venlafaxine)	No dependency Sufficient evidence from clinical studies Favorable side effect profile Relatively safe in overdose	Latency of effect 2–6 weeks Initial jitteriness, nausea, restlessness, sexual dysfunctions, increase in blood pressure at high doses, and other side effects Withdrawal symptoms possible
Tricyclic antidepressants	No dependency Sufficient evidence from clinical studies	Latency of effect 2–6 weeks Anticholinergic effects; cardiovascular, weight gain, and other side effects; and sexual dysfunctions May be lethal in overdose Withdrawal symptoms possible
Benzodiazepines	Rapid onset of action Sufficient evidence from clinical studies Favorable side effect profile (with the exception of addiction potential) Relatively safe in overdose	Dependency possible Sedation, slow reaction time, and other side effects Lack efficacy for comorbid depression

ment algorithm is provided in Table 22–3, and frequently asked questions about treatment are answered in Table 22–4.

Special Populations

Pregnancy and Breastfeeding

According to several studies, the use of antidepressants during pregnancy has been associated with adverse effects on the newborn. However, all of these studies relied on observational designs, and the impact of genetic factors and the environment is difficult to distinguish from that of prenatal medication exposure. Reviews came to the conclusion that the risks of drug treatment during pregnancy must be weighed against the risk of withholding treatment for panic disorder (Ornoy and Koren 2017; Rotem-Kohavi and Oberlander 2017). Cognitive-behavioral therapy (CBT) might be an alternative.

SSRIs and TCAs are excreted into breast milk, and low levels have been found in infant serum (Blier 2006). In mothers receiving TCAs, it seems unwarranted to recommend discontinuing breastfeeding. Fluoxetine should probably be avoided during lactation, but treatment with other SSRIs (citalopram, fluvoxamine, paroxetine, or sertraline) seems to be compatible with breastfeeding. Benzodiazepines should be avoided during breastfeeding.

TABLE 22–3.	Treatment algorithm for panic disorder
First-line treatments	Selective serotonin reuptake inhibitors (SSRIs) and the serotonin-norepinephrine reuptake inhibitor (SNRI) venlafaxine Cognitive-behavioral therapy
When to change treatments due to lack of efficacy	After 4–6 weeks
What to do after 4–6 weeks if partial response is seen	Treat another 4–6 weeks with increased dosage before changing the treatment strategy
Treatment options for resistant cases	Switch from one SSRI to another Switch from venlafaxine to an SSRI or vice versa Switch to a tricyclic antidepressant Switch to benzodiazepines, phenelzine, or moclobemide* Switch to drugs that have been effective in preliminary open studies or case reports: mirtazapine, valproate, inositol Switch to drugs that were effective in other anxiety disorders in double-blind placebo-controlled studies: pregabalin, duloxetine, quetiapine, buspirone
Options for treatment combinations	Monotherapy usually is the better option. Combinations of drugs may be used in treatment-resistant cases. The following combinations are supported by studies: Benzodiazepines in first weeks before onset of efficacy of antidepressant Augmentation with olanzapine

Note.   Not all drugs mentioned here are licensed in every country; please refer to local prescribing information and consider drug labeling.
*Not available in the United States.

Treating Children and Adolescents

Most studies have found an age at onset of panic disorder between 23 and 28 years (Bandelow and Michaelis 2015). Therefore, panic disorder in children and adolescents is relatively uncommon, and no double-blind treatment studies in this age group have been published. Experiences with pharmacological treatment in children and adolescents derive mainly from the controlled clinical studies conducted in patients with other anxiety disorders and OCD (Ipser et al. 2009). These data suggest that SS-RIs should be first-line treatment in children and adolescents. In the largest study in children and adolescents with separation anxiety disorder, generalized anxiety disorder, or social anxiety disorder (Walkup et al. 2008), the combination of CBT and sertraline was more effective than either treatment alone. However, treatment with SSRIs and SNRIs has been associated with suicidal ideation and attempted suicide (but not death from suicide) in adolescents with depression. Therefore, the risks and benefits of drug treatment should be weighed carefully in this age group, and it may be preferable to reserve pharmacological treatments for patients who do not respond to evidence-based psychological approaches.

Treatment of the Elderly

Symptoms of panic disorder tend to decrease after age 45–50 years, and new-onset panic disorder is relatively rare in elderly patients. However, panic attacks may occur

TABLE 22–4.   **Treatment of panic disorder: frequently asked questions**

Question	Answer
How can compliance be improved?	Inform patient about delayed onset of action and possible side effects that might occur in first weeks of treatment (e.g., insomnia or restlessness with SSRIs/SNRIs).
Can medication be stopped after onset of efficacy?	Expert consensus recommends extending treatment for at least 6–12 months to avoid relapses.
Will drug treatment be lifelong?	In most patients, symptoms of panic disorder usually lessen after age 40–45, and the disorder has a waxing and waning course. Therefore, only a few patients require long-term treatment over a few years.
Are irreversible side effects possible after year-long treatment?	No evidence has been found of irreversible side effects with SSRIs, SNRIs, or TCAs.
What dosages are used in maintenance treatment?	SSRIs should be used in the same dosages as in acute treatment; TCAs may be used in half the dosage recommended for acute treatment.
Should medication be stopped before starting CBT?	No evidence has been found that drugs may weaken the effects of CBT; by contrast, meta-analyses have shown that a combination of both treatment modalities is more effective than both monotherapies.

Note.   CBT=cognitive-behavioral therapy; SNRI=serotonin-norepinephrine reuptake inhibitor; SSRI= selective serotonin reuptake inhibitor; TCA=tricyclic antidepressant.

in elderly patients with major depression. Medical causes also need to be excluded. Few studies have investigated the treatment of anxiety disorders in the elderly, although escitalopram and citalopram appeared effective in reducing panic attack frequency in a small sample of elderly patients with recurrent panic attacks associated with a range of anxiety disorders (Rampello et al. 2006).

Factors to consider in the treatment of the elderly include an increased sensitivity to the anticholinergic properties of drugs and to extrapyramidal symptoms, an increased risk for orthostatic hypotension and electrocardiogram changes, and possible paradoxical reactions to benzodiazepines. Thus, treatment with TCAs or benzodiazepines is less favorable, whereas SSRIs and SNRIs appear to be relatively safe.

Management of Treatment-Resistant Panic Disorder

Many patients continue to experience recurrent panic attacks, agoraphobic avoidance, or distress and impairment. According to clinical studies, around 20%–40% of patients treated with standard treatments remain symptomatic (Bandelow et al. 2004). In naturalistic settings, this percentage may be even higher, because the patients selected in clinical studies often are younger and less severely ill and have fewer comorbid conditions than the general patient population.

A number of risk factors predicting poorer outcome of treatment have been identified, including long duration of illness; high baseline illness severity; severe agoraphobic avoidance; strong hypochondriacal fears; frequent emergency department visits; comorbidity with other anxiety disorders, depression, or personality disorders;

reduced general mental health; unemployment; delayed response to medication; and low treatment compliance with a CBT regimen. It should be ascertained that the diagnosis is correct, the patient is compliant with therapy, the dosage prescribed is therapeutic, and the trial period has been adequate. Concurrent prescription drugs (e.g., metabolic enhancers or inhibitors) may interfere with efficacy. Some patients metabolize drugs very quickly. Although determination of plasma levels is not used routinely because of the low correlation between oral dose and plasma levels or between plasma levels and clinical effect, this method might be helpful to identify patients who do not take their medication at all or who are fast metabolizers. Psychosocial factors may affect response, and depression, borderline personality disorder, and substance abuse are especially likely to complicate panic disorder.

Few studies are available to guide selection of treatment for patients with treatment-resistant panic disorder. Data from controlled clinical studies of patients with non-refractory panic disorder are not easily transferable to treatment-resistant cases. In a double-blind, placebo-controlled study of patients with treatment-resistant panic, pindolol had an augmenting effect on fluoxetine (Hirschmann et al. 2000), but this strategy is rarely used in practice. In a small study of patients with SSRI-resistant panic disorder, the addition of quetiapine to ongoing SSRI treatment (Goddard et al. 2015) was not effective. In a small open study, an augmentation strategy in which patients receiving a TCA had fluoxetine added and patients receiving fluoxetine had a TCA added was very successful (Tiffon et al. 1994). In some studies (e.g., Khaldi et al. 2003), the addition of olanzapine to various drug combinations led to relief of panic attacks. Some drugs that have been investigated in other anxiety disorders may also work in panic disorder. These include drugs that have shown efficacy in generalized anxiety disorder, such as the azapirone buspirone, the SNRI duloxetine, the calcium channel modulator pregabalin (Baldwin et al. 2013), and the atypical antipsychotic quetiapine (Bandelow et al. 2010).

Psychological treatments such as CBT have to be considered in all patients, regardless of whether they are nonresponders. The addition of group CBT may be beneficial in patients whose symptoms do not respond to pharmacological approaches (Heldt et al. 2003), whereas nonresponders to CBT may benefit from a switch to an SSRI (Payne et al. 2016).

Novel Treatment Approaches

Regrettably, no new pharmacological treatment approaches for panic disorder have emerged in recent years. Some studies indicate that the partial NMDA receptor agonist D-cycloserine potentially augments response to exposure therapy in panic disorder by enhancing extinction learning. Although a pilot trial suggested large effect sizes for the additive benefit of D-cycloserine augmentation of CBT (Otto et al. 2010), this finding could not be replicated in other studies (Leyfer et al. 2019; Pyrkosch et al. 2018).

Psychotherapy, Drugs, and Their Combination

All patients with panic disorder require supportive interviews and attention to emotional states. Also, psychoeducational methods, including information about the nature and etiology of panic disorder and agoraphobia and the mechanism of action of psychological and drug treatments, are essential. Many patients may require specific psychological treatment interventions (see Chapter 23, "Psychotherapy for Panic Disorder").

Psychological and pharmacological treatment modalities must be seen as partners, not alternatives, in the treatment of panic disorder. In a meta-analysis of the few studies that included both CBT and drug treatment, a combination of both modalities was more effective than either alone (Bandelow et al. 2007a). When the benefits of medication are compared to those of psychotherapy, it must be taken into account that medications are generally compared to a pill placebo, which usually generates relatively high effect sizes (Cohen's $d=1.3$ in studies on anxiety disorders), whereas psychological therapies are often compared with untreated waitlist control conditions, which are associated with minimal change ($d=0.2$). Thus, comparing medication to psychotherapy on the basis of treated versus control effect sizes could put medication approaches at a relative disadvantage. In a meta-analysis that included 234 studies of anxiety disorders (Bandelow et al. 2015b), effect sizes before and after all available treatments were compared. This analysis showed that medications were associated with a significantly higher average pre/post effect size ($d=2.02$) than were psychotherapies ($d=1.22$), meaning that only 60% of the symptom reduction obtained with drugs can be achieved with psychotherapy. The study also found that patients included in CBT studies were significantly less severely ill than those recruited for medication studies.

It is a widespread opinion that after treatment with psychotherapy, patients with anxiety disorders maintain their gains beyond the active treatment period, whereas those treated with medication experience a relapse soon after treatment termination. However, in a meta-analysis of all available follow-up studies, we found that patients remained stable after terminating psychotherapies and that patients who stopped medication did not show significantly less enduring effects (Bandelow et al. 2018).

Exercise

In the only controlled studies of exercise in panic disorder, aerobic exercise was less effective than clomipramine and paroxetine and was not superior to a relaxation control group, but it was more effective than placebo (Bandelow et al. 2000; Wedekind et al. 2010). Therefore, exercise can be recommended as an add-on to standard treatments.

Conclusion

The following case example represents a typical case of panic disorder with agoraphobia.

Mrs. S, a 36-year-old woman, started to have anxiety attacks after giving birth 5 years previously. During the attacks, which lasted for approximately half an hour, she experienced a fast and irregular heartbeat, trembling, dizziness, the feeling that she could faint at any moment, numb feelings in her face and on her left side, and a fear of dying. She was referred several times to emergency treatments in a hospital, where a complete checkup did not reveal any irregularities. She was on sick leave frequently because of her anxiety attacks. Around 6 months after her first attacks, she developed agoraphobia in crowded spaces. As a consequence, she tended to avoid going to parties, restaurants, shopping malls, or cinemas.

Her general practitioner started to treat her with St. John's wort tablets and homeopathic formulations, which did not change the course of illness. Mrs. S was referred to a hospital psychotherapy clinic, where she received individual and group psychodynamic psychotherapy for 3 months. Soon after discharge, her symptoms reappeared.

After 2 years of severe panic disorder, Mrs. S was referred to an academic specialty center for anxiety disorders. She received treatment with an SSRI, which showed efficacy after 3 weeks. Initial jitteriness disappeared after 10 days. Moreover, Mrs. S was also treated with individual outpatient CBT, which involved therapist-guided exposure to crowded places. She achieved a stable remission and could start work again.

Panic disorder is a common and disabling condition. Because of increased efforts in the systematic clinical evaluation of psychopharmacological agents for the treatment of anxiety, a comprehensive database has been collected so that precise recommendations can be provided for treating panic disorder.

Drugs recommended as the first-line treatment for panic disorder are the SSRIs or the SNRI venlafaxine. TCAs such as imipramine or clomipramine are effective in panic disorder; however, because of their more unfavorable side effect profile as compared to the SSRIs or SNRIs, TCAs remain second-line. In treatment-resistant cases, benzodiazepines such as alprazolam may be used when the patient does not have a history of substance use problems. Benzodiazepines can be combined with antidepressants in the first weeks of treatment before the onset of effect of the antidepressants.

A number of treatment options exist for patients with panic disorder that is nonresponsive to standard treatments.

In most cases, drug treatment and CBT may substantially improve quality of life in patients with panic disorder.

Key Points

- Selective serotonin reuptake inhibitors (SSRIs) or the serotonin-norepinephrine reuptake inhibitor (SNRI) venlafaxine is first-line treatment for panic disorder. Tricyclic antidepressants (TCAs) may be used as second-line treatments. Benzodiazepines are third-line treatments.

- Both pharmacotherapy and cognitive-behavioral therapy (CBT) appear to be effective for all levels of severity of panic disorder and are first-line treatments; however, according to meta-analytic data of clinical trials, pharmacotherapy appears more effective than psychotherapy. Meta-analytic data of a small number of combination studies suggest that the combination of pharmacotherapy and CBT may be more effective than monotherapy; however, initiating both treatments is not always feasible or acceptable to patients, and more research is needed. The choice of treatment modality should be based on patient preference, the risks and benefits of the two modalities, the patient's treatment history, co-occurring medical or psychiatric conditions, treatment availability, and costs.

- Compliance with SSRIs or SNRIs can be improved when the patient is informed about the late onset of action and possible side effects that might occur in the first weeks of treatment, such as insomnia or restlessness.

- In some patients, treatment may be started with half the recommended dosage in the first days or weeks. Patients with panic disorder are sensitive to antidepressants and may otherwise discontinue treatment because of initial jitteriness and nervousness.

- Expert opinion tends to recommend extending treatment for at least 6 months after remission of panic disorder to avoid relapse.

- In maintenance treatment, SSRIs should be used at the same dosages as in acute treatment, whereas TCAs may be used at half the dosage recommended for acute treatment.

References

Andrews G, Bell C, Boyce P, et al: Royal Australian and New Zealand College of Psychiatrists clinical practice guidelines for the treatment of panic disorder, social anxiety disorder and generalised anxiety disorder. Aust NZ J Psychiatry 52(12):1109–1172, 2018

Baldwin DS: Sexual dysfunction associated with antidepressant drugs. Expert Opin Drug Saf 3(5):457–470, 2004 15335301

Baldwin DS, Ajel K, Masdrakis VG, et al: Pregabalin for the treatment of generalized anxiety disorder: an update. Neuropsychiatr Dis Treat 9:883–892, 2013 23836974

Baldwin DS, Anderson IM, Nutt DJ, et al: Evidence-based pharmacological treatment of anxiety disorders, post-traumatic stress disorder and obsessive-compulsive disorder: a revision of the 2005 guidelines from the British Association for Psychopharmacology. J Psychopharmacol 28(5):403–439, 2014 24713617

Bandelow B, Michaelis S: Epidemiology of anxiety disorders in the 21st century. Dialogues Clin Neurosci 17(3):327–335, 2015 26487813

Bandelow B, Schüller K: Mean age and gender distribution of patients with major mental disorders participating in clinical trials. Eur Arch Psychiatry Clin Neurosci January 2, 2019 30600352 Epub ahead of print

Bandelow B, Broocks A, Pekrun G, et al: The use of the Panic and Agoraphobia Scale (P & A) in a controlled clinical trial. Pharmacopsychiatry 33(5):174–181, 2000 11071019

Bandelow B, Behnke K, Lenoir S, et al: Sertraline versus paroxetine in the treatment of panic disorder: an acute, double-blind noninferiority comparison. J Clin Psychiatry 65(3):405–413, 2004 15096081

Bandelow B, Seidler-Brandler U, Becker A, et al: Meta-analysis of randomized controlled comparisons of psychopharmacological and psychological treatments for anxiety disorders. World J Biol Psychiatry 8(3):175–187, 2007a 17654408

Bandelow B, Stein DJ, Dolberg OT, et al: Improvement of quality of life in panic disorder with escitalopram, citalopram, or placebo. Pharmacopsychiatry 40(4):152–156, 2007b 17694478

Bandelow B, Zohar J, Hollander E, et al: World Federation of Societies of Biological Psychiatry (WFSBP) guidelines for the pharmacological treatment of anxiety, obsessive-compulsive and post-traumatic stress disorders—first revision. World J Biol Psychiatry 9(4):248–312, 2008 18949648

Bandelow B, Chouinard G, Bobes J, et al: Extended-release quetiapine fumarate (quetiapine XR): a once-daily monotherapy effective in generalized anxiety disorder. Data from a randomized, double-blind, placebo- and active-controlled study. Int J Neuropsychopharmacol 13(3):305–320, 2010 19691907

Bandelow B, Lichte T, Rudolf S, et al: The German guidelines for the treatment of anxiety disorders. Eur Arch Psychiatry Clin Neurosci 265(5):363–373, 2015a 25404200

Bandelow B, Reitt M, Röver C, et al: Efficacy of treatments for anxiety disorders: a meta-analysis. Int Clin Psychopharmacol 30(4):183–192, 2015b 25932596

Bandelow B, Baldwin D, Abelli M, et al: Biological markers for anxiety disorders, OCD and PTSD—a consensus statement. Part I: neuroimaging and genetics. World J Biol Psychiatry 17(5):321–365, 2016 27403679

Bandelow B, Baldwin D, Abelli M, et al: Biological markers for anxiety disorders, OCD and PTSD: a consensus statement. Part II: neurochemistry, neurophysiology and neurocognition. World J Biol Psychiatry 18(3):162–214, 2017 27419272

Bandelow B, Sagebiel A, Belz M, et al: Enduring effects of psychological treatments for anxiety disorders: meta-analysis of follow-up studies. Br J Psychiatry 212(6):333–338, 2018 29706139

Blier P: Pregnancy, depression, antidepressants and breast-feeding. J Psychiatry Neurosci 31(4):226–228, 2006 16862240

Den Boer JA, Westenberg HG: Effect of a serotonin and noradrenaline uptake inhibitor in panic disorder; a double-blind comparative study with fluvoxamine and maprotiline. Int Clin Psychopharmacol 3(1):59–74, 1988 2833543

Goddard AW, Brouette T, Almai A, et al: Early coadministration of clonazepam with sertraline for panic disorder. Arch Gen Psychiatry 58(7):681–686, 2001 11448376

Goddard AW, Mahmud W, Medlock C, et al: A controlled trial of quetiapine XR coadministration treatment of SSRI-resistant panic disorder. Ann Gen Psychiatry 14:26, 2015 26379759

Heldt E, Manfor GG, Kipper L, et al: Treating medication-resistant panic disorder: predictors and outcome of cognitive-behaviour therapy in a Brazilian public hospital. Psychother Psychosom 71(1):43–48, 2003

Hirschmann S, Dannon PN, Iancu I, et al: Pindolol augmentation in patients with treatment-resistant panic disorder: a double-blind, placebo-controlled trial. J Clin Psychopharmacol 20(5):556–559, 2000 11001241

Ipser JC, Stein DJ, Hawkridge S, et al: Pharmacotherapy for anxiety disorders in children and adolescents. Cochrane Database Syst Rev (3):CD005170, 2009 19588367

Khaldi S, Kornreich C, Dan B, et al: Usefulness of olanzapine in refractory panic attacks. J Clin Psychopharmacol 23(1):100–101, 2003 12544382

Klein DF, Fink M: Psychiatric reaction patterns to imipramine. Am J Psychiatry 119:432–438, 1962 14033346

Lecrubier Y, Judge R: Long-term evaluation of paroxetine, clomipramine and placebo in panic disorder. Acta Psychiatr Scand 95(2):153–160, 1997 9065681

Lepola U, Arató M, Zhu Y, et al: Sertraline versus imipramine treatment of comorbid panic disorder and major depressive disorder. J Clin Psychiatry 64(6):654–662, 2003 12823079

Leyfer O, Carpenter A, Pincus D: N-methyl-D-aspartate partial agonist enhanced intensive cognitive-behavioral therapy of panic disorder in adolescents. Child Psychiatry Hum Dev 50(2):268–277, 2019 30078111

National Institute for Health and Clinical Excellence: Generalised anxiety disorder and panic disorder in adults: management. London, National Institute for Health and Clinical Excellence, January 2011. Available at: https://www.nice.org.uk/guidance/cg113. Accessed June 27, 2019.

Ornoy A, Koren G: Selective serotonin reuptake inhibitors during pregnancy: do we have now more definite answers related to prenatal exposure? Birth Defects Res 109(12):898–908, 2017 28714608

Otto MW, Tolin DF, Simon NM, et al: Efficacy of d-cycloserine for enhancing response to cognitive-behavior therapy for panic disorder. Biol Psychiatry 67(4):365–370, 2010 19811776

Payne LA, White KS, Gallagher MW, et al: Second-stage treatments for relative nonresponders to cognitive behavioral therapy (CBT) for panic disorder with or without agoraphobia—continued CBT versus SSRI: a randomized controlled trial. Depress Anxiety 33(5):392–399, 2016 26663632

Pyrkosch L, Mumm J, Alt I, et al: Learn to forget: does post-exposure administration of d-cycloserine enhance fear extinction in agoraphobia? J Psychiatr Res 105:153–163, 2018 30237105

Rampello L, Alvano A, Raffaele R, et al: New possibilities of treatment for panic attacks in elderly patients: escitalopram versus citalopram. J Clin Psychopharmacol 26(1):67–70, 2006 16415709

Rickels K: Benzodiazepines in the treatment of anxiety. Am J Psychother 36(3):358–370, 1982 6128929

Rotem-Kohavi N, Oberlander TF: Variations in neurodevelopmental outcomes in children with prenatal SSRI antidepressant exposure. Birth Defects Res 109(12):909–923, 2017 28714603

Schweizer E, Rickels K, De Martinis N, et al: The effect of personality on withdrawal severity and taper outcome in benzodiazepine dependent patients. Psychol Med 28(3):713–720, 1998 9626727

Sheehan DV, Ballenger J, Jacobsen G: Treatment of endogenous anxiety with phobic, hysterical, and hypochondriacal symptoms. Arch Gen Psychiatry 37(1):51–59, 1980 7352840

Spiegel DA: Psychological strategies for discontinuing benzodiazepine treatment. J Clin Psychopharmacol 19(6 suppl 2):17S–22S, 1999 10587280

Taylor CB, Hayward C, King R, et al: Cardiovascular and symptomatic reduction effects of alprazolam and imipramine in patients with panic disorder: results of a double-blind, placebo-controlled trial. J Clin Psychopharmacol 10(2):112–118, 1990 2187912

Tiffon L, Coplan JD, Papp LA, et al: Augmentation strategies with tricyclic or fluoxetine treatment in seven partially responsive panic disorder patients. J Clin Psychiatry 55(2):66–69, 1994 8077156

Walkup JT, Albano AM, Piacentini J, et al: Cognitive behavioral therapy, sertraline, or a combination in childhood anxiety. N Engl J Med 359(26):2753–2766, 2008 18974308

Wedekind D, Broocks A, Weiss N, et al: A randomized, controlled trial of aerobic exercise in combination with paroxetine in the treatment of panic disorder. World J Biol Psychiatry 11(7):904–913, 2010 20602575

Recommended Readings

Baldwin DS, Anderson IM, Nutt DJ, et al: Evidence-based pharmacological treatment of anxiety disorders, post-traumatic stress disorder and obsessive-compulsive disorder: a revision of the 2005 guidelines from the British Association for Psychopharmacology. J Psychopharmacol 28:403–39, 2014

Bandelow B, Sher L, Bunevicius R, et al: Guidelines for the pharmacological treatment of anxiety disorders, obsessive-compulsive disorder and posttraumatic stress disorder in primary care. Int J Psychiatry Clin Pract 16:77–84, 2012

CHAPTER 23

Psychotherapy for Panic Disorder

Abigail L. Barthel, M.A.

Simona Stefan, Ph.D.

Stefan G. Hofmann, Ph.D.

Traditionally, explanatory models and psychological treatments for panic disorder have focused on dismantling the physiological and cognitive mechanisms of panic attacks and the intense preoccupation and avoidance behaviors associated with subsequent attacks. Although panic disorder can be conceptualized according to various theoretical models, cognitive and behavioral models provide the best empirically supported approach to its understanding and treatment. Cognitive models that inform treatment include anxiety sensitivity and catastrophizing or misinterpreting symptoms. Behavioral models center on avoidance of bodily sensation, locations associated with having a panic attack, or emotions associated with panic (Clark and Beck 2010; Craske and Barlow 2007; Depreeuw et al. 2018). A combination of cognitive and behavioral models informs the gold standard treatment for panic disorder, cognitive-behavioral therapy (CBT), which is discussed in more detail in the following sections.

Fear of Bodily Sensations

Fear of bodily sensations is a common feature of panic disorder, contributing to the vicious circle of panic attacks. Individuals tend to interpret benign bodily sensations (e.g., increased heart rate, shallow breathing, sweating, dizziness, blurry vision, nausea) as signs of danger and harm, as potential symptoms of severe illnesses, or as being dangerous (i.e., not necessarily as signs of an underlying condition). Similarly, a key concept in current models of panic disorder is anxiety sensitivity—the tendency to fear and respond fearfully to anxiety-related sensations because of arousal beliefs that they will cause harm or danger (McNally 2002; Reiss and McNally 1985). Therefore, if someone is especially sensitive to one or more of these physical feelings, he or she may experience states of high arousal, which lead to arousal beliefs about potential negative outcomes such as a heart attack or fainting (Reiss and McNally 1985). As such, someone with low anxiety sensitivity may also experience high arousal or physical symptoms but will not believe these feelings to be harmful, whereas someone with high anxiety sensitivity will believe that harm is inevitable (Reiss and McNally 1985). Furthermore, Gallagher et al. (2013) provided evidence that anxiety sensitivity is a main mechanism of change in CBT for panic disorder.

Cognitive Distortions and Catastrophic Misinterpretations

Individuals with panic disorder tend to show a hypervigilance and attentional bias toward interoceptive cues, despite evidence that they do not experience more symptoms than individuals without panic disorder (Beck et al. 1992; Clark and Beck 2010; Depreeuw et al. 2018; Ehlers and Breuer 1992; Pergamin-Hight et al. 2015). As a result of this attentional bias and heightened interoceptive awareness, people with panic disorder often overestimate their physical sensations, thinking that these symptoms will cause them to die, go crazy, or lose control. However, whether on its own or coupled with other physical symptoms, an increased heart rate is not dangerous in itself, so the reactions to the physical sensations of a panic attack are out of proportion with the nature of the actual situation or threat.

Individuals who engage in catastrophizing and who show cognitive distortions often view physical symptoms as being indicative of something harmful (e.g., signs of an underlying heart condition) rather than being symptoms of anxiety. In contrast, the concept of *anxiety sensitivity* refers to the tendency to perceive arousal symptoms as dangerous in themselves, not necessarily as signs of something else (e.g., high arousal itself can cause a heart condition; Hofmann 2010). However, both catastrophic misinterpretations and anxiety sensitivity work to perpetuate the cycle of panic attacks because engaging in hyperawareness and overestimation further increases anxious arousal and symptomatology.

Avoidance

Barlow (2002) distinguished four types of avoidance: distraction, interoceptive avoidance, safety behaviors, and agoraphobic avoidance. *Distraction* allows people to avoid their panic disorder symptoms by diverting attention away from those symptoms to something else that is unassociated. *Interoceptive avoidance* refers to avoiding activities that might naturally induce physical symptoms similar to those experienced during a panic attack (e.g., drinking caffeine, taking hot baths). *Safety behaviors* (e.g., carrying medication everywhere, not leaving the house alone) are meant to keep a person safe in case a panic attack occurs, but such behaviors maintain anxiety in the long run. Finally, *agoraphobic avoidance* occurs when someone with panic disorder avoids places associated with previous panic attacks or places in which escape is difficult. Over time, these avoidance behaviors tend to become habitual and prevent individuals from confronting their fears, thus maintaining anxiety and apprehension in the long run. Consequently, exposure to internal stimuli such as arousal-related sensations, as well as in vivo exposure to avoided situations, are key ingredients in CBT protocols for panic disorder (Barlow 2002; Depreeuw et al. 2018).

Despite the close association between agoraphobic avoidance and panic disorder, DSM-5 (American Psychiatric Association 2013) separated the two diagnoses, possibly introducing a high level of comorbidity. The cognitive-behavioral model of panic, comprising mechanisms and treatment targets, is depicted in Figure 23–1. A harmless trigger (e.g., increased heart rate) is misinterpreted as dangerous (e.g., sign of an underlying heart condition) because of deeply held beliefs that anxiety symptoms are harmful (i.e., anxiety sensitivity) and an implicit tendency to focus on bodily symptoms. Furthermore, this misinterpretation triggers a vicious circle of subjective experience of fear leading to increased physiological arousal (enhancing the experience of fear), which then primes avoidance behaviors (e.g., sitting down, taking medication). These avoidance behaviors, in turn, strengthen the perception of arousal as dangerous, and thus fear and physiological arousal increase further. This vicious circle strengthens beliefs about the dangerousness of arousal symptoms. Each component in the model is subject to specific intervention strategies (shown in italics in Figure 23–1). Attention bias modification targets the implicit focus on body sensations, and cognitive restructuring aims to challenge beliefs associated with arousal, as well as misinterpretations of bodily symptoms, as dangerous. Breathing retraining is helpful in controlling the increased physiological arousal associated with fear, and exposure techniques and acceptance address the overall circle of fear-arousal-avoidance.

Models of Exposure Therapy

Exposure therapy is widely used and supported in the treatment of panic disorder, and several theoretical and experimental models have been proposed, with somewhat different techniques (for a review, see Craske et al. 2014). By earlier accounts, exposure is effective primarily because of the mechanism of fear habituation (Foa and Kozak 1986): when a person is confronted with a feared stimulus, anxiety peaks, reaches a plateau, and then naturally begins to decrease (after approximately 60–90 minutes), thus leading to a deconstruction of the fear memory structure or conditioned response, with no cognitive mediation necessary. High initial levels of physiological arousal, within-session habituation (significant decreases in anxiety during the exposure session), and between-session habituation (initial levels of anxiety becoming lower from one session to the next) are considered markers of successful treatment according to this approach (Foa and Kozak 1986).

In addition to habituation, cognitive models of exposure have advanced the idea that successful extinction is cognitively mediated by modifying *expectancies* about the occurrence of the unconditioned, feared stimuli or the consequences of their occurrence. That is, fear drops because, through exposure, the individual learns that the feared consequence either does not occur or does occur but is less aversive and easier to control than previously expected (Hofmann 2008). In the case of panic disorder, for

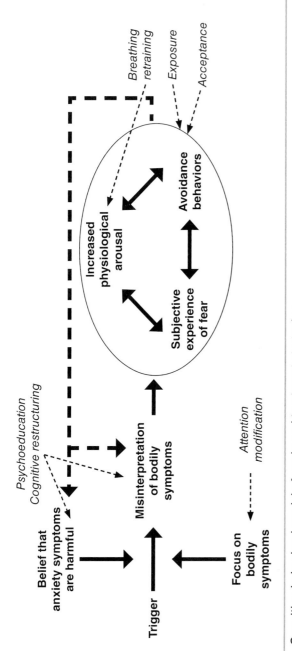

FIGURE 23–1.   Cognitive-behavioral model of panic and treatment strategies.

Source.   Reprinted from Hofmann 2012. Copyright © 2012 John Wiley & Sons, Ltd. Used with permission.

example, interoceptive exposure to arousal sensations allows the individual to notice that feared consequences of panic-like symptoms (e.g., going crazy) do not occur, and this begins to break the association between these panic symptoms and fear.

Finally, the *inhibitory learning model of extinction* posits that the fear structure is not really deconstructed but that exposure provides new learning experiences that lead to the formation of a new, inhibitory memory structure in which the unconditioned stimulus is no longer predicted by the conditioned stimulus. Thus, the inhibitory approach does not require an immediate reduction in subjective distress for the exposure to be successful. Rather, the inhibitory learning approach seeks to violate the person's automatic expectancies or feared outcomes about a situation, which can be accomplished even if distress is still heightened following an exposure.

This model also elaborates on why within-session habituation is not always a good predictor of fear extinction and why the fear response can reoccur at later times after the initial fear has habituated (Craske et al. 2014). Specifically, for conducting exposure in panic disorder, some clinical implications of the inhibitory learning model include violations of expectancies (i.e., perceived consequences of experiencing feared sensations), deepened exposure (i.e., combining multiple types of feared stimuli), and removal of safety behaviors. Recent advances in exposure therapy for panic disorder also include the use of D-cycloserine, a partial agonist of the glutamatergic NMDA receptor, as adjunctive to exposure-based CBT. Research indicates that D-cycloserine speeds treatment response at posttreatment compared to placebo (Hofmann et al. 2015; Otto et al. 2016).

Panic Control Theory

The most popular and effective psychotherapy technique for treating panic disorder is CBT. One common CBT treatment manual used for treating panic disorder is Craske and Barlow's (2007) *Mastery of Your Anxiety and Panic* therapist guide, based on panic control theory (PCT). This treatment has a wide array of empirical evidence to support its use for panic disorder with or without agoraphobia, with one study showing that it is more effective than relaxation training protocols (Barlow et al. 1989) and similarly effective to medication (Barlow et al. 2000). The PCT protocol includes three sections, as described in the following discussion.

Section 1

The first section of Craske and Barlow's (2007) PCT protocol calls for one or two sessions of psychoeducation about the nature and function of panic disorder and treatment components. CBT educates patients and targets their hypersensitivity to threat by teaching them to engage in more accurate and flexible emotional awareness. The PCT protocol emphasizes the cyclical nature of thoughts, physical sensations, and behaviors using the three-component model of emotions. Patients complete homework and are actively involved in planning their own behavioral experiments, otherwise known as exposures, in which they engage in real-world situations that tend to elicit the physical symptoms, thoughts, or behaviors of their panic disorder to learn to tolerate these negative emotional experiences and behaviors.

Section 2

Section two of the PCT manual targets skill building in the form of slowed breathing and cognitive restructuring. In the third session, the diaphragmatic breathing technique is introduced. This breathing skill encourages deep, slow breathing that moves the stomach instead of over-breathing or shallow breathing that is quick and engages only the chest and lungs. When learning diaphragmatic breathing, patients typically undergo a hyperventilation test first to emphasize the contrast between breathing during a panic attack and normal breathing. The therapist models hyperventilation activity, breathing fast and shallowly through the chest for 60 seconds, which often induces panic symptoms such as shortness of breath, sweating, dizziness, and blurred vision. After practice with diaphragmatic breathing, patients are told to count their breaths and focus on relaxing while breathing slowly for a full cycle of 6 seconds. Patients practice these skills in sessions three and four and engage in further practice and monitoring for homework by doing these breathing activities several times a day.

The second skill, which targets the cognitive nature of panic disorder and anxiety, is cognitive restructuring (thinking skills). As Craske and Barlow (2007) outlined, the main goal of cognitive skill building is to teach patients that thoughts are not definitive and are not actions. Patients are asked to identify their negative thought patterns, which tend to be cognitive errors that often contrast with the reality of the situation or the odds (i.e., probability overestimation and catastrophizing). Therapists work with patients to counter these thoughts through cognitive challenging or restructuring. Typical exercises for reevaluating automatic negative thoughts include 1) inquiring if the feared outcome has ever happened, 2) recognizing incorrect reasons for continued anxiety, 3) identifying the evidence for and against the feared outcome, 4) using a scale to rate the odds of a particular feared outcome occurring, and 5) examining alternative possibilities or explanations.

Section 3

The final segment of Craske and Barlow's (2007) PCT treatment targets patients' fear and avoidance of negative symptoms through interoceptive and situational exposure exercises. This approach of repetitive exposure to feared situations, physical sensations, and outcomes has been shown to be one of the most important components of anxiety disorder treatment, based in fear extinction theories (Barlow 2002; Depreeuw et al. 2018; Vervliet et al. 2013). Exposures help patients learn to manage their thoughts, feelings, and behaviors associated with panic attacks and work to remove their safety behaviors and avoidance strategies so that they are able to manage and recover from a panic attack in the future without needing to use buffers to escape the full experience.

Interoceptive exposures target the physical sensations that are contributing to patients' fear and avoidance around panic attacks. Common interoceptive exposure exercises include hyperventilating, spinning in a chair, running in place, and straw breathing through a slender coffee stirrer. Patients often are asked to rate their anxiety after engaging in one of these exposures as well as the level of similarity that exists between the simulated exposure and a real panic attack. With increased experiencing of symptoms through subsequent exposures, patients' distress and anxiety related to those symptoms decrease over time. In addition to or as an alternative to interoceptive exposures, some patients may benefit from in vivo situational exposure exercises that may involve other people, safety behaviors, or locations in which panic attacks typically occur. This section of the manual should be used for individuals who report frequent agoraphobic avoidance and safety behaviors. Situational exposures may include circumstances or places that someone avoids because of fear of having a panic attack, fear of embarrassment, or fear of not being able to escape the situation.

Emerging Treatments

Unified Protocol

Another form of CBT with recent evidence of effectiveness in treating anxiety disorders, including panic disorder, is the *Unified Protocol for the Transdiagnostic Treatment of Emotional Disorders*, developed by Barlow and colleagues in 2010, with a second edition released in 2017 (Barlow et al. 2017). This approach to treatment deemphasizes one's specific diagnosis and seeks to provide a single manual for the treatment of all anxiety and related disorders by targeting common mechanisms among them. These common mechanisms include neuroticism, avoidance, negative evaluation, and emotion dysregulation (Barlow et al. 2017).

The Unified Protocol is broken into five core modules: 1) mindful emotion awareness, 2) cognitive flexibility, 3) emotional avoidance identification and prevention, 4) increasing tolerance of physical sensations, and 5) interoceptive and situational exposures. Mindful emotion awareness includes three skills: staying in the present moment and noticing emotions in a nonjudgmental manner; mindful mood induction, which is an exercise aimed at learning to tolerate negative emotions or thoughts when induced in session, while continuing to stay present and nonjudgmental of emotions; and anchoring in the present moment. Cognitive flexibility, prevention of avoidance, and exposure exercises operate similarly to the PCT approach in this protocol. A recent randomized controlled trial (RCT) concluded that the Unified Protocol performed equally as well as single-disorder protocols from baseline to 6-month follow-up, and both were superior to the waitlist control group (Barlow et al. 2017).

Applied Relaxation

According to the American Psychological Association's Division 12 Society of Clinical Psychology, applied relaxation therapy for panic disorder has only modest research support. As Depreeuw et al. (2018) noted, the common technique associated with applied relaxation is progressive muscle relaxation (Jacobson 1938), which is the process of slowly and deliberately tensing and releasing different muscles to gain control over them and to feel more relaxed. In essence, progressive muscle relaxation acts to give patients more autonomy and familiarity with their physical sensations while teaching them to act this way when symptoms of a panic attack come up (Öst 1986). Research evidence in support of applied relaxation reveals mixed findings (for reviews, see Depreeuw et al. 2018 and Öst and Westling 1995), and it is not generally recommended as a stand-alone treatment for panic disorder.

Mindfulness

The concept of *mindfulness* refers to present, nonjudgmental awareness of emotions, thoughts, behaviors, internal sensations, and circumstances by approaching these situations with acceptance and curiosity (Allen et al. 2006; Bishop et al. 2004; Kabat-Zinn 2003). Although mindfulness is not specifically targeted to panic disorder, several studies support the effectiveness of mindfulness interventions for the treatment of anxiety and related disorders (Hofmann et al. 2010; Khoury et al. 2013; Kim et al. 2016). Moreover, Kabat-Zinn et al. (1992), Miller et al. (1995), and Kim et al. (2010) found that mindfulness for panic disorder is beneficial in group formats and in addition to medication treatments. As such, preliminary evidence has shown mindfulness to be successful for treating panic disorder, but more controlled trials looking specifically at panic disorder are needed.

Computer-Based and Online Interventions

In recent years, CBT protocols for panic disorder and other anxiety and related disorders have been developed in internet-based (iCBT) and mobile application formats. Some of these online protocols have been tested in RCTs and shown to be effective and potentially cheaper interventions (Andrews et al. 2010; National Institute for Health and Clinical Excellence 2011). For instance, a recent meta-analysis (Andrews et al. 2018) found iCBT interventions to be effective in treating anxiety disorders and depression, with a large effect size when compared with control conditions, specifically for panic disorder trials (12 trials, $g=1.31$; 95% CI 0.85–1.76). The authors concluded that iCBT interventions are similarly effective as face-to-face interventions (Andrews et al. 2018).

Addressing Comorbidities in Treatment

For panic disorder, comorbidity is the rule rather than the exception, with studies indicating comorbidity prevalence reaching 80%–90% (Kessler et al. 2006; Tilli et al. 2012). The most frequently comorbid conditions are major depression and other anxiety disorders (about 50%–60%; Arch and Craske 2008), but other mood disorders, substance use disorders, and personality disorders are also frequent. Because panic disorder comorbidities are so frequent, randomized trials have not excluded patients with common comorbid disorders, such as major depression or anxiety disorders; therefore, we can argue that current CBT protocols for panic disorder are also effective for patients with comorbid conditions (Brown et al. 1995; Tsao et al. 2002).

Newer, transdiagnostic approaches, such as the Unified Protocol (Barlow et al. 2017), acceptance and commitment therapy (ACT; Hayes 2016), and process-based CBT (Hayes and Hofmann 2018; Hofmann and Hayes 2019) can be particularly effective in the case of comorbidities. These treatments are based on the assumption that overarching pathological processes are leading to emotional dysregulation (Hofmann et al. 2012). For example, ACT promotes acceptance and cognitive diffusion in relation to maladaptive emotions and cognitions and emphasizes values-congruent behavior change, regardless of diagnosis. That is why some data indicate that patients with comorbid anxiety disorders may do better with ACT, whereas people with single diagnoses seem to achieve better results with traditional CBT (Wolitzky-Taylor et al. 2012).

Following a similar line, process-based CBT aims to find evidence-based procedures to target evidence-based processes (e.g., cognitive flexibility) as they manifest in particular individuals, not in the context of syndromes and disorders. In this sense, the model offers an alternative to the existing diagnostic systems (not only a transdiagnostic approach) based on functional analysis and evolutionary science (Hofmann and Hayes 2019). In brief, process-based CBT moves away from a nomothetic approach toward an idiographic approach and is a radical departure from the latent disease model of DSM-5 because it embraces and uses principles and techniques of functional analysis, dynamic complex network approaches, and evolutionary science (Hayes and Hofmann 2017, 2018; Hayes et al. 2019; Hofmann and Hayes 2019).

Agoraphobia

Panic disorder is often accompanied by agoraphobia. Accordingly, the presence of agoraphobia makes comorbidity with other disorders more likely (Kessler et al. 2006) and contributes largely to disability, especially through agoraphobic avoidance (Bonham and Uhlenhuth 2014). Having been designed for this configuration, the treatment models presented previously address agoraphobia mainly by employing in vivo exposure techniques in feared, avoided situations (Hofmann 2010). In this respect, a meta-analysis indicated that therapy is similarly effective for patients with panic disorder with and without agoraphobia (Sánchez-Meca et al. 2010).

Depression

When discussing comorbid panic disorder and depression in particular, depression can affect the course of panic disorder and its treatment in specific ways (Otto et al. 2008). For example, depression tends to enhance fears of anxiety sensations by making negative thoughts feel truer. Depression may cause someone to negatively evaluate the progress of therapy, which may indicate that patients with comorbid panic disorder and depression require more motivational techniques and closer guidance related to goals and homework completion (usually because of the low energy and negativity experienced in depression). Behavioral activation can also be adapted to address both panic disorder and depression by combining pleasant, values-congruent behaviors with exposure to the feared situations that patients avoid because of panic (Hopko et al. 2004).

Physical Illness

Finally, panic disorder can be comorbid with actual physical illness, such as respiratory diseases (e.g., asthma), cardiovascular conditions (e.g., hypertension, mitral valve prolapse), gastrointestinal conditions (e.g., irritable bowel syndrome), or diabetes (Meuret et al. 2017). When this is the case, therapy should provide additional psychoeducation about the distinction between panic and physical disease symptoms (e.g., palpitations are frequent in panic but medically only weakly associated with arrhythmia) and should avoid interoceptive exposure exercises that can exacerbate the physical conditions (e.g., hyperventilation exercises in patients with asthma) (Lehrer et al. 2008; Meuret et al. 2017).

Conclusion

CBT is currently considered the gold standard for treating panic disorder, with strong empirical support for both its practice and its theory (Carpenter et al. 2018; Depreeuw et al. 2018; Pompoli et al. 2016). Because panic disorder is often comorbid with other psychological disorders, psychotherapists should account for comorbidities and adapt protocols accordingly. Emerging treatments include transdiagnostic approaches, such as the Unified Protocol, mindfulness-based approaches, iCBT, exercise treatment, and process-based CBT (Hayes and Hofmann 2018). These emerging treatments have received various degrees of research support and, as such, require further investigation in the context of RCTs before being accepted as uniformly effective for panic disorder.

Key Points

- Cognitive-behavioral components of panic disorder include anxiety sensitivity, catastrophizing, and behavioral avoidance, which can be differentially targeted using cognitive-behavioral therapy (CBT) treatments. Common approaches to CBT include habituation and inhibitory learning models.

- CBT is the gold standard for treating panic disorder and typically encompasses skill building in the form of slow breathing, cognitive restructuring, interoceptive exposure, and situational exposures.

- Emerging treatments for panic disorder include the Unified Protocol, mindfulness interventions, applied relaxation, exercising, and online interventions. However, these treatments have varying degrees of research support and cannot yet be considered gold standards of treatment.

References

Allen NB, Chambers R, Knight W: Mindfulness-based psychotherapies: a review of conceptual foundations, empirical evidence and practical considerations. Aust N Z J Psychiatry 40(4):285–294, 2006 16620310

American Psychiatric Association: Diagnostic and Statistical Manual of Mental Disorders, 5th Edition. Arlington, VA, American Psychiatric Association, 2013

Andrews G, Cuijpers P, Craske MG, et al: Computer therapy for the anxiety and depressive disorders is effective, acceptable and practical health care: a meta-analysis. PLoS One 5(10):e13196, 2010 20967242

Andrews G, Basu A, Cuijpers P, et al: Computer therapy for the anxiety and depression disorders is effective, acceptable and practical health care: an updated meta-analysis. J Anxiety Disord 55:70–78, 2018 29422409

Arch J, Craske MG: Panic disorder, in Psychopathology: History, Diagnosis, and Empirical Foundations. Edited by Craighead W, Miklowitz DJ, Craighead LW. Hoboken, NJ, Wiley, 2008, pp 115–158

Barlow DH: Anxiety and Its Disorders: The Nature and Treatment of Anxiety and Panic, 2nd Edition. New York, Guilford, 2002

Barlow DH, Craske MG, Cerny JA, et al: Behavioral treatment of panic disorder. Behav Ther 20:261–282, 1989

Barlow DH, Gorman JM, Shear MK, et al: Cognitive-behavioral therapy, imipramine, or their combination for panic disorder: a randomized controlled trial. JAMA 283(19):2529–2536, 2000 10815116

Barlow DH, Farchione TJ, Bullis JR, et al: The Unified Protocol for Transdiagnostic Treatment of Emotional Disorders compared with diagnosis-specific protocols for anxiety disorders: a randomized clinical trial. JAMA Psychiatry 74(9):875–884, 2017 28768327

Beck JG, Stanley MA, Averill PM, et al: Attention and memory for threat in panic disorder. Behav Res Ther 30(6):619–629, 1992 1417687

Bishop SR, Lau M, Shapiro S, et al: Mindfulness: a proposed operational definition. Clin Psychol Sci Pract 11:230–241, 2004

Bonham CA, Uhlenhuth E: Disability and comorbidity: diagnoses and symptoms associated with disability in a clinical population with panic disorder. Psychiatry J 2014:619727, 2014 24829902

Brown TA, Antony MM, Barlow DH: Diagnostic comorbidity in panic disorder: effect on treatment outcome and course of comorbid diagnoses following treatment. J Consult Clin Psychol 63(3):408–418, 1995 7608353

Carpenter JK, Andrews LA, Witcraft SM, et al: Cognitive behavioral therapy for anxiety and related disorders: a meta-analysis of randomized placebo-controlled trials. Depress Anxiety 35(6):502–514, 2018 29451967

Clark DA, Beck AT: Cognitive theory and therapy of anxiety and depression: convergence with neurobiological findings. Trends Cogn Sci 14(9):418–424, 2010 20655801

Craske MG, Barlow DH: Mastery of Your Anxiety and Panic: Therapist Guide. New York, Oxford University Press, 2007

Craske MG, Treanor M, Conway CC, et al: Maximizing exposure therapy: an inhibitory learning approach. Behav Res Ther 58:10–23, 2014 24864005

Depreeuw B, Andrews LA, Eldar S, et al: Panic and phobias disorders, in Evidence-Based Psychotherapy: The State of the Science and Practice. Edited by David D, Lynn SJ, Montgomery GH. Hoboken, NJ, Wiley Blackwell, 2018, pp 63–78

Ehlers A, Breuer P: Increased cardiac awareness in panic disorder. J Abnorm Psychol 101(3):371–382, 1992 1500594

Foa EB, Kozak MJ: Emotional processing of fear: exposure to corrective information. Psychol Bull 99(1):20–35, 1986 2871574

Gallagher MW, Payne LA, White KS, et al: Mechanisms of change in cognitive behavioral therapy for panic disorder: the unique effects of self-efficacy and anxiety sensitivity. Behav Res Ther 51(11):767–777, 2013 24095901

Hayes SC: Acceptance and commitment therapy, relational frame theory, and the third wave of behavioral and cognitive therapies—republished article. Behav Ther 47(6):869–885, 2016 27993338

Hayes SC, Hofmann SG: The third wave of cognitive behavioral therapy and the rise of process-based care. World Psychiatry 16(3):245–246, 2017 28941087

Hayes SC, Hofmann SG: Process-Based CBT: The Science and Core Clinical Competencies of Cognitive Behavioral Therapy. Oakland, CA, Context Press, 2018

Hayes SC, Hofmann SG, Stanton CE, et al: The role of the individual in the coming era of process-based therapy. Behav Res Ther 117:40–53, 2019 30348451

Hofmann SG: Cognitive processes during fear acquisition and extinction in animals and humans: implications for exposure therapy of anxiety disorders. Clin Psychol Rev 28(2):199–210, 2008 17532105

Hofmann SG: Psychotherapy for panic disorder, in Textbook of Anxiety Disorders, 2nd Edition. Edited by Stein DJ, Hollander E, Rothbaum BO. Washington, DC, American Psychiatric Publishing, 2010, pp 417–433

Hofmann SG: An Introduction to Modern CBT: Psychological Solutions to Mental Health Problems. Malden, MA, Wiley Blackwell, 2012

Hofmann SG, Hayes SC: The future of intervention science: process-based therapy. Clin Psychol Sci 7(1):37–50, 2019 30713811

Hofmann SG, Sawyer AT, Witt AA, et al: The effect of mindfulness-based therapy on anxiety and depression: a meta-analytic review. J Consult Clin Psychol 78(2):169–183, 2010 20350028

Hofmann SG, Sawyer AT, Fang A, et al: Emotion dysregulation model of mood and anxiety disorders. Depress Anxiety 29(5):409–416, 2012 22430982

Hofmann SG, Otto MW, Pollack MH, et al: D-cycloserine augmentation of cognitive behavioral therapy for anxiety disorders: an update. Curr Psychiatry Rep 17(1):532, 2015 25413638

Hopko DR, Lejuez CW, Hopko SD: Behavioral activation as an intervention for coexistent depressive and anxiety symptoms. Clin Case Stud 3(1):37–48, 2004

Jacobson E: Progressive Relaxation, 2nd Edition. Chicago, IL, University of Chicago Press, 1938

Kabat-Zinn J: Mindfulness-based interventions in context: past, present, and future. Clin Psychol Sci Pract 10:144–156, 2003

Kabat-Zinn J, Massion AO, Kristeller J, et al: Effectiveness of a meditation-based stress reduction program in the treatment of anxiety disorders. Am J Psychiatry 149(7):936–943, 1992 1609875

Kessler RC, Chiu WT, Jin R, et al: The epidemiology of panic attacks, panic disorder, and agoraphobia in the National Comorbidity Survey Replication. Arch Gen Psychiatry 63(4):415–424, 2006 16585471

Khoury B, Lecomte T, Fortin G, et al: Mindfulness-based therapy: a comprehensive meta-analysis. Clin Psychol Rev 33(6):763–771, 2013 23796855

Kim B, Lee SH, Kim YW, et al: Effectiveness of a mindfulness-based cognitive therapy program as an adjunct to pharmacotherapy in patients with panic disorder. J Anxiety Disord 24(6):590–595, 2010 20427148

Kim MK, Lee KS, Kim B, et al: Impact of mindfulness-based cognitive therapy on intolerance of uncertainty in patients with panic disorder. Psychiatry Investig 13(2):196–202, 2016 27081380

Lehrer PM, Karavidas MK, Lu S-E, et al: Psychological treatment of comorbid asthma and panic disorder: a pilot study. J Anxiety Disord 22(4):671–683, 2008 17693054

McNally RJ: Anxiety sensitivity and panic disorder. Biol Psychiatry 52(10):938–946, 2002 12437935

Meuret AE, Kroll J, Ritz T: Panic disorder comorbidity with medical conditions and treatment implications. Annu Rev Clin Psychol 13:209–240, 2017 28375724

Miller JJ, Fletcher K, Kabat-Zinn J: Three-year follow-up and clinical implications of a mindfulness meditation-based stress reduction intervention in the treatment of anxiety disorders. Gen Hosp Psychiatry 17(3):192–200, 1995 7649463

National Institute for Health and Clinical Excellence: Generalised anxiety disorder and panic disorder in adults: management. London, National Institute for Health and Clinical Excellence, January 2011. Available at: https://www.nice.org.uk/guidance/cg113. Accessed June 27, 2019.

Öst L: Antidepressants and the treatment of agoraphobia and panic: an evaluative overview (in Swedish). Lakartidningen 83(41):3421–3422, 3424–3425, 1986 3537591

Öst LG, Westling BE: Applied relaxation vs cognitive behavior therapy in the treatment of panic disorder. Behav Res Ther 33(2):145–158, 1995 7887873

Otto MW, Powers MB, Stathopoulou G, et al: Panic disorder and social phobia, in Adapting Cognitive Therapy for Depression: Managing Complexity and Comorbidity. Edited by Whisman MA. New York, Guilford, 2008, pp 185–208

Otto MW, Pollack MH, Dowd SM, et al: Randomized trial of d-cycloserine enhancement of cognitive-behavioral therapy for panic disorder. Depress Anxiety 33(8):737–745, 2016 27315514

Pergamin-Hight L, Naim R, Bakermans-Kranenburg MJ, et al: Content specificity of attention bias to threat in anxiety disorders: a meta-analysis. Clin Psychol Rev 35:10–18, 2015 25462110

Pompoli A, Furukawa TA, Imai H, et al: Psychological therapies for panic disorder with or without agoraphobia in adults: a network meta-analysis. Cochrane Database Syst Rev 4:CD011004, 2016 27071857

Reiss S, McNally RJ: The expectancy model of fear, in Theoretical Issues in Behavior Therapy. Edited by Reiss S, Bootzin RR. Cambridge, MA, Academic Press, 1985, pp 107–121

Sánchez-Meca J, Rosa-Alcázar AI, Marín-Martínez F, et al: Psychological treatment of panic disorder with or without agoraphobia: a meta-analysis. Clin Psychol Rev 30(1):37–50, 2010 19775792

Tilli V, Suominen K, Karlsson H: Panic disorder in primary care: comorbid psychiatric disorders and their persistence. Scand J Prim Health Care 30(4):247–253, 2012 23113695

Tsao JCI, Mystkowski JL, Zucker BG, et al: Effects of cognitive-behavioral therapy for panic disorder on comorbid conditions: replication and extension. Behav Ther 33(4):493–509, 2002

Vervliet B, Craske MG, Hermans D: Fear extinction and relapse: state of the art. Annu Rev Clin Psychol 9:215–248, 2013 23537484

Wolitzky-Taylor KB, Arch JJ, Rosenfield D, et al: Moderators and non-specific predictors of treatment outcome for anxiety disorders: a comparison of cognitive behavioral therapy to acceptance and commitment therapy. J Consult Clin Psychol 80(5):786–799, 2012 22823858

Recommended Readings

Craske MG, Barlow DH: Mastery of Your Anxiety and Panic: Therapist Guide. New York, Oxford University Press, 2007

Craske MG, Treanor M, Conway CC, et al: Maximizing exposure therapy: an inhibitory learning approach. Behav Res Ther 58:10–23, 2014 24864005

Hofmann SG: Psychotherapy for panic disorder, in Textbook of Anxiety Disorders, 2nd Edition. Edited by Stein DJ, Hollander E, Rothbaum BO. Washington, DC, American Psychiatric Publishing, 2010, pp 417–433

Hofmann SG: An Introduction to Modern CBT: Psychological Solutions to Mental Health Problems. Malden, MA, Wiley Blackwell, 2012

PART VI

Social Anxiety Disorder
(Social Phobia)

CHAPTER 24

Phenomenology of Social Anxiety Disorder

Murray B. Stein, M.D., M.P.H.

Charles T. Taylor, Ph.D.

The history of social phobia (social anxiety disorder) as a diagnostic category is relatively brief. Although the term *social phobia* was coined in the early 1900s to describe individuals with performance-related anxieties (Janet 1903), it was not included in the first two versions of the DSM nomenclature (American Psychiatric Association 1952, 1968). Instead, symptoms resembling social phobia were subsumed under the rubric of phobic disorders. It was not until the advent of DSM-III (American Psychiatric Association 1980) and findings suggesting that certain phobias were qualitatively distinct (Marks and Gelder 1966) that social phobia was given its own diagnostic category.

Social phobia has long been referred to as a "neglected anxiety disorder" (Liebowitz et al. 1985). In its first appearance in DSM-III, social phobia was defined as an excessive fear of observation or scrutiny in performance-related situations (e.g., public speaking, eating in front of others, writing in front of others). Exposure to these situations typically resulted in panic-like symptoms (e.g., heart palpitations, tremors, blushing, sweating), leading many individuals to avoid such situations or to endure them with a great deal of distress. DSM-III criteria also specified that individuals experiencing these symptoms recognize that their fears are unreasonable or excessive. In cases in which the patient avoided multiple social situations, an Axis II diagnosis of avoidant personality disorder was to supersede a social phobia diagnosis. As a result, many individuals received a diagnosis of avoidant personality disorder rather than social phobia. Although the diagnostic criteria for these two disorders overlapped considerably, avoidant personality disorder was differentiated from social phobia by its pervasiveness, the intense feelings of inferiority it produced, and its earlier age at onset.

In DSM-III-R (American Psychiatric Association 1987), an attempt was made to improve the classification criteria by expanding the social phobia category to include individuals who feared many social situations. With this revision, avoidant personality disorder was dropped as an exclusionary criterion. Such inclusiveness resulted in a very heterogeneous diagnostic group; for example, an individual who feared only public speaking situations was given the same diagnosis as one who feared most social interactions. Consequently, DSM-III-R created a generalized subtype for persons who feared "most" social situations, including both performance (e.g., giving speeches, speaking at a meeting) and interactional (e.g., talking to strangers, interacting at a party) situations (Kessler et al. 1998). Those who did not fit this subtype were informally termed "nongeneralized"; however, such labels as "circumscribed," "discrete," "limited," and "specific" were also applied.

Subsequently, the DSM-IV (American Psychiatric Association 1994) diagnostic criteria for social phobia (social anxiety disorder) remained largely consistent with those put forth in DSM-III-R. With regard to the subtyping system, the generalized subtype was once again included to distinguish individuals with fears of "most" social situations from those with specific fears. DSM-IV extended the criteria for social phobia to apply to children, specifically advising that anxiety might be expressed differently in children (e.g., by children's crying, tantrums, freezing, or withdrawal) than in adults. It was also noted that children, unlike adults, might not perceive their reactions to social situations as being unreasonable or excessive.

In DSM-5 (American Psychiatric Association 2013), the term *social anxiety disorder* is the preferred diagnostic nomenclature (rather than social phobia), emphasizing that this is, for most patients, more than just a circumscribed phobia. DSM-IV used *social phobia* but emphasized the existence of a substantial subgroup of patients with pervasive social fears and avoidance, which was termed "generalized" social phobia. The developers of DSM-5 elected to abolish the "generalized" subtype, instead coining the specifier "performance only" to encompass such situations as public speaking or other types of performing (Heimberg et al. 2014). Accordingly, the performance-only specifier codifies the most delimited form of social anxiety disorder.

Additional revisions to the social anxiety disorder criteria in DSM-5 include more detailed mention of the types of social situations avoided to include social interaction, observation, and performance, with examples of each provided. Fear of negative evaluation is now explicitly emphasized in the diagnostic criteria—encompassing the individual's concerns that he or she will act in a way or show anxiety symptoms that result in embarrassment or humiliation. To increase the cultural sensitivity of the diagnosis (see cross-national and cultural findings in the section "Epidemiology"), the feared consequence of offending others has been added as an example of fear of negative evaluation. The criteria no longer require the individual to recognize that the fear is excessive but do require the fear to be out of proportion to the actual threat posed. This acknowledges that when patients do not see their fear as excessive but are clearly not psychotic, it is sufficient for the clinician to confirm the excessiveness of the fear for a diagnosis of social anxiety disorder.

Another important change in DSM-5 was modification of the medical exclusion criterion. Prior to DSM-5, the diagnostic criteria for social anxiety disorder specified that it not be diagnosed if the social anxiety was exclusively about symptoms of a medical condition, such as tremor. This restriction was removed in DSM-5, largely because it was recognized that social anxiety symptoms are very common among patients with observable medical conditions such as Parkinson's disease or obesity (Dalrymple et al. 2017), and those symptoms may be amenable to treatment. When social fears or avoidance is judged to be unrelated to or "excessive" in relation to the individual's physical illness, a DSM-5 diagnosis of social anxiety disorder is now permitted (American Psychiatric Association 2013).

Clinical Features

Social anxiety disorder is characterized by a marked fear of social and performance situations in which scrutiny by others is possible. The individual fears being negatively evaluated by others and, as result, being embarrassed, being humiliated or rejected, or offending others (Box 24–1; American Psychiatric Association 2013). These fears lead the individual to avoid social situations or, if situational avoidance is not possible, to engage in subtle avoidance (safety) behaviors within social situations that are intended to prevent feared outcomes and maintain a sense of safety (e.g., remaining quiet during a social gathering to avoid the possibility of saying something that could be criticized or made fun of by others). Safety behaviors often have the unintended consequence of perpetuating social fears, either by exacerbating feared outcomes (e.g., increasing anxiety through excessive self-monitoring or eliciting negative responses from others) or by preventing the individual from learning that the feared outcome would not have happened or would have been tolerable even if the safety behavior had not been used (Piccirillo et al. 2016).

Box 24–1.   DSM-5 diagnostic criteria for social anxiety disorder

A. Marked fear or anxiety about one or more social situations in which the individual is exposed to possible scrutiny by others. Examples include social interactions (e.g., having a conversation, meeting unfamiliar people), being observed (e.g., eating or drinking), and performing in front of others (e.g., giving a speech).

   Note: In children, the anxiety must occur in peer settings and not just during interactions with adults.

B. The individual fears that he or she will act in a way or show anxiety symptoms that will be negatively evaluated (i.e., will be humiliating or embarrassing; will lead to rejection or offend others).

C. The social situations almost always provoke fear or anxiety.

   Note: In children, the fear or anxiety may be expressed by crying, tantrums, freezing, clinging, shrinking, or failing to speak in social situations.

D. The social situations are avoided or endured with intense fear or anxiety.

E. The fear or anxiety is out of proportion to the actual threat posed by the social situation and to the sociocultural context.

F. The fear, anxiety, or avoidance is persistent, typically lasting for 6 months or more.

G. The fear, anxiety, or avoidance causes clinically significant distress or impairment in social, occupational, or other important areas of functioning.

H. The fear, anxiety, or avoidance is not attributable to the physiological effects of a substance (e.g., a drug of abuse, a medication) or another medical condition.

I. The fear, anxiety, or avoidance is not better explained by the symptoms of another mental disorder, such as panic disorder, body dysmorphic disorder, or autism spectrum disorder.

J. If another medical condition (e.g., Parkinson's disease, obesity, disfigurement from burns or injury) is present, the fear, anxiety, or avoidance is clearly unrelated or is excessive.

Specify if:
   Performance only: If the fear is restricted to speaking or performing in public.

Source.   Reprinted from American Psychiatric Association: *Diagnostic and Statistical Manual of Mental Disorders*, 5th Edition. Arlington, VA, American Psychiatric Association, 2013. Copyright © 2013 American Psychiatric Association. Used with permission.

The clinical presentation of social anxiety disorder can vary considerably from person to person. Although many individuals with social anxiety disorder are characterized by prototypical expressions of anxiousness and inhibited behavior, other clinical presentations include hostile and angry behavior (Erwin et al. 2003; Kachin et al. 2001) as well as high novelty seeking and impulsiveness (Kashdan and Hofmann 2008). This heterogeneity in expression has been associated with distinct demographic (e.g., gender) and clinical characteristics (e.g., depression, substance use disorders), as well as response to treatment (e.g., patients characterized by higher pretreatment anger suppression displayed worse response to group cognitive-behavioral therapy; Erwin et al. 2003).

Differential Diagnosis

Social anxiety disorder is not especially difficult to diagnose in a clinical context, once an index of suspicion is high enough (Stein and Stein 2008). Patients may not spontaneously report symptoms but, when asked, will endorse fear and avoidance of social situations because of concerns about embarrassment, humiliation, or rejection. When such an individual reports experiencing functional impairment or distress in relation to these concerns, a diagnosis of social anxiety disorder is highly likely. However, the differential diagnosis can be somewhat more challenging in some areas.

Shyness is a personality trait that can range from normative to extreme and is not in and of itself an indicator of psychopathology. Many persons with social anxiety disorder do consider themselves to be shy, and many report that they were extremely socially inhibited and withdrawn as children (Biederman et al. 2001). Shyness, then, may be a precursor to social anxiety disorder for some individuals, although most shy children will "outgrow" their shyness. It has been suggested that a stable pattern of behavioral inhibition in childhood that merges into social avoidance and withdrawal is a risk indicator for subsequent social anxiety disorder that may merit early intervention (Chronis-Tuscano et al. 2018).

Panic attacks often occur in individuals with social anxiety disorder when they are in feared social situations or even anticipating such situations. Directly asking about the cognitions patients experience during or in anticipation of their anxiety symptoms or feared situations (e.g., "What were you thinking about when you felt anxious and uncomfortable?") is essential in differential diagnosis. Patients with social anxiety disorder attribute their symptoms to the situation and its evaluative characteristics, whereas those with panic disorder experience their anxiety symptoms as occurring "out of the blue" (at least in the initial stages of illness, after which panic attacks may become more common in certain situations than in others). Differential diagnosis of social anxiety disorder from panic and other anxiety disorders, including separation anxiety disorder and generalized anxiety disorder, is summarized in Table 24–1.

Social anxiety disorder is frequently comorbid with major depression but should not be diagnosed if social avoidance is confined to depressive episodes. However, considerable comorbidity exists between social anxiety disorder and major depressive disorder, discussed in more detail later in this chapter (see "Comorbidity").

Social anxiety (and more extensive interpersonal dysfunction) can occur with schizophrenia and can, especially in young adults in the prodromal stages of illness, be difficult to distinguish from social anxiety disorder. However, other evidence of psychotic symptoms will eventually surface.

Eating disorders or OCD may be associated with social evaluative anxiety. For example, individuals may be concerned that others will observe and judge them on the basis of their abnormal eating or checking behaviors or that they may act on an unwanted impulse, such as shouting obscenities in public. However, a diagnosis of social anxiety disorder should be made only if social anxiety symptoms co-occur independent of those disorder-specific fears.

Body dysmorphic disorder, which is classified with the obsessive-compulsive and related disorders in DSM-5, may be accompanied by social concerns and avoidance. However, in the case of body dysmorphic disorder, the concern is that others will negatively evaluate perceived defects or flaws in the individual's physical appearance, whereas in social anxiety disorder the concern is that others will negatively evaluate the individual's behavior and internal self (e.g., personality, intelligence). Studies suggest considerable comorbidity between social anxiety disorder and body dysmorphic disorder (Fang and Hofmann 2010).

Selective mutism, a childhood disorder now classified among the anxiety disorders in DSM-5, is characterized by failure to speak among unfamiliar people (e.g., in school), despite having the capacity for normal speech as evidenced in other settings (e.g., at home with parents). Selective mutism may be very difficult to distinguish from social anxiety disorder; this overlap is an artifact of the DSM-5 diagnostic criteria, wherein it is acknowledged that most children with the former diagnosis also meet criteria for the latter (American Psychiatric Association 2013).

Avoidant personality disorder will be diagnosable as a comorbid disorder in many patients with social anxiety disorder, particularly those with diagnoses that do *not* have the performance-only specifier. Therefore, avoidant personality disorder is not considered to be an alternative diagnosis but rather is an additional diagnosis that may represent a marker of increased social anxiety disorder severity. These two disorders are thought to share several genetic and environmental risk factors (Welander-Vatn et al. 2019).

Epidemiology

In the United States, epidemiological and community-based studies have reported lifetime prevalence rates of social anxiety disorder ranging from 2.4% to 13.0% (Hasin and Grant 2015; Kessler et al. 1994, 2005; Ruscio et al. 2008), making it one of the most common psychiatric disorders (after major depressive disorder and alcohol use disorder). Variations in diagnostic rates can be attributed to changes in diagnostic criteria,

TABLE 24–1.   Differential diagnosis of social anxiety disorder and other anxiety disorders

Diagnosis	Characteristics	Description
Separation anxiety disorder	Marked fear of separation from attachment figure(s) (e.g., parents)	In adolescents and adults, concerns about negative evaluation are paramount in social anxiety disorder, although individuals may prefer to have attachment figures nearby in such situations. In separation anxiety disorder, concerns pertain mainly to worries that attachment figures will come to harm or be lost. It may be very difficult to disentangle separation anxiety from social fears among young children, given similar behavioral patterns (e.g., refusal to go to school).
Selective mutism	Consistent failure to speak in certain social situations (e.g., school) where there is an expectation to speak, despite speaking in other situations	Selective mutism is not limited to interactions with adults. Most children with selective mutism will exhibit behaviors (and when they are old enough, describe cognitions) consistent with social anxiety disorder through avoidance not only of speaking but also of interacting with peers in other situations. Accordingly, most (but not all) children with selective mutism will also meet DSM-5 criteria for social anxiety disorder.
Specific phobia	Marked fear, anxiety, or avoidance of circumscribed objects or situations	Common fears are of insects, heights, or flying. By definition, if fears involve negative evaluation in social situations, even if very specific to certain situations (e.g., public speaking), the DSM-5 diagnosis of social anxiety disorder applies.
Panic disorder	Recurrent unexpected (i.e., occur without an apparent cue) panic attacks	Panic attacks may occur in social anxiety disorder but are not spontaneous or unexpected. Rather, they occur in—or in advance of—feared social situations.
Agoraphobia	Marked fear, anxiety, or avoidance of two or more situations such as public transportation, open spaces, enclosed places, lines or crowds, or being outside the home alone	In agoraphobia, individuals fear that escape might be difficult or help not available in the event of panic-like symptoms. These same situations may be feared and avoided in social anxiety disorder but would be avoided because of social-evaluative fears, not because of fears of being incapacitated by panic-like symptoms. Most patients are able to distinguish between these two concerns when questioned. In some cases, the concerns (cognitions) cannot be disambiguated, and both diagnoses may apply.
Generalized anxiety disorder	Marked anxiety and worry (more days than not) about various domains, such as work and school performance, that the individual finds difficult to control	In social anxiety disorder, although individuals may report anxiety and worry about multiple situations, these situations involve social interaction and perceived possibility of negative evaluation. For generalized anxiety disorder, the concerns would need to be broader and cover additional domains of function.

required level of impairment, and differing assessment methodologies. The 12-month prevalence of social anxiety disorder in the United States is reported to be approximately 8% in adolescents and adults (Kessler et al. 2012). Epidemiological data reporting on the relative distribution of the new DSM-5 performance-only specifier versus more pervasive expressions of social anxiety disorder involving multiple situations are not currently available.

The World Mental Health Survey Initiative, with 142,405 respondents, assessed the prevalence of social anxiety disorder across a range of 29 countries in different geographical regions of the world. The 30-day, 12-month, and lifetime prevalence estimates across countries were 1.3%, 2.4%, and 4.0%, respectively. Prevalence rates were lowest in low- and lower-middle-income countries and highest in high-income countries. Age at onset is early across the globe, and persistence is highest in upper-middle-income countries, Africa, and the eastern Mediterranean. The study found consistent global patterns of early age at onset, functional impairment, and comorbidity (Stein et al. 2017).

Cultural variations of social anxiety disorder do exist. An Asian pattern of social anxiety called *taijin kyofusho* is seen in such countries as Japan and Korea. Unlike the traditional conceptualization of social phobia in Western nations, which involves the fear of humiliating oneself, *taijin kyofusho* involves the fear of offending others by embarrassing them or by making them uncomfortable through a personal flaw or short-coming (e.g., blushing in front of others, emitting an unpleasant body odor, exposing an unsightly body part). It has been suggested that these fears of offending others actually may not be uncommon among U.S. patients (Choy et al. 2008) but are typically not considered or asked about by clinicians. As noted earlier, the feared consequence of offending others has been added in DSM-5 as an example of fear of negative evaluation, with the intent of increasing the cultural sensitivity of the criteria in this regard.

Epidemiological findings presenting prevalence rates of social anxiety disorder across ethnic groups within the United States have been scant. Some data suggest that African, Asian, and Hispanic race or ethnicity is associated with lower lifetime prevalence in U.S. samples compared with their white counterparts (Asnaani et al. 2010; Grant et al. 2005; Ruscio et al. 2008). Epidemiological studies have also found that individuals with social anxiety disorder are more likely to be female, single, and unemployed and to have lower income and education compared with those without the disorder (Grant et al. 2005; Ruscio et al. 2008). In treatment-seeking samples, however, the disorder seems to be equally distributed among males and females (Turk et al. 1998). Overall, social phobia and simple phobias typically have an earlier age at onset than do other anxiety disorders (Grant et al. 2005; Kessler et al. 2005; Scheibe and Albus 1992). Epidemiological and patient sample studies suggest the typical age at onset of social anxiety disorder is early to middle adolescence and onset after age 25 is relatively uncommon (Kessler et al. 2005). Some evidence suggests that a bimodal distribution in onset, with one group beginning in early childhood (as behavioral inhibition and extreme shyness) and persisting into adolescence and adulthood and another group reporting de novo onset of symptoms in adolescence.

Course

Few studies have examined the longitudinal course of social phobia (Steinert et al. 2013). Data from the Harvard/Brown Anxiety Research Project (HARP), a naturalistic longitudinal study of anxiety disorders, suggest that social phobia has a chronic and unremitting course (Ramsawh et al. 2009). A study from the HARP group found that in comparison with generalized anxiety disorder and panic disorder, individuals with social phobia had the smallest probability of recovery over 12 years (Bruce et al. 2005).

Comorbidity

It is well established that most individuals with social anxiety disorder have one or more comorbid conditions and that the presence of psychiatric comorbidity is associated with a poorer prognosis (Stein and Stein 2008; Vriends et al. 2007). Mental disorders most frequently comorbid with social anxiety disorder are major depression, bipolar disorder (Simon et al. 2004), other anxiety disorders, substance use disorders (Lemyre et al. 2019), sexual dysfunction (Corretti et al. 2006), and eating disorders (Kaye et al. 2004). Given its typical early onset in childhood or adolescence, social anxiety disorder frequently precedes the onset of these comorbid conditions, suggesting that it may increase the risk for development of subsequent psychopathology. Persons with social anxiety disorder have an increased risk of attempted suicide and death from suicide compared to persons in the general population without social anxiety disorder (Kanwar et al. 2013).

Epidemiological studies suggest an association between anxiety disorders and medical illness (Roy-Byrne et al. 2008; Sareen et al. 2005). Although few studies have examined the relationship between medical illness and social anxiety in particular, social anxiety disorder has been linked to heart disease, autoimmune disorders, and Parkinson's disease (Stein and Stein 2008). Some reports suggest social phobia estimates as high as 29% among individuals with Parkinson's disease (Stein et al. 1990); other studies suggest that the rate may be closer to 15% (Broen et al. 2016). As noted earlier, the DSM-5 criteria for social anxiety disorder were changed to permit the diagnosis in persons with medical illness whose concerns pertained to the visibility of their symptoms (e.g., tremor in Parkinson's disease); under DSM-IV criteria, the diagnosis would not have been made. Prior to DSM-5, then, it is likely that social anxiety disorder was underdiagnosed among persons with medical illness. Additional examples of specific conditions in which it may appear include stuttering (Iverach and Rapee 2014) and obesity (Dalrymple et al. 2017).

Evaluation

Several reliable and valid clinician- and self-rated instruments are available to assess the diagnostic status, symptom severity, and associated features (e.g., physiological symptoms) of social anxiety disorder. The Structured Clinical Interview for DSM-5 (SCID-5; First et al. 2015) and the Anxiety Disorders Interview for DSM-5 (ADIS-5; Brown and Barlow 2014) are commonly used semistructured clinical interviews that assess symptoms required to assign a DSM-5 diagnosis of social anxiety disorder. The SCID-5 is brief and focuses on establishing the presence or absence of symptoms as described in DSM-5. The ADIS-5 assesses symptoms beyond DSM-5 criteria (e.g., severity of fear, avoidance pertaining to a range of social and performance situations) and provides a clinical severity rating based on the clinician's judgment across fear, avoidance, distress, and impairment ratings. Although lengthier to administer, the ADIS-5 can be used for treatment planning and evaluation of treatment response.

The Liebowitz Social Anxiety Scale (LSAS; Liebowitz 1987) is the gold standard clinician-administered dimensional rating scale of social anxiety symptoms. The LSAS comprises 24 items that separately assess level of fear and level of avoidance of 24 social situations, including interaction (e.g., attending a social gathering) and performance (e.g., eating in public). A score of 30 or higher on the LSAS distinguishes people with a diagnosis of social anxiety disorder from control subjects without a current psychiatric diagnosis, and a score of 60 or greater identifies people with social anxiety disorder who endorse fearing "most" social situations (formerly the generalized subtype as in DSM-IV) (Rytwinski et al. 2009). A self-report version of the LSAS (Fresco et al. 2001) demonstrates high convergence with the clinician-administered version.

The most well-established self-report scales assessing social anxiety symptoms and associated features include the Social Interaction Anxiety Scale (SIAS) and the Social Phobia Scale (SPS; Mattick and Clarke 1998), the Social Phobia and Anxiety Inventory (SPAI; Turner et al. 1989), the Fear of Negative Evaluation Scale (FNE; Watson and Friend 1969), the Brief Fear of Negative Evaluation Scale (BFNE; Leary 1983), and the Social Phobia Inventory (SPIN; Connor et al. 2000). These measures are reliable, valid, and sensitive to documenting treatment response. The 20-item SIAS measures anxiety when engaging in social interactions with different types of people, whereas the 20-item SPS reflects fears of being observed by others in social situations. The 30-item FNE and 12-item BFNE measure apprehension about being negatively evaluated by others—a core defining feature of social anxiety disorder. The SPAI comprises 45 items that measure somatic, cognitive, and behavioral expressions of social anxiety across a range of social and performance situations; it also includes items assessing panic disorder and agoraphobia. The 17-item SPIN assesses symptoms of fear, avoidance, and physiological arousal. Because each self-report measure assesses somewhat different features of social anxiety disorder and varies in length of administration, the choice of which measure to use often comes down to the specific intent of the clinician or researcher.

Even in the absence of comorbidity, social anxiety disorder has been associated with significant distress and interference, as manifested by financial problems, work impairment and days missed from work, impaired school performance and dropout, weakened social support systems, increased use of psychotropic medication, and more help-seeking from medical and mental health professionals (Merikangas et al. 2007). The relationship between quality of life and social anxiety disorder appears to be even more pronounced in the generalized type than it is in persons who meet criteria for the performance-only specifier (Aderka et al. 2012).

Conclusion

Social anxiety disorder is a common and disabling condition that begins in early adolescence and, in the absence of treatment, runs a chronic course associated with significant functional impairment and diminished quality of life. Characterized by a marked fear of social and performance situations in which the individual is concerned about negative evaluation, the clinical presentation is heterogeneous and can range from prototypical anxious, inhibited behavior to anger, hostility, or impulsivity. Social anxiety disorder frequently co-occurs with and often precedes the onset of several psychiatric conditions and increases the risk for suicide; it also co-occurs with several medical illnesses. Detection and monitoring can be aided by a number of available clinical interview and self-report assessments.

Key Points

- Social anxiety disorder is highly prevalent in the general population, in primary care medical settings, and in mental health clinic settings. Although performance-only (mostly public speaking) fears are more common in the general population, individuals with more pervasive social fears and avoidance are more likely to present for treatment and to experience greater severity, impairment, and comorbidity relative to persons with the performance-only specifier.

- Social anxiety disorder is common worldwide, and cultural variations of the disorder may exist that influence its presentation.

- Social anxiety disorder typically first appears in early to middle adolescence, and it has been shown to have a chronic and unremitting course without treatment. Psychiatric comorbidity further worsens prognosis.

- Social anxiety disorder is especially common in association with certain medical conditions in which symptoms of the condition may be visible to others (e.g., stuttering, tremor, obesity).

References

Aderka IM, Hofmann SG, Nickerson A, et al: Functional impairment in social anxiety disorder. J Anxiety Disord 26(3):393–400, 2012 22306132

American Psychiatric Association: Diagnostic and Statistical Manual: Mental Disorders. Washington, DC, American Psychiatric Association, 1952

American Psychiatric Association: Diagnostic and Statistical Manual of Mental Disorders, 2nd Edition. Washington, DC, American Psychiatric Association, 1968

American Psychiatric Association: Diagnostic and Statistical Manual of Mental Disorders, 3rd Edition. Washington, DC, American Psychiatric Association, 1980

American Psychiatric Association: Diagnostic and Statistical Manual of Mental Disorders, 3rd Edition, Revised. Washington, DC, American Psychiatric Association, 1987

American Psychiatric Association: Diagnostic and Statistical Manual of Mental Disorders, 4th Edition. Washington, DC, American Psychiatric Association, 1994

American Psychiatric Association: Diagnostic and Statistical Manual of Mental Disorders, 5th Edition. Arlington, VA, American Psychiatric Association, 2013

Asnaani A, Richey JA, Dimaite R, et al: A cross-ethnic comparison of lifetime prevalence rates of anxiety disorders. J Nerv Ment Dis 198(8):551–555, 2010 20699719

Biederman J, Hirshfeld-Becker DR, Rosenbaum JF, et al: Further evidence of association between behavioral inhibition and social anxiety in children. Am J Psychiatry 158(10):1673–1679, 2001 11579001

Broen MP, Narayen NE, Kuijf ML, et al: Prevalence of anxiety in Parkinson's disease: a systematic review and meta-analysis. Mov Disord 31(8):1125–1133, 2016 27125963

Brown TA, Barlow DH: Anxiety Disorders Interview Schedule for DSM-5 (ADIS-5)—Lifetime Version. New York, Oxford University Press, 2014

Bruce SE, Yonkers KA, Otto MW, et al: Influence of psychiatric comorbidity on recovery and recurrence in generalized anxiety disorder, social phobia, and panic disorder: a 12-year prospective study. Am J Psychiatry 162(6):1179–1187, 2005 15930067

Choy Y, Schneier FR, Heimberg RG, et al: Features of the offensive subtype of taijin-kyofu-sho in US and Korean patients with DSM-IV social anxiety disorder. Depress Anxiety 25(3):230–240, 2008 17340609

Chronis-Tuscano A, Danko CM, Rubin KH, et al: Future directions for research on early intervention for young children at risk for social anxiety. J Clin Child Adolesc Psychol 47(4):655–667, 2018 29405747

Connor KM, Davidson JR, Churchill LE, et al: Psychometric properties of the Social Phobia Inventory (SPIN). New self-rating scale. Br J Psychiatry 176:379–386, 2000 10827888

Corretti G, Pierucci S, De Scisciolo M, et al: Comorbidity between social phobia and premature ejaculation: study on 242 males affected by sexual disorders. J Sex Marital Ther 32(4):183–187, 2006 16418108

Dalrymple KL, Walsh E, Rosenstein L, et al: Modification of the medical exclusion criterion in DSM-5 social anxiety disorder: comorbid obesity as an example. J Affect Disord 210:230–236, 2017 28064111

Erwin BA, Heimberg RG, Schneier FR, et al: Anger experience and expression in social anxiety disorder: pretreatment profile and predictors of attrition and response to cognitive-behavioral treatment. Behav Ther 34:331–350, 2003

Fang A, Hofmann SG: Relationship between social anxiety disorder and body dysmorphic disorder. Clin Psychol Rev 30(8):1040–1048, 2010 20817336

First MB, Williams JB, Karg RS, et al: Structured Clinical Interview for DSM-5 (SCID-5). Arlington, VA, American Psychiatric Publishing, 2015

Fresco DM, Coles ME, Heimberg RG, et al: The Liebowitz Social Anxiety Scale: a comparison of the psychometric properties of self-report and clinician-administered formats. Psychol Med 31(6):1025–1035, 2001 11513370

Grant BF, Hasin DS, Blanco C, et al: The epidemiology of social anxiety disorder in the United States: results from the National Epidemiologic Survey on Alcohol and Related Conditions. J Clin Psychiatry 66(11):1351–1361, 2005 16420070

Hasin DS, Grant BF: The National Epidemiologic Survey on Alcohol and Related Conditions (NESARC) Waves 1 and 2: review and summary of findings. Soc Psychiatry Psychiatr Epidemiol 50(11):1609–1640, 2015 26210739

Heimberg RG, Hofmann SG, Liebowitz MR, et al: Social anxiety disorder in DSM-5. Depress Anxiety 31(6):472–479, 2014 24395386

Iverach L, Rapee RM: Social anxiety disorder and stuttering: current status and future directions. J Fluency Disord 40:69–82, 2014 24929468

Janet P: Les Obsessions et la Psychasthenie. Paris, France, Felix Alcan, 1903

Kachin KE, Newman MG, Pincus AL: An interpersonal problem approach to the division of social phobia subtypes. Behav Ther 32:479–501, 2001

Kanwar A, Malik S, Prokop LJ, et al: The association between anxiety disorders and suicidal behaviors: a systematic review and meta-analysis. Depress Anxiety 30(10):917–929, 2013 23408488

Kashdan TB, Hofmann SG: The high-novelty-seeking, impulsive subtype of generalized social anxiety disorder. Depress Anxiety 25(6):535–541, 2008 17935217

Kaye WH, Bulik CM, Thornton L, et al: Comorbidity of anxiety disorders with anorexia and bulimia nervosa. Am J Psychiatry 161(12):2215–2221, 2004 15569892

Kessler RC, McGonagle KA, Zhao S, et al: Lifetime and 12-month prevalence of DSM-III-R psychiatric disorders in the United States: results from the National Comorbidity Survey. Arch Gen Psychiatry 51(1):8–19, 1994 8279933

Kessler RC, Stein MB, Berglund P: Social phobia subtypes in the National Comorbidity Survey. Am J Psychiatry 155(5):613–619, 1998 9585711

Kessler RC, Berglund P, Demler O, et al: Lifetime prevalence and age-of-onset distributions of DSM-IV disorders in the National Comorbidity Survey Replication. Arch Gen Psychiatry 62(6):593–602, 2005 15939837

Kessler RC, Petukhova M, Sampson NA, et al: Twelve-month and lifetime prevalence and lifetime morbid risk of anxiety and mood disorders in the United States. Int J Methods Psychiatr Res 21(3):169–184, 2012 22865617

Leary M: A brief version of the Fear of Negative Evaluation Scale. Pers Soc Psychol Bull 9(3):371–375, 1983

Lemyre A, Gauthier-Legare A, Belanger RE: Shyness, social anxiety, social anxiety disorder, and substance use among normative adolescent populations: a systematic review. Am J Drug Alcohol Abuse 45(3):230–247, 2019 30422012

Liebowitz MR: Social phobia. Mod Probl Pharmacopsychiatry 22:141–173, 1987 2885745

Liebowitz MR, Gorman JM, Fyer AJ, et al: Social phobia: review of a neglected anxiety disorder. Arch Gen Psychiatry 42(7):729–736, 1985 2861796

Marks IM, Gelder MG: Different ages of onset in varieties of phobia. Am J Psychiatry 123(2):218–221, 1966 5944004

Mattick RP, Clarke JC: Development and validation of measures of social phobia scrutiny fear and social interaction anxiety. Behav Res Ther 36(4):455–470, 1998 9670605

Merikangas KR, Ames M, Cui L, et al: The impact of comorbidity of mental and physical conditions on role disability in the US adult household population. Arch Gen Psychiatry 64(10):1180–1188, 2007 17909130

Piccirillo ML, Taylor Dryman M, Heimberg RG: Safety behaviors in adults with social anxiety: review and future directions. Behav Ther 47(5):675–687, 2016 27816080

Ramsawh HJ, Raffa SD, Edelen MO, et al: Anxiety in middle adulthood: effects of age and time on the 14-year course of panic disorder, social phobia and generalized anxiety disorder. Psychol Med 39(4):615–624, 2009 18667095

Roy-Byrne PP, Davidson KW, Kessler RC, et al: Anxiety disorders and comorbid medical illness. Gen Hosp Psychiatry 30(3):208–225, 2008 18433653

Ruscio AM, Brown TA, Chiu WT, et al: Social fears and social phobia in the USA: results from the National Comorbidity Survey Replication. Psychol Med 38(1):15–28, 2008 17976249

Rytwinski NK, Fresco DM, Heimberg RG, et al: Screening for social anxiety disorder with the self-report version of the Liebowitz Social Anxiety Scale. Depress Anxiety 26(1):34–38, 2009 18781659

Sareen J, Cox BJ, Clara I, Asmundson GJ: The relationship between anxiety disorders and physical disorders in the U.S. National Comorbidity Survey. Depress Anxiety 21(4):193–202, 2005 16075453

Scheibe G, Albus M: Age at onset, precipitating events, sex distribution, and co-occurrence of anxiety disorders. Psychopathology 25(1):11–18, 1992 1603905

Simon NM, Otto MW, Wisniewski SR, et al: Anxiety disorder comorbidity in bipolar disorder patients: data from the first 500 participants in the Systematic Treatment Enhancement Program for Bipolar Disorder (STEP-BD). Am J Psychiatry 161(12):2222–2229, 2004 15569893

Stein DJ, Lim CCW, Roest AM, et al: The cross-national epidemiology of social anxiety disorder: data from the World Mental Health Survey Initiative. BMC Med 15(1):143, 2017 28756776

Stein MB, Stein DJ: Social anxiety disorder. Lancet 371(9618):1115–1125, 2008 18374843

Stein MB, Heuser IJ, Juncos JL, et al: Anxiety disorders in patients with Parkinson's disease. Am J Psychiatry 147(2):217–220, 1990 2301664

Steinert C, Hofmann M, Leichsenring F, et al: What do we know today about the prospective long-term course of social anxiety disorder? A systematic literature review. J Anxiety Disord 27(7):692–702, 2013 24176803

Turk CL, Heimberg RG, Orsillo SM, et al: An investigation of gender differences in social phobia. J Anxiety Disord 12(3):209–223, 1998 9653680

Turner SM, Beidel DC, Dancu CV, et al: An empirically derived inventory to measure social fears and anxiety: the Social Phobia and Anxiety Inventory. Psychol Assess 1:35–40, 1989

Vriends N, Becker ES, Meyer A, et al: Recovery from social phobia in the community and its predictors: data from a longitudinal epidemiological study. J Anxiety Disord 21(3):320–337, 2007 16919416

Watson D, Friend R: Measurement of social-evaluative anxiety. J Consult Clin Psychol 33(4):448–457, 1969 5810590

Welander-Vatn A, Torvik FA, Czajkowski N, et al: Relationships among avoidant personality disorder, social anxiety disorder, and normative personality traits: a twin study. J Pers Disord 33(3):289–309, 2019 29505386

Recommended Readings

Hofmann SG, DiBartolo, PM (eds): Social Anxiety: Clinical, Developmental, and Social Perspectives, 3rd Edition. Oxford, UK, Elsevier/Academic Press, 2014

Stein MB, Stein DJ: Social anxiety disorder. Lancet 371(9618):1115–1125, 2008 18374843

Weeks JW (ed): The Wiley Blackwell Handbook of Social Anxiety Disorder. New York, John Wiley and Sons, 2014

CHAPTER 25

Pathogenesis of Social Anxiety Disorder

Janna Marie Bas-Hoogendam, M.Sc.

Eline F. Roelofs, M.D.

P. Michiel Westenberg, Ph.D.

Nic J.A. van der Wee, M.D., Ph.D.

Although social anxiety disorder is a highly prevalent condition that has received increasing attention over the past few decades, its pathogenesis has not yet been fully elucidated. Insight into the development and maintenance of the disorder is of utmost importance given its typical onset during adolescence (Miers et al. 2013) and its often chronic, unremitting course (Steinert et al. 2013), a combination not usually found in other anxiety disorders. Furthermore, social anxiety disorder is associated with high levels of comorbid psychopathology (Beesdo et al. 2007) and substantial negative personal and societal consequences (Hendriks et al. 2014). With regard to its pathogenesis, various putative key elements have been identified in neurobiological, developmental, and psychological domains, but the complex interactions between (epi)genetic factors, neurobiological vulnerability, and especially developmental trajectories, temperament, and environmental factors that characterize this disorder still warrant further research (Poole et al. 2018a).

In this chapter we give an overview of the progress of the research into biological, developmental, and psychological factors relevant to the pathogenesis of social anxiety disorder. We discuss findings in the context of etiological models and outline future research approaches.

Biological Factors

Genetics

Studies involving families and twins indicate that social anxiety disorder has a genetic component (Scaini et al. 2014). In addition, animal studies revealed that extreme early life anxiety in nonhuman primates is heritable (Fox and Kalin 2014). Nevertheless, research on the specific genetic variations related to anxiety disorders, and social anxiety disorder in particular, is still scarce (Smoller 2017). Two large studies related genetic variants on chromosome 3 and alterations in the gene *PDE4B* on chromosome 1 to anxiety (Meier et al. 2018; Otowa et al. 2016), but these results are still preliminary and not specific for social anxiety disorder.

A handful of studies specifically focused on the genetic background of social anxiety disorder reported divergent results. Early studies examining two serotonin genes and genes involved in the dopamine system failed to find significant linkage results (Kennedy et al. 2001; Stein et al. 1998), whereas a more recent genetic linkage study related variations on chromosome 16 to the disorder (Gelernter et al. 2004). The first genome-wide association study on social anxiety disorder pointed to genetic risk variants on chromosomes 1 and 6 (Stein et al. 2017).

Another line of related genetic research focused on (epi)genetic variations in the oxytocin system because oxytocin is a modulating neuropeptide known to facilitate prosocial behavior (Neumann and Slattery 2015). A multilevel study indicated a relationship between decreased methylation of the oxytocin receptor and social anxiety disorder–related traits (Ziegler et al. 2015); another study of healthy participants indicated a gene–environment interaction effect between the oxytocin genotype and attachment style on the level of social anxiety (Notzon et al. 2016). More research (e.g., using an endophenotype approach) is needed to gain advanced insight into the genetic vulnerability for the disorder (Bas-Hoogendam et al. 2016).

Neurochemistry and Neuropharmacology

Research on the neurochemistry and neuropharmacology specifically involved in social anxiety disorder has used various approaches. Apart from investigating the efficacy of specific classes of medication, early, often small, studies in this field typically have used challenge paradigms such as carbon dioxide or cholecystokinin to provoke symptoms or studied peripheral markers in blood, urine, or cerebrospinal fluid or on blood cells. Taken together, these studies in adult patients suggest involvement of the serotonergic system but have generated negative or unequivocal results on the involvement of dopaminergic, noradrenergic, and GABAergic systems and that of neuropeptides such as cholecystokinin/pentagastrin and neurokinins (Morreale et al. 2010).

Recent studies on the neurochemistry of social anxiety disorder often employ radioactive ligands to assess transporter or receptor densities in specific brain regions or use magnetic resonance spectroscopy to assess concentrations of metabolites or neurotransmitters, sometimes in combination with a pharmacological challenge paradigm or a pharmacological treatment.

A considerable body of research in humans and animals suggests the involvement of the serotonergic system in normal and pathological fear and anxiety, including social anxiety (Bandelow et al. 2016). Together with the therapeutic efficacy of selective serotonin reuptake inhibitors (SSRIs), human radiotracer studies in social anxiety disorder point to the involvement of serotonin type 1A receptors and serotonin transporters in limbic areas (Frick et al. 2015).

Furthermore, although antipsychotics are not efficacious, several radiotracer studies have identified abnormalities in striatal dopamine transporter densities in adult patients with social anxiety disorder, as well as altered striatal dopamine D_2 receptor binding capacity, although it should be noted that these results are not unequivocal (Bandelow et al. 2016). Interestingly, escitalopram administration altered striatal dopamine transporter densities in patients with social anxiety disorder, illustrating the close interaction between dopaminergic and serotonergic systems in this disorder (Warwick et al. 2012).

So far, only a small number of magnetic resonance spectroscopy studies have been performed, with unequivocal results for creatine and GABA levels and two studies reporting elevated glutamate levels (Phan et al. 2005; Pollack et al. 2008). Other neuroimaging studies have examined changes in blood flow, brain activation, or connectivity after a pharmacological challenge or pharmacological treatment. Examples of this approach are some interesting studies on the effects of oxytocin. These studies showed that oxytocin attenuated the abnormal amygdala reactivity to fearful faces and changed amygdala-prefrontal functional connectivity in social anxiety disorder (Gorka et al. 2015; Labuschagne et al. 2010).

Neuroanatomy, Pathophysiology, and Brain Imaging

In the 2010s, neuroimaging research on the neurobiological background of social anxiety disorder has expanded: whereas early imaging studies focused on key emotional structures in the brain, more recent studies aimed to characterize related changes in the anatomy and function of the whole brain. Structural MRI studies demonstrated several gray-matter alterations: changes were found in the frontal lobe, temporal lobe, and parietal cortex as well as in subcortical areas such as the amygdala, thalamus, and putamen (Bas-Hoogendam et al. 2017, 2018b; Brühl et al. 2014). However, it should be noted that the results of these studies are heterogeneous and often lack reproducibility, probably because of small sample sizes and variations in analysis methods (Brühl et al. 2014). See also the meta-analysis by Wang et al. (2018) and the accompanying commentary (Bas-Hoogendam 2019).

In addition to these structural MRI studies, functional MRI (fMRI) studies yielded important insights into neurobiological characteristics related to social anxiety disorder. Most fMRI studies use stimuli that are anxiety provoking for patients. Examples of stimuli include photographs of faces with negative or neutral expressions, stories describing social situations, and sentences involving personal feedback (Brühl et al. 2014). Such stimuli lead to increased brain activation in several areas, including the amygdala, insula, and prefrontal cortex; in addition, enhanced brain responsivity of the parietal cortex has been associated with social anxiety disorder (Miskovic and Schmidt 2012). The involvement of these areas in the pathophysiology of the disorder has been confirmed by the results of a meta-analysis on fMRI findings (Brühl et al. 2014). Interestingly, several fMRI studies provided evidence for correlations between these alterations in brain responsivity and the severity of social anxiety (Frick et al.

2013). Such associations support the hypothesis that neurobiological brain alterations underlie the thoughts and behavior associated with social anxiety disorder. This idea is also substantiated by studies investigating treatment effects. To illustrate, Phan et al. (2013) reported that the exaggerated amygdala response to fearful faces was significantly reduced after a 12-week treatment with the SSRI sertraline.

Another line of neuroimaging research investigates changes in functional and anatomical connectivity. Brain networks can be examined using fMRI and diffusion tensor imaging. In this context, fMRI studies estimate functional connections by exploring temporal correlations in brain activation patterns (Damoiseaux et al. 2006). Diffusion tensor imaging scans map connections between areas by enabling reconstruction of white matter tracts (Chanraud et al. 2010). Previous work, summarized more extensively elsewhere (Brühl et al. 2014; Cremers and Roelofs 2016), suggested that social anxiety disorder is characterized by changes in subcortical networks typically involved in social cognition and self-reflection (Pannekoek et al. 2013) as well as in the uncinate fasciculus, the white matter tract that connects the amygdala and the prefrontal cortex.

Autonomic Dysregulation

Anxiety disorders, including social anxiety disorder, are associated with cardiovascular risk factors and diseases (Vogelzangs et al. 2010). Heart rate variability (HRV), the extent to which the interval between beats varies with time, is thought to be closely linked to autonomic nervous system activity; reduced HRV is seen in cardiovascular diseases and is a predictor of mortality. Shared dysfunctions in the autonomic nervous system underlying both anxiety disorders and cardiovascular diseases have been hypothesized, suggesting HRV as a possible biomarker for social anxiety disorder. Indeed, one meta-analysis showed a significant decrease of resting-state time-domain and high-frequency HRV in subjects with social anxiety disorder compared to healthy control subjects, suggesting parasympathetic underactivity (Chalmers et al. 2014). However, resting-state HRV did not co-segregate with social anxiety disorder within families genetically enriched for the diagnosis (Harrewijn et al. 2018).

Autonomic arousal in children at risk for social anxiety disorder has been an emerging topic in recent years, because early physiological hyperarousal may be a risk factor for later social anxiety. However, results are few and contradictory. Some findings reported autonomic hyperarousal, such as increased blushing and increased electrodermal activity, during socially challenging tasks in children of parents diagnosed with the disorder. Furthermore, increased electrodermal activity and blushing and reduced HRV were associated with greater social anxiety (Nikolic et al. 2016). However, another study in children suggested increased resting-state and task-related state anxiety, rather than social anxiety, as an explanation for decreased autonomic function (Alkozei et al. 2015). More research is needed to clarify these relationships.

Neuroendocrinology

An increasing number of studies have examined neuroendocrinological abnormalities in social anxiety disorder. As with research in other affective disorders, the first focus has been on (reactivity of) the hypothalamic-pituitary-adrenal (HPA) axis, with later studies also examining the role of testosterone and the balance between cortisol and testosterone. Studies have been performed at rest, after behavioral challenges such as a public speaking task, or using the dexamethasone suppression test. Early studies found no abnormal baseline cortisol levels as measured in urine and saliva, suggesting no global HPA axis dysfunction. Also, these studies found no abnormal results of the dexamethasone suppression test in social anxiety disorder (Morreale et al. 2010), but some studies identified abnormalities in salivary α-amylase in baseline conditions, suggesting involvement of the autonomic nervous system (see also the previous subsection, "Autonomic Dysregulation") (van Veen et al. 2008).

Another picture with regard to the HPA axis, however, emerged from a series of studies examining stress reactivity to a public performance paradigm, typically the Trier Social Stress Task, although comparison of studies is often hampered by methodological issues. Zorn et al. (2017) performed a meta-analysis with data from several studies using the Trier Social Stress Task and found that, in particular, men with social anxiety disorder showed an increased cortisol response to psychosocial stress. High cortisol responses to the paradigm were also associated with increased social avoidance tendencies in approach-avoidance paradigms (Cremers and Roelofs 2016). Interestingly, single-dose administration of cortisol resulted in increased avoidance tendencies in patients with social anxiety disorder in this type of paradigm.

Of relevance, recent studies have started to explore the effects of the interaction between child cortisol reactivity and environmental factors on trajectories of child social anxiety. For instance, Poole et al. (2018b) found that, in children, having a socially anxious parent and an increased cortisol reactivity predicted the highest levels of clinically significant social anxiety over a 3-year period.

More recently, the hypothalamic-pituitary-gonadal (HPG) axis has become a topic of study because the gonadal hormone testosterone has been shown to reduce submissive and avoidance behavior in animals and healthy participants (Cremers and Roelofs 2016). Giltay et al. (2012), for instance, found basal testosterone salivary levels to be low in female patients with social anxiety disorder. Interestingly, single-dose testosterone administration in patients with social anxiety disorder and socially anxious participants seems to result in a shift from avoidance to approach tendency and reduced subordinate behavior (Terburg et al. 2016). In addition to behavioral effects, studies have demonstrated the effects of cortisol and testosterone administration on emotion-processing brain circuitry typically implicated in social anxiety disorder; these changes could underlie the behavioral effects. In particular, the testosterone/cortisol ratio may influence functional connectivity of the amygdala with prefrontal regulation regions and the striatum (Cremers and Roelofs 2016).

The effects of oxytocin on a range of social cognitive and emotional processes have been investigated in healthy participants as well as in patients with various psychiatric disorders. For instance, in patients with social anxiety disorder, intranasal administration of oxytocin was found to influence reward sensitivity and functional connectivity in the emotion-processing circuitry, but randomized controlled trials have not yet demonstrated a clear effect on clinical symptoms (De Cagna et al. 2019).

Immunology

Because immune function has been linked to stress, inflammatory parameters in anxiety disorders have become a focus in medical research, although reports on social anxiety disorder are few (Vogelzangs et al. 2013). Several hypotheses have been proposed and are reviewed elsewhere (Glaser and Kiecolt-Glaser 2005). In general, hypotheses suggest that prolonged stressful situations, such as are experienced in anxiety, lead to continuous activation of the sympathetic nervous system and insufficient parasympathetic counteraction. This could eventually result in increased levels of proinflammatory cytokines. In line with this hypothesis, increased baseline C-reactive protein and interleukin-6 levels in patients with social anxiety disorder compared to healthy control subjects have been reported, but these levels seem to be lower when compared with those of patients with other anxiety disorders (Naudé et al. 2018). More research with a specific focus on social anxiety disorder is needed to further investigate these findings.

Another emerging topic in mental health is the microbiome. Thought to be linked to numerous processes in the body, the microbiome interacts with gut peptides to regulate microbiota-gut-brain signaling and is involved in the immune system. In rodent studies, germ-free mice have shown impaired social skills, indicating that the microbiome may be a contributing factor in the development of social behavior. Interestingly, reconstitution of microbiota in time improves this impaired social interaction. In human research, treatment with probiotics was found to positively affect anxiety and depressive symptoms (for further review, see Pirbaglou et al. 2016).

Psychosocial and Psychological Factors

Childhood and Developmental Factors

Several developmental factors are associated with an increased risk for developing social anxiety disorder. A systematic summary of these factors indicated that, besides the genetic predispositions discussed earlier in this chapter, ample evidence exists for inhibited temperament as an early risk factor. Furthermore, specific parental factors as well as negative peer experiences increase the risk (Wong and Rapee 2016).

Behavioral inhibition refers to the relatively stable tendency to withdraw from new and unfamiliar objects, situations, and people; this temperamental trait is already measurable in young children, as well as in young animals, offering opportunities for cross-species research and the development of preventive interventions (Fox and Kalin 2014). A meta-analysis indicated that extreme behavioral inhibition is present in 15% of all children, of which almost 50% will develop social anxiety disorder later in life (Clauss and Blackford 2012).

Another factor is the influence of parents. Interactions between parental anxiety and infant behavioral inhibition, leading to anxiety or anxious behavior in the child, have been reported (Aktar et al. 2013). Other studies indicated a contributing role of general parental psychopathology, parenting style, and parents' responsiveness to the development of anxiety in their children (Natsuaki et al. 2013); furthermore, specific maternal and paternal effects have been reported (Aktar et al. 2018; Bynion et al. 2017). These findings suggest a complex interplay between the temperament of the child and parental factors in the development of (vulnerability for) social anxiety disorder (Knappe et al. 2010).

The typical age at onset is during late childhood and early adolescence, a period of life in which important changes in social-affective and social-cognitive processes occur (Crone and Dahl 2012). Examples of such changes are increased importance of the opinion of peers, heightened self-awareness, and increased self-evaluation (Caouette and Guyer 2014). Furthermore, adolescence is characterized by increasing HPA-axis responsivity to social-evaluative stressors due to pubertal and sociocognitive maturation (van den Bos et al. 2016). In addition, numerous studies have indicated that negative peer experiences, in particular peer victimization, increase the risk for future social anxiety disorder (Spence and Rapee 2016). These changes in social information processing and social environment, in addition to maturational effects in the adolescent brain, add to the vulnerability for developing the disorder (Haller et al. 2015).

Personality Factors

Most studies on the relationship between personality factors and social anxiety disorder examined the personality traits of extraversion and neuroticism. On the basis of this work, neuroticism is considered to be a vulnerability factor for the development of social anxiety, and extraversion is considered to be a protective factor (Cremers and Roelofs 2016). Furthermore, genetic variations contributing to individual differences in these personality traits also account for the genetic vulnerability to develop social anxiety disorder (Bienvenu et al. 2007). However, it should be noted that these relationships are not specific for social anxiety but rather are predictive of anxiety disorders in general. Findings on the relationship between social anxiety and perfectionism are mixed (Newby et al. 2017).

Cognitive-Behavioral Factors

Much research has been conducted on the cognitive-behavioral factors involved in the development and maintenance of social anxiety disorder, mostly focusing on specific cognitive biases in information processing, such as memory biases and disturbed social learning of self-related information, and on the behavioral consequences of the social fear (see also Chapter 27, "Psychotherapy for Social Anxiety Disorder," and Spence and Rapee 2016). These cognitive biases lead to maladaptive changes in behavior, among which avoidance of social situations and specific safety behaviors are prominent. Adolescence is an important developmental period for the progression of social avoidance among youth with higher levels of social anxiety, indicating this as a key period for preventive interventions (Miers et al. 2014). It is interesting to note that the use of safety behaviors by socially anxious individuals is not restricted to real-life social encounters; although research on this topic is still in its infancy, a first study demonstrated that students with higher levels of social anxiety preferred online communication tools that enabled them to control how they presented themselves (Kamalou et al. 2019). Clearly, more research on this topic is important for increasing our knowledge about the factors that play a role in the development and maintenance of social anxiety in the modern-day social world.

Etiological Models

The complex etiology of social anxiety disorder is well captured by Wong and Rapee (2016), who attempted to integrate two sets of etiological models—one focusing on the origin and developmental course of social anxiety (Rapee and Spence 2004) and the other focusing on factors that drive the persistence of the disorder (Heimberg et al. 2010). Developmental factors such as genetic and environmental influences, as well as maintenance factors such as negative cognitions and safety behaviors, have been mentioned in previous sections of this chapter. On the basis of a systematic review of the recent literature, Wong and Rapee (2016) proposed an *integrated etiological and maintenance* model of social anxiety disorder (Figure 25–1). It is a comprehensive model, and a full description is beyond the scope of this chapter. In brief, the main thesis of their model revolves around the social-evaluative threat principle—in short, the *threat value* of social-evaluative situations. This principle is the connecting thread between developmental factors on one hand and maintenance factors on the other hand. Social stimuli acquire a particular threat value early in life because of the interaction of genetic and environmental risk factors, and this is grounded in neurobiological processes. During the course of development, this threat value is elaborated through cognitive and behavioral characteristics, such as an attentional bias toward threat in the environment and the failure to develop social skills caused by the avoidance of social interactions. In turn, maintenance factors strengthen the threat value of particular social situations.

It is plausible that, over time, this vicious circle of threat value and maintaining factors starts to operate independently of its developmental roots and creates a self-fulfilling prophecy. Several studies have shown that there is a kernel of truth to the socially anxious person's negative expectations regarding social situations (Miers et al. 2010). Socially anxious youth are regarded as less competent, less attractive, and less likable and are treated more negatively than their nonanxious counterparts (Blöte et al. 2015). The expectation of an unfavorable evaluation by peers may not be just a figment of their distorted imagination. Treatment should pay attention to cognitive distortions as well as to the restoration of social skills and confidence in social situations (Beidel et al. 2003). It may not be sufficient to remove negative cognitions while paying insufficient attention to social skills, because this may lead to disappointing social interactions and rebounding negative cognitions.

Wong and Rapee (2016) recommended various research avenues for a more in-depth understanding of the mutual interaction of developmental and maintenance factors, two of which are particularly urgent. First, although early risk factors are highlighted in the model, much less research has been devoted to the influence of maturational processes during late childhood and adolescence. For instance, a longitudinal study of social anxiety in a community sample of 196 participants, ages 8–17 years at time 1, showed that the relation between social anxiety and the cortisol response to a social-evaluative stressor varies with pubertal development: socially anxious individuals showed *higher* responses at low levels of pubertal development but *lower* responses at high levels of pubertal development (van den Bos et al. 2017). Attenuation of the stress response in socially anxious individuals may be due to protective mechanisms (Del Giudice et al. 2011), and these mechanisms may contribute to the persistence of social anxiety over time.

A second avenue for further research concerns the question of modifiability. Although much research has shown a relationship between cognitive operations and neurobiological processes, experimental manipulations and other interventions are needed to study causal relationships. For example, neurofeedback with real-time fMRI

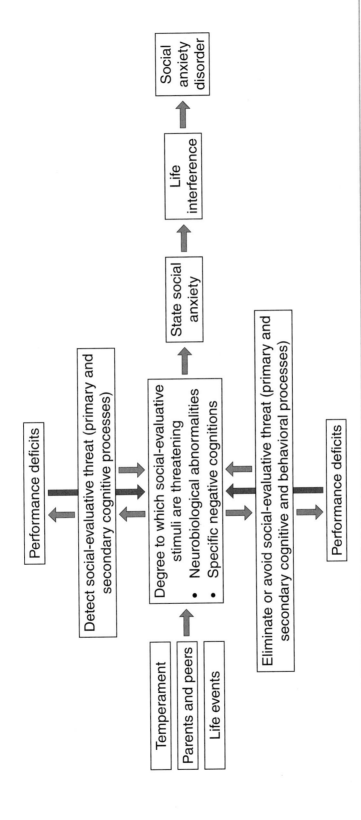

FIGURE 25–1. Simplified overview of the integrated etiological and maintenance model for social anxiety disorder proposed by Wong and Rapee (2016).

is a new and promising method that can be used to train participants in modulating activation in specific brain regions (Haller et al. 2015), and repetitive transcranial magnetic stimulation can also be used to alter brain activation levels (Hoogendam et al. 2010). Furthermore, family studies, preferably with a longitudinal design and in families genetically enriched for social anxiety disorder, may yield unique insights into the genetic susceptibility for social anxiety, as well as into the interactions between genetic factors and environmental influences (Bas-Hoogendam et al. 2018a).

Conclusion

Recent research on the pathogenesis of social anxiety disorder has further elucidated or corroborated the involvement of several biological, developmental, psychological, and psychosocial factors, but data on the roles of other factors, such as genetics and epigenetics, are still scarce. For instance, progress has been made in discerning putative disorder-specific patterns of neural reactivity and connectivity and HPA axis reactivity. The roles of oxytocin, the HPG axis, the autonomic nervous system, and the microbiome need further study. Previous studies have already provided ample evidence for inhibited temperament as an early risk factor, and more recent studies stress the interaction of specific parental factors with negative peer experiences, such as peer victimization, and its impact on the development and maintenance of social anxiety disorder. Finally, given the typical onset of social anxiety disorder during adolescence and its often chronic and unremitting course, there is a clear need for (longitudinal) studies examining the interaction not only between factors involved in the development but also between those involved in the maintenance of social anxiety disorder.

Key Points

- The pathogenesis of social anxiety disorder is multifactorial, with recent studies suggesting complex interactions among (epi)genetic factors; neurobiological vulnerability; and developmental trajectories, temperament, and environmental factors.

- Genetic and epigenetic mechanisms are implicated in social anxiety disorder but need further study.

- Compelling evidence has been found for involvement of the serotonergic system and, to a lesser extent, the dopaminergic system in social anxiety disorder.

- Neuroimaging data point to increased reactivity of, among others, the amygdala and prefrontal cortex and parietal areas in response to faces and anxiety-provoking stimuli that diminishes with treatment. Other imaging data suggest that patients are characterized by changes in large-scale subcortical functional networks as well as in the white matter tract that connects the amygdala and the regulating prefrontal cortex.

- Baseline functioning of the hypothalamic-pituitary-adrenal axis seems normal in social anxiety disorder, but an increased response has been shown after public speaking challenge paradigms. Testosterone/cortisol ratio may also be important.

- The role of the affiliative neuropeptide oxytocin needs further study.

- Findings on autonomic dysfunction and immune dysregulation are few and contradictory.

- Ample evidence exists for inhibited temperament as an early risk factor, interacting with specific parental factors and negative peer experiences.

- Specific negative cognitive biases in social information processing and the behavioral consequences of social fear are important in the development and maintenance of social anxiety disorder.

- Adolescence is an important developmental period for the progression and maintenance of social avoidance among youth with higher levels of social anxiety, indicating that this is a key period for preventive interventions.

- It is important to study the development and maintenance of social anxiety in the modern-day digitalized social world.

References

Aktar E, Majdandžić M, de Vente W, et al: The interplay between expressed parental anxiety and infant behavioural inhibition predicts infant avoidance in a social referencing paradigm. J Child Psychol Psychiatry 54(2):144–156, 2013 22924437

Aktar E, Van Bockstaele B, Perez-Edgar K, et al: Intergenerational transmission of attentional bias and anxiety. Dev Sci 22(3):e12772, 2018 30428152

Alkozei A, Creswell C, Cooper PJ, et al: Autonomic arousal in childhood anxiety disorders: associations with state anxiety and social anxiety disorder. J Affect Disord 175:25–33, 2015 25590763

Bandelow B, Baldwin D, Abelli M, et al: Biological markers for anxiety disorders, OCD and PTSD—a consensus statement. Part I: neuroimaging and genetics. World J Biol Psychiatry 17(5):321–365, 2016 27403679

Bas-Hoogendam JM: Commentary: gray matter structural alterations in social anxiety disorder: a voxel-based meta-analysis. Front Psychiatry 10:1–3, 2019

Bas-Hoogendam JM, Blackford JU, Brühl AB, et al: Neurobiological candidate endophenotypes of social anxiety disorder. Neurosci Biobehav Rev 71:362–378, 2016 27593443

Bas-Hoogendam JM, van Steenbergen H, Nienke Pannekoek J, et al: Voxel-based morphometry multi-center mega-analysis of brain structure in social anxiety disorder. Neuroimage Clin 16:678–688, 2017 30140607

Bas-Hoogendam JM, Harrewijn A, Tissier RL, et al: The Leiden Family Lab study on social anxiety disorder: a multiplex, multigenerational family study on neurocognitive endophenotypes. Int J Methods Psychiatr Res 27(2):e1616, 2018a 29700902

Bas-Hoogendam JM, van Steenbergen H, Tissier RLM, et al: Subcortical brain volumes, cortical thickness and cortical surface area in families genetically enriched for social anxiety disorder—a multiplex multigenerational neuroimaging study. EBioMedicine 36:410–428, 2018b 30266294

Beesdo K, Bittner A, Pine DS, et al: Incidence of social anxiety disorder and the consistent risk for secondary depression in the first three decades of life. Arch Gen Psychiatry 64(8):903–912, 2007 17679635

Beidel DC, Turner SM, Morris TL: Social Effectiveness Therapy for Children and Adolescents (SET-C): Therapist Guide. North Tonawanda, NY, Multi Health Systems, 2003

Bienvenu OJ, Hettema JM, Neale MC, et al: Low extraversion and high neuroticism as indices of genetic and environmental risk for social phobia, agoraphobia, and animal phobia. Am J Psychiatry 164(11):1714–1721, 2007 17974937

Blöte AW, Miers AC, Westenberg PM: The role of social performance and physical attractiveness in peer rejection of socially anxious adolescents. J Res Adolesc 25(1):189–200, 2015

Brühl AB, Delsignore A, Komossa K, et al: Neuroimaging in social anxiety disorder—a meta-analytic review resulting in a new neurofunctional model. Neurosci Biobehav Rev 47:260–280, 2014 25124509

Bynion T-M, Blumenthal H, Bilsky SA, et al: Dimensions of parenting among mothers and fathers in relation to social anxiety among female adolescents. J Adolesc 60:11–15, 2017 28738315

Caouette JD, Guyer AE: Gaining insight into adolescent vulnerability for social anxiety from developmental cognitive neuroscience. Dev Cogn Neurosci 8:65–76, 2014 24239049

Chalmers JA, Quintana DS, Abbott MJ-A, et al: Anxiety disorders are associated with reduced heart rate variability: a meta-analysis. Front Psychiatry 5:80, 2014 25071612

Chanraud S, Zahr N, Sullivan EV, et al: MR diffusion tensor imaging: a window into white matter integrity of the working brain. Neuropsychol Rev 20(2):209–225, 2010 20422451

Clauss JA, Blackford JU: Behavioral inhibition and risk for developing social anxiety disorder: a meta-analytic study. J Am Acad Child Adolesc Psychiatry 51(10):1066–1075, 2012 23021481

Cremers HR, Roelofs K: Social anxiety disorder: a critical overview of neurocognitive research. Wiley Interdiscip Rev Cogn Sci 7(4):218–232, 2016 27240280

Crone EA, Dahl RE: Understanding adolescence as a period of social-affective engagement and goal flexibility. Nat Rev Neurosci 13(9):636–650, 2012 22903221

Damoiseaux JS, Rombouts SA, Barkhof F, et al: Consistent resting-state networks across healthy subjects. Proc Natl Acad Sci USA 103(37):13848–13853, 2006 16945915

De Cagna F, Fusar-Poli L, Damiani S, et al: The role of intranasal oxytocin in anxiety and depressive disorders: a systematic review of randomized controlled trials. Clin Psychopharmacol Neurosci 17(1):1–11, 2019 30690935

Del Giudice M, Ellis BJ, Shirtcliff EA: The Adaptive Calibration Model of stress responsivity. Neurosci Biobehav Rev 35(7):1562–1592, 2011 21145350

Fox AS, Kalin NH: A translational neuroscience approach to understanding the development of social anxiety disorder and its pathophysiology. Am J Psychiatry 171(11):1162–1173, 2014 25157566

Frick A, Howner K, Fischer H, et al: Altered fusiform connectivity during processing of fearful faces in social anxiety disorder. Transl Psychiatry 3:e312, 2013 24105443

Frick A, Åhs F, Engman J, et al: Serotonin synthesis and reuptake in social anxiety disorder: a positron emission tomography study. JAMA Psychiatry 72(8):794–802, 2015 26083190

Gelernter J, Page GP, Stein MB, et al: Genome-wide linkage scan for loci predisposing to social phobia: evidence for a chromosome 16 risk locus. Am J Psychiatry 161(1):59–66, 2004 14702251

Giltay EJ, Enter D, Zitman FG, et al: Salivary testosterone: associations with depression, anxiety disorders, and antidepressant use in a large cohort study. J Psychosom Res 72(3):205–213, 2012 22325700

Glaser R, Kiecolt-Glaser JK: Stress-induced immune dysfunction: implications for health. Nat Rev Immunol 5(3):243–251, 2005 15738954

Gorka SM, Fitzgerald DA, Labuschagne I, et al: Oxytocin modulation of amygdala functional connectivity to fearful faces in generalized social anxiety disorder. Neuropsychopharmacology 40(2):278–286, 2015 24998619

Haller SPW, Cohen Kadosh K, Scerif G, et al: Social anxiety disorder in adolescence: how developmental cognitive neuroscience findings may shape understanding and interventions for psychopathology. Dev Cogn Neurosci 13:11–20, 2015 25818181

Harrewijn A, Van der Molen MJW, Verkuil B, et al: Heart rate variability as candidate endophenotype of social anxiety: a two-generation family study. J Affect Disord 237:47–55, 2018 29763849

Heimberg RG, Brozovich FA, Rapee RM: A cognitive behavioral model of social anxiety disorder: update and extension, in Social Anxiety, 2nd Edition. Edited by Hofmann SG, DiBartolo PMBT. San Diego, CA, Academic Press, 2010, pp 395–422

Hendriks SM, Spijker J, Licht CMM, et al: Disability in anxiety disorders. J Affect Disord 166:227–233, 2014 25012435

Hoogendam JM, Ramakers GMJ, Di Lazzaro V: Physiology of repetitive transcranial magnetic stimulation of the human brain. Brain Stimul 3(2):95–118, 2010 20633438

Kamalou S, Shaughnessy K, Moscovitch DA: Social anxiety in the digital age: the measurement and sequelae of online safety-seeking. Comput Human Behav 90:10–17, 2019

Kennedy JL, Neves-Pereira M, King N, et al: Dopamine system genes not linked to social phobia. Psychiatr Genet 11(4):213–217, 2001 11807412

Knappe S, Beesdo-Baum K, Wittchen H-U: Familial risk factors in social anxiety disorder: calling for a family oriented approach for targeted prevention and early intervention. Eur Child Adolesc Psychiatry 19(12):857–871, 2010 20922550

Labuschagne I, Phan KL, Wood A, et al: Oxytocin attenuates amygdala reactivity to fear in generalized social anxiety disorder. Neuropsychopharmacology 35(12):2403–2413, 2010 20720535

Meier S, Trontti K, Als TD, et al: Genome-wide association study of anxiety and stress-related disorders in the iPSYCH cohort. bioRxiv, February 12, 2018. Available at: https://www.biorxiv.org/content/10.1101/263855v1.article-info. Accessed July 6, 2019.

Miers AC, Blöte AW, Westenberg PM: Peer perceptions of social skills in socially anxious and nonanxious adolescents. J Abnorm Child Psychol 38(1):33–41, 2010 19680804

Miers AC, Blöte AW, de Rooij M, et al: Trajectories of social anxiety during adolescence and relations with cognition, social competence, and temperament. J Abnorm Child Psychol 41(1):97–110, 2013 22723078

Miers AC, Blöte AW, Heyne DA, et al: Developmental pathways of social avoidance across adolescence: the role of social anxiety and negative cognition. J Anxiety Disord 28(8):787–794, 2014 25265547

Miskovic V, Schmidt LA: Social fearfulness in the human brain. Neurosci Biobehav Rev 36(1):459–478, 2012 21855571

Morreale M, Tancer ME, Uhde TW: Pathogenesis of social anxiety disorder, in Textbook of Anxiety Disorders, 2nd Edition. Edited by Stein DJ, Hollander E, Rothbaum BO. Washington, DC, American Psychiatric Publishing, 2010, pp 453–470

Natsuaki MN, Leve LD, Neiderhiser JM, et al: Intergenerational transmission of risk for social inhibition: the interplay between parental responsiveness and genetic influences. Dev Psychopathol 25(1):261–274, 2013 23398764

Naudé PJW, Roest AM, Stein DJ, et al: Anxiety disorders and CRP in a population cohort study with 54,326 participants: the LifeLines study. World J Biol Psychiatry 19(6):461–470, 2018 29376460

Neumann ID, Slattery DA: Oxytocin in general anxiety and social fear: a translational approach. Biol Psychiatry 79(3):213–221, 2015 26208744

Newby J, Pitura VA, Penney AM, et al: Neuroticism and perfectionism as predictors of social anxiety. Pers Individ Dif 106:263–267, 2017

Nikolic M, de Vente W, Colonnesi C, et al: Autonomic arousal in children of parents with and without social anxiety disorder: a high-risk study. J Child Psychol Psychiatry 57(9):1047–1055, 2016 27133173

Notzon S, Domschke K, Holitschke K, et al: Attachment style and oxytocin receptor gene variation interact in influencing social anxiety. World J Biol Psychiatry 17(1):76–83, 2016 26488131

Otowa T, Hek K, Lee M, et al: Meta-analysis of genome-wide association studies of anxiety disorders. Mol Psychiatry 21:1391–1399, 2016

Pannekoek JN, Veer IM, van Tol M-J, et al: Resting-state functional connectivity abnormalities in limbic and salience networks in social anxiety disorder without comorbidity. Eur Neuropsychopharmacol 23(3):186–195, 2013 22749355

Phan KL, Fitzgerald DA, Cortese BM, et al: Anterior cingulate neurochemistry in social anxiety disorder: 1H-MRS at 4 Tesla. Neuroreport 16(2):183–186, 2005 15671874

Phan KL, Coccaro EF, Angstadt M, et al: Corticolimbic brain reactivity to social signals of threat before and after sertraline treatment in generalized social phobia. Biol Psychiatry 73(4):329–336, 2013 23164370

Pirbaglou M, Katz J, de Souza RJ, et al: Probiotic supplementation can positively affect anxiety and depressive symptoms: a systematic review of randomized controlled trials. Nutr Res 36(9):889–898, 2016 27632908

Pollack MH, Jensen JE, Simon NM, et al: High-field MRS study of GABA, glutamate and glutamine in social anxiety disorder: response to treatment with levetiracetam. Prog Neuropsychopharmacol Biol Psychiatry 32(3):739–743, 2008 18206286

Poole KL, Tang A, Schmidt LA: The temperamentally shy child as the social adult: an exemplar of multifinality, in Behavioral Inhibition: Integrating Theory, Research, and Clinical Perspectives. Edited by Pérez-Edgar K, Fox NA. New York, Springer, 2018a, pp 185–212

Poole KL, Van Lieshout RJ, McHolm AE, et al: Trajectories of social anxiety in children: influence of child cortisol reactivity and parental social anxiety. J Abnorm Child Psychol 46(6):1309–1319, 2018b 29256026

Rapee RM, Spence SH: The etiology of social phobia: empirical evidence and an initial model. Clin Psychol Rev 24(7):737–767, 2004 15501555

Scaini S, Belotti R, Ogliari A: Genetic and environmental contributions to social anxiety across different ages: a meta-analytic approach to twin data. J Anxiety Disord 28(7):650–656, 2014 25118017

Smoller JW: Anxiety genetics: dispatches from the frontier. Am J Med Genet B Neuropsychiatr Genet 174(2):117–119, 2017 28224734

Spence SH, Rapee RM: The etiology of social anxiety disorder: an evidence-based model. Behav Res Ther 86:50–67, 2016 27406470

Stein MB, Chartier MJ, Kozak MV, et al: Genetic linkage to the serotonin transporter protein and 5HT2A receptor genes excluded in generalized social phobia. Psychiatry Res 81(3):283–291, 1998 9925179

Stein MB, Chen C-Y, Jain S, et al: Genetic risk variants for social anxiety. Am J Med Genet B Neuropsychiatr Genet 174(2):120–131, 2017 28224735

Steinert C, Hofmann M, Leichsenring F, et al: What do we know today about the prospective long-term course of social anxiety disorder? A systematic literature review. J Anxiety Disord 27(7):692–702, 2013 24176803

Terburg D, Syal S, Rosenberger LA, et al: Testosterone abolishes implicit subordination in social anxiety. Psychoneuroendocrinology 72:205–211, 2016 27448713

van den Bos E, van Duijvenvoorde ACK, Westenberg PM: Effects of adolescent sociocognitive development on the cortisol response to social evaluation. Dev Psychol 52(7):1151–1163, 2016 27177160

van den Bos E, Tops M, Westenberg PM: Social anxiety and the cortisol response to social evaluation in children and adolescents. Psychoneuroendocrinology 78:159–167, 2017 28209542

van Veen JF, van Vliet IM, Derijk RH, et al: Elevated alpha-amylase but not cortisol in generalized social anxiety disorder. Psychoneuroendocrinology 33(10):1313–1321, 2008 18757137

Vogelzangs N, Seldenrijk A, Beekman ATF, et al: Cardiovascular disease in persons with depressive and anxiety disorders. J Affect Disord 125(1–3):241–248, 2010 20223521

Vogelzangs N, Beekman ATF, de Jonge P, et al: Anxiety disorders and inflammation in a large adult cohort. Translational Psychiatry 3:e249, 2013

Wang X, Cheng B, Luo Q, et al: Gray matter structural alterations in social anxiety disorder: a voxel-based meta-analysis. Front Psychiatry 9:449, 2018

Warwick JM, Carey PD, Cassimjee N, et al: Dopamine transporter binding in social anxiety disorder: the effect of treatment with escitalopram. Metab Brain Dis 27(2):151–158, 2012 22350963

Wong QJJ, Rapee RM: The aetiology and maintenance of social anxiety disorder: a synthesis of complimentary theoretical models and formulation of a new integrated model. J Affect Disord 203:84–100, 2016 27280967

Ziegler C, Dannlowski U, Bräuer D, et al: Oxytocin receptor gene methylation: converging multilevel evidence for a role in social anxiety. Neuropsychopharmacology 40(6):1528–1538, 2015 25563749

Zorn JV, Schür RR, Boks MP, et al: Cortisol stress reactivity across psychiatric disorders: a systematic review and meta-analysis. Psychoneuroendocrinology 77:25–36, 2017 28012291

Recommended Readings

Bas-Hoogendam JM, Blackford JU, Brühl AB, et al: Neurobiological candidate endophenotypes of social anxiety disorder. Neurosci Biobehav Rev 71:362–378, 2016

Bas-Hoogendam JM, Harrewijn A, Tissier RLM, et al: The Leiden Family Lab study on social anxiety disorder: a multiplex, multigenerational family study on neurocognitive endophenotypes. Int J Methods Psychiatr Res 27:e1616, 2018

Brühl AB, Delsignore A, Komossa K, et al: Neuroimaging in social anxiety disorder: a meta-analytic review resulting in a new neurofunctional model. Neurosci Biobehav Rev 47:260–280, 2014

Spence SH, Rapee RM: The etiology of social anxiety disorder: an evidence-based model. Behav Res Ther 86:50–67, 2016

Wong QJJ, Rapee RM: The aetiology and maintenance of social anxiety disorder: a synthesis of complimentary theoretical models and formulation of a new integrated model. J Affect Disord 203:84–100, 2016

CHAPTER 26

Pharmacotherapy for Social Anxiety Disorder

Franklin R. Schneier, M.D.

Social anxiety disorder is among the most common anxiety disorders, with a prevalence of 5%–13% (Grant et al. 2005). It typically has an early age at onset in adolescence and a chronic course. The best-established treatments are cognitive-behavioral therapy (CBT) and pharmacotherapy. This chapter reviews the literature on medication treatment of social anxiety disorder, focusing on randomized controlled trials (RCTs) of marketed medications and meta-analytic or systematic reviews of the literature, supplemented with findings from open trials and clinical experience. For a more comprehensive listing and description of individual RCTs, which is beyond the scope of this chapter, we refer the reader to a Cochrane review (Williams et al. 2017).

When interpreting the clinical trial literature in social anxiety disorder, one should keep several issues in mind. First, the definition of the disorder has shifted over recent decades, particularly with respect to the scope of situations feared. Most treatment studies, however, have required the generalized form or an equivalent severity score threshold to include subjects who fear most social situations, and they therefore have often excluded individuals with what DSM-5 (American Psychiatric Association 2013) calls the "performance-only" subtype. Second, despite the chronic nature of the disorder, most studies have limited assessments to an 8- to 12-week timeframe of acute response to treatment, with a smaller body of work addressing long-term outcomes. Third, although social anxiety disorder is most commonly comorbid with other anxiety, depressive, or substance use disorders, most trials have excluded patients with comorbid major depression or active substance use disorders. The most common primary outcome measure in these trials has been the Liebowitz Social Anxiety Scale (LSAS), which totals anxiety and avoidance ratings (each scored 0–3) in 24 common interpersonal and performance situations, yielding a total score of 0–144 (Liebowitz 1987). Responder status has most commonly been defined by a Clinical Global Impression Scale–Improvement (Guy 1976) score of 1 or 2, much to very much improved.

First-Line Treatments

Selective serotonin reuptake inhibitors (SSRIs) and serotonin-norepinephrine re-uptake inhibitors (SNRIs) have been established as the first-line pharmacological treatments of social anxiety disorder on the basis of more than 30 randomized clinical trials involving more than 6,000 patients. Almost all SSRIs and SNRIs have been stud-ied in at least one RCT, but only paroxetine, sertraline, controlled-release fluvoxamine, and extended-release venlafaxine have received FDA approval for this indication. Meta-analytic reviews have consistently documented efficacy for these classes (Curtiss et al. 2017; de Menezes et al. 2011; Williams et al. 2017); their findings, along with the medications' favorable side effect profiles and efficacy for comorbid depression, have supported their use as first-line pharmacotherapy for social anxiety disorder. The SNRI venlafaxine is grouped here with the SSRIs because fixed-dose studies have re-ported no general advantage for dosing greater than 75–150 mg/day, a range in which venlafaxine is believed to act primarily as a serotonergic agent without much noradrenergic effect (Stein et al. 2005).

Effect Size and Response Rates

Meta-analyses of placebo-controlled clinical trials have estimated that, relative to placebo, SSRIs and SNRIs further reduce the mean severity of social anxiety disorder as scored on the LSAS by 10.14 points (95% CI 6.22–14.05) and 11.91 points (95% CI 7.76–16.06), respectively (Williams et al. 2017), or effect sizes of $g=0.44$ (95% CI 0.37–0.51) and $g=0.45$ (95% CI 0.35–0.55), respectively (Curtiss et al. 2017), representing moderate effect. Individual trials have typically reported response rates of 40%–80%, compared with mean placebo group response rates averaging ~23.5% (Oosterbaan et al. 2001). Vilazodone, which combines SSRI activity with activity at serotonin type 1A (5-HT_{1A}) receptors, has also been reported as efficacious in a single RCT (Careri et al. 2015).

Across SSRI trials, secondary outcome measures, such as assessments of quality of life, have tended to show improvements in concert with social anxiety symptomatol-ogy, but with somewhat smaller effects. SSRIs are generally well tolerated in patients with social anxiety disorder, with no difference in clinical trial dropout rates for SSRIs versus placebo (Williams et al. 2017). The most common adverse events include nau-sea, insomnia, sexual dysfunction, sweating, and weight gain. No well-replicated pre-dictors of individual response to SSRIs in patients with social anxiety disorder have been identified.

Dosing and Time Course of Response

Dosing for social anxiety disorder is similar to the dosing used for depression. For ex-ample, sertraline might be initiated at 50 mg/day and increased during week 1 or 2 to 100 mg/day. After 4 weeks, nonresponders can have their dosage increased to 150 mg/day for 2 weeks and then to 200 mg/day, as tolerated (see Table 26–1 for more information on individual medications in each class). Improvement often begins early; by the end of 4 weeks of treatment, patients who had shown no benefit from treatment

TABLE 26–1. **Recommendations for drug treatment of social anxiety disorder**

Treatment class and examples	Usual daily dosage, *mg*	Key advantages	Key disadvantages
Selective serotonin reuptake inhibitors (SSRIs)		Best studied, well tolerated, efficacious for comorbid depression	Sexual side effects, insomnia, sweating, weight gain, nausea; delayed response
*Paroxetine	10–60		
*Paroxetine CR	12.5–75		
*Sertraline	50–200		
*Fluvoxamine CR	100–300		
Serotonin-norepinephrine reuptake inhibitor (SNRI)		Same as for SSRIs	Same as for SSRIs but riskier in overdose and may increase blood pressure
*Venlafaxine XR	75–150		
Benzodiazepines		Rapid effect, can be used together with antidepressants	Abuse potential; sedation and impairment of cognition or balance; lacks efficacy for comorbid depression; usually requires greater than once-daily dosing
Clonazepam	0.5–3.0		
$\alpha_2\delta$ Ligands		Can be used together with antidepressants	Similar to benzodiazepines; weight gain
Pregabalin	600		
Gabapentin	900–3,600		
Noradrenergic and specific serotonergic antidepressant		Efficacious for comorbid depression; low rate of sexual side effects	Sedation, weight gain, dry mouth; mixed evidence for efficacy
Mirtazapine	15–45		
Monoamine oxidase inhibitor		May be highly efficacious for social anxiety disorder and depression	Need for low-tyramine diet to prevent hypertensive reactions; weight gain, sedation, hypotension
Phenelzine	30–90		
Reversible inhibitor of monoamine oxidase		Well tolerated, efficacious for comorbid depression	Not available in United States; may be less efficacious than SSRIs
Moclobemide	300–600		

Note. CR=controlled release; XR=extended release.
*FDA approved for social anxiety disorder.

with the SSRI escitalopram had only a 20% chance of ultimately responding (Baldwin et al. 2009). However, late responses are also not uncommon; in a report of pooled trials of paroxetine, 28% of subjects who were nonresponders (which includes minimal responders) after 8 weeks of treatment became responders during an additional 4 weeks of continued treatment (Stein et al. 2002a).

Differences in Response to Individual SSRIs and SNRIs

Across SSRIs and SNRIs, no consistent differences in efficacy have been demonstrated for particular medications, although adverse effect profiles may influence treatment selection. Among FDA-approved medications for social anxiety disorder, paroxetine has the potential disadvantages of being the only SSRI to be classified in pregnancy risk class D and of possibly manifesting higher rates of weight gain and withdrawal symptoms (Aberg-Wistedt et al. 2000), whereas venlafaxine carries greater risk of toxicity in overdose (Thase 2006). Withdrawal effects occur in a subset of persons discontinuing SSRIs and SNRIs but are less common for drugs with longer elimination half-lives (e.g., fluoxetine) and can be minimized by gradually tapering medication dosage prior to discontinuation.

Other Treatments

Non-SSRI/SNRI Antidepressants

Various other antidepressants have been studied with RCTs in patients with social anxiety disorder. Mirtazapine, a non-SSRI with activity at several serotonin and norepinephrine receptors, was efficacious in one of two placebo-controlled trials (Muehlbacher et al. 2005; Schutters et al. 2010). Relatively high rates of sedation and weight gain sometimes limit its use. Bupropion, a widely used antidepressant, has not been studied in any RCTs and appeared ineffective in an open trial (Emmanuel et al. 2000), as did the tricyclic antidepressant imipramine (Simpson et al. 1998). Nefazodone lacked efficacy in a single RCT (Van Ameringen et al. 2007).

Classic monoamine oxidase inhibitors (MAOIs) are possibly the most efficacious medication class for treating social anxiety disorder, with four RCTs of phenelzine yielding a differential improvement of 16.39 points (95% CI 0.51–32.27) on the LSAS, yet they see only rare usage in clinical practice (Williams et al. 2017). These medications are of historical importance because early trials initiated before the advent of SSRIs helped establish the proof of principle that pharmacotherapy could be efficacious for social anxiety and that patients were willing to pursue such treatments. MAOIs are now generally reserved for use in treatment-refractory cases because they require patients to adhere strictly to a low-tyramine diet to prevent dangerous hypertensive reactions and have a relatively high rate of other adverse events, such as weight gain and postural hypotension. Moclobemide, a reversible inhibitor of monoamine oxidase A, is safer and is marketed widely outside the United States. It has appeared efficacious for social anxiety disorder in six RCTs. Meta-analyses report an overall symptom reduction superiority of 12.17 points (95% CI 0.84–23.51) on the LSAS, but this was reduced to 7.59 points (95% CI 3.84–11.35) after one outlier study was removed (Williams et al. 2017), suggesting that moclobemide may generally be somewhat less efficacious than SSRIs.

Benzodiazepines

An RCT of clonazepam reported one of the largest effects in patients with social anxiety disorder, with a response rate of 78% versus 20% for placebo (Davidson et al. 1993).

RCTs of bromazepam (not marketed in the United States; Versiani et al. 1997) and alprazolam (Gelernter et al. 1991), along with studies of clonazepam compared to CBT (Otto et al. 2000) and clonazepam open trials, have also supported efficacy of benzodiazepines for this disorder. Clonazepam has been well tolerated in studies using standing dosages in the range of 2–3 mg/day. Benzodiazepines have advantages of rapid onset and good tolerability but drawbacks that include lack of efficacy for comorbid depression, sedation, incoordination, and potential for abuse. Although physical dependency develops with daily use, a long-term double-blind discontinuation trial in clonazepam responders found that tapering over several months resulted in low rates of withdrawal symptoms (28%) and of relapse (21%) over the next 5 months (Connor et al. 1998). Benzodiazepines also are reported anecdotally to be helpful when used as needed for managing anticipatory anxiety prior to specific social or performance situations, although as-needed dosing is generally insufficient as monotherapy for the generalized form of social anxiety disorder. Additionally, benzodiazepines taken during CBT exposure exercises may interfere with the therapeutic process.

Gabapentin and Pregabalin

Three RCTs support the efficacy of gabapentin or pregabalin, medications that bind to the $\alpha_2\delta$ subunit of voltage-sensitive calcium channels. Pregabalin appeared efficacious at a 600-mg/day dosage in two RCTs (Feltner et al. 2011; Pande et al. 2004). A drawback of these two medications, like benzodiazepines, is their lack of efficacy for comorbid depression, as well as their abuse potential, particularly for persons with a history of substance abuse (Bonnet and Scherbaum 2017). Somnolence and dizziness were the most common adverse effects.

Beta-Adrenergic Blockers

β-Blockers are widely used on an as-needed basis for performance-only-type social anxiety disorder, yet no clinical trials have tested the efficacy of such use. Evidence for their efficacy is based on a series of small RCTs in analogue samples of anxious performers (Liebowitz et al. 1985) and widespread anecdotal clinical reports. In the only two RCTs of a β-blocker for social anxiety disorder, atenolol was prescribed on a daily basis in samples that consisted predominantly of persons with the generalized form and was found to lack efficacy for this use (Liebowitz et al. 1992; Turner et al. 1994). It is plausible, however, that β-blockers are ineffective for generalized social anxiety disorder but efficacious for the performance-only subtype when given on an as-needed basis prior to performances.

Antipsychotics

Two small studies of olanzapine and quetiapine in patients with social anxiety disorder found no significant differences on primary outcome measures but some evidence of efficacy for secondary outcomes (Williams et al. 2017). Notably, however, several case reports have been made of social anxiety disorder symptoms emerging as an adverse effect during antipsychotic treatment of other disorders (Scahill et al. 2003). Quetiapine also appeared ineffective in an RCT of its as-needed use for public speaking anxiety in patients with social anxiety disorder (Donahue et al. 2009).

Other Medications

In one small RCT, the cannabis derivative cannabidiol reduced anxiety during simulated public speaking in patients with social anxiety disorder (Bergamaschi et al. 2011). In a small crossover study, a single intravenous ketamine infusion was superior to placebo in reducing symptoms over 2 weeks, although clinicians rated only 33% of participants as responders (Taylor et al. 2018). Medications with only negative outcomes in RCTs, in addition to nefazodone as discussed earlier (see "Non-SSRI/SNRI Antidepressants"), include the anticonvulsants tiagabine, levetiracetam, and sodium valproate; the norepinephrine reuptake inhibitor atomoxetine; and doses up to 30 mg/day of the 5-HT$_{1A}$ partial agonist buspirone (Williams et al. 2017). The herbal preparation St. John's wort also was ineffective in one RCT (Kobak et al. 2005).

Long-Term Efficacy Data

The long-term efficacy of medications for social anxiety disorder has been examined in a small number of studies, including naturalistic and double-blind discontinuation studies in which responders to an acute course of treatment were randomized to continuation treatment or to taper with a switch to placebo. Several discontinuation RCTs of SSRIs or venlafaxine have shown that responders to a 12- to 20-week course benefit significantly from 6 months of continued treatment, with relapse rates under 25% for continuation versus 36%–50% after switching to placebo (Montgomery et al. 2005; Stein et al. 1996, 2002b; Walker et al. 2000). A single RCT supports the efficacy of pregabalin maintenance treatment in preventing relapse (Greist et al. 2011). Open trials also suggest long-term efficacy for moclobemide (Stein et al. 2002c) and clonazepam (Davidson et al. 1991).

Treatment-Refractory Illness

Few studies have addressed the important problem of how best to treat the subset of patients for whom social anxiety disorder does not respond adequately to one or more courses of treatment. One controlled trial in nonresponders to 10 weeks of sertraline treatment found that patients randomized to augmentation with clonazepam (up to 3 mg/day), but not to a switch to venlafaxine (up to 225 mg/day), had superior rates of remission after 12 weeks relative to augmentation with placebo (Pollack et al. 2014). In another RCT, nonresponders to medication treatment who were then randomized to CBT (either augmentation or switch) improved more than patients randomized to continuing treatment as usual (Campbell-Sills et al. 2016).

Small open trials in SSRI nonresponders have suggested possible efficacy for augmenting treatment with buspirone (Van Ameringen et al. 1996) or risperidone (Simon et al. 2006) or for switching to citalopram (Simon et al. 2002), venlafaxine (Altamura et al. 1999), or phenelzine (Aarre 2003). Switching treatment from an SSRI to an MAOI requires a washout period of at least 2 weeks (5 weeks for fluoxetine). In another open trial, 48% of nonresponders to paroxetine subsequently responded to escitalopram (Pallanti and Quercioli 2006).

Combined Treatments

Two RCTs involving patients with social anxiety disorder have studied combined treatment with medications having potentially complementary mechanisms of action. In a small study, Seedat and Stein (2004) found that paroxetine combined with 1–2 mg/day of clonazepam for 10 weeks did not accelerate response relative to paroxetine combined with placebo, although it did result in a trend toward greater overall response rates (79% vs. 43%). Another very small RCT found that pindolol, a 5-HT$_{1A}$ receptor agonist and β-adrenergic blocker, did not augment the efficacy of paroxetine (Stein et al. 2001).

Other RCTs have combined the two best-established first-line treatments for social anxiety disorder, SSRIs and CBT, which presumably have distinct mechanisms of action and the potential for additive or synergistic effects. One study compared 16 weeks of clinician-led CBT to self-exposure plus medication (fluoxetine) and self-exposure plus placebo. CBT was superior to both other treatments at posttreatment and at 12-month follow-up, but fluoxetine efficacy was not different from placebo (Clark et al. 2003). A second study randomized patients to a different form of CBT, fluoxetine, placebo, combined CBT plus fluoxetine, or CBT plus placebo. Each active treatment was superior to placebo but not different from the other active treatments after 14 weeks (Davidson et al. 2004). One other study randomized patients to an SSRI (sertraline) with or without exposure therapy or to a placebo with or without exposure therapy. After 24 weeks, the sertraline and combined sertraline plus exposure groups improved more than the exposure or placebo monotherapy groups. At 1-year follow-up, however, the exposure plus placebo group had deteriorated less than either of the sertraline groups (Blomhoff et al. 2001; Haug et al. 2003). Most recently, an RCT assigned patients to treatment with paroxetine, cognitive therapy, combined treatments, or pill placebo (Nordahl et al. 2016). At posttreatment, cognitive therapy was equivalent to combined treatment and superior to monotherapy with paroxetine or placebo. At 12-month follow-up, cognitive therapy was significantly better than paroxetine or placebo monotherapy, and the combined-treatment group had an intermediate outcome. In contrast, a single study comparing phenelzine or CBT with combined treatment and placebo found advantages for combined treatment over CBT alone (Blanco et al. 2010). In summary, combined medication plus CBT from the outset of treatment is not generally advantageous, but further study is needed to identify whether a subgroup of patients might benefit from combined treatment. CBT appears advantageous particularly with respect to long-term persistence of benefits after treatment discontinuation, and even patients receiving pharmacotherapy alone should be encouraged to enter feared situations in order to assess efficacy and overcome habitual avoidance (see Figure 26–1 for an algorithm summarizing key treatment decisions in social anxiety disorder).

A different approach to combined medication and psychotherapy treatments has aimed to use medication in conjunction with sessions of exposure therapy, with the aim of enhancing fear-extinction learning processes. Best studied has been use of the NMDA receptor partial agonist D-cycloserine. Although two small RCTs initially suggested that D-cycloserine enhanced efficacy of an abbreviated (four- or five-session) course of CBT, a large-scale RCT found that it accelerated improvement but did not

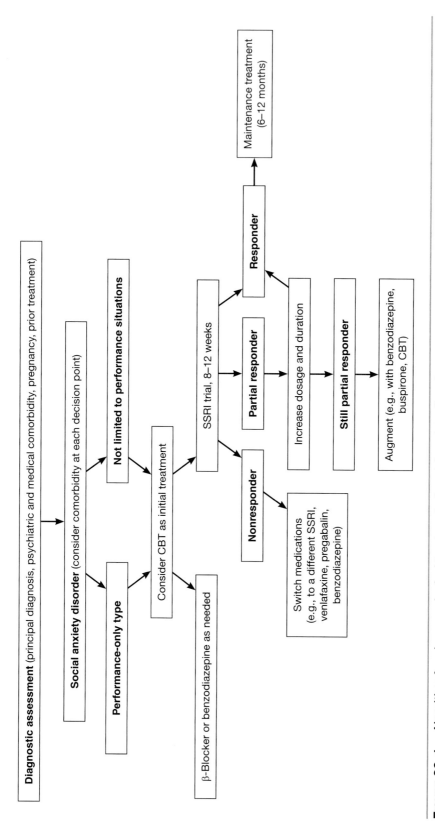

FIGURE 26–1.   Algorithm for pharmacological treatment of social anxiety disorder.

CBT=cognitive-behavioral therapy; SSRI=selective serotonin reuptake inhibitor.

increase efficacy (Hofmann et al. 2013). In one RCT of another putative cognitive enhancer, the α_2-adrenoceptor antagonist yohimbine, given prior to four exposure sessions, accelerated and enhanced symptomatic improvement more than placebo (Smits et al. 2014). Study of cognitive enhancers of CBT remains an area of active investigation.

Addressing Comorbidity

Social anxiety disorder is commonly comorbid with a host of disorders, particularly other anxiety disorders and depression, but most RCTs have not reported the impact of comorbidity on outcome, and many studies excluded patients with significant depression or substance use disorders. In one RCT of patients with social anxiety disorder and comorbid major depression, Liebowitz et al. (2017) found evidence of efficacy for vortioxetine, an SSRI with additional activity at other serotonin receptors. This study also replicated a prior open trial finding that depressive symptoms respond more rapidly than social anxiety symptoms to SSRI (citalopram) treatment in patients with comorbid diagnoses (Schneier et al. 2003).

In one RCT of adults with comorbid ADHD, the norepinephrine reuptake inhibitor atomoxetine—which did not appear useful in the treatment of social anxiety disorder without comorbidity in another study (Williams et al. 2017)—was efficacious in reducing the severity of symptoms of each disorder, although the magnitude of mean drug–placebo difference in change on the LSAS (8.5 points) was modest (Adler et al. 2009).

A series of three RCTs by one research group assessed the efficacy of the SSRI paroxetine in patients with social anxiety disorder and comorbid alcohol use disorders. In a very small trial ($N=15$), Randall et al. (2001) found that 8 weeks of treatment with paroxetine significantly improved social anxiety and global measures of alcohol abuse (but not alcohol quantity or frequency of use) more than placebo. A larger RCT ($N=42$) in a sample of patients with the same comorbidity who reported drinking to cope with anxiety replicated the superiority of paroxetine for social anxiety disorder symptoms and the absence of significant change in alcohol consumption. However, paroxetine did decrease the amount of drinking specifically ascribed to coping (Book et al. 2008). In the third study, Book et al. (2013) randomized a similar comorbid sample ($N=83$) to paroxetine alone or paroxetine with a behavioral intervention (brief alcohol intervention). Paroxetine again significantly decreased social anxiety symptoms and drinking to cope, but alcohol use did not decrease in either group. In sum, these studies support the safety of SSRI treatment for social anxiety disorder in the context of alcohol use disorders and indicate its efficacy for social anxiety disorder without improvement of alcohol consumption.

Another RCT examined combined medication treatments in patients with social anxiety disorder comorbid with pathological sweating (hyperhidrosis), finding that both disorders improved more with combined SSRI and botulinum toxin treatment for sweating than with SSRI alone (Connor et al. 2006). Novel treatments for sweating in patients with social anxiety disorder and those with comorbid hyperhidrosis that have been studied only in open trials include topical aluminum chloride (Bohn and Sternbach 1996) and a surgical procedure, endoscopic thoracic sympathectomy, which has also been advocated as a treatment for severe blushing (Jadresic et al. 2011).

Children

SSRIs and SNRIs are the best-studied medications for social anxiety disorder in children. They have appeared efficacious in two studies limited to the disorder alone and in several other RCTs that included it among other childhood anxiety disorders. Wagner et al. (2004) found paroxetine to be efficacious in children ages 8–17 years, with response rates of 78% for paroxetine and 38% for placebo in a large multicenter RCT. In another multicenter RCT involving the same age group, March et al. (2007) reported efficacy for venlafaxine, with a response rate of 56% versus 37% for placebo. RCTs for childhood anxiety disorders have also shown efficacy for fluoxetine (Birmaher et al. 2003), for fluvoxamine (Research Unit on Pediatric Psychopharmacology Anxiety Study Group 2001), and for sertraline alone and in combination with CBT (Walkup et al. 2008). The α_2-adrenergic agonist guanfacine appeared promising for childhood anxiety disorders in a pilot study (Strawn et al. 2017).

Conclusion

Social anxiety disorder is a very common and often disabling condition that can be treated effectively with CBT and a variety of medications. SSRIs and the SNRI venlafaxine are the best-established first-line pharmacotherapies, according to more than 30 RCTs. Moclobemide has also been widely studied, but it is unavailable in the United States and may be less efficacious than the SSRIs. Benzodiazepines and pregabalin have also appeared efficacious in more than one RCT. One of the most highly efficacious medications is the MAOI phenelzine, but it is generally reserved for highly refractory cases because of its unfavorable side effect profile. Pharmacotherapy for the performance-only subtype of social anxiety disorder has received little study, but limited evidence supports use of β-blockers and benzodiazepines on an as-needed basis.

Key Points

- Selective serotonin reuptake inhibitors (SSRIs) are the first-line pharmacotherapy option for social anxiety disorder based on their efficacy in more than 30 randomized controlled trials (RCTs), benign side effect profile, and efficacy for commonly comorbid depression.

- Multiple RCTs support the efficacy of the serotonin-norepinephrine reuptake inhibitor (SNRI) venlafaxine, pregabalin, the monoamine oxidase inhibitor phenelzine, and the reversible inhibitor of monoamine oxidase moclobemide (marketed outside the United States).

- Multiple RCTs also support the efficacy of benzodiazepines, with the strongest evidence for clonazepam.

- Single RCTs suggest possible efficacy for mirtazapine and gabapentin.

- Responders to an acute course of treatment have a high likelihood of maintaining response if treatment is continued for an additional 6 months, but the optimal duration of treatment has not been established.

- Performance-only social anxiety disorder has not been studied with RCTs of pharmacotherapy, but evidence from analogue studies of performance anxiety suggest efficacy for as-needed use of β-adrenergic blockers.

- SSRIs and SNRIs are the only medication class with multiple RCTs documenting efficacy for social anxiety disorder in children and adolescents.

References

Aarre TF: Phenelzine efficacy in refractory social anxiety disorder: a case series. Nord J Psychiatry 57(4):313–315, 2003 12888407

Aberg-Wistedt A, Agren H, Ekselius L, et al: Sertraline versus paroxetine in major depression: clinical outcome after six months of continuous therapy. J Clin Psychopharmacol 20(6):645–652, 2000 11106136

Adler LA, Liebowitz M, Kronenberger W, et al: Atomoxetine treatment in adults with attention-deficit/hyperactivity disorder and comorbid social anxiety disorder. Depress Anxiety 26(3):212–221, 2009 19194995

Altamura AC, Pioli R, Vitto M, et al: Venlafaxine in social phobia: a study in selective serotonin reuptake inhibitor non-responders. Int Clin Psychopharmacol 14(4):239–245, 1999 10468317

American Psychiatric Association: Diagnostic and Statistical Manual of Mental Disorders, 5th Edition. Arlington, VA, American Psychiatric Association, 2013

Baldwin DS, Stein DJ, Dolberg OT, et al: How long should a trial of escitalopram treatment be in patients with major depressive disorder, generalised anxiety disorder or social anxiety disorder? An exploration of the randomised controlled trial database. Hum Psychopharmacol 24(4):269–275, 2009 19334042

Bergamaschi MM, Queiroz RH, Chagas MH, et al: Cannabidiol reduces the anxiety induced by simulated public speaking in treatment-naïve social phobia patients. Neuropsychopharmacology 36(6):1219–1226, 2011 21307846

Birmaher B, Axelson DA, Monk K, et al: Fluoxetine for the treatment of childhood anxiety disorders. J Am Acad Child Adolesc Psychiatry 42(4):415–423, 2003 12649628

Blanco C, Heimberg RG, Schneier FR, et al: A placebo-controlled trial of phenelzine, cognitive behavioral group therapy, and their combination for social anxiety disorder. Arch Gen Psychiatry 67(3):286–295, 2010 20194829

Blomhoff S, Haug TT, Hellström K, et al: Randomised controlled general practice trial of sertraline, exposure therapy and combined treatment in generalised social phobia. Br J Psychiatry 179:23–30, 2001 11435264

Bohn P, Sternbach H: Topical aluminum chloride for social phobia-related hyperhidrosis. Am J Psychiatry 153(10):1368, 1996 8831456

Bonnet U, Scherbaum N: How addictive are gabapentin and pregabalin? A systematic review. Eur Neuropsychopharmacol 27(12):1185–1215, 2017 28988943

Book SW, Thomas SE, Randall PK, et al: Paroxetine reduces social anxiety in individuals with a co-occurring alcohol use disorder. J Anxiety Disord 22(2):310–318, 2008 17448631

Book SW, Thomas SE, Smith JP, et al: Treating individuals with social anxiety disorder and at-risk drinking: phasing in a brief alcohol intervention following paroxetine. J Anxiety Disord 27(2):252–258, 2013 23523988

Campbell-Sills L, Roy-Byrne PP, Craske MG, et al: Improving outcomes for patients with medication-resistant anxiety: effects of collaborative care with cognitive behavioral therapy. Depress Anxiety 33(12):1099–1106, 2016 27775823

Careri JM, Draine AE, Hanover R, et al: A 12-week double-blind, placebo-controlled, flexible-dose trial of vilazodone in generalized social anxiety disorder. Prim Care Companion CNS Disord 17(6), 2015 27057414

Clark DM, Ehlers A, McManus F, et al: Cognitive therapy versus fluoxetine in generalized social phobia: a randomized placebo-controlled trial. J Consult Clin Psychol 71(6):1058–1067, 2003 14622081

Connor KM, Davidson JR, Potts NL, et al: Discontinuation of clonazepam in the treatment of social phobia. J Clin Psychopharmacol 18(5):373–378, 1998 9790154

Connor KM, Cook JL, Davidson JR: Botulinum toxin treatment of social anxiety disorder with hyperhidrosis: a placebo-controlled double-blind trial. J Clin Psychiatry 67(1):30–36, 2006 16426085

Curtiss J, Andrews L, Davis M, et al: A meta-analysis of pharmacotherapy for social anxiety disorder: an examination of efficacy, moderators, and mediators. Expert Opin Pharmacother 18(3):243–251, 2017 28110555

Davidson JR, Ford SM, Smith RD, et al: Long-term treatment of social phobia with clonazepam. J Clin Psychiatry 52(suppl):16–20, 1991 1757453

Davidson JR, Potts N, Richichi E, et al: Treatment of social phobia with clonazepam and placebo. J Clin Psychopharmacol 13(6):423–428, 1993 8120156

Davidson JR, Foa EB, Huppert JD, et al: Fluoxetine, comprehensive cognitive behavioral therapy, and placebo in generalized social phobia. Arch Gen Psychiatry 61(10):1005–1013, 2004 15466674

de Menezes GB, Coutinho ES, Fontenelle LF, et al: Second-generation antidepressants in social anxiety disorder: meta-analysis of controlled clinical trials. Psychopharmacology (Berl) 215(1):1–11, 2011 21181129

Donahue CB, Kushner MG, Thuras PD, et al: Effect of quetiapine vs. placebo on response to two virtual public speaking exposures in individuals with social phobia. J Anxiety Disord 23(3):362–368, 2009 19157776

Emmanuel NP, Brawman-Mintzer O, Morton WA, et al: Bupropion-SR in treatment of social phobia. Depress Anxiety 12(2):111–113, 2000 11091936

Feltner DE, Liu-Dumaw M, Schweizer E, et al: Efficacy of pregabalin in generalized social anxiety disorder: results of a double-blind, placebo-controlled, fixed-dose study. Int Clin Psychopharmacol 26(4):213–220, 2011 21368587

Gelernter CS, Uhde TW, Cimbolic P, et al: Cognitive-behavioral and pharmacological treatments of social phobia. A controlled study. Arch Gen Psychiatry 48(10):938–945, 1991 1929764

Grant BF, Hasin DS, Blanco C, et al: The epidemiology of social anxiety disorder in the United States: results from the National Epidemiologic Survey on Alcohol and Related Conditions. J Clin Psychiatry 66(11):1351–1361, 2005 16420070

Greist JH, Liu-Dumaw M, Schweizer E, et al: Efficacy of pregabalin in preventing relapse in patients with generalized social anxiety disorder: results of a double-blind, placebo-controlled 26-week study. Int Clin Psychopharmacol 26(5):243–251, 2011 21734588

Guy W: ECDEU Assessment Manual for Psychopharmacology—Revised (DHEW Publ No ADM 76–338). Rockville, MD, U.S. Government Printing Office, 1976

Haug TT, Blomhoff S, Hellstrøm K, et al: Exposure therapy and sertraline in social phobia: 1-year follow-up of a randomised controlled trial. Br J Psychiatry 182:312–318, 2003 12668406

Hofmann SG, Smits JA, Rosenfield D, et al: d-Cycloserine as an augmentation strategy with cognitive-behavioral therapy for social anxiety disorder. Am J Psychiatry 170(7):751–758, 2013 23599046

Jadresic E, Súarez C, Palacios E, et al: Evaluating the efficacy of endoscopic thoracic sympathectomy for generalized social anxiety disorder with blushing complaints: a comparison with sertraline and no treatment—Santiago de Chile 2003–2009. Innov Clin Neurosci 8(11):24–35, 2011 22191086

Kobak KA, Taylor LV, Warner G, et al: St. John's wort versus placebo in social phobia: results from a placebo-controlled pilot study. J Clin Psychopharmacol 25(1):51–58, 2005 15643100

Liebowitz MR: Social phobia. Mod Probl Pharmacopsychiatry 22:141–173, 1987 2885745

Liebowitz MR, Gorman JM, Fyer AJ, et al: Social phobia: review of a neglected anxiety disorder. Arch Gen Psychiatry 42(7):729–736, 1985 2861796

Liebowitz MR, Schneier F, Campeas R, et al: Phenelzine vs atenolol in social phobia: a placebo-controlled comparison. Arch Gen Psychiatry 49(4):290–300, 1992 1558463

Liebowitz MR, Careri J, Blatt K, et al: Vortioxetine versus placebo in major depressive disorder comorbid with social anxiety disorder. Depress Anxiety 34(12):1164–1172, 2017 29166552

March JS, Entusah AR, Rynn M, et al: A randomized controlled trial of venlafaxine ER versus placebo in pediatric social anxiety disorder. Biol Psychiatry 62(10):1149–1154, 2007 17553467

Montgomery SA, Nil R, Dürr-Pal N, et al: A 24-week randomized, double-blind, placebo-controlled study of escitalopram for the prevention of generalized social anxiety disorder. J Clin Psychiatry 66(10):1270–1278, 2005 16259540

Muehlbacher M, Nickel MK, Nickel C, et al: Mirtazapine treatment of social phobia in women: a randomized, double-blind, placebo-controlled study. J Clin Psychopharmacol 25(6):580–583, 2005 16282842

Nordahl HM, Vogel PA, Morken G, et al: Paroxetine, cognitive therapy or their combination in the treatment of social anxiety disorder with and without avoidant personality disorder: a randomized clinical trial. Psychother Psychosom 85(6):346–356, 2016 27744447

Oosterbaan DB, van Balkom AJ, Spinhoven P, et al: The placebo response in social phobia. J Psychopharmacol 15(3):199–203, 2001 11565629

Otto MW, Pollack MH, Gould RA, et al: A comparison of the efficacy of clonazepam and cognitive-behavioral group therapy for the treatment of social phobia. J Anxiety Disord 14(4):345–358, 2000 11043885

Pallanti S, Quercioli L: Resistant social anxiety disorder response to escitalopram. Clin Pract Epidemiol Ment Health 2:35, 2006 17166264

Pande AC, Feltner DE, Jefferson JW, et al: Efficacy of the novel anxiolytic pregabalin in social anxiety disorder: a placebo-controlled, multicenter study. J Clin Psychopharmacol 24(2):141–149, 2004 15206660

Pollack MH, Van Ameringen M, Simon NM, et al: A double-blind randomized controlled trial of augmentation and switch strategies for refractory social anxiety disorder. Am J Psychiatry 171(1):44–53, 2014 24399428

Randall CL, Johnson MR, Thevos AK, et al: Paroxetine for social anxiety and alcohol use in dual-diagnosed patients. Depress Anxiety 14(4):255–262, 2001 11754136

Research Unit on Pediatric Psychopharmacology Anxiety Study Group: Fluvoxamine for the treatment of anxiety disorders in children and adolescents. N Engl J Med 344(17):1279–1285, 2001 11323729

Scahill L, Leckman JF, Schultz RT, et al: A placebo-controlled trial of risperidone in Tourette syndrome. Neurology 60(7):1130–1135, 2003 12682319

Schneier FR, Blanco C, Campeas R, et al: Citalopram treatment of social anxiety disorder with comorbid major depression. Depress Anxiety 17(4):191–196, 2003 12820174

Schutters SI, Van Megen HJ, Van Veen JF, et al: Mirtazapine in generalized social anxiety disorder: a randomized, double-blind, placebo-controlled study. Int Clin Psychopharmacol 25(5):302–304, 2010 20715300

Seedat S, Stein MB: Double-blind, placebo-controlled assessment of combined clonazepam with paroxetine compared with paroxetine monotherapy for generalized social anxiety disorder. J Clin Psychiatry 65(2):244–248, 2004 15003080

Simon NM, Korbly NB, Worthington JJ, et al: Citalopram for social anxiety disorder: an open-label pilot study in refractory and nonrefractory patients. CNS Spectr 7(9):655–657, 2002 15097929

Simon NM, Hoge EA, Fischmann D, et al: An open-label trial of risperidone augmentation for refractory anxiety disorders. J Clin Psychiatry 67(3):381–385, 2006 16649823

Simpson HB, Schneier FR, Campeas RB, et al: Imipramine in the treatment of social phobia. J Clin Psychopharmacol 18(2):132–135, 1998 9555598

Smits JA, Rosenfield D, Davis ML, et al: Yohimbine enhancement of exposure therapy for social anxiety disorder: a randomized controlled trial. Biol Psychiatry 75(11):840–846, 2014 24237691

Stein DJ, Cameron A, Amrein R, et al: Moclobemide is effective and well tolerated in the long-term pharmacotherapy of social anxiety disorder with or without comorbid anxiety disorder. Int Clin Psychopharmacol 17(4):161–170, 2002a 12131599

Stein DJ, Stein MB, Pitts CD, et al: Predictors of response to pharmacotherapy in social anxiety disorder: an analysis of 3 placebo-controlled paroxetine trials. J Clin Psychiatry 63(2):152–155, 2002b 11874217

Stein DJ, Versiani M, Hair T, et al: Efficacy of paroxetine for relapse prevention in social anxiety disorder: a 24-week study. Arch Gen Psychiatry 59(12):1111–1118, 2002c 12470127

Stein MB, Chartier MJ, Hazen AL, et al: Paroxetine in the treatment of generalized social phobia: open-label treatment and double-blind placebo-controlled discontinuation. J Clin Psychopharmacol 16(3):218–222, 1996 8784653

Stein MB, Sareen J, Hami S, Chao J: Pindolol potentiation of paroxetine for generalized social phobia: a double-blind, placebo-controlled, crossover study. Am J Psychiatry 158(10):1725–1727, 2001 11579011

Stein MB, Pollack MH, Bystritsky A, et al: Efficacy of low and higher dose extended-release venlafaxine in generalized social anxiety disorder: a 6-month randomized controlled trial. Psychopharmacology (Berl) 177(3):280–288, 2005 15258718

Strawn JR, Compton SN, Robertson B, et al: Extended release guanfacine in pediatric anxiety disorders: a pilot, randomized, placebo-controlled trial. J Child Adolesc Psychopharmacol 27(1):29–37, 2017 28165762

Taylor JH, Landeros-Weisenberger A, Coughlin C, et al: Ketamine for social anxiety disorder: a randomized, placebo-controlled crossover trial. Neuropsychopharmacology 43(2):325–333, 2018 28849779

Thase ME: Treatment of anxiety disorders with venlafaxine XR. Expert Rev Neurother 6(3):269–282, 2006 16533131

Turner SM, Beidel DC, Jacob RG: Social phobia: a comparison of behavior therapy and atenolol. J Consult Clin Psychol 62(2):350–358, 1994 8201073

Van Ameringen M, Mancini C, Wilson C: Buspirone augmentation of selective serotonin reuptake inhibitors (SSRIs) in social phobia. J Affect Disord 39(2):115–121, 1996 8827420

Van Ameringen M, Mancini C, Oakman J, et al: Nefazodone in the treatment of generalized social phobia: a randomized, placebo-controlled trial. J Clin Psychiatry 68(2):288–295, 2007 17335328

Versiani M, Nardi AE, Figueira I, et al: Double-blind placebo controlled trials with bromazepam. J Bras Psiquiatr 46:167–171, 1997

Wagner KD, Berard R, Stein MB, et al: A multicenter, randomized, double-blind, placebo-controlled trial of paroxetine in children and adolescents with social anxiety disorder. Arch Gen Psychiatry 61(11):1153–1162, 2004 15520363

Walker JR, Van Ameringen MA, Swinson R, et al: Prevention of relapse in generalized social phobia: results of a 24-week study in responders to 20 weeks of sertraline treatment. J Clin Psychopharmacol 20(6):636–644, 2000 11106135

Walkup JT, Albano AM, Piacentini J, et al: Cognitive behavioral therapy, sertraline, or a combination in childhood anxiety. N Engl J Med 359(26):2753–2766, 2008 18974308

Williams T, Hattingh CJ, Kariuki CM, et al: Pharmacotherapy for social anxiety disorder (SAnD). Cochrane Database Syst Rev 10:CD001206, 2017 29048739

Recommended Readings

Liebowitz MR, Gorman JM, Fyer AJ, et al: Social phobia: review of a neglected anxiety disorder. Arch Gen Psychiatry 42(7):729–736, 1985 2861796

Williams T, Hattingh CJ, Kariuki CM, et al: Pharmacotherapy for social anxiety disorder (SAnD). Cochrane Database Syst Rev 10:CD001206, 2017 29048739

CHAPTER 27

Psychotherapy for Social Anxiety Disorder

Arielle Horenstein, M.A.

Michaela B. Swee, M.A.

Simona C. Kaplan, M.A.

Richard G. Heimberg, Ph.D.

In the four decades since the publication of DSM-III (American Psychiatric Association 1980), researchers have gathered significant empirical support for the efficacy of psychotherapy for social anxiety disorder. Cognitive-behavioral therapies (CBTs) are the most well-studied psychological treatments for the disorder and demonstrate efficacy and effectiveness in both individual and group formats. Other effective treatments include mindfulness and acceptance-based therapies, psychodynamic therapy, interpersonal psychotherapy (IPT), and technology-based interventions. In this chapter, we review and summarize existing empirical support for these psychotherapeutic treatments as well as other factors that may be important to consider for treatment.

Cognitive-Behavioral Therapy

Theoretical Model

Social anxiety disorder is characterized by pervasive and chronic fear of negative evaluation by others, often leading to significant interpersonal and occupational impairment (American Psychiatric Association 2013). Clark and Wells (1995) and Rapee and Heimberg (1997) proposed that individuals with social anxiety disorder hold negative assumptions about themselves and others that lead them to be hypervigilant for threat cues in social situations, subsequently initiating a set of cognitive and behavioral processes that further enhance perceived threat and associated anxiety. For instance, Rapee and Heimberg (1997) suggested that when these individuals perceive an evaluative audience, a negative image/representation of the self is initiated, and they begin to attend to both internal cues (e.g., racing heart, heat in the face) and external cues (e.g., others' facial expressions, body language) that, even if ambiguous, are interpreted as signs that they are performing poorly or being negatively evaluated. Individuals might also use "safety behaviors" (e.g., standing at the periphery of a group) in a maladaptive attempt to reduce anxiety and prevent negative evaluation (Clark and Wells 1995; Piccirillo et al. 2016). These behaviors may reduce anxiety in the short term but ultimately prevent individuals from fully engaging in social interactions and gathering evidence that the negative evaluation they fear may not occur. In a revised model, Heimberg et al. (2014) proposed that individuals also engage in both anticipatory and postevent processing of social events (Brozovich and Heimberg 2008; Clark and Wells 1995), such that they anticipate social events with trepidation and engage in negatively biased post-hoc review of their performance, leading to the maintenance of a negative self-image and increased likelihood that future social situations will be avoided or viewed as threatening.

Hofmann (2007) additionally emphasized that perceived and actual social skills difficulties among patients with social anxiety disorder contribute to the anticipation of social failures and avoidance of social situations. Wong and Rapee's (2016) model emphasized etiological factors (e.g., inherited tendencies, family and peer experiences) that contribute to the degree of threat an individual assigns to social-evaluative stimuli and the subsequent development of the cognitive and behavioral processes described. Consistent with these and earlier cognitive-behavioral models, CBTs include various combinations of cognitive restructuring (i.e., identifying and questioning maladaptive thought patterns) and exposure (i.e., engagement with feared situations) to help patients reduce avoidance and modify negative schemas related to social situations. CBT has been delivered in both individual and group formats; although some studies have demonstrated greater benefit with individual CBT than group CBT (Mörtberg et al. 2007; Stangier et al. 2003), the overwhelming evidence suggests little difference in efficacy between these modalities (Barkowski et al. 2016).

Exposure-Only Treatment

Exposure therapy is designed to allow patients to engage with feared situations in a systematic, graduated fashion, typically through imaginal exposures, in-session/role-play-based exposures, or in vivo exposures (i.e., in the patient's real life). In doing so, patients are given the opportunity to habituate to feared stimuli and to modify previously held dysfunctional beliefs about social situations. Inhibitory learning has been proposed as one of the primary mechanisms of action in exposures, during which a new learned response to the social situation competes with the previously learned fear response (Bouton 2002). Achieving inhibitory learning within exposure therapy necessitates violating the patient's expectation of aversive outcomes, preventing or removing safety behaviors and safety signals, and completing exposures across multiple contexts (Craske et al. 2014b). Other exposure-based approaches include interoceptive exposure (i.e., repeated exposure to anxiety-related bodily sensations; Dixon et al. 2015) and virtual reality exposure (VRE; e.g., exposure in a computer-generated virtual environment), as well as the addition of video feedback procedures (Warnock-

Parkes et al. 2017). In comparative studies, exposure as a stand-alone treatment has proven superior to both waitlist control conditions (Newman et al. 1994) and progressive muscle relaxation training (Al-Kubaisy et al. 1992). Studies have demonstrated significant reductions in social anxiety following non-therapist-aided in vivo exposure "homework" that were maintained after 1 year (Fava et al. 1989) and at 2-, 5-, and 10-year follow-ups (Fava et al. 2001).

Combined Cognitive Restructuring and Exposure Therapy

Cognitive restructuring—or the process of identifying, disputing, and modifying maladaptive thought patterns and beliefs—is based on the notion that anxiety arises because of a person's thoughts about a situation, not situation itself (Beck and Emery 1985). Cognitive restructuring in combination with exposure techniques ("combined CBT") is the most common and most well researched form of CBT. Many studies have examined the efficacy of combined CBT protocols based on the work of Clark and Wells (1995) or Heimberg and colleagues (Heimberg and Becker 2002; Hope et al. 2010).

Combined CBT has compared favorably to waitlist conditions. Gains have been maintained in combined CBT at 3-month (Ledley et al. 2009), 6-month (Mörtberg et al. 2006; Stangier et al. 2003), and 1-year (Goldin et al. 2012) follow-ups. Combined CBT has also compared favorably to more rigorous control conditions, such as in two studies that compared group CBT to educational-supportive psychotherapy (Heimberg et al. 1990, 1998). In a follow-up of the first study, gains made by those in group CBT were maintained at 5-year follow-up (Heimberg et al. 1993). However, one study found that group CBT was not superior to a control group psychotherapy (based on the educational/supportive control used in Heimberg et al. 1990 and Heimberg et al. 1998) (Bjornsson et al. 2011); this finding may have been due to use of an abbreviated version of Heimberg and Becker's (2002) protocol. Several studies have also found combined CBT superior to pill placebo (Clark et al. 2003; Heimberg et al. 1998).

Despite the theoretical benefit of a combined CBT approach over exposure therapy alone, several meta-analyses have found no significant differences between combined CBT and exposure-only treatment for social anxiety disorder (Acarturk et al. 2009; Feske and Chambless 1995; Powers et al. 2008). The meta-analysis by Mayo-Wilson et al. (2014) found that across studies, both combined CBT in either individual or group modalities and exposure-only treatments were superior to waitlist conditions; however, only individual combined CBT was superior to psychological placebos.

Cognitive-Behavioral Therapy Compared to or Combined With Medication

Relative Efficacy of Cognitive-Behavioral Therapy and Medication

Some studies indicate that CBT is as efficacious as medication for social anxiety disorder but that the two treatment modalities may differ in their rates of improvement and relapse. Heimberg et al. (1998) randomized 133 patients to receive group CBT, educational/supportive psychotherapy, the monoamine oxidase inhibitor (MAOI) phenelzine, or pill placebo. Individuals in the group CBT and phenelzine cohorts demonstrated better response rates and symptom reduction than those in the educational/supportive therapy and placebo groups. The phenelzine cohort had more midtreatment responders than the group CBT cohort and improved more on several measures of social anxiety at 12 weeks. However, in a follow-up study (Liebowitz et al. 1999), individuals who had received phenelzine were more likely to relapse compared to those who had received group CBT. Otto et al. (2000) somewhat similarly found that group CBT, compared to clonazepam, was equally efficacious but slower acting; although clonazepam was superior to group CBT on a few outcome measures at 12 weeks, no differences were found between the treatments in remission rates or several measures of social anxiety at 24 weeks.

Several studies have demonstrated that CBT is superior to medication for individuals with social anxiety disorder. Clark et al. (2003) randomized patients to one of three conditions: cognitive therapy (CT; based on Clark and Wells's [1995] model), self-exposure (instructions and homework for completing in vivo exposures at home) plus the selective serotonin reuptake inhibitor (SSRI) fluoxetine, or self-exposure plus pill placebo. Patients in all conditions improved, but those who received CT improved more than those who received self-exposure with fluoxetine or placebo, and CT was superior to fluoxetine with self-exposure after 12 months. Turner et al. (1994) randomized 72 patients to receive exposure therapy (both in vivo and imaginal exposure exercises), atenolol (a β-blocker), or pill placebo. Only the exposure therapy yielded greater improvements than placebo, and individuals in that group performed significantly better than those given atenolol on measures of global impairment, avoidance of social situations, behavioral measures from a speech task, with rates of at least moderate improvement (88.9% vs. 46.6%). In another randomized controlled trial (RCT), Oosterbaan et al. (2001) assigned 82 patients to receive CT, the reversible MAOI moclobemide, or pill placebo. CT patients improved more than those who received moclobemide—but not pill placebo—at posttreatment and significantly more than both groups at 2-month follow-up.

Combined Cognitive-Behavioral Therapy and Medication

Overall, evidence for the added benefit of combining psychiatric and psychological treatment for social anxiety disorder is limited and inconclusive. One study that compared CBT plus the SSRI fluoxetine to either CBT plus placebo or CBT alone found these treatment variations to be equally efficacious (Davidson et al. 2004). Some studies have found that combining phenelzine with group CBT (Blanco et al. 2010) or the SSRI escitalopram with internet-delivered CBT (iCBT; Gingnell et al. 2016) leads to better outcomes compared to group CBT alone or iCBT combined with pill placebo, respectively. Other studies suggest that CBT without medication is superior in the longer term, showing greater improvements after 1-year follow-up in those who did not take medication in combination with CBT than in those who did (Nordahl et al. 2016).

Social Skills Training or a Relational Focus

Social skills training (SST) is a behavioral intervention focused on teaching the social skills necessary to achieve desired social outcomes. The principles of SST generally assume that individuals with social anxiety disorder exhibit certain social skills difficulties, such as poor eye contact and difficulty with conversation maintenance, that may be perceived negatively by others and lead to worse interpersonal outcomes (Lucock and Salkovskis 1988). Common techniques used in SST include therapist modeling, behavioral rehearsal, corrective feedback, social reinforcement, and homework assignments. However, whether the social skills deficits observed in patients should be attributed to a true deficit or to anxiety-induced behavioral inhibition has been debated, because many individuals report a lack of social skills due to underestimation of their own performance (Rapee and Lim 1992), suggesting that at least self-reported deficits are an issue of self-perception rather than true lack of skill. There seems to be limited empirical support for SST as a stand-alone intervention (Ponniah and Hollon 2008), although one study showed that group SST and group CT both led to improvements in social anxiety among adults with social anxiety disorder and did not differ from each other (Bögels and Voncken 2008). SST, however, has been shown to be useful as an add-on to CBT (rather than as a stand-alone intervention): studies have demonstrated that group CBT (Herbert et al. 2005) and exposure therapy (Beidel et al. 2014) yield better outcomes when augmented with SST. A similar line of research has examined the addition of a "relational" focus to CBT. A relational focus emphasizes social skills such as openness and self-disclosure, emotional expression, reciprocity, and responsivity within conversations with others (Alden et al. 2018). Two studies have demonstrated that CBT with a relational focus leads to better outcomes compared to a waitlist condition (Alden and Taylor 2011) and to a graduated exposure–applied relaxation treatment regimen (Alden et al. 2018). However, no studies have directly compared CBT with and CBT without a relational focus, limiting any conclusions regarding its efficacy as a true augmentation to CBT.

Negative Self-Imagery and Imagery Rescripting

Research has shown that many of the negative self-images patients with social anxiety disorder hold of themselves in social situations are often linked to early and socially traumatic events (Hackmann et al. 2000). A technique termed "imagery rescripting" has been developed to address these self-images through procedures focused on changing the original unpleasant memory. The rescripting technique involves repeating the memory while inserting corrective information and compassionate imagery into new iterations of the memory (Stopa 2009). Imagery rescripting has been found to reduce social anxiety and negative social beliefs (Wild et al. 2007), and a single session of imagery rescripting led to greater reductions in social anxiety and negative appraisal of autobiographical memories than a nonintervention control (Reimer and Moscovitch 2015). Norton and Abbott (2016) found imagery rescripting and cognitive restructuring to be equally efficacious.

Effectiveness Trials

Although controlled trials of CBT and its variations have provided substantial support for the efficacy of these treatments, the generalizability and transportability of CBT can be better understood through an examination of effectiveness trials, which are conducted in less controlled settings and among more diverse patient populations. Several of these trials have demonstrated the effectiveness of CBT in outpatient

(Lincoln et al. 2003), private (Gaston et al. 2006), and community settings (McEvoy et al. 2012), with many of these studies yielding improvements in social anxiety with large effect sizes comparable to those found in most efficacy trials.

Mindfulness and Acceptance-Based Treatments

Mindfulness and acceptance-based treatments have been utilized as treatments for social anxiety disorder since the early 2000s. Overall, the goal of mindfulness and acceptance-based treatments is to assist patients in reducing attempts to control unwanted internal experiences in social situations, which in turn can help end a vicious circle of increased self-focused attention, greater control efforts, and heightened social anxiety (Herbert and Cardaciotto 2005).

Acceptance and Commitment Therapy

Acceptance and commitment therapy (ACT; Hayes et al. 2011) helps patients foster acceptance of unwanted thoughts and feelings and simultaneously engage in meaningful behavior change. ACT includes the use of techniques such as cognitive defusion (i.e., separating oneself from inner experiences), mindfulness and acceptance, identification of values or areas of meaning in one's life, and committed action (i.e., engaging in behavior in line with one's values). The application of ACT to treatment of social anxiety disorder has produced promising results. An early study examining the efficacy of a 12-week integrated ACT and exposure therapy among 19 patients found significant decreases in social anxiety, fear of negative evaluation, and experiential avoidance, as well as a significant increase in quality of life at posttreatment and at 3-month follow-up (Dalrymple and Herbert 2007). In a study examining mindfulness- and acceptance-based group therapy, which is largely based on ACT, 137 subjects with social anxiety disorder were randomly assigned to group CBT, mindfulness and acceptance-based group therapy, or a waitlist control condition. Mindfulness and acceptance-based group therapy and group CBT were both superior to the waitlist condition and did not differ from each other on any outcome measures (Kocovski et al. 2013). Another study compared the relative efficacy of individual ACT, CBT, and a waitlist control condition among 87 patients with social anxiety disorder and also found no differences in outcomes between active treatments, although both were superior to the waitlist condition (Craske et al. 2014a).

Mindfulness-Based Stress Reduction

Mindfulness-based stress reduction (MBSR; Kabat-Zinn 1990) uses intensive training in mindfulness meditation as its core intervention. It typically includes training in body scan meditation, sitting meditation, mindful stretching, and mindfulness as a method for noticing reactions and responding in new ways in social situations. Koszycki et al. (2016) compared 12 weeks of an intervention based on MBSR, with additional explicit training in self-compassion and exposure procedures, to a waitlist condition among 39 adults with social anxiety disorder and found that patients in the MBSR group had greater reductions in social anxiety, depression, and social adjustment and gains were maintained at 3-month follow-up. In a study comparing MBSR (completed in eight group sessions, a 1-day meditation retreat, and daily home practice) to an aerobic exercise control condition, both groups showed significant improvements in social anxiety, depression, and subjective well-being at posttreatment and 3-month follow-up; overall, MBSR did not outperform the control condition, and the effect sizes in MBSR were smaller than those typically found in CBT trials (Jazaieri et al. 2012).

Other trials directly comparing MBSR to CBT have yielded mixed results. Koszycki et al. 2007 compared 8 weeks of MBSR to 12 weeks of group CBT (based on Heimberg and Becker 2002) among 53 patients with social anxiety disorder and found that MBSR was similar to group CBT in reducing depression and improving quality of life, but group CBT was superior to MBSR in reducing social anxiety symptom severity and had higher response and remission rates. Goldin et al. (2016) compared 12 weekly sessions of group CBT (based on Heimberg and Becker 2002 and Hope et al. 2010) to MBSR and a waitlist condition and found that the reduction in social anxiety was significantly greater in both treatment conditions compared to the waitlist condition and not significantly different from each other at posttreatment, with gains maintained for both treatments at 1-year follow-up.

Psychodynamic Therapy

Several psychodynamic models of social anxiety disorder have been proposed over the years. One model (Leichsenring et al. 2007) focuses on the "Core Conflictual Relationship Theme" (CCRT; Luborsky 1984) and proposes that the CCRT in social anxiety disorder comprises three main components: the wish or desire of the individual (e.g., a wish to be affirmed), the anticipated response from others to that desire or wish (e.g., others will reject me), and the response from the self (e.g., "I won't expose my true self to others"). The therapist focuses on identifying the CCRT for the patient, considering how it arises within the patient–therapist relationship as well as other relationships and supporting the patient in confronting anxiety-producing situations.

In a multicenter controlled noninferiority trial conducted in Germany in 495 adults with social anxiety disorder, patients were randomized to 25 sessions of CT (Clark and Wells 1995), psychodynamic therapy (Leichsenring et al. 2007), or a waitlist. Both treatments were superior to the waitlist condition and did not differ in their response rates, but significantly more CT patients (36%) than psychodynamic psychotherapy patients (26%) remitted and improved on measures of social anxiety and interpersonal symptoms (Leichsenring et al. 2013); however, no differences were found between treatments at 6-month follow-up, and response and remission rates at 2-year follow-up were similar (Leichsenring et al. 2014). Therefore, it seems that although CBT may be more effective than psychodynamic therapy immediately posttreatment, few differences exist between the treatments in the long term. Bögels et al. (2014) compared the efficacy of up to 36 sessions of either psychodynamic psychotherapy or CBT in 47 adults with social anxiety disorder and found that both treatments demonstrated large reductions in social anxiety, with no difference in rates of clinically significant change between the two conditions at either posttreatment or 1-year follow-up. However, CBT required fewer sessions to yield the same outcomes as psychodynamic therapy. Therefore, CBT may lead to a faster, although not necessarily greater, rate of improvement compared to psychodynamic treatments. A meta-analysis by Mayo-

Wilson et al. (2014) also demonstrated that individual CBT was generally more effective in treating social anxiety disorder than psychodynamic psychotherapy.

Interpersonal Psychotherapy

IPT (Klerman et al. 1984) is based on a model in which symptoms of psychological disorders occur and are maintained within an interpersonal context; therefore, IPT aims to reduce symptoms by targeting interpersonal difficulties. Treatment includes review and identification of symptoms as part of a known treatable disorder, assessment of current and past relationships (the "interpersonal inventory"), and a focus on specific interpersonal problem areas linked to social anxiety, using techniques that help patients express their full range of feelings regarding interpersonal problem areas and develop ways to fix or adaptively cope with them (Lipsitz et al. 2008).

In a study comparing IPT to a supportive therapy control, both conditions led to significant improvements in social anxiety, but they did not differ significantly from each other (Lipsitz et al. 2008). However, due to the supportive and interpersonally focused elements of the control condition, it was not clear whether IPT did not outperform the control condition because of its limited efficacy or because of the potentially active nature of the control condition. In a study conducted by Borge et al. (2008), 80 patients with treatment-refractory social anxiety disorder were randomly assigned to 10 weeks of residential CT (based on Clark and Wells 1995) or residential IPT, both adapted to be more intensive and include both individual and group elements. Individuals in both the IPT and CT groups demonstrated significant improvements that did not differ from each other at posttreatment. Both groups also continued to improve at a 1-year follow-up. Stangier et al. (2011) randomized 117 adults to 16 sessions over 20 weeks, plus one booster session of CT (based on Clark and Wells 1995) or IPT, or to a waitlist control condition. CT was superior to the IPT and waitlist conditions on one social anxiety outcome measure, and these differences were maintained at 1-year follow-up. In addition, more CT patients than IPT patients and control subjects were categorized as responders at posttreatment and 1-year follow-up. Overall, evidence seems to suggest that IPT is efficacious in treating social anxiety disorder but may be less so relative to CBT.

Technology-Based Interventions

As technology proliferates, novel technology-assisted therapeutic interventions for social anxiety have emerged, including internet-delivered therapies, computer programs, and VRE. Given that approximately one-third of people with lifetime social anxiety disorder never seek treatment (Ruscio et al. 2008), these interventions may be especially important given their potential utility in assisting those who face barriers to in-person care.

Internet- or Computer-Assisted Interventions

Numerous studies have examined the efficacy of iCBT. Typically, iCBT requires patients to work through treatment modules and complete homework assignments (e.g., exposures) independently. Some protocols offer online forums, discussion groups, or opportunities to consult with a therapist or coach via phone, text, or email. A study comparing 9 weeks of iCBT to a waitlist condition demonstrated favorable outcomes in social anxiety, avoidance, general anxiety, and depression at posttreatment and 12-month follow-up (Carlbring et al. 2007), with gains maintained 30 months later (Carlbring et al. 2009). Meta-analytic results support the superiority of iCBT over several other control interventions, as well as its equivalence to face-to-face CBT (Andrews et al. 2018). Other trials have found iCBT comparable to group CBT at posttreatment and at 6-month and 4-year follow-ups (Hedman et al. 2011, 2014). An integrated acceptance-based iCBT either with or without 10–15 minutes of weekly therapist videoconferencing and daily text message support resulted in significant improvement in social anxiety symptoms and reported quality of life across both groups (Gershkovich et al. 2017), although patients who received therapist support showed less attrition. iCBT for social anxiety disorder has also been examined in effectiveness trials. El Alaoui et al. (2015) found that in an outpatient clinic, therapist-guided iCBT resulted in a reduction of social anxiety and depressive symptoms, and improvements were comparable to those demonstrated in efficacy trials of face-to-face CBT.

Mobile or Application-Based Interventions

iCBT delivered via smartphone applications ("apps") is a modernized alternative to iCBT delivered via computer and allows patients more mobility as they engage in interventions. In an RCT comparing 12 weeks of mobile CBT to both iCBT on a desktop computer and a waitlist condition, researchers found that both active treatments were superior to the waitlist condition and equivalent to one another in reducing social anxiety and increasing overall well-being (Stolz et al. 2018). Dagöö et al. (2014) compared 9 weeks of a mobile version of CBT with a mobile version of IPT for patients with social anxiety disorder and found that more patients were classified as responders in mobile CBT (55.6%) than in mobile IPT (8.0%), although both groups evinced significant reductions in social anxiety at posttreatment. Boettcher et al. (2018) examined the efficacy of pairing a cognitive-behavioral self-help program with an app that guides patients in completing exposure exercises and offers the opportunity for patients to seek anonymous feedback from other users, compared to the efficacy of a sequential treatment (i.e., the self-help program followed by app use) or a waitlist condition. Both interventions resulted in equivalent and large decreases in social anxiety that were maintained at 4- and 12-month follow-ups. However, the sequential group evidenced larger decreases in social anxiety at 12-month follow-up, suggesting a potential long-term benefit of using the app after completing the self-help program.

Virtual Reality Exposure

VRE allows patients to immerse themselves in feared environments with sights and sounds that realistically simulate in vivo social situations. VRE can be structured around a patient's specific feared situations, and therapists can use voiceover and computer manipulations in real time to alter the course of the exposure (Anderson et al. 2013). In an RCT comparing VRE to in vivo exposure therapy (iVET) and a waitlist control condition, VRE and iVET both led to significant decreases in social anxiety, although iVET was superior and maintained gains at 3-month follow-up (Kampmann et al. 2016a). However, another RCT comparing CBT plus VRE to both iVET and a waitlist control group found that both interventions led to significant reductions in social anxiety but that VRE was slightly superior and that therapists rated it as more practical (Bouchard et al. 2017). In a study of individuals with social anxiety disorder and a primary fear of public speaking, VRE was compared to group exposure therapy and a waitlist condition (Anderson et al. 2013). Both treatments were superior to the waitlist condition and equally efficacious, and gains were maintained after 6 months (Anderson et al. 2017). Overall, the literature suggests that VRE is comparably efficacious to iCBT for social anxiety disorder (Kampmann et al. 2016b).

Factors Affecting Treatment Outcome and Other Important Considerations

Comorbidity With Other Disorders

Approximately half of patients with social anxiety disorder meet diagnostic criteria for at least one additional anxiety disorder, 39% meet criteria for a comorbid mood disorder, and about 50% have a comorbid alcohol or substance use disorder (Grant et al. 2005). Therefore, understanding the impact of these common comorbidities on treatment outcome is crucial. In a study of individuals with social anxiety disorder with no comorbid disorders, those with a comorbid anxiety disorder, and those with a comorbid mood disorder, the comorbid anxiety disorder condition responded to group CBT similarly to those with no comorbid disorders, whereas those with a comorbid mood disorder had more severe symptoms at pre- and posttreatment (Erwin et al. 2002), suggesting that comorbid mood disorders may complicate treatment of social anxiety disorder more so than comorbid anxiety disorders. Research has also indicated that comorbidity between social anxiety disorder and substance use disorders is associated with greater severity of both disorders and decreased treatment seeking (Schneier et al. 2010). These findings are important for clinicians to keep in mind as they treat clients who have social anxiety disorder and common comorbid conditions.

Therapeutic Alliance

The therapeutic or working alliance can also affect treatment outcome, although the literature is mixed on this topic. Some studies have shown that patient-rated alliance predicts posttreatment reductions in social anxiety (Hayes et al. 2007), whereas other research suggests it does not (Adler et al. 2018; Haug et al. 2016). A study comparing group CBT and group MBSR found that the patient-rated working alliance was significantly predictive of social anxiety reductions in the short and long term for those in MBSR but not for those in CBT (Jazaieri et al. 2018).

Moderators and Mediators of Treatment Outcome

Research has identified several moderators and mediators of treatment outcome for social anxiety disorder; a few notable findings are summarized briefly here. Cognitive reappraisal self-efficacy—that is, the belief that one can successfully reframe circumstances in a manner that promotes emotion regulation—is a mediator of social anxiety reduction in CBT (Goldin et al. 2012), and cognitive reappraisal mediates improvement in mindfulness and acceptance-based group therapy (Kocovski et al. 2015). Goldin et al. (2016) examined mediators of group CBT and MBSR and found that cognitive reappraisal, attention focusing and shifting, mindfulness skills, and reductions in safety behaviors and cognitive distortions all mediated the effect of either treatment on social anxiety. Another study found that changes in negative thinking predict reductions in social anxiety and depression in both CBT and ACT (Niles et al. 2014). Diverting attention away from oneself toward external stimuli has also been shown to mediate improvements in CT (Mörtberg et al. 2015).

Additionally, patient traits and experiences moderate treatment outcome and, in some cases, differentially predict outcomes in distinct treatments for social anxiety disorder. Individuals with lower distress tolerance and higher intolerance of uncertainty exhibit higher symptom severity across multiple time points in CBT (Katz et al. 2017). Individuals with poorer psychological flexibility and stronger fears of negative evaluation achieve better outcomes in CBT than in ACT (Craske et al. 2014a). In contrast, more rapid changes in experiential avoidance toward the beginning of treatment are associated with reductions in social anxiety and depression at the end of ACT but not CBT (Niles et al. 2014). The effect of attentional bias may also interact with treatment type, with individuals who exhibit more severe attentional bias exhibiting greater reduction in therapist-rated fear and avoidance in CBT than in ACT (Niles et al. 2013).

Conclusion and Future Directions

To date, most efficacy research has focused on CBT for social anxiety disorder; overall, evidence suggests that exposure-only treatment is as efficacious as combined CBT and that individual and group formats are equally beneficial. Furthermore, CBT seems to be as efficacious as pharmacological treatments; although CBT may take longer to reduce symptoms in some cases, it seems to be associated with lower relapse risk and longer-term gains. Additionally, effectiveness trials have demonstrated CBT's utility in a variety of mental health settings.

Although other treatments have a smaller evidence base than CBT, ACT and MBSR seem to be efficacious treatments. Evidence indicates that IPT and psychodynamic therapy are also efficacious, but with some indication that they are neither as efficacious nor as fast-acting as CBT. Finally, technology-assisted CBT has evolved over the years and proven to be a novel treatment approach, with many of these technology-based interventions being as efficacious as face-to-face interventions.

Future research on psychotherapy for social anxiety disorder is warranted in several areas. Perhaps one of the most notable gaps in the literature is evidence for the efficacy and effectiveness of empirically supported treatments among minority populations. Some research suggests that racial and ethnic minorities often experience a more chronic course (Sibrava et al. 2013) and report more barriers to treatment (Goetter et al. 2018), and one study found that Latinx patients with anxiety disorders attended fewer sessions and scored lower on perceived understanding of CBT principles

(Chavira et al. 2014). Studies such as these indicate a need for more diverse treatment research and development of clinical practice that is sensitive to minority stressors and needs. The need to tailor interventions to patients who experience social anxiety disorder in the context of marginalization or discrimination should also be explored.

More work is also needed in refining treatments to simultaneously address psychological conditions that are commonly comorbid with social anxiety disorder. Although people with social anxiety disorder and comorbid anxiety disorders may respond to treatment as well as individuals with no comorbid disorders, comorbid mood symptoms may complicate treatment and warrant a supplemental approach. Additionally, limited research is available on the concurrent treatment of social anxiety disorder and substance use disorders. More work is needed to understand how substance use, which is common among individuals with social anxiety disorder, might affect treatment outcome.

Finally, not all patients achieve symptom reduction or remission, suggesting room for improvement in tailoring interventions for social anxiety disorder so they can adequately address the needs of a larger percentage of patients. Using research on patient characteristics that affect treatment outcome to refine treatments or assign patients to specific treatments that are based on these individual characteristics may be one route to increasing rates of improvement. A better understanding of how patient characteristics affect outcome as well as research on the feasibility of routing individuals to appropriate care based on these characteristics could also be important future goals for the field.

Key Points

- Overall, cognitive-behavioral therapy has the most evidence for the treatment of social anxiety disorder, and other promising treatment approaches may also be efficacious. Taking each of these approaches into consideration, the following treatment components seem to be important:

    - Providing patients with psychoeducation and a conceptualization of social anxiety disorder through a cognitive-behavioral, acceptance-based, interpersonal, or psychodynamic framework

    - Helping patients develop alternative methods or strategies for managing anxiety in social situations (e.g., cognitive restructuring, imagery rescripting, mindfulness, cognitive defusion, interpersonal problem solving)

    - Exposing patients to feared social situations, either in imagery, in session, in vivo, or via technology-assisted interventions, with the aim of generalizing learning across contexts

    - Providing patients training in other skills or approaches that can facilitate social approach and reductions in anxiety

References

Acarturk C, Cuijpers P, van Straten A, et al: Psychological treatment of social anxiety disorder: a meta-analysis. Psychol Med 39(2):241–254, 2009 18507874

Adler G, Shahar B, Dolev T, et al: The development of the working alliance and its ability to predict outcome in emotion-focused therapy for social anxiety disorder. J Nerv Ment Dis 206(6):446–454, 2018 29782423

Al-Kubaisy T, Marks IM, Logsdail S, et al: Role of exposure homework in phobia reduction: a controlled study. Behav Ther 23:599–621, 1992

Alden LE, Taylor CT: Relational treatment strategies increase social approach behaviors in patients with generalized social anxiety disorder. J Anxiety Disord 25(3):309–318, 2011 21094019

Alden LE, Buhr K, Robichaud M, et al: Treatment of social approach processes in adults with social anxiety disorder. J Consult Clin Psychol 86(6):505–517, 2018 29781649

American Psychiatric Association: Diagnostic and Statistical Manual of Mental Disorders, 3rd Edition. Washington, DC, American Psychiatric Association, 1980

American Psychiatric Association: Diagnostic and Statistical Manual of Mental Disorders, 5th Edition. Arlington, VA, American Psychiatric Association, 2013

Anderson PL, Price M, Edwards SM, et al: Virtual reality exposure therapy for social anxiety disorder: a randomized controlled trial. J Consult Clin Psychol 81(5):751–760, 2013 23796315

Anderson PL, Edwards SM, Goodnight JR: Virtual reality and exposure group therapy for social anxiety disorder: results from a 4–6 year follow-up. Cognit Ther Res 41:230–236, 2017

Andrews G, Basu A, Cuijpers P, et al: Computer therapy for the anxiety and depression disorders is effective, acceptable and practical health care: an updated meta-analysis. J Anxiety Disord 55:70–78, 2018 29422409

Barkowski S, Schwartze D, Strauss B, et al: Efficacy of group psychotherapy for social anxiety disorder: a meta-analysis of randomized-controlled trials. J Anxiety Disord 39:44–64, 2016 26953823

Beck AT, Emery G: Anxiety Disorders and Phobias: A Cognitive Perspective. New York, Basic Books, 1985

Beidel DC, Alfano CA, Kofler MJ, et al: The impact of social skills training for social anxiety disorder: a randomized controlled trial. J Anxiety Disord 28(8):908–918, 2014 25445081

Bjornsson AS, Bidwell LC, Brosse AL, et al: Cognitive-behavioral group therapy versus group psychotherapy for social anxiety disorder among college students: a randomized controlled trial. Depress Anxiety 28(11):1034–1042, 2011 22076970

Blanco C, Heimberg RG, Schneier FR, et al: A placebo-controlled trial of phenelzine, cognitive behavioral group therapy, and their combination for social anxiety disorder. Arch Gen Psychiatry 67(3):286–295, 2010 20194829

Boettcher J, Magnusson K, Marklund A, et al: Adding a smartphone app to internet-based self-help for social anxiety: a randomized controlled trial. Comput Human Behav 87:98–108, 2018

Bögels SM, Voncken M: Social skills training versus cognitive therapy for social anxiety disorder characterized by fear of blushing, trembling, or sweating. Int J Cogn Ther 1:138–150, 2008

Bögels SM, Wijts P, Oort FJ, et al: Psychodynamic psychotherapy versus cognitive behavior therapy for social anxiety disorder: an efficacy and partial effectiveness trial. Depress Anxiety 31(5):363–373, 2014 24577880

Borge FM, Hoffart A, Sexton H, et al: Residential cognitive therapy versus residential interpersonal therapy for social phobia: a randomized clinical trial. J Anxiety Disord 22(6):991–1010, 2008 18035519

Bouchard S, Dumoulin S, Robillard G, et al: Virtual reality compared with in vivo exposure in the treatment of social anxiety disorder: a three-arm randomised controlled trial. Br J Psychiatry 210(4):276–283, 2017 27979818

Bouton ME: Context, ambiguity, and unlearning: sources of relapse after behavioral extinction. Biol Psychiatry 52(10):976–986, 2002 12437938

Brozovich F, Heimberg RG: An analysis of post-event processing in social anxiety disorder. Clin Psychol Rev 28(6):891–903, 2008 18294745

Carlbring P, Gunnarsdóttir M, Hedensjö L, et al: Treatment of social phobia: randomised trial of internet-delivered cognitive-behavioural therapy with telephone support. Br J Psychiatry 190:123–128, 2007 17267928

Carlbring P, Nordgren LB, Furmark T, et al: Long-term outcome of internet-delivered cognitive-behavioural therapy for social phobia: a 30-month follow-up. Behav Res Ther 47(10):848–850, 2009 19631312

Chavira DA, Golinelli D, Sherbourne C, et al: Treatment engagement and response to CBT among Latinos with anxiety disorders in primary care. J Consult Clin Psychol 82(3):392–403, 2014 24660674

Clark DM, Wells A: A cognitive model of social phobia, in Social Phobia: Diagnosis, Assessment and Treatment. Edited by Heimberg RG, Liebowitz MR, Hope DA, et al. New York, Guilford, 1995, pp 69–93

Clark DM, Ehlers A, McManus F, et al: Cognitive therapy versus fluoxetine in generalized social phobia: a randomized placebo-controlled trial. J Consult Clin Psychol 71(6):1058–1067, 2003 14622081

Craske MG, Niles AN, Burklund LJ, et al: Randomized controlled trial of cognitive behavioral therapy and acceptance and commitment therapy for social phobia: outcomes and moderators. J Consult Clin Psychol 82(6):1034–1048, 2014a 24999670

Craske MG, Treanor M, Conway CC, et al: Maximizing exposure therapy: an inhibitory learning approach. Behav Res Ther 58:10–23, 2014b 24864005

Dagöö J, Asplund RP, Bsenko HA, et al: Cognitive behavior therapy versus interpersonal psychotherapy for social anxiety disorder delivered via smartphone and computer: a randomized controlled trial. J Anxiety Disord 28(4):410–417, 2014 24731441

Dalrymple KL, Herbert JD: Acceptance and commitment therapy for generalized social anxiety disorder: a pilot study. Behav Modif 31(5):543–568, 2007 17699117

Davidson JRT, Foa EB, Huppert JD, et al: Fluoxetine, comprehensive cognitive behavioral therapy, and placebo in generalized social phobia. Arch Gen Psychiatry 61(10):1005–1013, 2004 15466674

Dixon LJ, Kemp JJ, Farrell NR, et al: Interoceptive exposure exercises for social anxiety. J Anxiety Disord 33:25–34, 2015 25988536

El Alaoui S, Hedman E, Kaldo V, et al: Effectiveness of internet-based cognitive-behavior therapy for social anxiety disorder in clinical psychiatry. J Consult Clin Psychol 83(5):902–914, 2015 26009780

Erwin BA, Heimberg RG, Juster H, et al: Comorbid anxiety and mood disorders among persons with social anxiety disorder. Behav Res Ther 40(1):19–35, 2002 11762424

Fava GA, Grandi S, Canestrari R: Treatment of social phobia by homework exposure. Psychother Psychosom 52(4):209–213, 1989 2577258

Fava GA, Grandi S, Rafanelli C, et al: Long-term outcome of social phobia treated by exposure. Psychol Med 31(5):899–905, 2001 11459387

Feske U, Chambless DL: Cognitive behavioral versus exposure only treatment for social phobia: a meta-analysis. Behav Ther 26:695–720, 1995

Gaston JE, Abbott MJ, Rapee RM, et al: Do empirically supported treatments generalize to private practice? A benchmark study of a cognitive-behavioural group treatment programme for social phobia. Br J Clin Psychol 45(Pt 1):33–48, 2006 16480565

Gershkovich M, Herbert JD, Forman EM, et al: Internet-delivered acceptance-based cognitive-behavioral intervention for social anxiety disorder with and without therapist support: a randomized trial. Behav Modif 41(5):583–608, 2017 28776431

Gingnell M, Frick A, Engman J, et al: Combining escitalopram and cognitive-behavioural therapy for social anxiety disorder: randomised controlled fMRI trial. Br J Psychiatry 209(3):229–235, 2016 27340112

Goetter EM, Frumkin MR, Palitz SA, et al: Barriers to mental health treatment among individuals with social anxiety disorder and generalized anxiety disorder. Psychol Serv August 2, 2018 30070552 Epub ahead of print

Goldin PR, Ziv M, Jazaieri H, et al: Cognitive reappraisal self-efficacy mediates the effects of individual cognitive-behavioral therapy for social anxiety disorder. J Consult Clin Psychol 80(6):1034–1040, 2012 22582765

Goldin PR, Morrison A, Jazaieri H, et al: Group CBT versus MBSR for social anxiety disorder: a randomized controlled trial. J Consult Clin Psychol 84(5):427–437, 2016 26950097

Grant BF, Hasin DS, Blanco C, et al: The epidemiology of social anxiety disorder in the United States: results from the National Epidemiologic Survey on Alcohol and Related Conditions. J Clin Psychiatry 66(11):1351–1361, 2005 16420070

Hackmann A, Clark DM, McManus F: Recurrent images and early memories in social phobia. Behav Res Ther 38(6):601–610, 2000 10846808

Haug T, Nordgreen T, Öst LG, et al: Working alliance and competence as predictors of outcome in cognitive behavioral therapy for social anxiety and panic disorder in adults. Behav Res Ther 77:40–51, 2016 26708332

Hayes SA, Hope DA, VanDyke MM, et al: Working alliance for clients with social anxiety disorder: relationship with session helpfulness and within-session habituation. Cogn Behav Ther 36(1):34–42, 2007 17364650

Hayes SC, Strosahl K, Wilson KG: Acceptance and Commitment Therapy: The Process and Practice of Mindful Change, 2nd Edition. New York, Guilford, 2011

Hedman E, Andersson G, Ljótsson B, et al: Internet-based cognitive behavior therapy vs. cognitive behavioral group therapy for social anxiety disorder: a randomized controlled noninferiority trial. PLoS One 6(3):e18001, 2011 21483704

Hedman E, El Alaoui S, Lindefors N, et al: Clinical effectiveness and cost-effectiveness of internet- vs. group-based cognitive behavior therapy for social anxiety disorder: 4-year follow-up of a randomized trial. Behav Res Ther 59:20–29, 2014 24949908

Heimberg RG, Becker RE: Cognitive-Behavioral Group Therapy for Social Phobia: Basic Mechanisms and Clinical Strategies. New York, Guilford, 2002

Heimberg RG, Dodge CS, Hope DA, et al: Cognitive-behavioral group treatment of social phobia: comparison to a credible placebo control. Cognit Ther Res 14:1–23, 1990

Heimberg RG, Salzman DG, Holt CS, et al: Cognitive-behavioral group treatment for social phobia: effectiveness at five-year follow-up. Cognit Ther Res 17:325–339, 1993

Heimberg RG, Liebowitz MR, Hope DA, et al: Cognitive behavioral group therapy vs phenelzine therapy for social phobia: 12-week outcome. Arch Gen Psychiatry 55(12):1133–1141, 1998 9862558

Heimberg RG, Brozovich FA, Rapee RM: A cognitive-behavioral model of social anxiety disorder, in Social Anxiety: Clinical, Developmental, and Social Perspectives, 3rd Edition. Edited by SG Hofmann, DiBartolo PM. Waltham, MA, Academic Press, 2014, pp 705–728

Herbert JD, Cardaciotto LA: An Acceptance and Mindfulness-Based Perspective on Social Anxiety Disorder. New York, Springer, 2005

Herbert JD, Gaudiano BA, Rheingold AA, et al: Social skills training augments the effectiveness of cognitive behavioral group therapy for social anxiety disorder. Behav Ther 36:125–138, 2005

Hofmann SG: Cognitive factors that maintain social anxiety disorder: a comprehensive model and its treatment implications. Cogn Behav Ther 36(4):193–209, 2007 18049945

Hope DA, Heimberg RG, Turk CL: Managing Social Anxiety: A Cognitive-Behavioral Therapy Approach (Client Workbook), 2nd Edition. New York, Oxford University Press, 2010

Jazaieri H, Goldin PR, Werner K, et al: A randomized trial of MBSR versus aerobic exercise for social anxiety disorder. J Clin Psychol 68(7):715–731, 2012 22623316

Jazaieri H, Goldin PR, Gross JJ: The role of working alliance in CBT and MBSR for social anxiety disorder. Mindfulness 9:1381–1389, 2018

Kabat-Zinn J: Full Catastrophe Living: Using the Wisdom of Your Body and Mind to Face Stress, Pain, and Illness. New York, Dell Publishing, 1990

Kampmann IL, Emmelkamp PM, Hartanto D, et al: Exposure to virtual social interactions in the treatment of social anxiety disorder: a randomized controlled trial. Behav Res Ther 77:147–156, 2016a 26752328

Kampmann IL, Emmelkamp PM, Morina N: Meta-analysis of technology-assisted interventions for social anxiety disorder. J Anxiety Disord 42:71–84, 2016b 27376634

Katz D, Rector NA, Laposa JM: The interaction of distress tolerance and intolerance of uncertainty in the prediction of symptom reduction across CBT for social anxiety disorder. Cogn Behav Ther 46(6):459–477, 2017 28641047

Klerman GL, Weissman MM, Rounsaville B, et al: Interpersonal Psychotherapy of Depression. New York, Basic Books, 1984

Kocovski NL, Fleming JE, Hawley LL, et al: Mindfulness and acceptance-based group therapy versus traditional cognitive behavioral group therapy for social anxiety disorder: a randomized controlled trial. Behav Res Ther 51(12):889–898, 2013 24220538

Kocovski NL, Fleming JE, Hawley LL, et al: Mindfulness and acceptance-based group therapy and traditional cognitive behavioral group therapy for social anxiety disorder: mechanisms of change. Behav Res Ther 70:11–22, 2015 25938187

Koszycki D, Benger M, Shlik J, et al: Randomized trial of a meditation-based stress reduction program and cognitive behavior therapy in generalized social anxiety disorder. Behav Res Ther 45(10):2518–2526, 2007 17572382

Koszycki D, Thake J, Mavounza C, et al: Preliminary investigation of a mindfulness-based intervention for social anxiety disorder that integrates compassion meditation and mindful exposure. J Altern Complement Med 22(5):363–374, 2016 27070853

Ledley DR, Heimberg RG, Hope DA, et al: Efficacy of a manualized and workbook-driven individual treatment for social anxiety disorder. Behav Ther 40(4):414–424, 2009 19892086

Leichsenring F, Beutel M, Leibing E: Psychodynamic psychotherapy for social phobia: a treatment manual based on supportive-expressive therapy. Bull Menninger Clin 71(1):56–83, 2007 17484670

Leichsenring F, Salzer S, Beutel ME, et al: Psychodynamic therapy and cognitive-behavioral therapy in social anxiety disorder: a multicenter randomized controlled trial. Am J Psychiatry 170(7):759–767, 2013 23680854

Leichsenring F, Salzer S, Beutel ME, et al: Long-term outcome of psychodynamic therapy and cognitive-behavioral therapy in social anxiety disorder. Am J Psychiatry 171(10):1074–1082, 2014 25016974

Liebowitz MR, Heimberg RG, Schneier FR, et al: Cognitive-behavioral group therapy versus phenelzine in social phobia: long-term outcome. Depress Anxiety 10(3):89–98, 1999 10604081

Lincoln TM, Rief W, Hahlweg K, et al: Effectiveness of an empirically supported treatment for social phobia in the field. Behav Res Ther 41(11):1251–1269, 2003 14527526

Lipsitz JD, Gur M, Vermes D, et al: A randomized trial of interpersonal therapy versus supportive therapy for social anxiety disorder. Depress Anxiety 25(6):542–553, 2008 17941096

Luborsky L: Principles of Psychoanalytic Psychotherapy: Manual for Supportive Expressive Treatment. New York, Basic Books, 1984

Lucock MP, Salkovskis PM: Cognitive factors in social anxiety and its treatment. Behav Res Ther 26(4):297–302, 1988 3214394

Mayo-Wilson E, Dias S, Mavranezouli I, et al: Psychological and pharmacological interventions for social anxiety disorder in adults: a systematic review and network meta-analysis. Lancet Psychiatry 1(5):368–376, 2014 26361000

McEvoy PM, Nathan P, Rapee RM, et al: Cognitive behavioural group therapy for social phobia: evidence of transportability to community clinics. Behav Res Ther 50(4):258–265, 2012 22394493

Mörtberg E, Karlsson A, Fyring C, et al: Intensive cognitive-behavioral group treatment (CBGT) of social phobia: a randomized controlled study. J Anxiety Disord 20(5):646–660, 2006 16169185

Mörtberg E, Clark DM, Sundin O, et al: Intensive group cognitive treatment and individual cognitive therapy vs. treatment as usual in social phobia: a randomized controlled trial. Acta Psychiatr Scand 115(2):142–154, 2007 17244178

Mörtberg E, Hoffart A, Boecking B, et al: Shifting the focus of one's attention mediates improvement in cognitive therapy for social anxiety disorder. Behav Cogn Psychother 43(1):63–73, 2015 23981858

Newman MG, Hofmann SG, Trabert W, et al: Does behavioral treatment of social phobia lead to cognitive changes? Behav Ther 25:503–517, 1994

Niles AN, Mesri B, Burklund LJ, et al: Attentional bias and emotional reactivity as predictors and moderators of behavioral treatment for social phobia. Behav Res Ther 51(10):669–679, 2013 23933107

Niles AN, Burklund LJ, Arch JJ, et al: Cognitive mediators of treatment for social anxiety disorder: comparing acceptance and commitment therapy and cognitive-behavioral therapy. Behav Ther 45(5):664–677, 2014 25022777

Nordahl HM, Vogel PA, Morken G, et al: Paroxetine, cognitive therapy or their combination in the treatment of social anxiety disorder with and without avoidant personality disorder: a randomized clinical trial. Psychother Psychosom 85(6):346–356, 2016 27744447

Norton AR, Abbott MJ: The efficacy of imagery rescripting compared to cognitive restructuring for social anxiety disorder. J Anxiety Disord 40:18–28, 2016 27070386

Oosterbaan DB, Balkom AJV, Spinhoven P, et al: Cognitive therapy versus moclobemide in social phobia: a controlled study. Clin Psychol Psychother 8(4):263–273, 2001

Otto MW, Pollack MH, Gould RA, et al: A comparison of the efficacy of clonazepam and cognitive-behavioral group therapy for the treatment of social phobia. J Anxiety Disord 14(4):345–358, 2000 11043885

Piccirillo ML, Taylor Dryman M, Heimberg RG: Safety behaviors in adults with social anxiety: review and future directions. Behav Ther 47(5):675–687, 2016 27816080

Ponniah K, Hollon SD: Empirically supported psychological interventions for social phobia in adults: a qualitative review of randomized controlled trials. Psychol Med 38(1):3–14, 2008 17640438

Powers MB, Sigmarsson SR, Emmelkamp PM: A meta-analytic review of psychological treatments for social anxiety disorder. Int J Cogn Ther 1(2):94–113, 2008

Rapee RM, Heimberg RG: A cognitive-behavioral model of anxiety in social phobia. Behav Res Ther 35(8):741–756, 1997 9256517

Rapee RM, Lim L: Discrepancy between self- and observer ratings of performance in social phobics. J Abnorm Psychol 101(4):728–731, 1992 1430614

Reimer SG, Moscovitch DA: The impact of imagery rescripting on memory appraisals and core beliefs in social anxiety disorder. Behav Res Ther 75:48–59, 2015 26555157

Ruscio AM, Brown TA, Chiu WT, et al: Social fears and social phobia in the USA: results from the National Comorbidity Survey Replication. Psychol Med 38(1):15–28, 2008 17976249

Schneier FR, Foose TE, Hasin DS, et al: Social anxiety disorder and alcohol use disorder comorbidity in the National Epidemiologic Survey on Alcohol and Related Conditions. Psychol Med 40(6):977–988, 2010 20441690

Sibrava NJ, Beard C, Bjornsson AS, et al: Two-year course of generalized anxiety disorder, social anxiety disorder, and panic disorder in a longitudinal sample of African American adults. J Consult Clin Psychol 81(6):1052–1062, 2013 24041233

Stangier U, Heidenreich T, Peitz M, et al: Cognitive therapy for social phobia: individual versus group treatment. Behav Res Ther 41(9):991–1007, 2003 12914803

Stangier U, Schramm E, Heidenreich T, et al: Cognitive therapy vs interpersonal psychotherapy in social anxiety disorder: a randomized controlled trial. Arch Gen Psychiatry 68(7):692–700, 2011 21727253

Stolz T, Schulz A, Krieger T, et al: A mobile app for social anxiety disorder: a three-arm randomized controlled trial comparing mobile and PC-based guided self-help interventions. J Consult Clin Psychol 86(6):493–504, 2018 29781648

Stopa L: How to use imagery in cognitive-behavioural therapy, in Imagery and the Threatened Self: Perspectives on Mental Imagery and the Self in Cognitive Therapy. Edited by Stopa L. New York, Routledge/Taylor and Francis Group, 2009, pp 65–93

Turner SM, Beidel DC, Jacob RG: Social phobia: a comparison of behavior therapy and atenolol. J Consult Clin Psychol 62(2):350–358, 1994 8201073

Warnock-Parkes E, Wild J, Stott R, et al: Seeing is believing: using video feedback in cognitive therapy for social anxiety disorder. Cognit Behav Pract 24(2):245–255, 2017 29033532

Wild J, Hackmann A, Clark DM: When the present visits the past: updating traumatic memories in social phobia. J Behav Ther Exp Psychiatry 38(4):386–401, 2007 17765865

Wong QJJ, Rapee RM: The aetiology and maintenance of social anxiety disorder: a synthesis of complementary theoretical models and formulation of a new integrated model. J Affect Disord 203:84–100, 2016 27280967

Recommended Readings

Antony MM, Swinson RP: The Shyness and Social Anxiety Workbook, 3rd Edition. Oakland, CA, New Harbinger, 2017

Heimberg RG, Becker RE: Cognitive-Behavioral Group Therapy for Social Phobia: Basic Mechanisms and Clinical Strategies. New York, Guilford, 2002

Hope DA, Heimberg RG, Turk CL: Managing Social Anxiety: A Cognitive-Behavioral Therapy Approach (Client Workbook), 3rd Edition. New York, Oxford University Press, 2019

Hope DA, Heimberg RG, Turk CL: Managing Social Anxiety: A Cognitive-Behavioral Therapy Approach (Therapist Guide), 3rd Edition. New York, Oxford University Press, 2019

Magee L, Heimberg RG: Social anxiety disorder, in Clinical Handbook of Psychological Disorders, 5th Edition. Edited by Barlow DH. New York, Guilford, 2014, pp 114–154

PART VII

Specific Phobia

CHAPTER 28

Specific Phobia

Ella L. Oar, Ph.D.
Ronald M. Rapee, Ph.D.

Phenomenology

Although specific phobias are highly prevalent (Wardenaar et al. 2017), relatively few individuals seek treatment (Stinson et al. 2007). This may be due to the circumscribed nature of specific phobias, which possibly leads to a misconception that phobias are less severe and complicated than other anxiety disorders (Ollendick and Sirbu 2012). However, many children and adults with phobias experience significant difficulties at school and work, interference in their social and family functioning, and poorer physical health (Wardenaar et al. 2017). Additionally, the diagnostic and symptom profile of phobias is complex. Phobias are highly comorbid and associated with unique physiological symptoms, extensive avoidance behaviors, and distorted cognitions (Hood and Antony 2012). They have been found to be a major psychopathological precursor for a range of other mental health disorders (Lieb et al. 2016). Consequently, clinicians and researchers must be aware of current issues relating to the nature, theory, and treatment of specific phobias.

Clinical Features

DSM-5 (American Psychiatric Association 2013) specifies that for a person to be diagnosed with a specific phobia, the person must have a marked and persistent fear or anxiety about a specific object or situation (Criterion A) that is disproportionate to any actual threat (Criterion D), and exposure to this object or situation immediately increases the person's fear or anxiety (Criterion B). The phobic object or situation must be avoided and, if this is not possible, endured with substantial distress (Criterion C). Most critically, the fear, anxiety, or avoidance must be associated with significant impairment in functioning (Criterion F). DSM-5 classifies phobias into five main subtypes: 1) animals (e.g., dogs, spiders, snakes), 2) natural environment (e.g., heights, thunderstorms, the dark, water), 3) blood-injection-injury (BII; e.g., seeing blood, experiencing injections and blood tests), 4) situational (e.g., flying, elevators, enclosed spaces), and 5) other (e.g., costumed characters, vomiting, choking, doctors or dentists, contracting an illness or disease).

Although most phobias are motivated primarily by fear, disgust also appears to play a role in the development and maintenance of particular phobia subtypes (Knowles et al. 2018). For example, patients with small-animal phobia, BII phobia, and emetophobia (fear of vomiting) report heightened disgust on exposure to fear-relevant stimuli (Tolin et al. 1997) and respond to phobic-related stimuli with disgust-specific facial expressions (de Jong et al. 2002). Moreover, individuals with phobias tend to show greater sensitivity to disgust (Tolin et al. 1997).

Epidemiology

Lifetime prevalence rates for phobias range from 7.4% to 12.5%, and 12-month prevalence rates from 2.0% to 8.8% (Alonso et al. 2004; Bijl et al. 2002; de Graaf et al. 2012; Grenier et al. 2011; Kessler et al. 2005; Stinson et al. 2007; Wardenaar et al. 2017; Wells et al. 2006). Findings have been mixed in relation to prevalence of distinct phobia subtypes. Animal phobia has generally been found to be the most common across all ages (LeBeau et al. 2010). Overall, phobias are more common in females than in males, with the exception of BII phobia, which appears to affect relatively equal proportions of females and males (LeBeau et al. 2010).

Phobias typically have their onset early in life, prior to age 10 years (LeBeau et al. 2010). Interestingly, differences have been observed in the emergence of phobia subtypes, with these following a similar pattern to the development of normal fears. For example, animal and natural environment phobias have been found to emerge in early childhood (Öst 1987); situational phobias tend to have a slightly later onset (LeBeau et al. 2010); and claustrophobic fears tend to have a relatively late onset (Öst 1987).

Many people with phobias experience significant impairment in functioning. Although some epidemiological studies have found that these individuals experience levels of impairment comparable to those in individuals with other anxiety disorder diagnoses (Stinson et al. 2007), other studies have found comparatively low levels of disability in those with specific phobias relative to other anxiety disorders (Wells et al. 2006). Across the phobia subtypes, some evidence suggests that BII and situational subtypes may be more impairing than animal and natural environment subtypes (Depla et al. 2008).

Differential Diagnosis and Comorbidity

Differential diagnosis between specific phobia and other disorders can be complex given their overlapping features and high rates of comorbidity. When differentiating between a specific phobia and another disorder, the clinician needs to consider the focus of the person's fear in addition to the presence of other associated symptoms. Table 28–1 describes key features to assist in differentiating specific phobia from other disorders.

As in other anxiety disorder presentations, high rates of comorbidity are found in those with specific phobia (lifetime prevalence of up to 83%; Magee et al. 1996). Phobias commonly co-occur alongside other phobias, other anxiety disorders, and affec-

TABLE 28–1.   **Common differential diagnoses for specific phobia**

Differential diagnosis	Shared features	Distinguishing features
Separation anxiety disorder	Situational avoidance (e.g., being alone in the dark)	If the person's fear is focused on being separated from a significant attachment figure, a diagnosis of separation anxiety disorder should be considered.
Panic disorder and/or agoraphobia	Situational avoidance (e.g., crowded spaces or flying) Fear of the physical sensations associated with anxiety Panic attacks	At times individuals with phobias may experience panic attacks in the presence of their feared stimuli. However, if panic attacks are unexpected and the person fears another panic attack, then a panic disorder diagnosis may be more appropriate. If the person fears only one agoraphobic situation, a situational-specific phobia is more likely. If, however, two or more situations are feared and avoided, a diagnosis of agoraphobia should be considered.
OCD	Fear of blood and illness Checking, reassurance seeking, and hand washing	If the person's fear focus (blood, illness, vomit, disease) is related to an obsession (e.g., fear of contamination from a range of sources), and if the person presents with a range of OCD symptoms, a diagnosis of OCD should be given.
Eating disorder	Fear and avoidance of food	An eating disorder diagnosis may be warranted if the person's fear and avoidance of food is driven by a fear of gaining weight or desire to control weight.
PTSD	Situational avoidance	If the person's fear develops after a traumatic event and the person experiences other symptoms of trauma (e.g., recurrent intrusive memories or thoughts), a diagnosis of PTSD should be considered.

tive disorders (Wardenaar et al. 2017). Most patients with specific phobia (up to 75%) meet criteria for multiple phobias during their lifetime (Wittchen et al. 2002).

Evaluation

A comprehensive assessment is needed not only for the purposes of diagnostic classification but also to inform treatment planning and evaluate outcome. Ideally, assessments should incorporate a range of methods, including clinical/diagnostic interviews, self-report measures, and behavioral approach tasks. Clinical interviews are an integral part of any specific phobia assessment. Interviews vary in their degree of structure, however; unstructured interviews are generally less reliable and valid than more structured diagnostic assessments due to their lack of standardization

(Schniering et al. 2000). In addition to clinical/diagnostic interviews, questionnaires should be administered as part of an evidence-based assessment of specific phobia. Recently, Ovanessian et al. (2019) evaluated the psychometric properties of the Specific Phobia Questionnaire (Fairbrother and Antony 2012), a screening tool for the assessment of DSM-5 phobias. The measure was found to have good convergent and discriminant validity and good test-retest reliability and was able to discriminate between clinical and nonclinical samples as well as between phobia subtypes. Additionally, several questionnaires are available to assess the different specific phobia subtypes (Olatunji et al. 2010; Vorstenbosch et al. 2012). Finally, behavioral avoidance tasks are an integral part of any phobia assessment because they allow for direct observation of a person's phobic response. A behavioral avoidance task is a standardized task that involves a person approaching a feared object or stimulus in a series of standard steps (Castagna et al. 2017). The degree to which the person approaches and interacts with the feared object or stimulus provides an observed measure of avoidance.

Pathogenesis

Biological Factors

Family aggregation and twin studies suggest a genetic contribution to phobias. First-degree relatives of adults with specific phobia are at significantly increased risk of developing a phobia (31%) compared with first-degree relatives of nonclinical control subjects (11%; Fyer et al. 1990). Interestingly, children of parents who have a phobia are at greater risk of developing the same type of phobia as their parent (Fredrikson et al. 1997). Although these studies suggest that phobias are highly familial, they do not distinguish between genetic and shared environmental factors (i.e., "nature vs. nurture"). In a systematic review and meta-analysis, Van Houtem et al. (2013) identified 10 adult twin studies of concordance for phobias. The authors concluded that phobias are moderately heritable, with mean estimates of 32% for animal phobia (range 22%–44%), 25% for situational phobia (range 0%–33%), and 33% for BII phobia (range 28%–63%). Hence, phobias appear to be have, in part, a genetic contribution.

Advances in neuroimaging have enabled an increasing number of studies to explore the neuropathophysiology of phobias. Two systematic reviews (Del Casale et al. 2012; Ipser et al. 2013) indicated that when confronted with feared stimuli, adults with phobias experience increased activation of brain regions associated with the emotional perception and early amplification of fear (e.g., left amygdala, left globus pallidus, left insula, right thalamus, cerebellum). Moreover, they appear to show reduced activation in brain regions that regulate fear (e.g., prefrontal, orbitofrontal, and visual cortices; Del Casale et al. 2012).

Conditioning

Direct Classical Conditioning

Early researchers conceptualized the etiology of specific phobias from a classical conditioning framework. According to this perspective, fear develops after a direct negative experience with an object or stimulus. Avoidance is believed to maintain that fear through negative reinforcement (i.e., reduction in fear and physiological arousal). Moreover, avoidance is thought to prevent the opportunity to disconfirm harm-related expectancies. The classical conditioning model continues to be one of the most influential models in the field of specific phobia; however, it is now recognized to have a number of shortcomings. First, classical conditioning theorists suggest that any stimuli can be feared; however, in large incidence studies, discrete categories of fears (e.g., animals, BII) emerge. Second, many people experience aversive conditioning events (e.g., a dog bite) but do not develop a phobia (Ehlers et al. 1994; Schindler et al. 2016). Third, many individuals with phobias have not had a direct negative experience with their feared stimuli (Menzies and Clarke 1995).

Indirect Conditioning

Rachman (1977) proposed that fears and phobias are acquired through three learning pathways: direct/classical conditioning, vicarious conditioning, and the transmission of negative information. As previously discussed, the classical conditioning model suggests that phobias are acquired through direct negative experiences with objects or situations. However, many children and adults develop phobias without ever having direct contact with their feared objects or stimuli (Menzies and Clarke 1995). Considerable support has been found for indirect learning pathways of fear acquisition in both nonclinical (Muris et al. 2010) and clinical samples (Öst 1985).

Preparedness Theory

In an attempt to address the limitations of the classical conditioning model, Seligman (1971) developed the preparedness theory of fear acquisition. When examining the objects or stimuli that become the targets of phobias, he noticed that these stimuli tended to be biologically threatening. Hence, he proposed that as a result of natural selection, humans are biologically prepared to fear stimuli (e.g., animals, blood) that pose a threat to personal safety. Although substantive evidence supports Seligman's central premise that phobias are "evolutionarily prepared," evidence for the key characteristics that Seligman proposed is limited (see McNally 1987 for a review).

Non-Associative Theory

The aforementioned pathways to fear acquisition are all based on an associative theory of phobias. Those theories suggest that the central mechanism underlying phobia development is the formation of an association between the feared stimulus (previously neutral) and a potentially threatening outcome. The non-associative theory suggests that phobias may be acquired without prior (direct or indirect) learning experiences (Menzies and Clarke 1995). Longitudinal studies provide support for the non-associative account. For example, in an examination of data from the Dunedin Longitudinal Study, Poulton et al. (1998) found that serious falls before age 9 were not predictive of a fear of heights at ages 11 and 18 years.

Cognitive Factors

Cognitive theories of specific phobia focus on the role of biases in attention and dysfunctional thoughts and beliefs related to the person's feared object or situation. Although some researchers have suggested that cognitive processes may mediate phobia acquisition (Rachman 1991), most research in the field has focused on the role of cognitions in the maintenance of the disorder. Experimental research indicates that individuals with phobias, in comparison with nonclinical control subjects, show attentional biases for threat (Armstrong and Olatunji 2012). Moreover, evidence suggests that, unlike nonclinical control subjects, individuals with specific phobias misinterpret ambiguous stimuli as threatening (Haberkamp and Schmidt 2014). Consequently, these early information processing biases are believed to result in exaggerated danger expectancies, which then lead to subsequent avoidance. For example, Jones and Menzies (2000) found that in comparison with nonclinical control subjects, individuals with spider phobias reported greater harm expectancies when confronted with their feared stimulus, including an increased likelihood of being bitten by a spider in addition to more severe consequences associated with being bitten. Additionally, these harm expectancies were found to predict greater avoidance during a spider behavioral avoidance task. Similar findings have been observed across multiple studies with a range of phobia subtypes (Marshall et al. 1992; Menzies et al. 1998).

Pharmacotherapy

Limited evidence is available for the efficacy of pharmacotherapy for specific phobia either as a stand-alone treatment or in combination with psychological therapy. For the acute treatment of specific phobia, anxiolytic medications often are prescribed (Hood and Antony 2012). Although in the short term benzodiazepines appear to reduce subjective and physiological symptoms, these benefits are not maintained (Jöhren et al. 2000; Wilhelm and Roth 1997). For example, in a sample of individuals with flight phobia ($N=28$), alprazolam (in comparison to a placebo) prior to a flight resulted in reduced subjective anxiety (Wilhelm and Roth 1997). However, on a repeat flight 1 week later, when no medication was given, those who had received alprazolam on the first flight reported greater subjective anxiety, physiological symptoms, and rates of panic attacks on the second flight. Similarly, in patients with dental phobia, midazolam decreased anxiety immediately; however, at 3-month and 1-year follow-ups, only a behavioral therapy group maintained treatment gains. Antidepressant medications have also been studied for treatment of specific phobia. Two randomized controlled trials (RCTs) with adults have examined the efficacy of selective serotonin reuptake inhibitor monotherapy for specific phobia (Alamy et al. 2008; Benjamin et al. 2000). In these two studies, modest treatment gains were found in favor of medications (paroxetine and escitalopram), but neither study included follow-up assessments.

Considerable interest has developed since the mid-2000s in the use of pharmacological agents such as D-cycloserine to enhance psychological therapy outcomes. These medications are purported to work by having an effect on the consolidation of extinction learning that underlies exposure therapy. Although several early trials showed promising results in adults with phobias and other anxiety disorders, more recent RCTs have reported mixed findings, and overall only small augmentation effects have been found (Mataix-Cols et al. 2017). In sum, support for the benefits of pharmacological approaches to treatment of specific phobia is limited.

Psychotherapy

Exposure

Exposure therapy is considered the treatment of choice for both children and adults with specific phobia (Choy et al. 2007). It involves having individuals repeatedly approach their feared objects or situations in a controlled and graduated manner. The guiding principle behind exposure is that the prevention of escape or avoidance will result in the individual learning that the feared outcome does not occur (i.e., it is "safe"; Lovibond et al. 2009) and that distress will decrease while still confronting the feared object. Exposure has consistently been found to be beneficial in comparison to a waitlist control condition and other active treatments and to result in reductions in subjective anxiety, phobic beliefs, and avoidance (Choy et al. 2007).

A number of factors need to be considered to maximize exposure therapy treatment outcome. For example, in vivo exposure has generally been found to outperform imaginal exposure (Wolitzky-Taylor et al. 2008). Findings relating to the optimal timing and spacing of exposure sessions for individuals with phobias have been mixed. Substantive support exists for treatment within a single session (Öst 1989). One-session treatment involves an intensive 3-hour massed exposure therapy session and has been found to produce outcomes comparable to those of multiple spaced exposure therapy sessions (totaling up to 5 hours; Öst et al. 1997). However, other studies comparing massed, spaced, and expanding exposure treatment schedules indicate that an expanding schedule, wherein exposure sessions are initially scheduled close together and then at gradually greater intervals, may be more effective at attenuating the return of fear (Rowe and Craske 1998; Tsao and Craske 2000).

Traditionally during exposure therapy, patients proceed from one exposure step in their hierarchy to the next, with steps repeated multiple times until their fear declines. Although graduated exposure is generally thought to be more tolerable and associated with fewer dropouts, some evidence suggests that varying the difficulty of exposure steps (e.g., completing exposure steps in random order) might enhance outcomes in the long term (Craske et al. 2014). Moreover, extinction learning is highly context dependent, meaning that if exposure therapy is not carried out in multiple settings and does not involve a variety of stimuli, learning may fail to generalize. Several studies have now shown that for adults with phobias, exposure carried out in multiple contexts diminishes return of fear (Bandarian-Balooch et al. 2015; Shiban et al. 2015).

Since the early 2000s, a substantive literature has explored the use of virtual reality to deliver exposure therapy (e.g., virtual reality exposure [VRE]; Carl et al. 2019). Several meta-analyses (Morina et al. 2015) have been conducted; the most recent by Carl et al. (2019) identified 14 controlled trials for specific phobia. Twelve of the studies compared VRE to waitlist conditions and five compared VRE to in vivo exposure. A large effect size was found in favor of VRE in comparison to the waitlist control ($g=0.95$); however, comparisons of VRE to in vivo exposure revealed small, nonsignificant effects in favor of in vivo exposure ($g=-0.08$). Support was also found for the long-term effectiveness of VRE (for up to 12 months; Carl et al. 2019).

Cognitive Therapy

Cognitive therapy involves helping patients learn to challenge the phobic beliefs that are involved in the maintenance of their fear. This is thought to lead to a subsequent decrease in anxiety and avoidance. Cognitive therapy has shown mixed outcomes as either a stand-alone or an adjunctive treatment for people with specific phobias. These mixed results may be due in part to considerable heterogeneity across interventions (Wolitzky-Taylor et al. 2008). Overall, cognitive therapy appears to be more effective than no treatment or a waitlist control but less effective than exposure (Craske and Rowe 1997). Moreover, as an adjunctive treatment, cognitive therapy results in limited added benefit above exposure alone (Choy et al. 2007; Wolitzky-Taylor et al. 2008).

Treatment of Blood-Injury-Injection Phobia

BII phobia has a unique clinical presentation relative to the other phobia subtypes in that many patients (56%–100%) report a history of fainting (e.g., vasovagal response) when confronted with their feared stimuli (Ayala et al. 2009), complicating the use of in vivo exposure. Hence, exposure for this disorder is often combined with applied tension, which utilizes a muscle tension/release technique along with in vivo exposure (Öst and Sterner 1987). The muscle tension is used to counteract the vasovagal response and has been delivered across multiple sessions or within a single session (maximized to 2 hours). Ayala et al. (2009) conducted a critical review of the BII phobia literature and identified five controlled treatment trials. Applied tension was found to outperform exposure therapy alone, applied relaxation (progressive muscle relaxation in combination with exposure), and a combination of applied tension and applied relaxation on measures of self-reported anxiety, in-session avoidance, and fainting, whereas exposure therapy alone outperformed all other treatments in terms of posttreatment effect sizes on BII phobia questionnaires. Contrary to expectations, applied tension did not appear to affect the physiological responses of patients. Across all treatments, fainting status did not affect treatment outcome (Ayala et al. 2009).

Research has highlighted the potential role of hyperventilation in BII phobia's vasovagal response (Ritz et al. 2010). Meuret et al. (2017) conducted a pilot RCT to evaluate the relative efficacy of two brief skills interventions (each involving a 12-minute training video) in comparison to a relaxation control condition. One intervention was a novel hypoventilation breathing program aimed at reducing hyperventilation, and the other was a brief muscle tension program. Greater reductions in self-reported physical symptoms and anxiety were found for the breathing and muscle tension training conditions than for the relaxation control condition (Meuret et al. 2017).

Conclusion

Specific phobias are highly prevalent and are often a precursor to more complex and debilitating mental health conditions (Lieb et al. 2016). The onset of specific phobia is believed to be multifactorial, including genetics, neurobiology, learning experiences, preparedness, and cognitions. The consensus in the literature is that exposure therapy is the treatment of choice for specific phobia, with little evidence for efficacy from pharmacological approaches. Significant evidence now supports the use of virtual reality to deliver exposure therapy. Promising brief treatments for BII phobia have recently been piloted and have the potential to provide a cost-effective alternative to traditional face-to-face therapy.

Key Points

- Specific phobias are one of the most common psychiatric conditions; however, many people do not seek treatment.

- DSM-5 specifies five different phobia subtypes: 1) animal, 2) natural environment (e.g., storms, water), 3) blood-injection-injury, 4) situational (e.g., flying, enclosed spaces), and 5) other (e.g., doctors and dentists, vomiting, choking, costumed characters).

- Although most phobias are motivated primarily by fear, disgust appears to play a role in phobias involving small animals, blood-injection-injury, and vomiting.

- Evidence has been found of genetic and neurological involvement in the development of specific phobia; however, precise contributions require further research.

- Conditioning models have emphasized learned associations between a feared stimulus (previously neutral) and a potentially threatening outcome, made via direct experiences, indirect experiences, or verbal transmission of information. Nonassociative accounts have suggested that phobias may be acquired without previous associative learning.

- Cognitive accounts of specific phobias have emphasized the importance of distorted negative thinking patterns and dysfunctional beliefs and attitudes.

- Exposure therapy (either face-to-face or virtual) is the treatment of choice for specific phobia, with limited evidence supporting the use of pharmacotherapy.

References

Alamy S, Wei Zhang, Varia I, et al: Escitalopram in specific phobia: results of a placebo-controlled pilot trial. J Psychopharmacol 22(2):157–161, 2008

Alonso J, Angermeyer MC, Bernert S, et al: 12-Month comorbidity patterns and associated factors in Europe: results from the European Study of the Epidemiology of Mental Disorders (ESEMeD) project. Acta Psychiatr Scand Suppl 109(s420):28–37, 2004 15128385

American Psychiatric Association: Diagnostic and Statistical Manual of Mental Disorders, 5th Edition. Arlington, VA, American Psychiatric Association, 2013

Armstrong T, Olatunji BO: Eye tracking of attention in the affective disorders: a meta-analytic review and synthesis. Clin Psychol Rev 32(8):704–723, 2012 23059623

Ayala ES, Meuret AE, Ritz T: Treatments for blood-injury-injection phobia: a critical review of current evidence. J Psychiatr Res 43(15):1235–1242, 2009 19464700

Bandarian-Balooch S, Neumann DL, Boschen MJ: Exposure treatment in multiple contexts attenuates return of fear via renewal in high spider fearful individuals. J Behav Ther Exp Psychiatry 47:138–144, 2015 25601294

Benjamin J, Ben-Zion IZ, Karbofsky E, et al: Double-blind placebo-controlled pilot study of paroxetine for specific phobia. Psychopharmacology (Berl) 149(2):194–196, 2000 10805616

Bijl RV, De Graaf R, Ravelli A, et al: Gender and age-specific first incidence of DSM-III-R psychiatric disorders in the general population. Results from the Netherlands Mental Health Survey and Incidence Study (NEMESIS). Soc Psychiatry Psychiatr Epidemiol 37(8):372–379, 2002 12195544

Carl E, Stein AT, Levihn-Coon A, et al: Virtual reality exposure therapy for anxiety and related disorders: a meta-analysis of randomized controlled trials. J Anxiety Disord 61:27–36, 2019 30287083

Castagna PJ, Davis TE 3rd, Lilly ME: The behavioral avoidance task with anxious youth: a review of procedures, properties, and criticisms. Clin Child Fam Psychol Rev 20(2):162–184, 2017 27995381

Choy Y, Fyer AJ, Lipsitz JD: Treatment of specific phobia in adults. Clin Psychol Rev 27(3):266–286, 2007 17112646

Craske MG, Rowe MK: A comparison of behavioral and cognitive treatments for phobias, in Phobias: A Handbook of Theory, Research, and Treatment. Edited by Davey GCL. New York, Wiley, 1997, pp 247–280

Craske MG, Treanor M, Conway CC, et al: Maximizing exposure therapy: an inhibitory learning approach. Behav Res Ther 58:10–23, 2014 24864005

de Graaf R, ten Have M, van Gool C, et al: Prevalence of mental disorders and trends from 1996 to 2009. Results from the Netherlands Mental Health Survey and Incidence Study–2. Soc Psychiatry Psychiatr Epidemiol 47(2):203–213, 2012 21197531

de Jong PJ, Peters M, Vanderhallen I: Disgust and disgust sensitivity in spider phobia: facial EMG in response to spider and oral disgust imagery. J Anxiety Disord 16(5):477–493, 2002

Del Casale A, Ferracuti S, Rapinesi C, et al: Functional neuroimaging in specific phobia. Psychiatry Res 202(3):181–197, 2012 22804970

Depla MF, ten Have ML, van Balkom AJ, et al: Specific fears and phobias in the general population: results from the Netherlands Mental Health Survey and Incidence Study (NEMESIS). Soc Psychiatry Psychiatr Epidemiol 43(3):200–208, 2008 18060338

Ehlers A, Hofmann SG, Herda CA, et al: Clinical characteristics of driving phobia. J Anxiety Disord 8(4):323–339, 1994

Fairbrother N, Antony MM: Specific Phobia Questionnaire. Unpublished scale, 2012

Fredrikson M, Annas P, Wik G: Parental history, aversive exposure and the development of snake and spider phobia in women. Behav Res Ther 35(1):23–28, 1997 9009040

Fyer AJ, Mannuzza S, Gallops MS, et al: Familial transmission of simple phobias and fears. A preliminary report. Arch Gen Psychiatry 47(3):252–256, 1990 2306167

Grenier S, Schuurmans J, Goldfarb M, et al: The epidemiology of specific phobia and subthreshold fear subtypes in a community-based sample of older adults. Depress Anxiety 28(6):456–463, 2011 21400642

Haberkamp A, Schmidt T: Enhanced visuomotor processing of phobic images in blood-injury-injection fear. J Anxiety Disord 28(3):291–300, 2014 24632074

Hood HK, Antony MM: Evidence-based assessment and treatment of specific phobias in adults, in Intensive One-Session Treatment of Specific Phobias. Edited by Davis TE III, Ollendick TH, Öst LG. New York, Springer, 2012, pp 19–42

Ipser JC, Singh L, Stein DJ: Meta-analysis of functional brain imaging in specific phobia. Psychiatry Clin Neurosci 67(5):311–322, 2013 23711114

Jöhren P, Jackowski J, Gängler P, et al: Fear reduction in patients with dental treatment phobia. Br J Oral Maxillofac Surg 38(6):612–616, 2000 11092778

Jones MK, Menzies RG: Danger expectancies, self-efficacy and insight in spider phobia. Behav Res Ther 38(6):585–600, 2000 10846807

Kessler RC, Berglund P, Demler O, et al: Lifetime prevalence and age-of-onset distributions of DSM-IV disorders in the National Comorbidity Survey Replication. Arch Gen Psychiatry 62(6):593–602, 2005 15939837

Knowles KA, Jessup SC, Olatunji BO: Disgust in anxiety and obsessive-compulsive disorders: recent findings and future directions. Curr Psychiatry Rep 20(9):68, 2018 30094516

LeBeau RT, Glenn D, Liao B, et al: Specific phobia: a review of DSM-IV specific phobia and preliminary recommendations for DSM-V. Depress Anxiety 27(2):148–167, 2010 20099272

Lieb R, Miché M, Gloster AT, et al: Impact of specific phobia on the risk of onset of mental disorders: a 10-year prospective longitudinal community study of adolescents and young adults. Depress Anxiety 33(7):667–675, 2016 26990012

Lovibond PF, Mitchell CJ, Minard E, et al: Safety behaviours preserve threat beliefs: protection from extinction of human fear conditioning by an avoidance response. Behav Res Ther 47(8):716–720, 2009 19457472

Magee WJ, Eaton WW, Wittchen HU, et al: Agoraphobia, simple phobia, and social phobia in the National Comorbidity Survey. Arch Gen Psychiatry 53(2):159–168, 1996 8629891

Marshall WL, Bristol D, Barbaree HE: Cognitions and courage in the avoidance behavior of acrophobics. Behav Res Ther 30(5):463–470, 1992 1520232

Mataix-Cols D, Fernández de la Cruz L, Monzani B, et al: d-Cycloserine augmentation of exposure-based cognitive behavior therapy for anxiety, obsessive-compulsive, and posttraumatic stress disorders: a systematic review and meta-analysis of individual participant data. JAMA Psychiatry 74(5):501–510, 2017 28122091

McNally RJ: Preparedness and phobias: a review. Psychol Bull 101(2):283–303, 1987 3562708

Menzies RG, Clarke JC: The etiology of phobias: a nonassociative account. Clin Psychol Rev 15(1):23–48, 1995

Menzies RG, Harris LM, Jones MK: Evidence from three fearful samples for a poor insight type in specific phobia. Depress Anxiety 8(1):29–32, 1998 9750977

Meuret AE, Simon E, Bhaskara L, et al: Ultra-brief behavioral skills trainings for blood injection injury phobia. Depress Anxiety 34(12):1096–1105, 2017 28294471

Morina N, Ijntema H, Meyerbröker K, et al: Can virtual reality exposure therapy gains be generalized to real-life? A meta-analysis of studies applying behavioral assessments. Behav Res Ther 74:18–24, 2015 26355646

Muris P, van Zwol L, Huijding J, et al: Mom told me scary things about this animal: parents installing fear beliefs in their children via the verbal information pathway. Behav Res Ther 48(4):341–346, 2010 20022590

Olatunji BO, Sawchuk CN, Moretz MW, et al: Factor structure and psychometric properties of the Injection Phobia Scale–Anxiety. Psychol Assess 22(1):167–179, 2010 20230163

Ollendick TH, Sirbu C: Handling difficult-to-treat cases of specific phobias in childhood and adolescence, in Intensive One-Session Treatment of Specific Phobias. Edited by Davis TE III, Ollendick TH, Öst LG. New York, Springer, 2012, pp 143–160

Öst LG: Ways of acquiring phobias and outcome of behavioral treatments. Behav Res Ther 23(6):683–689, 1985 4074284

Öst LG: Age of onset in different phobias. J Abnorm Psychol 96(3):223–229, 1987 3680761

Öst LG: One-session treatment for specific phobias. Behav Res Ther 27(1):1–7, 1989 2914000

Öst LG, Sterner U: Applied tension: a specific behavioral method for treatment of blood phobia. Behav Res Ther 25(1):25–29, 1987 3593159

Öst LG, Brandberg M, Alm T: One versus five sessions of exposure in the treatment of flying phobia. Behav Res Ther 35(11):987–996, 1997 9431728

Ovanessian MM, Fairbrother N, Vorstenbosch V, et al: Psychometric properties and clinical utility of the Specific Phobia Questionnaire in an anxiety disorders sample. J Psychopathol Behav Assess 41:36–52, 2019

Poulton R, Davies S, Menzies RG, et al: Evidence for a non-associative model of the acquisition of a fear of heights. Behav Res Ther 36(5):537–544, 1998 9648329

Rachman S: The conditioning theory of fear-acquisition: a critical examination. Behav Res Ther 15(5):375–387, 1977 612338

Rachman S: Neo-conditioning and the classical theory of fear acquisition. Clin Psychol Rev 11(2):155–173, 1991

Ritz T, Meuret AE, Ayala ES: The psychophysiology of blood-injection-injury phobia: looking beyond the diphasic response paradigm. Int J Psychophysiol 78(1):50–67, 2010 20576505

Rowe MK, Craske MG: Effects of varied-stimulus exposure training on fear reduction and return of fear. Behav Res Ther 36(7–8):719–734, 1998 9682527

Schindler B, Vriends N, Margraf J, et al: Ways of acquiring flying phobia. Depress Anxiety 33(2):136–142, 2016 26484616

Schniering CA, Hudson JL, Rapee RM: Issues in the diagnosis and assessment of anxiety disorders in children and adolescents. Clin Psychol Rev 20(4):453–478, 2000 10832549

Seligman MEP: Phobias and preparedness. Behav Ther 2(3):307–320, 1971 27816071

Shiban Y, Schelhorn I, Pauli P, et al: Effect of combined multiple contexts and multiple stimuli exposure in spider phobia: a randomized clinical trial in virtual reality. Behav Res Ther 71:45–53, 2015 26072451

Stinson FS, Dawson DA, Patricia Chou S, et al: The epidemiology of DSM-IV specific phobia in the USA: results from the National Epidemiologic Survey on Alcohol and Related Conditions. Psychol Med 37(7):1047–1059, 2007 17335637

Tolin DF, Lohr JM, Sawchuk CN, et al: Disgust and disgust sensitivity in blood-injection-injury and spider phobia. Behav Res Ther 35(10):949–953, 1997 9401135

Tsao JCI, Craske MG: Timing of treatment and return of fear: effects of massed, uniform-, and expanding-spaced exposure schedules. Behav Ther 31(3):479–497, 2000

Van Houtem CMHH, Laine ML, Boomsma DI, et al: A review and meta-analysis of the heritability of specific phobia subtypes and corresponding fears. J Anxiety Disord 27(4):379–388, 2013 23774007

Vorstenbosch V, Antony MM, Koerner N, et al: Assessing dog fear: evaluating the psychometric properties of the Dog Phobia Questionnaire. J Behav Ther Exp Psychiatry 43(2):780–786, 2012 22104660

Wardenaar KJ, Lim CCW, Al-Hamzawi AO, et al: The cross-national epidemiology of specific phobia in the World Mental Health Surveys. Psychol Med 47(10):1744–1760, 2017 28222820

Wells JE, Browne MA, Scott KM, et al: Prevalence, interference with life and severity of 12 month DSM-IV disorders in Te Rau Hinengaro: the New Zealand Mental Health Survey. Aust N Z J Psychiatry 40(10):845–854, 2006 16959010

Wilhelm FH, Roth WT: Acute and delayed effects of alprazolam on flight phobics during exposure. Behav Res Ther 35(9):831–841, 1997 9299803

Wittchen HU, Lecrubier Y, Beesdo K, et al: Relationships among anxiety disorders: patterns and implications, in Anxiety Disorders. Edited by Nutt DJ, Ballenger JC. Oxford, England, Blackwell Science, 2002, pp 25–37

Wolitzky-Taylor KB, Horowitz JD, Powers MB, et al: Psychological approaches in the treatment of specific phobias: a meta-analysis. Clin Psychol Rev 28(6):1021–1037, 2008 18410984

Recommended Readings

American Psychiatric Association: Diagnostic and Statistical Manual of Mental Disorders, 5th Edition. Arlington, VA, American Psychiatric Association, 2013

Ayala ES, Meuret AE, Ritz T: Treatments for blood-injury-injection phobia: a critical review of current evidence. J Psychiatr Res 43(15):1235–1242, 2009 19464700

Carl E, Stein AT, Levihn-Coon A, et al: Virtual reality exposure therapy for anxiety and related disorders: a meta-analysis of randomized controlled trials. J Anxiety Disord 61:27–36, 2019 30287083

LeBeau RT, Glenn D, Liao B, et al: Specific phobia: a review of DSM-IV specific phobia and preliminary recommendations for DSM-V. Depress Anxiety 27(2):148–167, 2010 20099272

Öst LG: One-session treatment for specific phobias. Behav Res Ther 27(1):1–7, 1989 2914000

Rachman S: The conditioning theory of fear-acquisition: a critical examination. Behav Res Ther 15(5):375–387, 1977 612338

PART VIII

Trauma- and Stressor-Related
Disorders

CHAPTER 29

Phenomenology of PTSD

Miranda Olff, Ph.D.
Alexander C. McFarlane, M.D.

Exposure to trauma is common throughout the world (Kessler et al. 2017). Media coverage of traumatic events such as natural disasters, accidents, and man-made violence and discussions about sexual violence (e.g., abuse in churches, #MeToo movement), have increased interest in psychological trauma and awareness of its impact. The recognition of trauma as a public health issue has led to more research, which has resulted in changes in clinical practice and public health policies (Magruder et al. 2017). This increased interest is reflected in exponential growth in the number of published articles in this field (Olff 2018). Increasingly, this body of work has emphasized that although trauma is common, PTSD is the exception rather than the rule following exposure to such events and that the stress response that underpins the condition is atypical in those who go on to develop PTSD (Yehuda and McFarlane 1995).

Several different diagnostic labels have been used to describe traumatic reactions in the past, including shell shock, war neurosis, and neurasthenia (Glass 1974). Although *traumatic neurosis* (Horowitz 1986) had been a widely accepted term since the nineteenth century, the term *posttraumatic stress disorder* came into use in the 1970s and was recognized in DSM-III in 1980 (American Psychiatric Association 1980). Controversies about the conceptualization of PTSD have continued in recent decades. For example, the American Psychiatric Association (2013) in DSM-5 and World Health Organization (WHO) in ICD-11 (World Health Organization 2018) have taken somewhat different approaches to the classification of PTSD (Vermetten et al. 2016).

This chapter was prepared with support of the Australian National Health and Medical Research Council—project grant number 201813 and program grant number 300403.

Epidemiology

Trauma Exposure

Careful definition of the stressor criterion (see "Clinical Features" later) has provided a benchmark for conducting epidemiological research on PTSD. Population-based research has identified that 50%–90% of adults have been exposed to traumatic experiences (de Vries and Olff 2009; Dückers et al. 2016). In the WHO World Mental Health Survey, trauma was found to be the norm rather than the exception worldwide (Kessler et al. 2017), with interpersonal-violence traumas carrying the highest PTSD risk. Likewise, Forbes et al. (2012) found that trauma types with the highest PTSD burden included those involving intimate partner sexual violence (relatively uncommon traumas associated with high PTSD risk) and the unexpected death of a loved one (a very common trauma associated with low PTSD risk).

The types of trauma exposure differ for men and women. The most common causes of PTSD in men are engaging in combat and witnessing death or severe injury, whereas the most common causes of PTSD in women are being raped or sexually molested. Exposure to trauma in childhood or prolonged trauma exposure are also associated with increased risk of developing PTSD or other disorders (Karam et al. 2014). Events that involve multiple, chronic, or repeated types of traumas that are of an interpersonal nature and from which escape is difficult or impossible, such as childhood abuse, domestic violence, genocide campaigns, and being a prisoner of war, are more frequently associated with a broader set of symptoms known as "complex PTSD" (see "Clinical Features" as well as Forbes et al. 2020 and International Society for Traumatic Stress Studies 2019).

Posttraumatic Stress Disorder

One of the striking findings from research is that generally only a minority—about 10%—of trauma-exposed individuals develop PTSD (de Vries and Olff 2009), a finding that emphasizes the importance of resilience in responding to trauma (Southwick et al. 2014). Population-based estimates have been made in many countries as part of the World Mental Health Survey (e.g., Karam et al. 2014). The replication of the National Comorbidity Study found a lifetime prevalence of 6.8% and a 12-month prevalence of 3.5% (Kessler et al. 2005).

The prevalence of PTSD has consistently been found to be two to three times higher in women than in men (de Vries and Olff 2009). Differences in PTSD prevalence are partly explained by differences in trauma exposure, with events carrying a higher conditional risk for PTSD, such as sexual violence and exposure at a younger age, being more common in women, but with other factors, such as differences in biological stress responses and coping styles, codetermining the differential prevalence rates between men and women (Olff et al. 2007).

Although socioeconomically disadvantaged individuals are ordinarily at heightened risk for developing PTSD in response to trauma, countries with fewer resources have been associated with a decreased, rather than increased, risk of PTSD, confirmed for both women and men (Dückers and Olff 2017). This can be explained by the hypothesis that traumatic events occurring in a particular societal context may moderate the pathogenic impact of a stressor (McNally 2018).

Clinical Features

Two differing diagnostic systems are currently in use. These operational definitions of PTSD have allowed a great deal of research to be conducted. The recent revisions of the diagnostic criteria in DSM-5 and ICD-11 draw on this accumulated body of knowledge.

Both DSM-5 and ICD-11 have new chapters on PTSD and related disorders. In DSM-5, PTSD is included in the category of "Trauma- and Stressor-Related Disorders." Similarly, ICD-11 has a category of disorders related to stress that includes both PTSD and complex PTSD.

Stressor Criterion

Traumatic events impose both an external and an internal reality on the individual. The external reality is of danger, because these events have the capacity to kill, maim, brutalize, and destroy. Examples of such events are disasters, wars, rape, assault, motor vehicle accidents, and predatory violence. The internal reality involves an attack on ideals and beliefs about safety, control, and freedom from pain. Victims are confronted with potentially overwhelming threats, and often their sense of powerlessness is compounded in the aftermath of the event by the recurring and involuntary memory of their perceptions and emotions. This state is magnified by memories of the trauma, which are triggered by often subtle and unrecognized reminders of the event.

One of the central issues for this field has been defining and observing a *traumatic event*. In DSM-5, the stressor criterion (Criterion A) includes traumatic events that are experienced directly, witnessed, or experienced indirectly (Box 29–1).

Diagnosis

For an individual to be diagnosed with PTSD according to DSM-5, one or more symptoms must be linked to the traumatic event—that is, symptoms must begin (Criteria A through E) or worsen (Criteria D and E) after the traumatic exposure. DSM-5 acknowledges the heterogeneity of symptoms by broadening the definition of PTSD to include a new symptom cluster (Criterion D: alterations of cognitions and mood) and the addition of a dissociative subtype.

The uniqueness of PTSD lies in Criterion B. Essentially, as van der Kolk and van der Hart (1991) stated, PTSD is a disorder of memory, in which the traumatic experience is not integrated normally. This is evident in the dominance of the traumatic memory in the victim's consciousness, with reexperiencing symptoms. Repeated involuntary memories may recur spontaneously or be triggered by various real and symbolic stimuli and may involve intense sensory and visual memories of the event that may or may not be accompanied by extreme physiological and psychological distress. They also may occur with a dissociative quality seen in flashbacks and in dreams.

Box 29–1.   DSM-5 diagnostic criteria for posttraumatic stress disorder

---

Posttraumatic Stress Disorder

Note: The following criteria apply to adults, adolescents, and children older than 6 years. For children 6 years and younger, see corresponding criteria below.

A. Exposure to actual or threatened death, serious injury, or sexual violence in one (or more) of the following ways:

1. Directly experiencing the traumatic event(s).
2. Witnessing, in person, the event(s) as it occurred to others.
3. Learning that the traumatic event(s) occurred to a close family member or close friend. In cases of actual or threatened death of a family member or friend, the event(s) must have been violent or accidental.
4. Experiencing repeated or extreme exposure to aversive details of the traumatic event(s) (e.g., first responders collecting human remains; police officers repeatedly exposed to details of child abuse).

   Note: Criterion A4 does not apply to exposure through electronic media, television, movies, or pictures, unless this exposure is work related.

B. Presence of one (or more) of the following intrusion symptoms associated with the traumatic event(s), beginning after the traumatic event(s) occurred:

1. Recurrent, involuntary, and intrusive distressing memories of the traumatic event(s).

   Note: In children older than 6 years, repetitive play may occur in which themes or aspects of the traumatic event(s) are expressed.

2. Recurrent distressing dreams in which the content and/or affect of the dream are related to the traumatic event(s).

   Note: In children, there may be frightening dreams without recognizable content.

3. Dissociative reactions (e.g., flashbacks) in which the individual feels or acts as if the traumatic event(s) were recurring. (Such reactions may occur on a continuum, with the most extreme expression being a complete loss of awareness of present surroundings.)

   Note: In children, trauma-specific reenactment may occur in play.

4. Intense or prolonged psychological distress at exposure to internal or external cues that symbolize or resemble an aspect of the traumatic event(s).
5. Marked physiological reactions to internal or external cues that symbolize or resemble an aspect of the traumatic event(s).

C. Persistent avoidance of stimuli associated with the traumatic event(s), beginning after the traumatic event(s) occurred, as evidenced by one or both of the following:

1. Avoidance of or efforts to avoid distressing memories, thoughts, or feelings about or closely associated with the traumatic event(s).
2. Avoidance of or efforts to avoid external reminders (people, places, conversations, activities, objects, situations) that arouse distressing memories, thoughts, or feelings about or closely associated with the traumatic event(s).

D. Negative alterations in cognitions and mood associated with the traumatic event(s), beginning or worsening after the traumatic event(s) occurred, as evidenced by two (or more) of the following:

1. Inability to remember an important aspect of the traumatic event(s) (typically due to dissociative amnesia and not to other factors such as head injury, alcohol, or drugs).

2. Persistent and exaggerated negative beliefs or expectations about oneself, others, or the world (e.g., "I am bad," "No one can be trusted," "The world is completely dangerous," "My whole nervous system is permanently ruined").

3. Persistent, distorted cognitions about the cause or consequences of the traumatic event(s) that lead the individual to blame himself/herself or others.

4. Persistent negative emotional state (e.g., fear, horror, anger, guilt, or shame).

5. Markedly diminished interest or participation in significant activities.

6. Feelings of detachment or estrangement from others.

7. Persistent inability to experience positive emotions (e.g., inability to experience happiness, satisfaction, or loving feelings).

E. Marked alterations in arousal and reactivity associated with the traumatic event(s), beginning or worsening after the traumatic event(s) occurred, as evidenced by two (or more) of the following:

1. Irritable behavior and angry outbursts (with little or no provocation) typically expressed as verbal or physical aggression toward people or objects

2. Reckless or self-destructive behavior

3. Hypervigilance

4. Exaggerated startle response

5. Problems with concentration

6. Sleep disturbance (e.g., difficulty falling or staying asleep or restless sleep)

F. Duration of the disturbance (Criteria B, C, D, and E) is more than 1 month.

G. The disturbance causes clinically significant distress or impairment in social, occupational, or other important areas of functioning.

H. The disturbance is not attributable to the physiological effects of a substance (e.g., medication, alcohol) or another medical condition.

Specify whether:

With dissociative symptoms: The individual's symptoms meet the criteria for posttraumatic stress disorder, and in addition, in response to the stressor, the individual experiences persistent or recurrent symptoms of either of the following:

1. **Depersonalization:** Persistent or recurrent experiences of feeling detached from, and as if one were an outside observer of, one's mental processes or body (e.g., feeling as though one were in a dream; feeling a sense of unreality of self or body or of time moving slowly).

2. **Derealization:** Persistent or recurrent experiences of unreality of surroundings (e.g., the world around the individual is experienced as unreal, dreamlike, distant, or distorted).

Note: To use this subtype, the dissociative symptoms must not be attributable to the physiological effects of a substance (e.g., blackouts, behavior during alcohol intoxication) or another medical condition (e.g., complex partial seizures).

Specify if:

With delayed expression: If the full diagnostic criteria are not met until at least 6 months after the event (although the onset and expression of some symptoms may be immediate).

Posttraumatic Stress Disorder for Children 6 Years and Younger

A. In children 6 years and younger, exposure to actual or threatened death, serious injury, or sexual violence in one (or more) of the following ways:

1. Directly experiencing the traumatic event(s).

2. Witnessing, in person, the event(s) as it occurred to others, especially primary caregivers.

Note: Witnessing does not include events that are witnessed only in electronic media, television, movies, or pictures.

3. Learning that the traumatic event(s) occurred to a parent or caregiving figure.

B. Presence of one (or more) of the following intrusion symptoms associated with the traumatic event(s), beginning after the traumatic event(s) occurred:

1. Recurrent, involuntary, and intrusive distressing memories of the traumatic event(s).

   Note: Spontaneous and intrusive memories may not necessarily appear distressing and may be expressed as play reenactment.

2. Recurrent distressing dreams in which the content and/or affect of the dream are related to the traumatic event(s).

   Note: It may not be possible to ascertain that the frightening content is related to the traumatic event.

3. Dissociative reactions (e.g., flashbacks) in which the child feels or acts as if the traumatic event(s) were recurring. (Such reactions may occur on a continuum, with the most extreme expression being a complete loss of awareness of present surroundings.) Such trauma-specific reenactment may occur in play.

4. Intense or prolonged psychological distress at exposure to internal or external cues that symbolize or resemble an aspect of the traumatic event(s).

5. Marked physiological reactions to reminders of the traumatic event(s).

C. One (or more) of the following symptoms, representing either persistent avoidance of stimuli associated with the traumatic event(s) or negative alterations in cognitions and mood associated with the traumatic event(s), must be present, beginning after the event(s) or worsening after the event(s):

Persistent Avoidance of Stimuli

1. Avoidance of or efforts to avoid activities, places, or physical reminders that arouse recollections of the traumatic event(s)

2. Avoidance of or efforts to avoid people, conversations, or interpersonal situations that arouse recollections of the traumatic event(s)

Negative Alterations in Cognitions

3. Substantially increased frequency of negative emotional states (e.g., fear, guilt, sadness, shame, confusion)

4. Markedly diminished interest or participation in significant activities, including constriction of play

5. Socially withdrawn behavior

6. Persistent reduction in expression of positive emotions

D. Alterations in arousal and reactivity associated with the traumatic event(s), beginning or worsening after the traumatic event(s) occurred, as evidenced by two (or more) of the following:

1. Irritable behavior and angry outbursts (with little or no provocation) typically expressed as verbal or physical aggression toward people or objects (including extreme temper tantrums)

2. Hypervigilance

3. Exaggerated startle response

4. Problems with concentration

5. Sleep disturbance (e.g., difficulty falling or staying asleep or restless sleep)

E. The duration of the disturbance is more than 1 month.

F. The disturbance causes clinically significant distress or impairment in relationships with parents, siblings, peers, or other caregivers or with school behavior.

G. The disturbance is not attributable to the physiological effects of a substance (e.g., medication or alcohol) or another medical condition.

Specify whether:

With dissociative symptoms: The individual's symptoms meet the criteria for post-traumatic stress disorder, and the individual experiences persistent or recurrent symptoms of either of the following:

1. **Depersonalization:** Persistent or recurrent experiences of feeling detached from, and as if one were an outside observer of, one's mental processes or body (e.g., feeling as though one were in a dream; feeling a sense of unreality of self or body or of time moving slowly).

2. **Derealization:** Persistent or recurrent experiences of unreality of surroundings (e.g., the world around the individual is experienced as unreal, dreamlike, distant, or distorted).

Note: To use this subtype, the dissociative symptoms must not be attributable to the physiological effects of a substance (e.g., blackouts) or another medical condition (e.g., complex partial seizures).

Specify if:

With delayed expression: If the full diagnostic criteria are not met until at least 6 months after the event (although the onset and expression of some symptoms may be immediate).

Source. Reprinted from American Psychiatric Association: *Diagnostic and Statistical Manual of Mental Disorders*, 5th Edition. Arlington, VA, American Psychiatric Association, 2013. Copyright © 2013 American Psychiatric Association. Used with permission.

The avoidance/numbing cluster described in DSM-IV (American Psychiatric Association 1994) has been divided into two distinct clusters in DSM-5: avoidance (Criterion C) and persistent negative alterations in cognitions and mood (Criterion D). The latter cluster, which retains most of the DSM-IV numbing symptoms, also includes new or reconceptualized symptoms, such as persistent negative emotional states and posttraumatic cognitions, that reflect the influence of cognitive-behavioral findings on DSM-5 criteria.

The final DSM-5 PTSD cluster—alterations in arousal and reactivity (Criterion E)—retains most of the DSM-IV arousal symptoms. It also includes irritable or aggressive behavior and reckless or self-destructive behavior.

PTSD criteria aim to be developmentally sensitive, with lower diagnostic thresholds for children and adolescents. Furthermore, separate criteria have been added for children ages 6 years and younger.

Complex PTSD

Although DSM-5 does not include a diagnosis of complex PTSD, ICD-11 defines both PTSD and complex PTSD. ICD-11 PTSD consists of three core elements or clusters: re-experiencing of the traumatic event in the present, avoidance of traumatic reminders, and a sense of current threat. Complex PTSD also includes three extra clusters that reflect the impact that trauma can have on systems of self-organization, specifically problems in emotion regulation, self-concept, and relational capacities under conditions of sustained, multiple, or repeated traumatic exposure (Ford 2015; Hansen et al. 2017; Karatzias et al. 2018).

Comorbidity

In a clinical setting, the existence of any psychiatric disorder without the co-occurrence of other disorders is the exception rather than the rule. Large epidemiological studies indicate that a range of other disorders, particularly affective disorders, panic disorder, and alcohol and substance abuse, frequently emerge comorbid with PTSD (Rytwinski et al. 2013) and that these comorbidities are not isolated to treatment-seeking populations. Patients with comorbid disorders are likely to have a worse long-term outcome than those without comorbidities and may require chronic maintenance therapy. Studies also have broadened attention to the range of psychiatric disorders that may arise as a consequence of trauma exposure.

Physical symptoms are very common in individuals with PTSD (Gupta 2013) and may be particularly problematic in combat veterans (Kelsall et al. 2009). Somatic presentations are also seen in several other clinical populations, including refugees (Van Ommeren et al. 2002). Chronic pain and disability due to traumatic injury (Pacella et al. 2013) represent another domain of somatic pathology in PTSD. The substantial and accumulating body of research evidence on comorbidities suggests the need to reconceptualize PTSD as a systemic disorder associated with a 4-year decreased life expectancy (Lohr et al. 2015).

Differential Diagnosis

The primary phenomenon that differentiates PTSD from other disorders is the centrality of the traumatic memories that drive the individual's arousal and affective dysphoria. This feature assists in differentiating PTSD from the unfocused anxiety of generalized anxiety disorder. In depression, the dysphoria is driven by a pervasive sense of negative appraisals rather than the more directed sense of powerlessness in a person who has been traumatized. Another differential diagnostic challenge is to ascertain whether panic attacks are indicative of a pattern of psychological and physiological distress triggered by a reminder of a traumatic event (symptoms B4 and B5) or whether these are more typical of the spontaneous attacks consistent with panic disorder.

Course

Acute stress disorder may develop for a period of 3 days to 1 month after exposure to one or more traumatic events. Based on evidence that acute posttraumatic reactions are very heterogeneous, diagnostic criteria in DSM-5 for acute stress disorder are met if individuals exhibit any 9 of 14 symptoms in these categories: intrusion, negative mood, dissociation, avoidance, and arousal. Important differences exist between the ICD-11 and DSM-5 definitions of acute stress reactions. ICD-11 considers an acute stress reaction to be a normal reaction to severe stress rather than a disorder. In contrast, DSM-5 highlights the risk that acute stress disorder might progress to PTSD after 1 month. Although acute stress disorder is a major risk factor for PTSD, most individuals with PTSD do not have a preceding acute stress disorder. Longitudinal research has found that delayed-onset PTSD is far more common than previously was recognized (Bryant et al. 2015).

A meta-analysis of the outcomes of PTSD (Morina et al. 2014) indicated that approximately 56% of individuals with this disorder have a chronic outcome. Longitudinal studies have found that between 18% and 50% of patients recover within 3–7 years (Steinert et al. 2015). The variability of the course of PTSD and the challenges that chronicity presents has led to the suggestion that a staging approach to PTSD should be used (McFarlane et al. 2017).

Impairment and Social and Cultural Issues

PTSD is often a chronic and disabling condition even in the absence of compensation, which highlights how the role of litigation and pensions in causing the chronicity of PTSD is exaggerated (Bruffaerts et al. 2012; Kessler and Frank 1997). An enduring pattern of chronic morbidity develops within this disorder, which is long-lasting and sometimes treatment resistant. Nearly 50% of individuals with PTSD have a lower probability of current employment (Savoca and Rosenheck 2000). In general, a relationship appears to exist between symptom severity and unemployment (Goldstein et al. 2016).

Identifying the symptoms of distress in refugee and war-torn populations (Knaevelsrud et al. 2017; Turner 2015) may support advocacy for the recognition of the suffering of these populations, rather than stigmatizing their distress (Silove et al. 1998). Ultimately, the human psyche, independent of culture, can react to extreme events in a limited number of ways, given the nature of the brain's biology. To argue that PTSD applies in one culture but not another is to ignore this basic commonality (McFarlane and Hinton 2009).

Evaluation

Several rating scales have been developed for use in the trauma field. These include measures for assessing the numbers or types of traumatic events to which individuals have been exposed, the symptoms of PTSD using self-report measures, and the presence of the diagnosis of PTSD. The most commonly reported prevalence estimates of the number of traumatic exposures employ the Composite International Diagnostic Interview, which has been used in most large national epidemiology studies. Comparison between different and traumatic events is important. However, this is inhibited if copyrighted measures are used. Attempts have been made to develop a common methodology of measures that are in the open domain (Olff 2015).

Structured clinical interviews play an important role in the assessment of PTSD in clinical and research settings. Instruments have been developed for use in both children and adults. Perhaps the most widely accepted instrument is the Clinician-Administered PTSD Scale for DSM-5 (Boeschoten et al. 2018; Weathers et al. 2018), which provides both current and lifetime diagnoses of PTSD according to DSM-5 criteria, as well as a rigorous estimation of symptom severity.

Various instruments also have been developed for measuring exposure to specific traumatic events, such as the Life Events Checklist for DSM-5 (Weathers et al. 2013a) and the PTSD Checklist for DSM-5 (Weathers et al. 2013b), developed by the U.S. Department of Veterans Affairs National Center for PTSD. The latter has been used extensively and is in the public domain; it has been shown to correlate highly with clinician-administered measures. A collaboration of traumatic stress societies around the world (Schnyder et al. 2017) developed a brief tool, the Global Psychotrauma Screen, to screen for a wide range of consequences of trauma exposure (www.global-psychotrauma.net/gps). This scale has now been translated into 17 languages (available through M.O.). Recently, the International Trauma Questionnaire was developed as a self-report measure of ICD-11 PTSD and complex PTSD (Cloitre et al. 2018; Shevlin et al. 2018).

Conclusion

PTSD is associated with substantial decreases in individuals' quality of life and work capacity. Accurate diagnosis plays a central role in instigating treatment, highlighting the importance of systematically assessing individuals who have experienced traumatic events for the symptoms of PTSD. Although diagnostic criteria will continue to undergo further revision as more information emerges about the patterns of adaptation to traumatic events, this diagnosis has done much to create a focus on and interest in the effects of psychological trauma.

Key Points

- Trauma is the norm rather than the exception worldwide and a public health concern.

- PTSD is often a chronic and disabling condition that is two to three times more prevalent in women compared to men.

- PTSD is associated with comorbidity.

- Accurate screening and diagnosis of trauma-related symptoms is essential.

References

American Psychiatric Association: Diagnostic and Statistical Manual of Mental Disorders, 3rd Edition. Washington, DC, American Psychiatric Association, 1980

American Psychiatric Association: Diagnostic and Statistical Manual of Mental Disorders, 4th Edition. Washington, DC, American Psychiatric Association, 1994

American Psychiatric Association: Diagnostic and Statistical Manual of Mental Disorders, 5th Edition. Arlington, VA, American Psychiatric Association, 2013

Boeschoten MA, Van der Aa N, Bakker A, et al: Development and evaluation of the Dutch Clinician-Administered PTSD Scale for DSM-5 (CAPS-5). Eur J Psychotraumatol 9(1):1546085, 2018 30510643

Bruffaerts R, Vilagut G, Demyttenaere K, et al: Role of common mental and physical disorders in partial disability around the world. Br J Psychiatry 200(6):454–461, 2012 22539779

Bryant RA, Nickerson A, Creamer M, et al: Trajectory of post-traumatic stress following traumatic injury: 6-year follow-up. Br J Psychiatry 206(5):417–423, 2015 25657356

Cloitre M, Shevlin M, Brewin CR, et al: The International Trauma Questionnaire: development of a self-report measure of ICD-11 PTSD and complex PTSD. Acta Psychiatr Scand 138(6):536–546, 2018 30178492

de Vries GJ, Olff M: The lifetime prevalence of traumatic events and posttraumatic stress disorder in the Netherlands. J Trauma Stress 22(4):259–267, 2009 19645050

Dückers ML, Olff M: Does the vulnerability paradox in PTSD apply to women and men? An exploratory study. J Trauma Stress 30(2):200–204, 2017 28329423

Dückers ML, Alisic E, Brewin CR: A vulnerability paradox in the cross-national prevalence of post-traumatic stress disorder. Br J Psychiatry 209(4):300–305, 2016 27445357

Forbes D, Fletcher S, Parslow R, et al: Trauma at the hands of another: longitudinal study of differences in the posttraumatic stress disorder symptom profile following interpersonal compared with noninterpersonal trauma. J Clin Psychiatry 73(3):372–376, 2012 22154900

Forbes D, Bisson JI, Monson C, et al (eds): Effective Treatments for PTSD: Practice Guidelines From the International Society for Traumatic Stress Studies, 3rd Edition. New York, Guilford, 2020

Ford JD: Complex PTSD: research directions for nosology/assessment, treatment, and public health. Eur J Psychotraumatol 6:27584, 2015 25994023

Glass AJ: Mental health programs in the armed forces, in American Handbook of Psychiatry, 2nd Edition. Edited by Arieti S. New York, Basic Books, 1974, pp 800–809

Goldstein RB, Smith SM, Chou SP, et al: The epidemiology of DSM-5 posttraumatic stress disorder in the United States: results from the National Epidemiologic Survey on Alcohol and Related Conditions-III. Soc Psychiatry Psychiatr Epidemiol 51(8):1137–1148, 2016 27106853

Gupta MA: Review of somatic symptoms in post-traumatic stress disorder. Int Rev Psychiatry 25(1):86–99, 2013 23383670

Hansen M, Smith SM, Chou SP, et al: Does size really matter? A multisite study assessing the latent structure of the proposed ICD-11 and DSM-5 diagnostic criteria for PTSD. Eur J Psychotraumatol 8(suppl 7):1398002, 2017 29201287

Horowitz MJ: Stress Response Syndromes, 2nd Edition. New York, Plenum, 1986

International Society for Traumatic Stress Studies: ISTSS PTSD Prevention and Treatment Guidelines. Oakbrook Terrace, IL, International Society for Traumatic Stress Studies 2015. Available at: https://istss.org/clinical-resources/treating-trauma/new-istss-prevention-and-treatment-guidelines. Accessed November 14, 2019.

Karam EG, Friedman MJ, Hill ED, et al: Cumulative traumas and risk thresholds: 12-month PTSD in the World Mental Health (WMH) surveys. Depress Anxiety 31(2):130–142, 2014 23983056

Karatzias T, Friedman MJ, Hill ED, et al: PTSD and complex PTSD: ICD-11 updates on concept and measurement in the UK, USA, Germany and Lithuania. Eur J Psychotraumatol 8(suppl 7):1418103, 2018 29372010

Kelsall HL, McKenzie DP, Sim MR, et al: Physical, psychological, and functional comorbidities of multisymptom illness in Australian male veterans of the 1991 Gulf War. Am J Epidemiol 170(8):1048–1056, 2009 19762370

Kessler RC, Frank RG: The impact of psychiatric disorders on work loss days. Psychol Med 27(4):861–873, 1997 9234464

Kessler RC, Chiu WT, Demler O, et al: Prevalence, severity, and comorbidity of 12-month DSM-IV disorders in the National Comorbidity Survey Replication. Arch Gen Psychiatry 62(6):617–627, 2005 15939839

Kessler RC, Aguilar-Gaxiola S, Alonso J, et al: Trauma and PTSD in the WHO World Mental Health surveys. Eur J Psychotraumatol 8(suppl 5):1353383, 2017 29075426

Knaevelsrud C, Stammel N, Olff M: Traumatized refugees: identifying needs and facing challenges for mental health care. Eur J Psychotraumatol 8(suppl 2):1388103, 2017 29152160

Lohr JB, Palmer BW, Eidt CA, et al: Is post-traumatic stress disorder associated with premature senescence? A review of the literature. Am J Geriatr Psychiatry 23(7):709–725, 2015 25959921

Magruder KM, McLaughlin KA, Elmore Borbon DL: Trauma is a public health issue. Eur J Psychotraumatol 8(1):1375338, 2017 29435198

McFarlane AC, Hinton D: Ethnocultural issues, in Post Traumatic Stress Disorder: Diagnosis, Management and Treatment, 2nd Edition. Edited by Nutt DJ, Stein MB, Zohar J. London, Informa, 2009, pp 163–175

McFarlane AC, Lawrence-Wood E, Van Hooff M, et al: The need to take a staging approach to the biological mechanisms of PTSD and its treatment. Curr Psychiatry Rep 19(2):10, 2017 28168596

McNally R: Resolving the vulnerability paradox in the cross-national prevalence of posttraumatic stress disorder. J Anxiety Disord 54:33–35, 2018 29421370

Morina N, Wicherts JM, Lobbrecht J, et al: Remission from post-traumatic stress disorder in adults: a systematic review and meta-analysis of long term outcome studies. Clin Psychol Rev 34(3):249–255, 2014 24681171

Olff M: Choosing the right instruments for psychotrauma related research. Eur J Psychotraumatol 6:30585, 2015 26714933

Olff M: Psychotraumatology on the move. Eur J Psychotraumatol 9(1):1439650, 2018 29535846

Olff M, Langeland W, Draijer N, et al: Gender differences in posttraumatic stress disorder. Psychol Bull 133(2):183–204, 2007 17338596

Pacella ML, Hruska B, Delahanty DL: The physical health consequences of PTSD and PTSD symptoms: a meta-analytic review. J Anxiety Disord 27(1):33–46, 2013 23247200

Rytwinski NK, Scur MD, Feeny NC, et al: The co-occurrence of major depressive disorder among individuals with posttraumatic stress disorder: a meta-analysis. J Trauma Stress 26(3):299–309, 2013 23696449

Savoca E, Rosenheck R: The civilian labor market experiences of Vietnam-era veterans: the influence of psychiatric disorders. J Ment Health Policy Econ 3(4):199–207, 2000 11967456

Schnyder U, Schäfer I, Aakvaag HF, et al: The global collaboration on traumatic stress. Eur J Psychotraumatol 8(suppl 7):1403257, 2017 29435201

Shevlin M, Hyland P, Roberts NP, et al: A psychometric assessment of Disturbances in Self-Organization symptom indicators for ICD-11 complex PTSD using the International Trauma Questionnaire. Eur J Psychotraumatol 9(1):1419749, 2018 29372014

Silove D, Steel Z, McGorry P, et al: Trauma exposure, postmigration stressors, and symptoms of anxiety, depression and post-traumatic stress in Tamil asylum-seekers: comparison with refugees and immigrants. Acta Psychiatr Scand 97(3):175–181, 1998 9543304

Southwick SM, Bonanno GA, Masten AS, et al: Resilience definitions, theory, and challenges: interdisciplinary perspectives. Eur J Psychotraumatol 5, 2014 25317257

Steinert C, Hofmann M, Leichsenring F, Kruse J: The course of PTSD in naturalistic long-term studies: high variability of outcomes. A systematic review. Nord J Psychiatry 69(7):483–496, 2015 25733025

Turner S: Refugee blues: a UK and European perspective. Eur J Psychotraumatol 6:29328, 2015 26514159

van der Kolk BA, van der Hart O: The intrusive past: the flexibility of memory and the engraving of trauma. Imago 48:425–454, 1991

Van Ommeren M, Sharma B, Sharma GK, et al: The relationship between somatic and PTSD symptoms among Bhutanese refugee torture survivors: examination of comorbidity with anxiety and depression. J Trauma Stress 15(5):415–421, 2002 12392230

Vermetten M, Baker DG, Jetly R, et al: Concerns over divergent approaches in the diagnostics of posttraumatic stress disorder. Psychiatr Ann 46(9):498–509, 2016

Weathers FW, Blake DD, Schnurr PP, et al: The Life Events Checklist for DSM-5 (LEC-5). Washington, DC, U.S. Department of Veterans Affairs, 2013a. Available at: https://www.ptsd.va.gov/professional/assessment/te-measures/life_events_checklist.asp#obtain. Accessed July 8, 2019.

Weathers FW, Litz BT, Keane TM, et al: The PTSD Checklist for DSM-5 (PCL-5). Washington, DC, U.S. Department of Veterans Affairs, 2013b. Available at: https://www.ptsd.va.gov/professional/assessment/adult-sr/ptsd-checklist.asp#obtain. Accessed July 8, 2019.

Weathers FW, Blake DD, Schnurr PP, et al: The Clinician-Administered PTSD Scale for DSM-5. Washington, DC, National Center for PTSD, April 16, 2018. Available at: https://www.ptsd.va.gov/professional/assessment/documents/CAPS_5_Past_Week.pdf. Accessed June 12, 2019.

World Health Organization: International Statistical Classification of Diseases and Related Health Problems, 11th Revision (advance preview). Geneva, World Health Organization, 2018

Yehuda R, McFarlane AC: Conflict between current knowledge about posttraumatic stress disorder and its original conceptual basis. Am J Psychiatry 152(12):1705–1713, 1995 8526234

Recommended Readings

Schnyder U, Cloitre M (eds): Evidence-based treatments for trauma-related psychological disorders: a practical guide for clinicians. New York, Springer International Publishing, 2015

CHAPTER 30

Pathogenesis of PTSD

Richard A. Bryant, Ph.D.

Since its beginnings more than 100 years ago, conceptualizations of what is now known as *posttraumatic stress disorder* have recognized that trauma memories, in which a person repeatedly experiences distress associated with a traumatic experience, are a key factor of this diagnosis. The central role of trauma memories is also seen in nearly all models of the pathogenesis of PTSD. In this chapter, I review the factors that underpin the development and maintenance of PTSD, beginning with a review of biological factors and then an outline of the psychological mechanisms of PTSD. I then overview the prevailing etiological frameworks for PTSD, including fear conditioning and cognitive-behavioral models.

Biological Bases of PTSD

Genetic Factors

The vast majority of people exposed to trauma do not develop PTSD (Galatzer-Levy et al. 2018). This well-documented fact highlights that key individual differences exist in one's propensity to develop PTSD following trauma. Overwhelming evidence indicates that genetic factors play an important role in one's susceptibility to PTSD, accounting for 30%–72% of the vulnerability to developing the disorder (Sartor et al. 2011; True et al. 1993).

Many studies have attempted to link PTSD with candidate genes, and not surprisingly, genes associated with PTSD are also linked with other common psychiatric disorders, including major depression, generalized anxiety disorder, panic disorder, and substance use (Koenen et al. 2008). For example, numerous studies have pointed to the functional polymorphism in the promoter region of the serotonin transporter gene *SLC6A4* across many disorders. The short allele of 5-HTTLPR is a repeat polymorphic region in *SLC6A4* that reduces serotonergic expression and uptake by nearly

50% (Lesch et al. 1996). A greater incidence of the short allele has been found in patients with PTSD (Lee et al. 2005). Moreover, this allele has been linked with impaired extinction learning in both mice and humans (Galatzer-Levy et al. 2017). Much attention has also focused on *FKBP5* because it modulates the glucocorticoid receptor, and gene × environment association studies indicate that FKBP5 alleles increase risk for PTSD (Binder et al. 2008). Overall, more than 50 gene variants have been linked with PTSD, including hypothalamic-pituitary-adrenal (HPA) axis functions, noradrenergic systems, dopaminergic and serotonin systems, and neurotrophins (Sheerin et al. 2017). This field of study is characterized by poor replication of studies, and accordingly there is convergent agreement that the most promising avenue for understanding a genetic basis of PTSD is via polygenetic approaches. The largest genome-wide study performed to date was conducted by the PTSD Working Group of the Psychiatric Genomics Consortium, which recently reported an analysis of 20,730 people; although no single-nucleotide polymorphism was found to be significantly associated with PTSD, this study did find a polygenetic risk profile that overlapped with risk for schizophrenia (Duncan et al. 2018).

The genetic influences on PTSD appear to be moderated by the type and timing of environmental factors. Early life stress appears to be particularly relevant; numerous studies have indicated that childhood trauma or adversity modifies the genetic risk for PTSD (Binder et al. 2008). This conclusion has led to the potential utility of epigenetic regulation to increase understanding of how genetic factors can modulate risk for PTSD. Most epigenetic studies in PTSD have focused on DNA methylation, with investigations assessing peripheral indicators of candidate genes (Zannas et al. 2015). Arguably, most of this work has narrowed on epigenetic regulation of the HPA axis because of the well-documented role of this stress system in moderating PTSD (Golier et al. 2007). Distinctive methylation in PTSD has been documented in a number of genes, including *NR3C1, CRHR1,* and *FKBP5* (Sheerin et al. 2017). Although increasing evidence indicates that trauma has the potential to induce epigenetic changes, and that these have been shown to be distinctive in PTSD, the evidence to date has been drawn from peripheral blood assessments, which represent proxy measurements. One must recognize that such evidence does not reflect central mechanisms occurring in neural circuits.

Neuroanatomy

Initial neuroimaging studies of PTSD focused on the hippocampus because of animal research indicating that it is susceptible to the adverse effects of stress. Many studies have since found that PTSD is characterized by a smaller hippocampus, with meta-analyses indicating that this effect is observed bilaterally (Smith 2005). Reinforcing this conclusion is a recent study of the Psychiatric Genomics Consortium's PTSD Working Group—a study comprising 1,868 participants (794 with PTSD)—in which smaller hippocampi were found in those with PTSD (Logue et al. 2018). The extent to which a smaller hippocampus is a function of PTSD or a risk factor has yet to be definitively addressed. The possibility that smaller hippocampal volume may represent a risk factor for PTSD was raised by a study that compared monozygotic co-twins who either did or did not serve in Vietnam (Gilbertson et al. 2002). This study found that Vietnam veterans with PTSD were characterized by smaller hippocampi than were Vietnam veterans without PTSD, but that the co-twins of those with PTSD who had not served in Vietnam had hippocampi that were just as small. Evidence has also been found of reduced volume in the prefrontal regions in individuals with PTSD (Kitayama et al. 2006), which is consistent with proposals that patients with PTSD are deficient in emotion regulation.

At a functional level, many studies have been conducted that have used fear provocation tasks to elicit the threat network in patients with PTSD. For many years, the prominent neurobiological theory of PTSD has revolved around the notion that the prefrontal cortex (PFC) inadequately regulates amygdala-based emotional reactivity (Rauch and Drevets 2009). Although findings across studies vary considerably, findings from a meta-analytic study generally support this conclusion, with evidence of underactivation of medial PFC regions and overengagement of the amygdala (Patel et al. 2012).

Increasingly, evidence shows that diverse networks are involved in the pathogenesis of PTSD that extend beyond this traditional "fear circuitry network." Recent commentaries have also noted the roles of dysfunctions in threat detection, executive functioning, emotion regulation, and contextual processing (Shalev et al. 2017). In terms of threat detection, a great deal of evidence has been found of hypervigilance and attentional bias to potentially threatening stimuli in PTSD (Block and Liberzon 2016), and numerous studies indicate overreactivity in regions associated with salience detection, including the amygdala, dorsal anterior cingulate cortex, and insula (Shalev et al. 2017). PTSD is also characterized by memory and concentration deficits, impoverished attentional control over intrusive memories, and deficits in ability to regulate emotions in a top-down manner (Block and Liberzon 2016). Accordingly, neuroimaging studies have documented reduced connectivity of frontoparietal networks with executive function networks (Sripada et al. 2012b). Considerable attention has also focused on contextual processing because of the tendency in patients with PTSD to overgeneralize fear to many contexts beyond what is actually dangerous. Whereas contextual processing can rely on optimal functioning in the hippocampus and medial PFC (Lang et al. 2009), abundant evidence has been reported of hippocampal dysfunction in PTSD (Patel et al. 2012) and of impaired medial PFC recruitment in PTSD during extinction recall and contextual processing (Milad et al. 2007).

Neurochemistry and Neuroendocrinology

A large body of evidence indicates neuroendocrinological abnormalities associated with PTSD. Much attention has focused on the overactivity of the noradrenergic system because this is associated with arousal, reexperiencing symptoms, and reactivity to trauma reminders (Pitman et al. 2012). At a preclinical level, abundant evidence has shown that noradrenergic activation is pivotal in the consolidation of emotional memories (McGaugh 2000). This finding led to early theories that the increased noradrenergic surge at the time of a traumatic event was pivotal to the strong consolidation of trauma memories, which subsequently formed the basis of reexperiencing, reactivity, and persistent fear (Pitman 1989). As a result, numerous attempts have been made to limit PTSD development using early administration of propranolol (a β-adrenergic antagonist) in the very acute period after trauma; although this treatment showed promise in reducing subsequent reactivity to trauma reminders (Pitman et al. 2002), it has not proven to reliably reduce PTSD symptoms (Stein et al. 2007). Indirect evidence for the role of noradrenergic processes emerges from the relationship between the development of PTSD and the use of morphine in the acute phase after trauma, because morphine inhibits the production of norepinephrine. In this context, it is interesting that a greater morphine dose in the acute period after trauma is associated with reduced PTSD (Bryant et al. 2009). None of these studies represent controlled trials, however, so any causal inferences regarding morphine and noradrenergic inhibition are tentative.

Arguably one of the most studied systems in PTSD, and perhaps one of the most controversial, has been the glucocorticoid system. Although increased cortisol levels are typically associated with chronic stress, PTSD has been somewhat surprisingly associated with *lower* cortisol levels (Yehuda et al. 1990). Furthermore, lower cortisol levels shortly after trauma predict subsequent PTSD severity (Delahanty et al. 2000), although evidence for this pattern is mixed (Shalev et al. 2008). This somewhat paradoxical finding has been interpreted in terms of cortisol binding to the glucocorticoid receptors in a negative feedback loop that promotes homeostasis of the stress response (Yehuda 1997). This proposal posits that lower cortisol in PTSD may result in elevated ongoing HPA activity, leading to exaggerated catecholamine response and consequent overconsolidation of trauma memories, a proposition that has received some support from early intervention studies in animal models that found administration of hydrocortisone shortly after stressor exposure results in reduced subsequent PTSD-like reactions (Cohen et al. 2008). Tentative evidence has indicated that this procedure also limits subsequent PTSD symptoms following trauma in humans (Zohar et al. 2011).

A major focus of attention in recent years is the role of sex hormones, because of the robust finding that females are twice as likely to develop PTSD as males (Olff et al. 2007). At a preclinical level, evidence indicates that females have greater noradrenergic response to aversive stimuli (Lithari et al. 2010), display greater startle modulation in threatening contexts (Grillon 2008), are more likely to have a noradrenergic response to a stressor (Segal and Cahill 2009), and have greater amygdala reactivity in response to threatening stimuli (Williams et al. 2005) compared with males. Furthermore, females retain emotional memories better than males over time (Andreano and Cahill 2009). It appears that menstrual phase plays an important role in adaptation to trauma because of the cycling levels of progesterone and estradiol. These hormones affect a range of neurobiological processes implicated in PTSD, including fear conditioning and extinction (Milad et al. 2009). Females with PTSD, relative to those without PTSD, showed impaired extinction learning in the midluteal phase (when progesterone and estradiol levels are high) (Pineles et al. 2016). Women are more likely to experience intrusive memories of a trauma film if they encode it in the midluteal phase (Ferree et al. 2011). They are also more likely to experience flashback memories if they are exposed to traumatic events during the midluteal phase (Bryant et al. 2011). One reason progesterone may facilitate emotional memories is that progesterone binds to glucocorticoid receptors, affects glucocorticoid's receptivity, and results in a marked increase in endogenous glucocorticoids in the midluteal phase (Kirschbaum et al. 1999). Although much is still not understood about the sex differences in trauma response, the emerging data are certainly pointing to hormonal factors playing an important role in how males and females may consolidate trauma memories differently.

Psychophysiological Indicators

A frequently reported finding in PTSD is the observation of enhanced psychophysiological reactivity to reminders of the trauma. In the most common form of this study, participants listen to prerecorded accounts of their trauma while heart rate, skin conductance response, or facial electromyography measurements are obtained. Many studies have shown that PTSD is distinguished from non-PTSD states by greater reactivity to memories of their trauma (Orr et al. 1993).

Heightened startle response is recognized in the definition of PTSD, so it is not surprising that elevated reactivity is repeatedly noted in experimental studies in response to startling stimuli (e.g., loud noises) (Pole 2007). Evidence is mixed regarding the extent to which this heightened reactivity is a risk factor for PTSD or is acquired after PTSD development. One study that assessed trainee firefighters prior to trauma exposure found that elevated startle response was associated with acute posttraumatic stress severity after exposure to a recent traumatic event (Guthrie and Bryant 2005). In contrast, a study of monozygotic twins (one of whom developed PTSD after serving in Vietnam) found greater heart rate in response to loud noises in the twin with PTSD, relative to the twin without PTSD, suggesting an acquired propensity for startle response (Orr et al. 2003). Furthermore, evidence indicates that elevated startle response develops over time with PTSD rather than being present immediately after trauma exposure (Shalev et al. 2000).

Psychosocial and Psychological Factors

Developmental Factors

Many studies have indicated that childhood trauma, particularly childhood abuse, is a major risk factor for PTSD development (Ozer et al. 2003). Childhood maltreatment is associated with structural deficits in the hippocampus, corpus callosum, anterior cingulate cortex, orbitofrontal cortex, and dorsolateral PFC (Teicher et al. 2012). The toxic effects of maltreatment can adversely impact neuronal development in core neural networks that underpin susceptibility to development of PTSD. It appears that the impact of these experiences on neuronal development may be dependent on the timing of the traumatic experience; for example, the strongest impact on hippocampal volume occurs at ages 3–5 years, whereas the greatest impact on the PFC appears to occur at ages 12–13 years (Teicher et al. 2016).

Neuropsychological Dysfunctions

Evidence strongly indicates that people with PTSD have deficits across a range of neuropsychological functions, including concentration, sustained attention, executive control, and working memory (Aupperle et al. 2012). These findings accord with evidence of alterations in attention-related neural networks in PTSD (Sripada et al. 2012a). Numerous symptoms of PTSD, as well as common problems associated with the disorder, are linked to altered attentional processes, including vigilance to threat (Buckley et al. 2000). For example, PTSD is characterized by strong bias to potentially threatening stimuli, as reflected in emotional Stroop (Bryant and Harvey 1995), dot probe (Bryant and Harvey 1997), and eye-tracking (Felmingham et al. 2011) paradigms. In addition, patients with PTSD have difficulties with disengagement from threat, response inhibition, and orienting (Block and Liberzon 2016). These diverse deficits in attentional focus and control can contribute to ongoing vigilance to potential threats in the environment, as well as the inability to control unwanted thoughts and memories, and they underpin many of the cognitive problems characterized by PTSD, such as memory and concentration deficits.

Catastrophic Appraisals

One of the most commonly observed cognitive dysfunctions in PTSD is the tendency to engage in excessively negative appraisals about oneself, the causes of the trauma, the ways in which one reacted to the event, or the likelihood of future harm. In terms of appraisals in the acute period after trauma exposure, extremely negative interpretations of the traumatic experience are associated with acute stress disorder (Warda and Bryant 1998) and are predictive of later PTSD (Dunmore et al. 2001). Catastrophic appraisals also are associated with maintenance of PTSD (Dunmore et al. 1999), and prospective studies suggest that this form of thinking is a risk factor for development of PTSD (Bryant and Guthrie 2005).

Etiological Models

Fear Conditioning

Arguably the most influential model of PTSD involves fear conditioning, in which the surge of stress hormones at the time of trauma results in strong associative learning with stimuli at the time of trauma and overconsolidation of the trauma memory; these associations lead to the intense memories and reactivity to trauma reminders (Pitman et al. 2000). The fear conditioning model of PTSD accords with the aforementioned alterations in key neural circuits in PTSD—the amygdala, PFC, and hippocampus—which are also implicated in fear learning, as well as with the robust findings of heightened reactivity in PTSD to trauma reminders (Orr et al. 1993). Evidence of elevated resting heart rate in the acute period after trauma in individuals who subsequently develop PTSD (Bryant et al. 2000), and particularly in response to trauma reminders (O'Donnell et al. 2007), provides more compelling support for this model. This model also posits that PTSD is maintained because of impoverished extinction of the initial conditioned fear response, which is supported by evidence of impaired extinction learning in PTSD (Peri et al. 2000), along with evidence of impoverished recruitment of neural networks implicated in extinction learning (Patel et al. 2012). Some evidence has shown that deficient capacity for extinction learning is a risk factor for PTSD (Guthrie and Bryant 2006). PTSD is also characterized by enhanced sensitization following trauma, such that individuals with PTSD are more susceptible to the effects of subsequent life stressors (Post et al. 1995).

Extinction learning requires synaptic plasticity, which may be impaired in PTSD and thereby contribute to difficulties in new safety learning. This logic has led to research into molecular mechanisms that may have an impact on recovery from trauma.

One example is brain-derived neurotrophic factor (BDNF), which underpins synaptic plasticity and has been shown to enhance extinction learning (Quirk and Mueller 2008). The Val66Met polymorphism in the *BDNF* gene results in diminished secretion of BDNF, impedes extinction learning, and has also been shown to increase risk for PTSD (Zhang et al. 2014). Moreover, carriers of the Val66Met polymorphism respond less successfully to extinction-based therapy for PTSD (exposure therapy), highlighting the role of BDNF in maintaining PTSD (Felmingham et al. 2013).

Cognitive-Behavioral Models

Although very consistent with biological models, cognitive-behavioral models place more emphasis on the roles of memory organization and appraisals (Figure 30–1). Cognitive-behavioral models propose that trauma memories are encoded in a fragmented manner because of the elevated arousal that occurs at the time of trauma, which limits how these memories can be consolidated in a coherent narrative; this in turn can impede processing of trauma memories and adaptation to the trauma experience (Ehlers and Clark 2000). According to these models, the predominantly sensory memories are typically visual (although other sensory modalities may also be represented), involving a mode of processing referred to as "data-driven processing," which is fragmented and impedes contextualization of memories into one's normal autobiographical memory narrative. One version posits that interference with the visual memory system during the consolidation phase after trauma exposure can limit subsequent PTSD symptoms (Iyadurai et al. 2018). Most cognitive-behavioral models recognize that trauma memories are strongly conditioned to the events that occurred at the time of the trauma, and in this sense these models overlap with fear conditioning models in their suggestion that conditioned stimuli at the time of trauma serve to trigger the sensory-based trauma memories.

Cognitive-behavioral models also place considerable emphasis on the extent to which people appraise the traumatic event, their responses to it, and their environment after the trauma. Specifically, these models emphasize how excessively negative appraisals after the trauma tend to exaggerate the individual's sense of threat, thereby maintaining the PTSD (Foa et al. 1999). Abundant evidence has been found of the predictive role of catastrophic appraisals in the development and maintenance of PTSD, as well as of their decline after successful therapy (Kleim et al. 2013). These models acknowledge that the exaggerated sense of threat perceived by patients with PTSD tends to result in strong avoidance of potential threats, which impedes emotional processing of trauma memories and extinction learning (Foa et al. 1989). Overall, there is considerable overlap between cognitive-behavioral and fear conditioning models. Drawing on both approaches, Figure 30–1 presents an overview of the factors that play etiological and maintaining roles in PTSD.

Conclusion

In summary, our understanding of the pathogenesis and maintenance of PTSD has advanced considerably thanks to the many technological advances in neuroscience and the surge of translational studies that bridge animal and human studies. One of

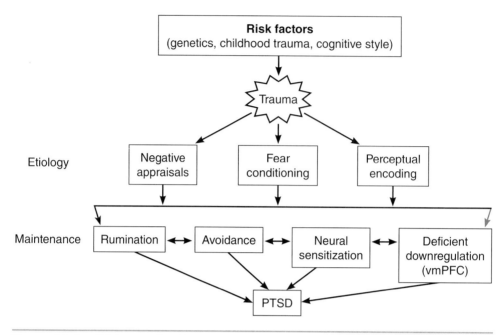

FIGURE 30–1. Etiology and maintenance of PTSD.

Note.   vmPFC=ventromedial prefrontal cortex.

the major challenges for the study of the pathogenesis of PTSD in the future is to understand the heterogeneity of the condition. Increasing recognition of factors beyond fear circuitry requires greater awareness of the roles of reward processing, affective and neutral attentional mechanisms, and varying forms of regulation. Better recognition of the diverse mechanisms that underpin the different forms of dysfunction in PTSD will shed more light on the diversity of problems underpinning the disorder.

Key Points

- Trauma memories are central to PTSD and reflect excessive noradrenergically driven overconsolidation of memories at the time of trauma.

- PTSD can be understood as failed extinction of the initial conditioned response to the traumatic experience, and impaired extinction learning capacity is a risk factor for PTSD.

- PTSD is characterized by lower cortisol levels, which may compromise the negative feedback loop that reduces arousal after a threat.

- Development and maintenance of PTSD is strongly predicted by excessively negative appraisals about the trauma and one's future, and these are reduced with resolution of the PTSD.

- Consistent with fear conditioning models, psychophysiological reactivity to trauma reminders is one of strongest markers of PTSD.

- Neural networks implicated in extinction learning, such as the medial prefrontal cortex, are insufficiently recruited in PTSD.

References

Andreano JM, Cahill L: Sex influences on the neurobiology of learning and memory. Learn Mem 16(4):248–266, 2009 19318467

Aupperle RL, Melrose AJ, Stein MB, et al: Executive function and PTSD: disengaging from trauma. Neuropharmacology 62(2):686–694, 2012 21349277

Binder EB, Bradley RG, Liu W, et al: Association of FKBP5 polymorphisms and childhood abuse with risk of posttraumatic stress disorder symptoms in adults. JAMA 299(11):1291–1305, 2008 18349090

Block SR, Liberzon I: Attentional processes in posttraumatic stress disorder and the associated changes in neural functioning. Exp Neurol 284(Pt B):153–167, 2016 27178007

Bryant RA, Guthrie RM: Maladaptive appraisals as a risk factor for posttraumatic stress: a study of trainee firefighters. Psychol Sci 16(10):749–752, 2005 16181434

Bryant RA, Harvey AG: Processing threatening information in posttraumatic stress disorder. J Abnorm Psychol 104(3):537–541, 1995 7673578

Bryant RA, Harvey AG: Attentional bias in posttraumatic stress disorder. J Trauma Stress 10(4):635–644, 1997 9391946

Bryant RA, Harvey AG, Guthrie RM, et al: A prospective study of psychophysiological arousal, acute stress disorder, and posttraumatic stress disorder. J Abnorm Psychol 109(2):341–344, 2000 10895573

Bryant RA, Creamer M, O'Donnell M, et al: A study of the protective function of acute morphine administration on subsequent posttraumatic stress disorder. Biol Psychiatry 65(5):438–440, 2009 19058787

Bryant RA, Felmingham KL, Silove D, et al: The association between menstrual cycle and traumatic memories. J Affect Disord 131(1–3):398–401, 2011 21093927

Buckley TC, Blanchard EB, Neill WT: Information processing and PTSD: a review of the empirical literature. Clin Psychol Rev 20(8):1041–1065, 2000 11098399

Cohen H, Matar MA, Buskila D, et al: Early post-stressor intervention with high-dose corticosterone attenuates posttraumatic stress response in an animal model of posttraumatic stress disorder. Biol Psychiatry 64(8):708–717, 2008 18635156

Delahanty DL, Raimonde AJ, Spoonster E: Initial posttraumatic urinary cortisol levels predict subsequent PTSD symptoms in motor vehicle accident victims. Biol Psychiatry 48(9):940–947, 2000 11074232

Duncan LE, Ratanatharathorn A, Aiello AE, et al: Largest GWAS of PTSD (N=20,070) yields genetic overlap with schizophrenia and sex differences in heritability. Mol Psychiatry 23(3):666–673, 2018 28439101

Dunmore E, Clark DM, Ehlers A: Cognitive factors involved in the onset and maintenance of posttraumatic stress disorder (PTSD) after physical or sexual assault. Behav Res Ther 37(9):809–829, 1999 10458046

Dunmore E, Clark DM, Ehlers A: A prospective investigation of the role of cognitive factors in persistent posttraumatic stress disorder (PTSD) after physical or sexual assault. Behav Res Ther 39(9):1063–1084, 2001 11520012

Ehlers A, Clark DM: A cognitive model of posttraumatic stress disorder. Behav Res Ther 38(4):319–345, 2000 10761279

Felmingham KL, Rennie C, Manor B, et al: Eye tracking and physiological reactivity to threatening stimuli in posttraumatic stress disorder. J Anxiety Disord 25(5):668–673, 2011 21477983

Felmingham KL, Dobson-Stone C, Schofield PR, et al: The brain-derived neurotrophic factor Val66Met polymorphism predicts response to exposure therapy in posttraumatic stress disorder. Biol Psychiatry 73(11):1059–1063, 2013 23312562

Ferree NK, Kamat R, Cahill L: Influences of menstrual cycle position and sex hormone levels on spontaneous intrusive recollections following emotional stimuli. Conscious Cogn 20(4):1154–1162, 2011 21353599

Foa EB, Steketee G, Rothbaum BO: Behavioral/cognitive conceptualizations of post-traumatic stress disorder. Behav Ther 20:155–176, 1989

Foa EB, Ehlers A, Clark DM, et al: The Posttraumatic Cognitions Inventory (PTCI): development and validation. Psychol Assess 11:303–314, 1999

Galatzer-Levy IR, Andero R, Sawamura T, et al: A cross species study of heterogeneity in fear extinction learning in relation to FKBP5 variation and expression: implications for the acute treatment of posttraumatic stress disorder. Neuropharmacology 116:188–195, 2017 28025095

Galatzer-Levy IR, Huang SH, Bonanno GA: Trajectories of resilience and dysfunction following potential trauma: a review and statistical evaluation. Clin Psychol Rev 63:41–55, 2018 29902711

Gilbertson MW, Shenton ME, Ciszewski A, et al: Smaller hippocampal volume predicts pathologic vulnerability to psychological trauma. Nat Neurosci 5(11):1242–1247, 2002 12379862

Golier JA, Schmeidler J, Legge J, et al: Twenty-four hour plasma cortisol and adrenocorticotropic hormone in Gulf War veterans: relationships to posttraumatic stress disorder and health symptoms. Biol Psychiatry 62(10):1175–1178, 2007 17612507

Grillon C: Greater sustained anxiety but not phasic fear in women compared to men. Emotion 8(3):410–413, 2008 18540756

Guthrie RM, Bryant RA: Auditory startle response in firefighters before and after trauma exposure. Am J Psychiatry 162(2):283–290, 2005 15677592

Guthrie RM, Bryant RA: Extinction learning before trauma and subsequent posttraumatic stress. Psychosom Med 68(2):307–311, 2006 16554398

Iyadurai L, Blackwell SE, Meiser-Stedman R, et al: Preventing intrusive memories after trauma via a brief intervention involving Tetris computer game play in the emergency department: a proof-of-concept randomized controlled trial. Mol Psychiatry 23(3):674–682, 2018 28348380

Kirschbaum C, Kudielka BM, Gaab J, et al: Impact of gender, menstrual cycle phase, and oral contraceptives on the activity of the hypothalamus-pituitary-adrenal axis. Psychosom Med 61(2):154–162, 1999 10204967

Kitayama N, Quinn S, Bremner JD: Smaller volume of anterior cingulate cortex in abuse-related posttraumatic stress disorder. J Affect Disord 90(2–3):171–174, 2006 16375974

Kleim B, Grey N, Wild J, et al: Cognitive change predicts symptom reduction with cognitive therapy for posttraumatic stress disorder. J Consult Clin Psychol 81(3):383–393, 2013 23276122

Koenen KC, Fu QJ, Ertel K, et al: Common genetic liability to major depression and posttraumatic stress disorder in men. J Affect Disord 105(1–3):109–115, 2008 17540456

Lang S, Kroll A, Lipinski SJ, et al: Context conditioning and extinction in humans: differential contribution of the hippocampus, amygdala and prefrontal cortex. Eur J Neurosci 29(4):823–832, 2009 19200075

Lee HJ, Lee MS, Kang RH, et al: Influence of the serotonin transporter promoter gene polymorphism on susceptibility to posttraumatic stress disorder. Depress Anxiety 21(3):135–139, 2005 15965993

Lesch KPBD, Bengel D, Heils A, et al: Association of anxiety-related traits with a polymorphism in the serotonin transporter gene regulatory region. Science 274(5292):1527–1531, 1996 8929413

Lithari C, Frantzidis CA, Papadelis C, et al: Are females more responsive to emotional stimuli? A neurophysiological study across arousal and valence dimensions. Brain Topogr 23(1):27–40, 2010 20043199

Logue MW, van Rooij SJH, Dennis EL, et al: Smaller hippocampal volume in posttraumatic stress disorder: a multisite ENIGMA-PGC study: subcortical volumetry results from Posttraumatic Stress Disorder Consortia. Biol Psychiatry 83(3):244–253, 2018 29217296

McGaugh JL: Memory—a century of consolidation. Science 287(5451):248–251, 2000 10634773

Milad MR, Wright CI, Orr SP, et al: Recall of fear extinction in humans activates the ventromedial prefrontal cortex and hippocampus in concert. Biol Psychiatry 62(5):446–454, 2007 17217927

Milad MR, Igoe SA, Lebron-Milad K, et al: Estrous cycle phase and gonadal hormones influence conditioned fear extinction. Neuroscience 164(3):887–895, 2009 19761818

O'Donnell ML, Creamer M, Elliott P, et al: Tonic and phasic heart rate as predictors of posttraumatic stress disorder. Psychosom Med 69(3):256–261, 2007 17420442

Olff M, Langeland W, Draijer N, et al: Gender differences in posttraumatic stress disorder. Psychol Bull 133(2):183–204, 2007 17338596

Orr SP, Pitman RK, Lasko NB, et al: Psychophysiological assessment of posttraumatic stress disorder imagery in World War II and Korean combat veterans. J Abnorm Psychol 102(1):152–159, 1993 8436691

Orr SP, Metzger LJ, Lasko NB, et al: Physiologic responses to sudden, loud tones in monozygotic twins discordant for combat exposure: association with posttraumatic stress disorder. Arch Gen Psychiatry 60(3):283–288, 2003 12622661

Ozer EJ, Best SR, Lipsey TL, et al: Predictors of posttraumatic stress disorder and symptoms in adults: a meta-analysis. Psychol Bull 129(1):52–73, 2003 12555794

Patel R, Spreng RN, Shin LM, et al: Neurocircuitry models of posttraumatic stress disorder and beyond: a meta-analysis of functional neuroimaging studies. Neurosci Biobehav Rev 36(9):2130–2142, 2012 22766141

Peri T, Ben-Shakhar G, Orr SP, et al: Psychophysiologic assessment of aversive conditioning in posttraumatic stress disorder. Biol Psychiatry 47(6):512–519, 2000 10715357

Pineles SL, Nillni YI, King MW, et al: Extinction retention and the menstrual cycle: different associations for women with posttraumatic stress disorder. J Abnorm Psychol 125(3):349–355, 2016 26866677

Pitman RK: Post-traumatic stress disorder, hormones, and memory. Biol Psychiatry 26(3):221–223, 1989 2545287

Pitman RK, Shalev AY, Orr SP: Posttraumatic stress disorder: emotion, conditioning and memory, in The New Cognitive Neuroscience, 2nd Edition. Edited by Corbetta MD, Gazzaniga M. New York, Plenum, 2000, pp 1133–1148

Pitman RK, Sanders KM, Zusman RM, et al: Pilot study of secondary prevention of posttraumatic stress disorder with propranolol. Biol Psychiatry 51(2):189–192, 2002 11822998

Pitman RK, Rasmusson AM, Koenen KC, et al: Biological studies of post-traumatic stress disorder. Nat Rev Neurosci 13(11):769–787, 2012 23047775

Pole N: The psychophysiology of posttraumatic stress disorder: a meta-analysis. Psychol Bull 133(5):725–746, 2007 17723027

Post RM, Weiss SRB, Smith MA: Sensitization and kindling: implications for the evolving neural substrates of post-traumatic stress disorder, in Neurobiological and Clinical Consequences of Stress: From Normal Adaptation to PTSD. Edited by Friedman MJ, Charney DS, Deutch AY. Philadelphia, PA, Lipincott-Raven, 1995, pp 203–224

Quirk GJ, Mueller D: Neural mechanisms of extinction learning and retrieval. Neuropsychopharmacology 33(1):56–72, 2008 17882236

Rauch SL, Drevets WC: Neuroimaging and neuroanatomy of stress-induced and fear circuitry disorders, in Stress-Induced and Fear Circuitry Disorders: Refining the Research Agenda for DSM-V. Edited by Andrews G, Charney DS, Sirovatka PJ. Arlington, VA, American Psychiatric Association, 2009, pp 215–254

Sartor CE, McCutcheon VV, Pommer NE, et al: Common genetic and environmental contributions to post-traumatic stress disorder and alcohol dependence in young women. Psychol Med 41(7):1497–1505, 2011 21054919

Segal SK, Cahill L: Endogenous noradrenergic activation and memory for emotional material in men and women. Psychoneuroendocrinology 34(9):1263–1271, 2009 19505766

Shalev AY, Peri T, Brandes D, et al: Auditory startle response in trauma survivors with posttraumatic stress disorder: a prospective study. Am J Psychiatry 157(2):255–261, 2000 10671396

Shalev AY, Videlock EJ, Peleg T, et al: Stress hormones and post-traumatic stress disorder in civilian trauma victims: a longitudinal study. Part I: HPA axis responses. Int J Neuropsychopharmacol 11(3):365–372, 2008 17971262

Shalev A, Liberzon I, Marmar C: Post-traumatic stress disorder. N Engl J Med 376(25):2459–2469, 2017 28636846

Sheerin CM, Lind MJ, Bountress KE, et al: The genetics and epigenetics of PTSD: overview, recent advances, and future directions. Curr Opin Psychol 14:5–11, 2017

Smith ME: Bilateral hippocampal volume reduction in adults with post-traumatic stress disorder: a meta-analysis of structural MRI studies. Hippocampus 15(6):798–807, 2005 15988763

Sripada RK, King AP, Garfinkel SN, et al: Altered resting-state amygdala functional connectivity in men with posttraumatic stress disorder. J Psychiatry Neurosci 37(4):241–249, 2012a 22313617

Sripada RK, King AP, Welsh RC, et al: Neural dysregulation in posttraumatic stress disorder: evidence for disrupted equilibrium between salience and default mode brain networks. Psychosom Med 74(9):904–911, 2012b 23115342

Stein MB, Kerridge C, Dimsdale JE, et al: Pharmacotherapy to prevent PTSD: results from a randomized controlled proof-of-concept trial in physically injured patients. J Trauma Stress 20(6):923–932, 2007 18157888

Teicher MH, Anderson CM, Polcari A: Childhood maltreatment is associated with reduced volume in the hippocampal subfields CA3, dentate gyrus, and subiculum. Proc Natl Acad Sci USA 109(9):E563–E572, 2012 22331913

Teicher MH, Samson JA, Anderson CM, et al: The effects of childhood maltreatment on brain structure, function and connectivity. Nat Rev Neurosci 17(10):652–666, 2016 27640984

True WR, Rice J, Eisen SA, et al: A twin study of genetic and environmental contributions to liability for posttraumatic stress symptoms. Arch Gen Psychiatry 50(4):257–264, 1993 8466386

Warda G, Bryant RA: Cognitive bias in acute stress disorder. Behav Res Ther 36(12):1177–1183, 1998 9745802

Williams LM, Barton MJ, Kemp AH, et al: Distinct amygdala-autonomic arousal profiles in response to fear signals in healthy males and females. Neuroimage 28(3):618–626, 2005 16081303

Yehuda R: Sensitization of the hypothalamic-pituitary-adrenal axis in posttraumatic stress disorder. Ann NY Acad Sci 821:57–75, 1997 9238194

Yehuda R, Southwick SM, Nussbaum G, et al: Low urinary cortisol excretion in patients with posttraumatic stress disorder. J Nerv Ment Dis 178(6):366–369, 1990 2348190

Zannas AS, Provençal N, Binder EB: Epigenetics of posttraumatic stress disorder: current evidence, challenges, and future directions. Biol Psychiatry 78(5):327–335, 2015 25979620

Zhang L, Benedek DM, Fullerton CS, et al: PTSD risk is associated with BDNF Val66Met and BDNF overexpression. Mol Psychiatry 19(1):8–10, 2014 23319005

Zohar J, Yahalom H, Kozlovsky N, et al: High dose hydrocortisone immediately after trauma may alter the trajectory of PTSD: interplay between clinical and animal studies. Eur Neuropsychopharmacol 21(11):796–809, 2011 21741804

Recommended Readings

Bryant RA: Acute Stress Disorder: What It Is, and How to Treat It. New York, Guilford, 2016

Fenster RJ, Lebois LA, Ressler KJ, et al: Brain circuit dysfunction in post-traumatic stress disorder: from mouse to man. Nat Rev Neurosci 19:535–551, 2018

Lopresto D, Schipper P, Homberg JR: Neural circuits and mechanisms involved in fear generalization: implications for the pathophysiology and treatment of posttraumatic stress disorder. Neurosci Biobehav Rev 60:31–42, 2016

Mahan AL, Ressler KJ: Fear conditioning, synaptic plasticity and the amygdala: implications for posttraumatic stress disorder. Trends Neurosci 35:24–35, 2012

Shalev A, Liberzon I, Marmar C: Post-traumatic stress disorder. N Engl J Med 376(25):2459–2469, 2017

Sheerin CM, Lind MJ, Bountress KE, et al: The genetics and epigenetics of PTSD: overview, recent advances, and future directions. Curr Opin Psychol 14:5–11, 2017

CHAPTER 31

Pharmacotherapy for PTSD

Boadie W. Dunlop, M.D.

Jonathan R.T. Davidson, M.D.

PTSD is a heterogeneous and complex disorder that may require a multi-faceted treatment approach. In Western nations, lifetime prevalence estimates for PTSD range from 6.4% to 9.2%, with current (past-year) prevalence estimates from 1.1% to 3.5% (Katzman et al. 2014). Internationally, the lifetime prevalence is estimated to be 3%–5% (Stein et al. 2014).

The complexity of PTSD is reflected in the DSM-5 criteria required for diagnosis, which include 20 symptoms across four symptom clusters (American Psychiatric Association 2013), making it the most complex DSM diagnosis. These four symptom clusters—intrusion, avoidance, negative alterations in cognitions and mood, and alterations of arousal and reactivity—reflect an expansion and subdivision of the three DSM-IV clusters—reexperiencing, avoidance/numbing, and hyperarousal (American Psychiatric Association 1994).

PTSD is associated with numerous alterations in CNS, endocrine, and inflammatory activity, which may be mediated via epigenetic changes and may differentially contribute to the various symptoms (Yehuda et al. 2015). Unfortunately, a large gap remains between the emerging biological models and their translation to treatments that specifically target pathophysiology. Consequently, the pharmacological treatment of PTSD continues to be a process of trial and error, built on evidence generated from clinical trials in which patients with PTSD are treated without consideration of biological subtyping that may allow for a more precision-based approach to treatment.

The trial-and-error approach has been the historical norm for the treatment of traumatic stress. More than a century ago, Weir Mitchell described the use of bromides, opium, chloral, and brandy for casualties from the American Civil War (Davidson and van der Kolk 1996). Wagner-Jauregg tried electrical stimulation for PTSD in Austrian soldiers in the early twentieth century, and treatments during World War II included barbiturates, insulin, stimulants, and ether (Davidson and van der Kolk 1996). Sargant and Slater (1972) administered carbon dioxide in the 1960s for chronic PTSD and later suggested that antidepressant drugs might be applicable to chronic PTSD. The monoamine oxidase inhibitor (MAOI) phenelzine was the first modern medication studied for PTSD, trialed in combat veterans from the Vietnam War (Hogben and Cornfield 1981).

When Should Pharmacotherapy Be Used?

More than 10 PTSD clinical practice guidelines have been published (Yehuda et al. 2015). The guidelines are consistent in recommending cognitive-behavioral therapy–based treatments, particularly trauma-focused therapies such as prolonged exposure therapy or cognitive processing therapy, as preferred first-line interventions. Trauma-focused therapies directly target core distressing memories and associated avoidance behavior. Successful exposure-based therapies can lead to substantial long-term gains and even resolve PTSD in certain cases.

A minority of guidelines also list pharmacotherapy as a first-line treatment option, usually to be administered in conjunction with psychotherapy. All guidelines recommend considering medication if the patient refuses or cannot access psychotherapy or attains inadequate improvement from a course of an evidence-based psychotherapy. An important consideration in pharmacological treatment selection is the presence of comorbid psychiatric and medical conditions; up to 75% of patients with PTSD have one or more comorbid psychiatric disorders, most often major depression, another anxiety disorder, or substance use disorder (Pietrzak et al. 2011). Comorbidity is likely a significant driver behind surveys that find that clinicians frequently deviate from practice guideline recommendations (Loeffler et al. 2018).

First-Line Treatments: Selective Serotonin Reuptake Inhibitors and Venlafaxine

The goals of pharmacotherapy are to reduce PTSD symptoms, improve functioning and quality of life, enhance resilience to stress and reduce relapse, and treat comorbid psychiatric conditions. Pharmacotherapy for PTSD, as for other complex psychiatric disorders, typically starts with a single agent to address the entire syndrome and then may move to more symptom-targeted interventions.

Only two medications have FDA approval for PTSD: the selective serotonin reuptake inhibitors (SSRIs) sertraline and paroxetine, approved in 1999 and 2001, respectively. PTSD clinical practice guidelines and meta-analyses recommend SSRIs or the serotonin-norepinephrine reuptake inhibitor (SNRI) venlafaxine as initial pharmacotherapy. Since the mid-2000s, treatment guidelines have moved from recommending SSRIs as a class to specifying specific agents within the class that have demonstrated efficacy in randomized controlled trials (RCTs) (typically one or more of sertraline, paroxetine, and fluoxetine) (Hoffman et al. 2018; Katzman et al. 2014). In contrast, treatment guidelines for major depressive disorder (MDD) recommend SSRIs—all of which have approved MDD indications—equally as a class without distinguishing between them. Venlafaxine is the only SNRI with placebo-controlled PTSD data; duloxetine has only been evaluated in small open-label trials (Walderhaug et al. 2010).

Sertraline has been evaluated in 10 placebo-controlled RCTs, fluoxetine in 6, paroxetine in 4, and venlafaxine (extended-release) in 2 (Cipriani et al. 2018). Both venlafaxine trials demonstrated efficacy over placebo. For the three SSRIs, however, at least 50% of the RCTs failed to demonstrate superiority over placebo on the primary outcome. Meta-analyses indicate small (Cohen's $d < 0.5$) but statistically significant effect sizes for these SSRIs (Cipriani et al. 2018; Hoskins et al. 2015). Overall, short-term PTSD SSRI response rates vary substantially, averaging roughly 55% for active medication versus 40% for placebo; around 30% of patients achieve full remission with a single psychotropic agent in short-term trials (Ipser and Stein 2012).

Pooled analyses of the SSRI and venlafaxine trials indicate that the medications significantly improve all three DSM-IV symptom clusters, although reexperiencing symptoms show less improvement than avoidance/numbing or hyperarousal symptoms (Davidson et al. 2006b; Stein et al. 2006). These agents also significantly reduce disability and comorbid depression in PTSD (Hoffman et al. 2018), with individual studies demonstrating improvements in anger (Davidson et al. 2002), resilience (Davidson et al. 2006a), and dissociation (Marshall et al. 2007). Other than lower symptom severity, consistent predictors of SSRI response in PTSD have not been identified, but these medications have shown a conspicuous absence of benefit compared to placebo among U.S. military veterans, despite proving efficacious in military veterans from other nations (Davidson 2015).

SSRI and venlafaxine dosing for PTSD has been consistent with that for MDD, although patients who experience panic attacks may better tolerate initiating at half the usual starting dosage for the first 4–7 days. Treatment effects can emerge within 2–4 weeks but may take 12 weeks or more to be fully realized (Ipser and Stein 2012). Effective treatment should continue for at least 1 year before a taper is considered (Bandelow et al. 2008).

Despite the demonstrated efficacy of paroxetine, sertraline, and fluoxetine for PTSD, efficacy cannot be assumed for other SSRIs. Vilazodone failed to beat placebo in an RCT of 59 civilians with PTSD (Ramaswamy et al. 2017). Citalopram was not superior to placebo in a three-armed RCT of 58 civilians with PTSD (Tucker et al. 2003); however, the active comparator, sertraline, also did not show superiority to placebo, indicating a failed trial. Five small open-label studies of fluvoxamine and one of escitalopram suggest possible efficacy (Katzman et al. 2014). One placebo-controlled RCT (NCT02637895) is evaluating the efficacy of vortioxetine, an SSRI with additional serotonin receptor modulating effects.

Whether the SSRIs differ sufficiently in efficacy for PTSD to warrant medication-specific recommendations remains unresolved. Important considerations when choosing an SSRI include differences in tolerability, discontinuation, safety in pregnancy, and drug interactions. These factors may lead a prescriber to use a non-established SSRI (e.g., escitalopram) over paroxetine, the SSRI that has the greatest pooled effect size and is the most consistently recommended by guidelines (Hoskins et al. 2015). In contrast, the SNRIs should not be considered equivalently efficacious for PTSD, given the absence of RCT data other than for venlafaxine and the meaningful differences between these drugs in their relative affinity for the serotonin and norepinephrine transporter (Auclair et al. 2013).

Other Treatments

PTSD treatment guidelines differ greatly with regard to second-level medication recommendations. Those medications with the greatest RCT support are tricyclic antidepressants (TCAs), MAOIs, nefazodone, and mirtazapine. Despite promising results
from small early trials with TCAs and MAOIs, the emergence of the FDA-approved
SSRIs for PTSD displaced research into use of the other medications, leading to their
likely underutilization in practice (Davidson 2015; Stein and Rothbaum 2018).

Tricyclic Antidepressants

Desipramine, amitriptyline, and imipramine have been evaluated for chronic PTSD in
RCTs involving military veteran samples. Although desipramine was not superior to
placebo among 18 veterans in a 4-week crossover trial (Reist et al. 1989), desipramine
subsequently proved as efficacious as paroxetine for PTSD symptoms in a 12-week
RCT of veterans with PTSD and alcohol dependence (Petrakis et al. 2012). In an 8-week
RCT, amitriptyline (50–300 mg/day) produced higher response rates than placebo
among 40 veterans who were treated for at least 4 weeks (50% vs. 17%, respectively;
$P=0.06$) (Davidson et al. 1990). In an 8-week RCT with military veterans, imipramine
(mean 225 mg/day) proved superior to placebo for PTSD, although 61% of the
23 imipramine-treated patients dropped out of the trial (Kosten et al. 1991).

Monoamine Oxidase Inhibitors

The irreversible MAOI phenelzine (45–75 mg/day) was not superior to placebo in a
5-week crossover study of 13 patients with PTSD (Shestatzky et al. 1988). In contrast,
a small 8-week RCT of veterans with PTSD found strongly positive effects for
phenelzine (mean 68 mg/day) compared to placebo (Kosten et al. 1991). Brofaromine,
a reversible inhibitor of monoamine oxidase A, failed to demonstrate efficacy in two
large RCTs and did not become commercially available (Lee et al. 2016). No RCT data
are available regarding the efficacy in PTSD of tranylcypromine, an irreversible
MAOI, or selegiline, which specifically inhibits monoamine oxidase B at low dosages.

Nefazodone

Nefazodone is a unique agent that acts primarily as a serotonin receptor 2A and 2C
($5\text{-}HT_{2A}$ and $5\text{-}HT_{2C}$) antagonist, although it also has weak serotonin, norepinephrine,
and dopamine reuptake blockade effects. One RCT demonstrated its efficacy for PTSD
among predominantly male combat veterans (Davis et al. 2004). In addition, two
small head-to-head RCTs found nefazodone to have roughly equal efficacy to sertraline in civilians with PTSD (McRae et al. 2004; Saygin et al. 2002). Nefazodone has
low rates of sexual dysfunction and beneficial effects on sleep. Nefazodone was commonly used for PTSD until the early 2000s, when hepatotoxicity was identified
(29 cases per 100,000 patient-years of exposure) (Lucena et al. 2003). The risk for severe liver failure resulting in death or transplant is estimated to be about 1 per 250,000
patient-years of use, and nefazodone is not recommended for patients with preexist-

ing liver disease (Voican et al. 2014). The branded versions of nefazodone were removed from the U.S. market by the manufacturer in 2004, but generic versions are available.

Mirtazapine

Mirtazapine is a dual-acting antidepressant with antagonism at 5-HT_2, 5-HT_3, and central presynaptic α_2 receptors. Mirtazapine was efficacious in a single small ($N=26$) 8-week RCT, with dramatically higher response rates than placebo (65% vs. 22%; $P=0.04$) (Davidson et al. 2003). Mirtazapine is also a potent antihistaminergic agent, leading to its frequent use as an adjunctive agent for insomnia.

Alpha$_1$-Receptor Antagonists and Alpha$_2$-Receptor Agonists

A large body of human and animal research implicates dysregulation of noradrenergic signaling as part of the pathophysiology of PTSD (Hendrickson and Raskind 2016). Excessive noradrenergic activity is believed to contribute to the symptoms of hyperarousal, insomnia, and nightmares. Diminishing noradrenergic effects through blocking α_1 receptors or by inhibiting norepinephrine release by α_2 autoreceptor agonism in the locus coeruleus has been explored for PTSD.

Prazosin, an α_1-receptor antagonist, has been evaluated in seven placebo-controlled RCTs of PTSD and sleep disturbances. The first six studies (including four military studies) all showed at least moderate effect sizes in favor of prazosin in reducing insomnia or nightmares, and three found benefit in overall PTSD symptoms (Khachatryan et al. 2016). The seventh and largest RCT, conducted with 304 U.S. military veterans with PTSD and nightmares, found no benefit with prazosin over placebo for recurrent distressing dreams, sleep quality, or overall PTSD symptoms (Raskind et al. 2018). Reasons for the failure of prazosin in this trial are unclear but may relate to the selection criteria, which may have reduced the number of patients with noradrenergic dysfunction. Based on this trial, the most recent Veterans Affairs/Department of Defense treatment guidelines dropped prazosin as a recommended medication due to "insufficient evidence" for PTSD-related nightmares and suggest against using it for global PTSD (U.S. Department of Veterans Affairs 2017).

Doxazosin, another α_1 antagonist, has a longer half-life than prazosin (15–22 hours vs. 2–3 hours), slower time to peak plasma concentration (2–3 hours vs. 1 hour), and likely longer duration of action (Elliott et al. 1987). One small ($N=8$) doxazosin RCT, involving only 16 days of active treatment in military veterans, had mixed results (Rodgman et al. 2016). Guanfacine, an α_2 receptor antagonist, failed to demonstrate efficacy for overall PTSD symptoms in two placebo-controlled RCTs (Lee et al. 2016).

Anticonvulsants

The rationale for the use of anticonvulsants is based on the affective instability in PTSD and that, via kindling, over time the brain becomes more sensitive to stressors, such that lower-intensity stressors are sufficient to trigger exaggerated reactions. Among the anticonvulsant medications, only topiramate has controlled data suggesting efficacy. Topiramate is a unique agent that inhibits carbonic anhydrase, blocks sodium channels, and modulates glutamate and some GABA receptors (Shank et al. 2000). One small topiramate RCT in civilians found global efficacy in PTSD (Yeh et al. 2011), but two other small RCTs using topiramate as monotherapy or augmentation did not. However, all three trials found that topiramate was helpful for reexperiencing symptoms. Although neurological side effects (e.g., drowsiness, vision changes, slowed cognition) often reduce the medication's tolerability, topiramate's ability to induce weight loss and its efficacy for alcohol dependence may make it a unique option for some patients with ongoing reexperiencing symptoms.

In the largest RCT (N=232) of an anticonvulsant for PTSD, tiagabine lacked efficacy (Davidson et al. 2007). Valproic acid also failed in two RCTs of veterans with PTSD (Lee et al. 2016). A small RCT of patients with PTSD (N=15) found nonstatistically significant improvement with lamotrigine over placebo for reexperiencing and avoidance/numbing (Hertzberg et al. 1999). In an RCT with 37 Iranian combat veterans, pregabalin (300 mg/day) augmentation given for 6 weeks to patients already taking both an SSRI and valproic acid achieved small but statistically significant effects (Baniasadi et al. 2014). The results of these small trials warrant efforts at replication. Although open-label studies and case reports with carbamazepine, oxcarbazepine, gabapentin, levetiracetam, and phenytoin exist, the efficacy of these agents in PTSD is unknown.

Bupropion

The antidepressant bupropion, in its sustained-release (SR) formulation, failed to show efficacy in two small RCTs, although bupropion SR was superior to placebo for smoking cessation among veterans with PTSD in one trial (Hertzberg et al. 2001).

Hypothalamic-Pituitary-Adrenal Axis Modulation

Substantial preclinical and clinical data implicate dysfunction of the hypothalamic-pituitary-adrenal (HPA) axis in PTSD, but few studies have evaluated interventions that directly modulate this hormonal system. Negative RCTs have been reported for 1) a glucocorticoid receptor agonist (hydrocortisone, 10 or 30 mg/day for 1 week); 2) a glucocorticoid receptor antagonist (mifepristone, 600 mg/day for 1 week); and 3) a corticotropin-releasing hormone type 1 receptor antagonist given for 6 weeks (Dunlop and Wong 2019). As described later in the chapter (see "Medication-Enhanced Psychotherapy"), HPA axis modulation with hydrocortisone or dexamethasone may have greater clinical utility when combined with psychotherapy than as a daily treatment.

Benzodiazepines

Benzodiazepines are the class of medications for which clinicians deviate most often from clinical practice guidelines for PTSD (Loeffler et al. 2018). These agents are commonly prescribed despite consistent recommendations against their use and very little controlled data evaluating their utility (Guina et al. 2015). Two very small RCTs of benzodiazepines in military veterans (N=10, N=6) found no benefit on core symptoms of PTSD or nightmares for either alprazolam (dosed up to 4.25 mg/day for 5 weeks) (Braun et al. 1990) or clonazepam (2 mg nightly for 2 weeks) (Cates et al. 2004).

Sleep-Focused Treatments

Targeted sleep interventions, including psychological, pharmacological, and mechanical (e.g., central positive airway pressure in patients with obstructive sleep apnea), can improve sleep symptoms of PTSD as well as comorbid sleep disorders that exacerbate other PTSD symptoms (Colvonen et al. 2018). Short-term use of eszopiclone, a nonbenzodiazepine $GABA_A$ receptor agonist, dosed at 3 mg nightly for 3 weeks, was efficacious for overall PTSD symptoms in a crossover trial of 24 civilians with chronic PTSD and sleep disturbance (Pollack et al. 2011). In contrast, in a 2-week RCT of 32 combat veterans receiving stable treatment with an SSRI, addition of zolpidem (10 mg nightly) proved less effective on sleep measures and overall PTSD symptoms than twice-weekly hypnotherapy sessions (Abramowitz et al. 2008).

Trazodone is an antagonist at the $5\text{-}HT_{2A}$ and α_1 receptors, with additional weak antagonist effects at histamine type 1 receptors and the serotonin transporter and partial agonism at $5\text{-}HT_{1A}$ receptors. Despite the absence of controlled trials in PTSD, trazodone is widely used adjunctively for sleep.

Relative Efficacy of Pharmacotherapy Treatments for PTSD

Only nine head-to-head RCTs of medications for PTSD have been conducted, none of which reported a significant difference between active treatments, although most were underpowered (Table 31–1).

A large meta-analysis evaluated 51 double-blind RCTs of pharmacotherapy for PTSD (Cipriani et al. 2018). Phenelzine emerged as the most efficacious agent, but this result was based on only one trial; differences between the other medications were small. Two other meta-analyses reached differing conclusions, with one finding sufficient evidence for fluoxetine, paroxetine, and venlafaxine (Hoskins et al. 2015) and the other asserting that only sertraline and venlafaxine were efficacious (Lee et al. 2016). These inconsistent meta-analyses demonstrate limitations in the existing PTSD pharmacotherapy trial data. Guidance for dosing selected medications for PTSD is provided in Table 31–2.

Prevention of PTSD After Trauma

Pharmacological treatments that have been evaluated in placebo-controlled RCTs to prevent the development of PTSD after traumatic events include β-blockers, glucocorticoids, temazepam, opiates, gabapentin, and SSRIs. In a meta-analysis, only hydrocortisone significantly prevented the development of PTSD after trauma (number needed to treat=7) (Sijbrandij et al. 2015). A single high dose of hydrocortisone (100–140 mg IV, based on weight) administered within 6 hours of a trauma to patients exhibiting symptoms of acute stress disorder effectively reduced PTSD development at 3-month follow-up (Zohar et al. 2011). Similarly, 10 days of oral hydrocortisone administered at 20 mg twice daily started within 12 hours of an injurious traumatic event produced lower PTSD symptoms at 3-month follow-up (Delahanty et al. 2013). Because most people who experience trauma do not go on to develop PTSD, addi-

TABLE 31–1.   Head-to-head randomized pharmacotherapy trials for adults with PTSD

Comparison	Sample (N)	PBO arm?	Mean dosage, mg/day	Treatment duration, weeks	Dropouts, n (%)	Reduction in PTSD symptoms*	Comment	Reference
Sertraline vs. venlafaxine XR	U.S. civilians (538)	Yes	SER: 110.2 VEN: 164.4	12	Overall: 181 (34)	SER: 46% VEN: 49%	VEN, but not SER, superior to PBO; VEN superior to PBO on avoidance/numbing and hyperarousal symptom clusters	Davidson et al. 2006b
Sertraline vs. venlafaxine SR	Traumatized refugees in Denmark (195)	No	SER: 96.2 VEN: 125.4	25	SER: 12 (15) VEN: 23 (25)	SER: 7% VEN: 4%	Open-label treatment and self-report outcome; 73% received adjunctive mianserin, 21% received antipsychotics	Sonne et al. 2016
Sertraline vs. mirtazapine	Korean veterans (100)	No	SER: 101.5 MIR: 34.1	6	SER: 6 (12) MIR: 7 (14)	SER: 37% MIR: 43%	Open-label treatment and unblinded assessment; More responders to MIR than SER (88% vs. 69%, $P=0.039$)	Chung et al. 2004
Paroxetine vs. desipramine	U.S. veterans with PTSD and alcohol dependence (88)	No	PAR: 39.7 DES: 187.2	12	PAR: 12 (29) DES: 9 (20)	PAR: 47% DES: 51%	DES significantly reduced number drinks per week compared with PAR	Petrakis et al. 2012
Imipramine vs. phenelzine	U.S. veterans (60)	Yes	IMI: 225 PHE: 68	8	IMI: 14 (61) PHE: 4 (21)	IMI: 25% PHE: 45%	PHE (68%) and IMI (65%) had significantly greater response rates than PBO (28%), $P<0.02$	Kosten et al. 1991
Sertraline vs. citalopram	U.S. civilians (58)	Yes	SER: 134.1 CIT: 36.2	10	SER: 6 (26) CIT: 5 (20)	SER: 50% CIT: 34%	Neither SER nor CIT statistically superior to PBO	Tucker et al. 2003

TABLE 31–1. Head-to-head randomized pharmacotherapy trials for adults with PTSD *(continued)*

Comparison	Sample (N)	PBO arm?	Mean dosage, mg/day	Treatment duration, weeks	Dropouts, n (%)	Reduction in PTSD symptoms*	Comment	Reference
Sertraline vs. nefazodone	Turkish civilians with PTSD after earthquake (54)	No	SER: 68.3 NEF: 332.4	20	SER: 0 (0) NEF: 6 (20)	SER: 73% NEF: 72%	Open-label treatment and unblinded assessment	Saygin et al. 2002
Fluvoxamine vs. reboxetine	Israeli civilians with PTSD after motor vehicle accident (28)	No	FLU: 150 REB: 8	8	FLU: 3 (15) REB: 9 (45)	FLU: 55 REB: 47	Analysis based on completers only	Spivak et al. 2006
Sertraline vs. nefazodone	U.S. civilians (26)	No	SER: 153 NEF: 463	12	Overall: 14 (38)	SER: 61 NEF: 58	Both medications significantly improved reexperiencing, avoidance/numbing, and hyperarousal symptom clusters	McRae et al. 2004

Note. CIT=citalopram; DES=desipramine; FLU=fluvoxamine; IMI=imipramine; MIR=mirtazapine; NEF=nefazodone; PAR=paroxetine; PBO=placebo; PHE= phenelzine; REB=reboxetine; SER=sertraline; SR=sustained release; VEN=venlafaxine; XR=extended release.
*Symptom change based on Clinician Administered PTSD Scale for all studies except the following: Kosten et al. 1991 (Impact of Events Scale), Saygin et al. 2002 (Treatment-Outcome Posttraumatic Stress Disorder Scale), and Sonne et al. 2016 (Part IV of the Harvard Trauma Questionnaire).

TABLE 31–2.   **Dosing guidance for selected medications for PTSD**

Medication	Initial dosing, *mg*	Dosing increments, *mg*	Target dosage, *mg/day*	Duration of trial, *weeks*
Mirtazapine	15 at bedtime	15 weekly	15–45	8
Nefazodone	100 twice daily	100 every 4 days	300–600	8
Prazosin	1 at bedtime	1 every 4 days	3–15	6
Quetiapine	25 at bedtime	50 weekly	50–400	4
Risperidone	0.5 at bedtime	0.5–1 weekly	0.5–4	4
Topiramate	25 twice daily	50 weekly	200–400	8

Note. Selective serotonin reuptake inhibitors, serotonin-norepinephrine reuptake inhibitors, tricyclic antidepressants, and monoamine oxidase inhibitors should be dosed similarly to their use for major depressive disorder.

tional research is necessary to identify those likely to benefit, as well as to better define hydrocortisone timing, dosing, and duration parameters (Dunlop and Wong 2019). Small trials suggest that administration of benzodiazepines in the aftermath of a traumatic event may increase the risk for developing PTSD, potentially interfering with natural recovery (Gelpin et al. 1996; Mellman et al. 2002).

Long-Term Efficacy Data

The benefits of longer-term pharmacotherapy for PTSD have been demonstrated in relapse-prevention RCTs, in which responders to open-label short-term treatment (up to 12 weeks) were randomly assigned to either continue the medication or be switched to placebo. Three 6-month relapse-prevention studies found that responders to fluoxetine or sertraline who were maintained on their SSRI had relapse rates less than half of those who were switched to placebo (Davidson et al. 2001, 2005; Martenyi et al. 2002), although one unpublished study of paroxetine did not find benefit from continued treatment (Batelaan et al. 2017). A meta-analysis of these four studies found an odds ratio for relapse of 2.45 (95% CI 0.86–6.97) with switch to placebo that could not be attributed to SSRI discontinuation/withdrawal symptoms (Batelaan et al. 2017). Open-label studies also support long-term treatment with SSRIs. With sertraline, 54% of nonresponders at 3 months became responders during 6 months of continuation treatment, and across all patients 20%–25% of the total 9-month improvement occurred during the continuation phase (Londborg et al. 2001). Similarly, remission rates continued to increase over 6 months in a large civilian PTSD trial of extended-release venlafaxine compared to placebo (Davidson et al. 2006a).

Treatment-Resistant PTSD

Response rates with short-term pharmacotherapy are approximately 60%, with remission rates of 30% or less (Ipser and Stein 2012). No specific definition for *treatment-*

resistant PTSD has been established, although efforts have been made to quantify the level of resistance to psychotherapy and pharmacotherapy (Dunlop et al. 2014). *Treatment resistance* should be distinguished from *treatment intolerance*, because side effects or poor adherence may lead to inadequate treatment duration or dosing. Patients who do not benefit from an SSRI or venlafaxine may switch or augment their initial medication, although no studies have established indicators for which patients should undergo switch versus augmentation.

Developing specific treatment algorithms for PTSD is particularly challenging due to the wide variety of symptom presentations. For example, a patient whose PTSD symptoms show response to an SSRI but who has persisting nightmares may benefit from augmentation with prazosin, whereas another patient whose symptoms show response to an SSRI and who has no sleep disturbance but does have ongoing negative alterations in cognitions and mood may benefit more from augmentation with a second antidepressant.

Antidepressant Combinations

The complementary pharmacological mechanisms of action of mirtazapine and the SSRIs, along with mirtazapine's salutary effects on sleep, have led practitioners to combine these medications for patients with treatment-resistant PTSD. In the only RCT of this combination, 36 civilians with PTSD were treated for 24 weeks with sertraline plus either mirtazapine or placebo (Schneier et al. 2015). The combination arm demonstrated a moderate, but not statistically significant, effect size ($d=0.51$, $P=0.17$) for PTSD symptom improvement but a significantly greater remission rate (39% vs. 11%, $P=0.042$) and lower depression. Appetite increase, but not weight gain, was significantly more common with the combination.

Antipsychotics

PTSD may be complicated by psychotic features, potentially related to reexperiencing phenomena or to secondary to comorbid disorders such as MDD or substance abuse. Risperidone was superior to placebo for psychotic symptoms in one RCT (Hamner et al. 2003), and in another olanzapine proved superior to fluphenazine (Pivac et al. 2004).

Atypical antipsychotics have been successfully used as SSRI augmentation agents in treatment-resistant PTSD without psychotic symptoms. Seven augmentation RCTs have evaluated risperidone (mean dosages ranging from 0.5 to 3 mg/day), with four reporting positive results (Ahearn et al. 2011). However, in the largest and longest RCT of an atypical antipsychotic, risperidone (mean dosage 2.74 mg/day) failed to demonstrate efficacy on overall PTSD scores during 24 weeks of treatment among 247 military veterans (97% male) with PTSD who had failed at least two SSRI trials. Post-hoc analyses did identify statistically significant improvement with risperidone in reexperiencing and hyperarousal (Krystal et al. 2011). Notably, this trial allowed initiation of other psychoactive medications, with 39% of patients doing so, which may have reduced differences in risperidone's effects versus placebo.

The atypical antipsychotics have also been evaluated as monotherapy in placebo-controlled RCTs that enrolled patients not specifically selected for treatment resistance. Quetiapine (mean dosage 258 mg/day) demonstrated a statistically significant effect size of 0.49 after 12 weeks among 80 veterans with PTSD (Villarreal et al. 2016). Similarly, risperidone (mean 2.6 mg/day) was efficacious on core PTSD symptoms in a 12-week study of civilian women (Padala et al. 2006). Olanzapine monotherapy for civilians with PTSD proved efficacious in one 8-week RCT of 28 patients (Carey et al. 2012) but failed to show benefit in another 10-week trial of 15 patients (Butterfield et al. 2001). Substantial weight gain with olanzapine was observed in both studies (mean 5.6 kg and 11.4 kg, respectively). An RCT that coinitiated sertraline plus ziprasidone had to be terminated due to adverse events (Kellner et al. 2010), indicating that sequential addition of an antipsychotic for patients not responding to an existing medication regimen is a more prudent clinical approach.

A meta-analysis of nine placebo-controlled RCTs of atypical antipsychotics found significant benefit for overall PTSD symptom scores, driven primarily by improvements in the reexperiencing cluster, with smaller, statistically nonsignificant benefits for hyperarousal or avoidance/numbing (Han et al. 2014). This analysis also found significantly greater response rates and reductions in depressive symptoms with atypical antipsychotic treatment. Taken together, existing results suggest that these agents work not only by improving insomnia but also by impacting core aspects of the illness.

The significant adverse general health effects of atypical antipsychotics, including weight gain, hyperlipidemia, hyperglycemia, and the potential for akathisia and tardive dyskinesia, are important factors to consider in determining when to use these medications. The importance of these considerations was evident in a large retrospective cohort analysis of veterans with PTSD who were treated with prazosin or quetiapine for nightmares. Both drugs were equally effective for the short term, but patients continued prazosin significantly longer and were less likely to discontinue due to side effects (Byers et al. 2010).

Ketamine

Ketamine has various pharmacological actions, including noncompetitive antagonism of the NMDA receptor, and it enhances synaptic plasticity and extinction of fear (Fortress et al. 2018). Subanesthetic doses of ketamine (typically 0.5 mg/kg IV) have been repeatedly shown to have rapid antidepressant effects for treatment-resistant MDD or bipolar disorder, leading to interest in its potential as an option for treatment-resistant PTSD. One midazolam-controlled RCT of 41 patients with PTSD found that a single dose of intravenous ketamine was highly efficacious (Feder et al. 2014), and an open-label study of 15 patients with PTSD and comorbid MDD found an 80% remission rate after six ketamine infusions over 12 days, with mean time to relapse of 41 days (Albott et al. 2018). Ongoing trials are exploring the efficacy and safety of repeated dosing of ketamine in military and civilian populations and its efficacy in medication-enhanced psychotherapy using ketamine in combination with prolonged exposure.

Cannabis and Related Compounds

Observational studies and anecdotal reports have identified potential therapeutic value for cannabis in patients with treatment-resistant PTSD. Activation of the endocannabinoid receptor CB_1 appears to help regulate fear and stress responses, and cannabidiol may enhance consolidation of fear extinction memories achieved through therapeutic exposure (Das et al. 2013). On the other hand, specific harms from chronic cannabis use are well established, including increased risk for substance use disorders, psychotic disorders, motor vehicle accidents, cognitive impairment, and adverse physical health outcomes (Steenkamp et al. 2017).

The cannabis plant contains more than 100 compounds, many of which may have psychoactive effects. However, only Δ^9-tetrahydrocannabinol (THC) and cannabidiol have been evaluated for therapeutic applications (Steenkamp et al. 2017). THC is a partial agonist at CB_1 receptors and produces the euphoric and potential anxiogenic and psychotic experiences associated with cannabis. Cannabidiol acts weakly at CB_1 receptors and has primarily anxiolytic actions. Individual responses to cannabis may vary based on genetics and the ratio of THC to cannabidiol in the cannabis (Steenkamp et al. 2017). Although extensive research into the therapeutic potential of cannabis is ongoing, no controlled data currently are available demonstrating the clinical efficacy of the plant or its components for PTSD. A synthetic CB_1 agonist, nabilone, is approved by the FDA for the treatment of nausea and vomiting associated with cancer chemotherapy. Two open-label trials suggested efficacy of nabilone for PTSD nightmares, and one small ($N=10$) crossover placebo-controlled RCT of active-duty military personnel with PTSD found nabilone (mean dosage 1.95 mg/day) to significantly reduce distressing dreams and enhance PTSD response (Jetly et al. 2015).

Combined Treatments

Psychotherapy-Pharmacotherapy Combination Treatments

Psychotherapy and pharmacotherapy may be combined either by starting both at the beginning of treatment or by adding one after nonremission with the other (sequential combination). As shown in Table 31–3, results have been mixed, with only one small trial ($N=23$; Simon et al. 2008) evaluating the guideline-recommended approach of initiating treatment with an evidence-based psychotherapy and adding medication for inadequate responders. The largest trial, which evaluated 207 military veterans, showed no benefit for combination treatment (Rauch et al. 2019), although the weight of the evidence from the civilian trials suggests that this approach is efficacious. Some researchers have shown concern that benzodiazepines, which impair attention and new memory formation (Tannenbaum et al. 2012), may act to diminish the efficacy of trauma-focused psychotherapies for PTSD. In two studies examining this question, short-term outcomes were not affected, but long-term gains were diminished when psychotherapy had been administered along with benzodiazepines (Rosen et al. 2013; Rothbaum et al. 2014). Importantly, although concern for impaired learning and memory has focused mostly on the benzodiazepines, anticholinergic agents and opiates may also disturb these cognitive systems (Tannenbaum et al. 2012).

Medication-Enhanced Psychotherapy

Another pharmacotherapy-psychotherapy combination treatment model is medication-enhanced psychotherapy (Dunlop et al. 2012). In this approach, a medication not believed to have efficacy for the disorder as a stand-alone treatment is administered

TABLE 31–3.   Randomized controlled trials evaluating combined pharmacotherapy and psychotherapy treatment for PTSD

Reference	Sample	Arms (n analyzed)	Therapy sessions, N	Mean dosage, mg/day	Combination duration, weeks	Dropouts, n (%)	Mean improvement in total PTSD symptoms, %*	Comment
Combination from initiation of treatment								
Otto et al. 2003	Cambodian refugees poorly responding to SSRI+CLO	CBT+SER (5) / SER alone (5)	10 / 0	100 / 125	n.r. / n.r.	n.r.	22 / –8	Large effect sizes favoring combination, but no between-group statistical test reported
Schneier et al. 2012	Post-9/11 U.S. civilians	PE+PAR (19) / PE+PBO (18)	10 / 10	32 / —	10	6 (32) / 5 (28)	70 / 46	Combination superior on PTSD symptoms ($P=0.01$) and remission rate (42% vs. 17%, $P=0.03$)
Rauch et al. 2019	U.S. combat veterans	PE+SER (69) / PE+PBO (67) / SER+EMM (71)	13 / 13 / 0	172 / — / 171	24	18 (26) / 25 (37) / 15 (21)	38 / 36 / 37	Nonsignificantly higher remission rates in SER+EMM (39%) and SER+PE (38%) than in PE+PBO arm (21%)
Combination by sequential addition								
Rothbaum et al. 2006	U.S. civilians responding at least partially to 10 weeks of SER	Continued SER +10 sessions of PE (34) / Continued SER alone (31)	10 / 0	173	5	6 (18) / 1 (3)	37 / –3	Significantly greater reduction in PTSD symptoms with combination ($P<0.001$), driven by patients with least benefit from open-label SER
Simon et al. 2008	U.S. civilians not remitting after 7–8 sessions of PE	PE+PAR (9) / PE+PBO (14)	5 / 5	46 / —	10	1 (11) / 2 (14)	14 / 27	Nonsignificantly higher remission rate in combination (33% vs. 14%)

Note. CBT=cognitive-behavioral therapy; CLO=clozapine; EMM=enhanced medication management; n.r.=not reported; PAR=paroxetine; PBO=placebo; PE=prolonged exposure; SER=sertraline; SSRI=selective serotonin reuptake inhibitor. —=not applicable.
*PTSD symptom improvement based on Clinician Administered PTSD Scale for all studies except Rothbaum et al. 2006 (Structured Interview for PTSD) and Simon et al. 2008 (Short PTSD Rating Interview).

either shortly before or after a psychotherapy session, with the aim of improving the magnitude or rate of benefit from the psychotherapy. The duration of treatment with the pharmacological agent is limited to the course of the psychotherapy. Medication-enhanced psychotherapy has been evaluated in RCTs with D-cycloserine, glucocorticoids, oxytocin, 3,4-methylenedioxymethamphetamine (MDMA), and propranolol.

D-Cycloserine is an antitubercular medication. It also acts as an NMDA receptor partial agonist that facilitates fear extinction when given shortly before or after extinction training, as was first demonstrated with acrophobia (Davis et al. 2006). Five placebo-controlled RCTs have evaluated D-cycloserine given prior to prolonged exposure sessions for PTSD, finding mixed results and weaker benefits than when used for phobic disorders (Baker et al. 2018). Glucocorticoids, which modulate the HPA axis, diminish retrieval of emotionally salient memories, and may facilitate extinction learning (de Quervain et al. 2017), have been studied in combination with prolonged exposure in two RCTs in military veterans. A trial using hydrocortisone found efficacy, but one using dexamethasone did not; the difference may be related to the timing of dosing or specific aspects of the two drugs (Dunlop and Wong 2019). Intranasal oxytocin (40 IU) delivered 45 minutes prior to eight prolonged exposure sessions in 17 civilians with PTSD produced nonsignificantly lower PTSD symptom scores compared to placebo (Flanagan et al. 2018).

MDMA consistently improves mood and affiliative behaviors, increases openness, and reduces neuroticism (Greer and Tolbert 1986). Acute MDMA administration increases serotonin, norepinephrine, and dopamine signaling and raises both cortisol and oxytocin concentrations (Mithoefer et al. 2018). The psychotherapy used thus far in MDMA-enhanced treatment studies has been specifically designed for PTSD and involves one, two, or three 8-hour sessions of therapy delivered after MDMA dosing, spaced approximately 1 month apart.

Four small RCTs (N=12–28) of MDMA-enhanced psychotherapy support its potential clinical utility when dosed at 75–125 mg, with two trials achieving statistical significance (Mithoefer et al. 2011, 2018). All trials included at least 1 year of follow-up and resulted in sustained benefits for most patients and no development of substance abuse. The FDA granted MDMA a "breakthrough therapy" designation for the treatment of PTSD in 2017, and MDMA is now under evaluation in phase-III trials (NCT03537014).

Another pharmacotherapy enhancement approach is to administer a drug immediately prior to a memory reactivation session, without providing psychotherapy, with the aim of weakening the reconsolidation of the trauma memory. Both high-dose oral dexamethasone (0.15 mg/kg) given over four sessions (Surís et al. 2017) and propranolol (0.67 mg/kg immediate release plus 1 mg/kg extended release) given over six sessions (Brunet et al. 2018) have demonstrated efficacy over placebo for PTSD symptoms in this paradigm.

Addressing Comorbidity

Comorbid MDD and anxiety disorders are highly prevalent among patients with PTSD, and pharmacological treatment of these patients should generally follow that used for patients with uncomplicated PTSD. The prevalence of PTSD among patients with schizophrenia spectrum disorders is 20%–30%, and although RCTs are lacking for this population, augmenting antipsychotics with an SSRI or venlafaxine is efficacious and safe (Helfer et al. 2016). Despite the high comorbidity between bipolar disorder and PTSD, no RCTs have been performed. Quetiapine may be the preferred initial option, given its demonstrated efficacy for both conditions, although valproic acid or olanzapine may also have utility (Rakofsky and Dunlop 2011). SSRIs started after effective mood stabilization may also be an option, particularly for non-rapid-cycling and non-mixed-state patients with bipolar disorder. Nine RCTs have evaluated pharmacotherapy treatments (SSRIs, desipramine, naltrexone, prazosin, and topiramate) for patients with comorbid PTSD and alcohol use disorder, with mixed results (Petrakis and Simpson 2017). The largest combination treatment trial found that naltrexone with either prolonged exposure or supportive therapy significantly improved alcohol use outcomes, with effects enduring for up to 6 months posttreatment (Foa et al. 2013). Improvement in PTSD symptoms appears to reduce alcohol use more than alcohol reduction improves PTSD symptoms, indicating that clinicians should not require a period of abstinence before instituting treatment for PTSD (Back et al. 2006). No RCTs have evaluated medication treatments for PTSD comorbid with other substance use disorders.

Conclusion

Although PTSD is increasingly diagnosed, only a minority of patients receive a minimally adequate course of treatment (Nobles et al. 2017). Pharmacological treatment should be individualized based on clinical presentation, comorbidity, and treatment history. Although many medications have been studied, trials are often small and of short duration. The exclusion from most RCTs of patients with complex comorbidity, including personality, bipolar, and substance use disorders, yields uncertainty about the generalizability of trial results to these patients.

Several medications, including the SSRIs (Davidson 2015), risperidone (Krystal et al. 2011), and prazosin (Raskind et al. 2018), have demonstrated efficacy in nonmilitary settings only to fail in large, unselective Veterans Affairs (VA) RCTs. The extent to which failure in a large VA trial should diminish the use of drugs that have otherwise shown efficacy remains unclear. Negative results may stem from certain characteristics of the VA study samples and trial designs, particularly chronicity of illness, failure of multiple prior drug and psychotherapy treatments, secondary gain, multiple permitted concomitant psychotropic medications, and broad inclusion criteria, including significant medical illnesses. Rather than being considered as proof of a medication's lack of efficacy, negative large VA trials may be better conceptualized as effectiveness trials within a specific chronically ill PTSD population. For patients without these negative predictors of outcome, judicious use of medications proven efficacious in other settings can have substantial clinical value.

The initial pharmacological intervention for most patients should be either an SSRI or venlafaxine, given the demonstrated efficacy of these medications in the short term (4–12 weeks), the long term (12 weeks and beyond), and for relapse prevention. Failure to achieve adequate benefit with one of these medications should be followed by at least one additional trial with another medication from this class. In addition to these agents, mirtazapine, nefazodone, TCAs, and MAOIs are worthy of consideration. Augmentation of antidepressant treatments should be tailored based on the patient's persisting symptoms. Nightmares can be treated with an α_1 receptor antagonist such as prazosin. Other reexperiencing symptoms in addition to nightmares may respond to topiramate, and reexperiencing and hyperarousal may respond to atypical antipsychotics (particularly quetiapine or risperidone). Before starting a medication, the relative benefits and potential adverse consequences of treatment should be discussed with the patient.

Key Points

- The first-line pharmacological choices for the treatment of PTSD are selective serotonin reuptake inhibitors (SSRIs), particularly fluoxetine, paroxetine, and sertraline, or the serotonin-norepinephrine reuptake inhibitor venlafaxine.

- An adequate medication trial with antidepressants when used for PTSD requires treatment with an adequate dosage for at least 6 weeks, and maximal benefit of the medication may take several months to emerge.

- Failure to respond to one SSRI should usually be followed by a trial with a second SSRI or venlafaxine before moving to other medication options.

- Although evidence is mixed, the combination of an evidence-based psychotherapy with pharmacological treatment for PTSD should be considered, combined either from the beginning of treatment or sequentially after nonremission to a single-modality intervention.

- When residual symptoms are present after treatment with a single medication, augmentation options should be selected based on the types of symptoms present. The combination of mirtazapine with an SSRI or venlafaxine can be helpful when residual symptoms cross multiple clusters.

- Medication-enhanced psychotherapy approaches may improve the efficacy of psychotherapeutic treatments for PTSD in the near future.

- Treatment should aim not only to reduce symptoms but also to enhance psychological resilience to stress or trauma, prevent relapse, and restore function and quality of life.

References

Abramowitz EG, Barak Y, Ben-Avi I, et al: Hypnotherapy in the treatment of chronic combat-related PTSD patients suffering from insomnia: a randomized, zolpidem-controlled clinical trial. Int J Clin Exp Hypn 56(3):270–280, 2008 18569138

Ahearn EP, Juergens T, Cordes T, et al: A review of atypical antipsychotic medications for posttraumatic stress disorder. Int Clin Psychopharmacol 26(4):193–200, 2011 21597381

Albott CS, Lim KO, Forbes MK, et al: Efficacy, safety, and durability of repeated ketamine infusions for comorbid posttraumatic stress disorder and treatment-resistant depression. J Clin Psychiatry 79(3):17m11634, 2018 29727073

American Psychiatric Association: Diagnostic and Statistical Manual of Mental Disorders, 4th Edition. Washington, DC, American Psychiatric Association, 1994

American Psychiatric Association: Diagnostic and Statistical Manual of Mental Disorders, 5th Edition. Arlington, VA, American Psychiatric Association, 2013

Auclair AL, Martel JC, Assié MB, et al: Levomilnacipran (F2695), a norepinephrine-preferring SNRI: profile in vitro and in models of depression and anxiety. Neuropharmacology 70:338–347, 2013 23499664

Back SE, Brady KT, Sonne SC, et al: Symptom improvement in co-occurring PTSD and alcohol dependence. J Nerv Ment Dis 194(9):690–696, 2006 16971821

Baker JF, Cates ME, Luthin DR: D-cycloserine in the treatment of posttraumatic stress disorder. Ment Health Clin 7(2):88–94, 2018 29955504

Bandelow B, Zohar J, Hollander E, et al: World Federation of Societies of Biological Psychiatry (WFSBP) guidelines for the pharmacological treatment of anxiety, obsessive-compulsive and post-traumatic stress disorders—first revision. World J Biol Psychiatry 9(4):248–312, 2008 18949648

Baniasadi M, Hosseini G, Fayyazi Bordbar MR, et al: Effect of pregabalin augmentation in treatment of patients with combat-related chronic posttraumatic stress disorder: a randomized controlled trial. J Psychiatr Pract 20(6):419–427, 2014 25406046

Batelaan NM, Bosman RC, Muntingh A, et al: Risk of relapse after antidepressant discontinuation in anxiety disorders, obsessive-compulsive disorder, and post-traumatic stress disorder: systematic review and meta-analysis of relapse prevention trials. BMJ 358:j3927, 2017 28903922

Braun P, Greenberg D, Dasberg H, et al: Core symptoms of posttraumatic stress disorder unimproved by alprazolam treatment. J Clin Psychiatry 51(6):236–238, 1990 2189869

Brunet A, Saumier D, Liu A, et al: Reduction of PTSD symptoms with pre-reactivation propranolol therapy: a randomized controlled trial. Am J Psychiatry 175(5):427–433, 2018 29325446

Butterfield MI, Becker ME, Connor KM, et al: Olanzapine in the treatment of post-traumatic stress disorder: a pilot study. Int Clin Psychopharmacol 16(4):197–203, 2001 11459333

Byers MG, Allison KM, Wendel CS, et al: Prazosin versus quetiapine for nighttime posttraumatic stress disorder symptoms in veterans: an assessment of long-term comparative effectiveness and safety. J Clin Psychopharmacol 30(3):225–229, 2010 20473055

Carey P, Suliman S, Ganesan K, et al: Olanzapine monotherapy in posttraumatic stress disorder: efficacy in a randomized, double-blind, placebo-controlled study. Hum Psychopharmacol 27(4):386–391, 2012 22730105

Cates ME, Bishop MH, Davis LL, et al: Clonazepam for treatment of sleep disturbances associated with combat-related posttraumatic stress disorder. Ann Pharmacother 38(9):1395–1399, 2004 15252193

Chung MY, Min KH, Jun YJ, et al: Efficacy and tolerability of mirtazapine and sertraline in Korean veterans with posttraumatic stress disorder: a randomized open label trial. Hum Psychopharmacol 19(7):489–494, 2004 15378676

Cipriani A, Williams T, Nikolakopoulou A, et al: Comparative efficacy and acceptability of pharmacological treatments for post-traumatic stress disorder in adults: a network meta-analysis. Psychol Med 48(12):1975–1984, 2018 29254516

Colvonen PJ, Straus LD, Stepnowsky C, et al: Recent advancements in treating sleep disorders in co-occurring PTSD. Curr Psychiatry Rep 20(7):48, 2018 29931537

Das RK, Kamboj SK, Ramadas M, et al: Cannabidiol enhances consolidation of explicit fear extinction in humans. Psychopharmacology (Berl) 226(4):781–792, 2013 23307069

Davidson JR: Vintage treatments for PTSD: a reconsideration of tricyclic drugs. J Psychopharmacol 29(3):264–269, 2015 25586404

Davidson JR, van der Kolk BA: The psychopharmacologic treatment of posttraumatic stress disorder, in Traumatic Stress: The Effects of Overwhelming Experience on Mind, Body, and Society. Edited by van der Kolk BA, McFarlane AC, Weisaeth L. New York, Guilford, 1996, pp 510–524

Davidson JR, Kudler H, Smith R, et al: Treatment of posttraumatic stress disorder with amitriptyline and placebo. Arch Gen Psychiatry 47(3):259–266, 1990 2407208

Davidson JR, Pearlstein T, Londborg P, et al: Efficacy of sertraline in preventing relapse of posttraumatic stress disorder: results of a 28-week double-blind, placebo-controlled study. Am J Psychiatry 158(12):1974–1981, 2001 11729012

Davidson JR, Landerman LR, Farfel GM, et al: Characterizing the effects of sertraline in post-traumatic stress disorder. Psychol Med 32(4):661–670, 2002 12102380

Davidson JR, Weisler RH, Butterfield MI, et al: Mirtazapine vs. placebo in posttraumatic stress disorder: a pilot trial. Biol Psychiatry 53(2):188–191, 2003 12547477

Davidson JR, Connor KM, Hertzberg MA, et al: Maintenance therapy with fluoxetine in post-traumatic stress disorder: a placebo-controlled discontinuation study. J Clin Psychopharmacol 25(2):166–169, 2005 15738748

Davidson JR, Baldwin D, Stein DJ, et al: Treatment of posttraumatic stress disorder with venlafaxine extended release: a 6-month randomized controlled trial. Arch Gen Psychiatry 63(10):1158–1165, 2006a 17015818

Davidson JR, Rothbaum BO, Tucker P, et al: Venlafaxine extended release in posttraumatic stress disorder: a sertraline- and placebo-controlled study. J Clin Psychopharmacol 26(3):259–267, 2006b 16702890

Davidson JR, Brady K, Mellman TA, et al: The efficacy and tolerability of tiagabine in adult patients with post-traumatic stress disorder. J Clin Psychopharmacol 27(1):85–88, 2007 17224720

Davis LL, Jewell ME, Ambrose S, et al: A placebo-controlled study of nefazodone for the treatment of chronic posttraumatic stress disorder: a preliminary study. J Clin Psychopharmacol 24(3):291–297, 2004 15118483

Davis M, Ressler K, Rothbaum BO, et al: Effects of d-cycloserine on extinction: translation from preclinical to clinical work. Biol Psychiatry 60(4):369–375, 2006 16919524

de Quervain D, Schwabe L, Roozendaal B: Stress, glucocorticoids and memory: implications for treating fear-related disorders. Nat Rev Neurosci 18(1):7–19, 2017 27881856

Delahanty DL, Gabert-Quillen C, Ostrowski SA, et al: The efficacy of initial hydrocortisone administration at preventing posttraumatic distress in adult trauma patients: a randomized trial. CNS Spectr 18(2):103–111, 2013 23557627

Dunlop BW, Wong A: The hypothalamic-pituitary-adrenal axis in PTSD: pathophysiology and treatment interventions. Prog Neuropsychopharmacol Biol Psychiatry 89:361–379, 2019 30342071

Dunlop BW, Mansson E, Gerardi M: Pharmacological innovations for posttraumatic stress disorder and medication-enhanced psychotherapy. Curr Pharm Des 18(35):5645–5658, 2012 22632469

Dunlop BW, Kaye JL, Youngner C, et al: Assessing treatment-resistant posttraumatic stress disorder: the Emory Treatment Resistance Interview for PTSD (E-TRIP). Behav Sci (Basel) 4(4):511–527, 2014 25494488

Elliott HL, Meredith PA, Reid JL: Pharmacokinetic overview of doxazosin. Am J Cardiol 59(14):78G–81G, 1987 2884857

Feder A, Parides MK, Murrough JW, et al: Efficacy of intravenous ketamine for treatment of chronic posttraumatic stress disorder: a randomized clinical trial. JAMA Psychiatry 71(6):681–688, 2014 24740528

Flanagan JC, Sippel LM, Wahlquist A, et al: Augmenting prolonged exposure therapy for PTSD with intranasal oxytocin: a randomized, placebo-controlled pilot trial. J Psychiatr Res 98:64–69, 2018 29294429

Foa EB, Yusko DA, McLean CP, et al: Concurrent naltrexone and prolonged exposure therapy for patients with comorbid alcohol dependence and PTSD: a randomized clinical trial. JAMA 310(5):488–495, 2013 23925619

Fortress AM, Smith IM, Pang KCH: Ketamine facilitates extinction of avoidance behavior and enhances synaptic plasticity in a rat model of anxiety vulnerability: implications for the pathophysiology and treatment of anxiety disorders. Neuropharmacology 137:372–381, 2018 29750979

Gelpin E, Bonne O, Peri T, et al: Treatment of recent trauma survivors with benzodiazepines: a prospective study. J Clin Psychiatry 57(9):390–394, 1996 9746445

Greer G, Tolbert R: Subjective reports of the effects of MDMA in a clinical setting. J Psychoactive Drugs 18(4):319–327, 1986 2880946

Guina J, Rossetter SR, DeRhodes BJ, et al: Benzodiazepines for PTSD: a systematic review and meta-analysis. J Psychiatr Pract 21(4):281–303, 2015 26164054

Hamner MB, Faldowski RA, Ulmer HG, et al: Adjunctive risperidone treatment in post-traumatic stress disorder: a preliminary controlled trial of effects on comorbid psychotic symptoms. Int Clin Psychopharmacol 18(1):1–8, 2003 12490768

Han C, Pae CU, Wang SM, et al: The potential role of atypical antipsychotics for the treatment of posttraumatic stress disorder. J Psychiatr Res 56:72–81, 2014 24882700

Helfer B, Samara MT, Huhn M, et al: Efficacy and safety of antidepressants added to antipsychotics for schizophrenia: a systematic review and meta-analysis. Am J Psychiatry 173(9):876–886, 2016 27282362

Hendrickson RC, Raskind MA: Noradrenergic dysregulation in the pathophysiology of PTSD. Exp Neurol 284(Pt B):181–195, 2016 27222130

Hertzberg MA, Butterfield MI, Feldman ME, et al: A preliminary study of lamotrigine for the treatment of posttraumatic stress disorder. Biol Psychiatry 45(9):1226–1229, 1999 10331117

Hertzberg MA, Moore SD, Feldman ME, et al: A preliminary study of bupropion sustained-release for smoking cessation in patients with chronic posttraumatic stress disorder. J Clin Psychopharmacol 21(1):94–98, 2001 11199956

Hoffman V, Middleton JC, Feltner C, et al: Psychological and pharmacological treatments for adults with posttraumatic stress disorder: a systematic review update. Comparative Effectiveness Review No 207 (AHRQ Publ No 18-EHC011-EF; PCORI Publ No 2018-SR-01). Rockville, MD, Agency for Healthcare Research and Quality, 2018

Hogben GL, Cornfield RB: Treatment of traumatic war neurosis with phenelzine. Arch Gen Psychiatry 38(4):440–445, 1981 7212974

Hoskins M, Pearce J, Bethell A, et al: Pharmacotherapy for post-traumatic stress disorder: systematic review and meta-analysis. Br J Psychiatry 206(2):93–100, 2015 25644881

Ipser JC, Stein DJ: Evidence-based pharmacotherapy of post-traumatic stress disorder (PTSD). Int J Neuropsychopharmacol 15(6):825–840, 2012 21798109

Jetly R, Heber A, Fraser G, et al: The efficacy of nabilone, a synthetic cannabinoid, in the treatment of PTSD-associated nightmares: a preliminary randomized, double-blind, placebo-controlled cross-over design study. Psychoneuroendocrinology 51:585–588, 2015 25467221

Katzman MA, Bleau P, Blier P, et al: Canadian clinical practice guidelines for the management of anxiety, posttraumatic stress and obsessive-compulsive disorders. BMC Psychiatry 14(suppl 1):S1, 2014 25081580

Kellner M, Muhtz C, Wiedemann K: Primary add-on of ziprasidone in sertraline treatment of posttraumatic stress disorder: lessons from a stopped trial? J Clin Psychopharmacol 30(4):471–473, 2010 20631571

Khachatryan D, Groll D, Booij L, et al: Prazosin for treating sleep disturbances in adults with posttraumatic stress disorder: a systematic review and meta-analysis of randomized controlled trials. Gen Hosp Psychiatry 39:46–52, 2016 26644317

Kosten TR, Frank JB, Dan E, et al: Pharmacotherapy for posttraumatic stress disorder using phenelzine or imipramine. J Nerv Ment Dis 179(6):366–370, 1991 2051152

Krystal JH, Rosenheck RA, Cramer JA, et al: Adjunctive risperidone treatment for antidepressant-resistant symptoms of chronic military service-related PTSD: a randomized trial. JAMA 306(5):493–502, 2011 21813427

Lee DJ, Schnitzlein CW, Wolf JP, et al: Psychotherapy versus pharmacotherapy for posttraumatic stress disorder: systematic review and meta-analysis to determine first-line treatments. Depress Anxiety 33(9):792–806, 2016 27126398

Loeffler G, Coller R, Tracy L, et al: Prescribing trends in U.S. active duty service members with posttraumatic stress disorder: a population-based study from 2007–2013. J Clin Psychiatry 79(4):17m11667, 2018 29985565

Londborg PD, Hegel MT, Goldstein S, et al: Sertraline treatment of posttraumatic stress disorder: results of 24 weeks of open-label continuation treatment. J Clin Psychiatry 62(5):325–331, 2001 11411812

Lucena MI, Carvajal A, Andrade RJ, et al: Antidepressant-induced hepatotoxicity. Expert Opin Drug Saf 2(3):249–262, 2003 12904104

Marshall RD, Lewis-Fernandez R, Blanco C, et al: A controlled trial of paroxetine for chronic PTSD, dissociation, and interpersonal problems in mostly minority adults. Depress Anxiety 24(2):77–84, 2007 16892419

Martenyi F, Brown EB, Zhang H, et al: Fluoxetine v. placebo in prevention of relapse in posttraumatic stress disorder. Br J Psychiatry 181:315–320, 2002 12356658

McRae AL, Brady KT, Mellman TA, et al: Comparison of nefazodone and sertraline for the treatment of posttraumatic stress disorder. Depress Anxiety 19(3):190–196, 2004 15129422

Mellman TA, Bustamante V, David D, et al: Hypnotic medication in the aftermath of trauma. J Clin Psychiatry 63(12):1183–1184, 2002 12530420

Mithoefer MC, Wagner MT, Mithoefer AT, et al: The safety and efficacy of ±3,4-methylenedioxymethamphetamine-assisted psychotherapy in subjects with chronic, treatment-resistant posttraumatic stress disorder: the first randomized controlled pilot study. J Psychopharmacol 25(4):439–452, 2011 20643699

Mithoefer MC, Mithoefer AT, Feduccia AA, et al: 3,4-methylenedioxymethamphetamine (MDMA)-assisted psychotherapy for post-traumatic stress disorder in military veterans, firefighters, and police officers: a randomised, double-blind, dose-response, phase 2 clinical trial. Lancet Psychiatry 5(6):486–497, 2018 29728331

Nobles CJ, Valentine SE, Zepeda ED, et al: Usual course of treatment and predictors of treatment utilization for patients with posttraumatic stress disorder. J Clin Psychiatry 78(5):e559–e566, 2017 28570794

Otto MW, Hinton D, Korbly NB, et al: Treatment of pharmacotherapy-refractory posttraumatic stress disorder among Cambodian refugees: a pilot study of combination treatment with cognitive-behavior therapy vs sertraline alone. Behav Res Ther 41(11):1271–1276, 2003 14527527

Padala PR, Madison J, Monnahan M, et al: Risperidone monotherapy for post-traumatic stress disorder related to sexual assault and domestic abuse in women. Int Clin Psychopharmacol 21(5):275–280, 2006 16877898

Petrakis IL, Simpson TL: Posttraumatic stress disorder and alcohol use disorder: a critical review of pharmacologic treatments. Alcohol Clin Exp Res 41(2):226–237, 2017 28102573

Petrakis IL, Ralevski E, Desai N, et al: Noradrenergic vs serotonergic antidepressant with or without naltrexone for veterans with PTSD and comorbid alcohol dependence. Neuropsychopharmacology 37(4):996–1004, 2012 22089316

Pietrzak RH, Goldstein RB, Southwick SM, et al: Prevalence and Axis I comorbidity of full and partial posttraumatic stress disorder in the United States: results from wave 2 of the National Epidemiologic Survey on Alcohol and Related Conditions. J Anxiety Disord 25(3):456–465, 2011 21168991

Pivac N, Kozaric-Kovacic D, Muck-Seler D: Olanzapine versus fluphenazine in an open trial in patients with psychotic combat-related post-traumatic stress disorder. Psychopharmacology (Berl) 175(4):451–456, 2004 15064916

Pollack MH, Hoge EA, Worthington JJ, et al: Eszopiclone for the treatment of posttraumatic stress disorder and associated insomnia: a randomized, double-blind, placebo-controlled trial. J Clin Psychiatry 72(7):892–897, 2011 21367352

Rakofsky JJ, Dunlop BW: Treating nonspecific anxiety and anxiety disorders in patients with bipolar disorder: a review. J Clin Psychiatry 72(1):81–90, 2011 21208580

Ramaswamy S, Driscoll D, Reist C, et al: A double-blind, placebo-controlled randomized trial of vilazodone in the treatment of posttraumatic stress disorder and comorbid depression. Prim Care Companion CNS Disord 19(4):17m02138, 2017 28858440

Raskind MA, Peskind ER, Chow B, et al: Trial of prazosin for post-traumatic stress disorder in military veterans. N Engl J Med 378(6):507–517, 2018 29414272

Rauch SA, Kim HM, Powell C, et al: Efficacy of prolonged exposure therapy, sertraline hydrochloride, and their combination among combat veterans with posttraumatic stress disorder. JAMA Psychiatry 76(2):117–126, 2019 30516797 Epub ahead of print

Reist C, Kauffmann CD, Haier RJ, et al: A controlled trial of desipramine in 18 men with posttraumatic stress disorder. Am J Psychiatry 146(4):513–516, 1989 2648867

Rodgman C, Verrico CD, Holst M, et al: Doxazosin XL reduces symptoms of posttraumatic stress disorder in veterans with PTSD: a pilot clinical trial. J Clin Psychiatry 77(5):e561–e565, 2016 27249080

Rosen CS, Greenbaum MA, Schnurr PP, et al: Do benzodiazepines reduce the effectiveness of exposure therapy for posttraumatic stress disorder? J Clin Psychiatry 74(12):1241–1248, 2013 24434093

Rothbaum BO, Cahill SP, Foa EB, et al: Augmentation of sertraline with prolonged exposure in the treatment of posttraumatic stress disorder. J Trauma Stress 19(5):625–638, 2006 17075912

Rothbaum BO, Price M, Jovanovic T, et al: A randomized, double-blind evaluation of d-cycloserine or alprazolam combined with virtual reality exposure therapy for posttraumatic stress disorder in Iraq and Afghanistan War veterans. Am J Psychiatry 171(6):640–648, 2014 24743802

Sargant WW, Slater E: The use of drugs in psychotherapy, in An Introduction to Physical Methods of Treatment in Psychiatry. Edited by Sargant WW, Slater E, Kelly D. New York, Science House, 1972, pp 142–162

Saygin MZ, Sungur MZ, Sabol EU, et al: Nefazodone versus sertraline in treatment of posttraumatic stress disorder. Klinik Psikofarmakol Bülteni 12:1–5, 2002

Schneier FR, Neria Y, Pavlicova M, et al: Combined prolonged exposure therapy and paroxetine for PTSD related to the World Trade Center attack: a randomized controlled trial. Am J Psychiatry 169(1):80–88, 2012 21908494

Schneier FR, Campeas R, Carcamo J, et al: Combined mirtazapine and SSRI treatment of PTSD: a placebo-controlled trial. Depress Anxiety 32(8):570–579, 2015 26115513

Shank RP, Gardocki JF, Streeter AJ, et al: An overview of the preclinical aspects of topiramate: pharmacology, pharmacokinetics, and mechanism of action. Epilepsia 41(suppl 1):S3–S9, 2000 10768292

Shestatzky M, Greenberg D, Lerer B: A controlled trial of phenelzine in posttraumatic stress disorder. Psychiatry Res 24(2):149–155, 1988 3406235

Sijbrandij M, Kleiboer A, Bisson JI, et al: Pharmacological prevention of post-traumatic stress disorder and acute stress disorder: a systematic review and meta-analysis. Lancet Psychiatry 2(5):413–421, 2015 26360285

Simon NM, Connor KM, Lang AJ, et al: Paroxetine CR augmentation for posttraumatic stress disorder refractory to prolonged exposure therapy. J Clin Psychiatry 69(3):400–405, 2008 18348595

Sonne C, Carlsson J, Bech P, et al: Treatment of trauma-affected refugees with venlafaxine versus sertraline combined with psychotherapy—a randomised study. BMC Psychiatry 16(1):383, 2016 27825327

Spivak B, Strous RD, Shaked G, et al: Reboxetine versus fluvoxamine in the treatment of motor vehicle accident-related posttraumatic stress disorder: a double-blind, fixed-dosage, controlled trial. J Clin Psychopharmacol 26(2):152–156, 2006 16633143

Steenkamp MM, Blessing EM, Galatzer-Levy IR, et al: Marijuana and other cannabinoids as a treatment for posttraumatic stress disorder: a literature review. Depress Anxiety 34(3):207–216, 2017 28245077

Stein DJ, Ipser JC, Seedat S: Pharmacotherapy for post traumatic stress disorder (PTSD). Cochrane Database Syst Rev (1):CD002795, 2006 16437445

Stein DJ, McLaughlin KA, Koenen KC, et al: DSM-5 and ICD-11 definitions of posttraumatic stress disorder: investigating "narrow" and "broad" approaches. Depress Anxiety 31(6):494–505, 2014 24894802

Stein MB, Rothbaum BO: 175 Years of progress in PTSD therapeutics: learning from the past. Am J Psychiatry 175(6):508–516, 2018 29869547

Surís A, Holliday R, Adinoff B, et al: Facilitating fear-based memory extinction with dexamethasone: a randomized controlled trial in male veterans with combat-related PTSD. Psychiatry 80(4):399–410, 2017 29466111

Tannenbaum C, Paquette A, Hilmer S, et al: A systematic review of amnestic and non-amnestic mild cognitive impairment induced by anticholinergic, antihistamine, GABAergic and opioid drugs. Drugs Aging 29(8):639–658, 2012 22812538

Tucker P, Potter-Kimball R, Wyatt DB, et al: Can physiologic assessment and side effects tease out differences in PTSD trials? A double-blind comparison of citalopram, sertraline, and placebo. Psychopharmacol Bull 37(3):135–149, 2003 14608246

U.S. Department of Veterans Affairs: VA/DOD Clinical Practice Guideline for the Management of posttraumatic stress disorder and acute stress disorder. Washington, DC, U.S. Department of Veterans Affairs, 2017. Available at https://www.healthquality.va.gov/guidelines/mh/ptsd. Accessed November 18, 2018.

Villarreal G, Hamner MB, Cañive JM, et al: Efficacy of quetiapine monotherapy in posttraumatic stress disorder: a randomized, placebo-controlled trial. Am J Psychiatry 173(12):1205–1212, 2016 27418378

Voican CS, Corruble E, Naveau S, et al: Antidepressant-induced liver injury: a review for clinicians. Am J Psychiatry 171(4):404–415, 2014 24362450

Walderhaug E, Kasserman S, Aikins D, et al: Effects of duloxetine in treatment-refractory men with posttraumatic stress disorder. Pharmacopsychiatry 43(2):45–49, 2010 20108200

Yeh MS, Mari JJ, Costa MC, et al: A double-blind randomized controlled trial to study the efficacy of topiramate in a civilian sample of PTSD. CNS Neurosci Ther 17(5):305–310, 2011 21554564

Yehuda R, Hoge CW, McFarlane AC, et al: Post-traumatic stress disorder. Nat Rev Dis Primers 1:15057, 2015 27189040

Zohar J, Yahalom H, Kozlovsky N, et al: High dose hydrocortisone immediately after trauma may alter the trajectory of PTSD: interplay between clinical and animal studies. Eur Neuropsychopharmacol 21(11):796–809, 2011 21741804

CHAPTER 32

Psychotherapy for PTSD

Lily A. Brown, Ph.D.

Monnica T. Williams, Ph.D.

Edna B. Foa, Ph.D.

The DSM-5 diagnosis of PTSD includes the following criteria: A) exposure to a traumatic event, including but not limited to actual or threatened loss of life or physical safety; B) intrusive symptoms; C) avoidance of internal or external stimuli; D) negative alterations in mood and cognition; and E) alterations in arousal and reactivity (American Psychiatric Association 2013). In this chapter, we briefly review empirically based PTSD treatments, introduce and review evidence for novel therapeutic approaches, and discuss the clinical management of comorbidities and other practical considerations for the treatment of PTSD.

Empirically Based Treatments

Following the release of DSM-5, several published studies improved the conceptual understanding of PTSD and its treatment. The Department of Veterans Affairs (VA) and the Department of Defense (DoD) released a clinical practice guideline for the treatment of PTSD in 2010 and revised the recommendations in 2017 (Department of Veterans Affairs and Department of Defense 2017). Similarly, in 2017, the American Psychological Association released *Clinical Practice Guideline for the Treatment of PTSD*. The goal of this chapter is to review recent findings on psychotherapy for PTSD, including treatments recommended in these clinical practice guidelines.

Cognitive-Behavioral Interventions for PTSD: An Overview

Cognitive-behavioral therapy (CBT) offers a broad approach across a range of techniques, the goals of which are to reduce the intensity and frequency of distressing negative emotional reactions, modify erroneous cognitions, and promote functioning. The best-supported treatments for PTSD are all forms of CBT. The proliferation of research on CBT for PTSD has resulted in a large body of knowledge on the efficacy of these treatments; at least 22 reviews or meta-analyses on CBT for PTSD have been conducted since 2008. A summary of key reviews or meta-analyses is presented in Tables 32–1 and 32–2.

Several important conclusions can be drawn from these reviews. First, CBT has substantial empirical evidence for the treatment of PTSD. Second, most studies on PTSD treatments have been conducted on exposure and cognitive therapies, and these treatments are equally efficacious. Third, more rigorous trials tend to result in smaller effect size differences between CBT modalities. In light of the impressive body of evidence in support of prolonged exposure (PE; Foa et al. 2007), cognitive processing therapy (CPT; Resick et al. 2016), eye movement desensitization and reprocessing (EMDR; Shapiro 1995), written exposure therapy (Sloan et al. 2013), and narrative exposure therapy (Schauer et al. 2011), we review these modalities in detail in the following sections.

Prolonged Exposure Therapy

Intrusive symptoms, including distressing memories, nightmares, and flashbacks, and arousal symptoms, including strong emotional and physiological reactions triggered by trauma-related reminders, are extremely common in PTSD. Most individuals with PTSD attempt to ward off these intrusive symptoms and avoid trauma reminders, even when such reminders are not inherently dangerous. Given that traumatic memories and external or internal reminders become feared stimuli in PTSD, the core components of PE for PTSD include

1. *Imaginal exposure*—revisiting the traumatic memory, repeatedly recounting it aloud, and processing the revisiting experience
2. *In vivo exposure*—repeated confrontation of trauma-related situations and objects that evoke excessive anxiety but are not inherently dangerous

The goal of this treatment is to reduce avoidance and promote processing of the traumatic memory, thereby reducing distress elicited by the trauma reminders. Additionally, individuals with pronounced symptoms of emotional numbing and depression are encouraged to engage in pleasurable activities.

Several interesting studies have been published that enhance the literature base on the efficacy of PE. A review of 207 articles found that exposure therapy (which mostly included PE) had the highest strength of evidence for treating PTSD compared to other psychosocial treatments (Forman-Hoffman et al. 2018). In a randomized controlled trial (RCT) of active-duty military personnel with PTSD, massed PE (i.e., 10 daily sessions over 2 weeks) was as effective as spaced PE (i.e., approximately weekly over 8 weeks) on PTSD outcomes (Foa et al. 2018). Although both weekly PE and present-centered therapy (PCT) were associated with significant and equivalent improvements in PTSD symptoms in active-duty military personnel, no differences were found between these conditions (Foa et al. 2018). However, additional analyses

TABLE 32–1. Support for exposure therapy or cognitive therapy for PTSD

Citation	Articles reviewed	Results summary
Forman-Hoffman et al. 2018	207	CBT, which included either exposure ($d=-1.23$) or mixed therapies, had high strength of evidence for reducing symptoms of PTSD vs. inactive control ($d=-1.24$), whereas CPT ($d=-1.35$), CT (only loss of diagnosis effect size reported, $d=0.55$), EMDR ($d=-1.08$), and NET ($d=-1.31$) had moderate strength of evidence. In contrast, imagery rehearsal training and trauma affect regulation therapy had low strength of evidence, and Seeking Safety had no strength of evidence. These findings were comparable when the outcome was changed to loss of PTSD diagnosis. When psychosocial treatments were directly compared, CBT that included exposure had moderate strength of evidence for superiority over relaxation in reducing PTSD and depression symptoms and in loss of PTSD diagnosis, but CBT with exposure performed comparably to EMDR. CBT that included mixed treatment components had low strength of evidence for outperforming relaxation for PTSD and depression. No other key differences between treatments emerged.
Kline et al. 2018	32	Significant differences were found between active CBT treatments (including exposure, CT, CBT-M, CPT, EMDR) and control treatments from pre- to posttreatment but disappeared by follow-up. During the follow-up period, the only advantage was for exposure therapy compared to an active control, but this effect was small ($d=0.27$).
Haagen et al. 2015	57	Exposure ($g=1.06$) and CPT ($g=1.33$) were more effective than EMDR ($g=0.38$) and stress management therapy ($g=0.16$). In addition, individual therapy was more effective than group therapy for veterans with PTSD. PTSD symptom outcome improved with more trauma-focused treatment sessions, whereas this association did not hold for increasing frequency of general therapy sessions.
Cusack et al. 2016	64	High strength of evidence found for exposure therapy, including PE (SMD -1.27; 95% CI -1.54 to -1.00); moderate strength of evidence for CT (-1.33; -1.99 to -0.67) and CPT (-1.40; -1.95 to -0.85); and low-moderate strength of evidence for EMDR (-1.08; -1.83 to -0.33) and NET (-1.25; -1.92 to -0.58).
Tran and Gregor 2016	22	Trauma-focused therapies had a small benefit ($g=0.14-0.17$) over non-trauma-focused therapies. In addition, PE and other exposure therapies had a small benefit ($g=0.19$) relative to other therapies, and PCT was slightly less efficacious than other treatments ($g=-0.20$).

Note. CBT=cognitive-behavioral therapy; CBT-M=mixed cognitive-behavioral therapy; CPT=cognitive processing therapy; CT=cognitive therapy; EMDR=eye movement desensitization and reprocessing; NET=narrative exposure therapy; PCT=present-centered therapy; PE=prolonged exposure.

TABLE 32–2.   **Support for cognitive-behavioral therapy (CBT) for PTSD**

Citation	Articles reviewed	Results summary
Montero-Marin et al. 2018	50	CBT had a medium effect size benefit for PTSD symptoms compared to relaxation (d=0.60).
Watts et al. 2013	112	Cognitive therapy (d=1.63), exposure therapy (d=1.08), and eye movement desensitization and reprocessing (d=1.01) all had large effect sizes on PTSD symptoms.
Otte 2011	56	CBT for PTSD had medium effect sizes (d=0.62) in placebo-controlled studies and large uncontrolled effect sizes (d=1.82). This meta-analysis also found large uncontrolled effect sizes for pre- to posttreatment changes in CBT effectiveness trials for PTSD (d=2.59).

suggested that patients with severe PTSD symptoms before treatment benefited more from PE than from PCT.

The VA/DoD clinical practice guidelines (Department of Veterans Affairs and Department of Defense 2017) indicated strong evidence in support of PE for PTSD. The American Psychological Association's (2017) practice guideline strongly recommended PE for PTSD as well.

Cognitive Therapy

The goal of cognitive therapy (CT) is to help patients identify trauma-related dysfunctional beliefs that influence emotional and behavioral responses to a situation. Once these dysfunctional beliefs are identified, patients are taught to evaluate their thoughts in a logical, evidence-based manner. Information that supports or refutes their belief is examined, as are alternative interpretations. The therapist helps patients weigh the evidence and consider alternative interpretations before deciding whether the belief accurately reflects reality and, if it does not, to replace or modify it. CT programs differ in their length and number of sessions. Moreover, some CT programs, such as that based on Ehlers and Clark's (2000) cognitive model of PTSD, include an exposure component.

Several important CT studies have been completed. A large review found that CPT had moderate strength of evidence for treating PTSD (Forman-Hoffman et al. 2018). In addition, a dismantling study demonstrated that the cognitive component of CPT outperformed the writing component of CPT, and therefore CPT is currently implemented without the written trauma narrative (Resick et al. 2008). CPT was less effective for veterans than for civilians (Morland et al. 2015) but more effective than PCT at reducing PTSD symptoms in veterans (Surís et al. 2013). Among military personnel, a group format of cognitive CPT was associated with significantly greater reductions in PTSD compared to a group format of PCT (Resick et al. 2015). However, group CPT was significantly less effective than individual CPT in active-duty military personnel (Resick et al. 2017). Both the VA/DoD and the American Psychological Association strongly recommended CPT for PTSD.

Eye Movement Desensitization and Reprocessing

In EMDR, patients generate images, thoughts, and feelings about the trauma; evaluate the aversive qualities of these stimuli; and make alternative cognitive appraisals of the trauma or their behavior during it. As the patient initially focuses on the distressing images and thoughts, and later focuses on the alternative cognition, the therapist elicits rapid, laterally alternating eye movements by instructing the patient to visually track the therapist's finger as it moves back and forth across the patient's visual field. Originally, Shapiro (1989) regarded these eye movements as essential to the processing of the traumatic memory, but the importance of the eye movements has not gained empirical support (for a review, see Spates et al. 2008). The VA/DoD guidelines indicated strong strength of evidence in support of EMDR for PTSD, but the American Psychological Association guidelines only conditionally recommended it.

Written and Narrative Exposure Therapies

Written exposure therapy involves writing about the details of the traumatic experience as well as the emotional response to it (Sloan et al. 2013). Specifically, participants are instructed to write about the trauma from a distanced perspective, "as you look back on it." The treatment program includes feedback on the writing, psychoeducation, and the treatment rationale, delivered in five 30-minute sessions. Evidence has accumulated in support of written exposure therapy for PTSD (van Emmerik et al. 2013). One RCT compared five sessions of written exposure therapy to 12 sessions of CPT and found equivalent outcomes on PTSD symptoms, with significantly less dropout from the written exposure group (6.4%) than from the CPT group (39.7%) (Sloan et al. 2018). Given the relative novelty of the written exposure intervention compared to traditional trauma-focused treatments, more research is necessary, particularly in terms of predictors and moderators of treatment.

Narrative exposure therapy is often used in community samples with refugees or survivors of violence (Schauer et al. 2011). Unlike written exposure therapy, the writing in narrative exposure therapy involves more than just the index trauma and can include positive experiences and a general narrative of each patient's life. As in written exposure therapy, the patient is guided to describe sensory and emotional experiences. As indicated in Table 32–1, sufficient evidence has shown that narrative exposure therapy is effective for the treatment of PTSD. The VA/DoD reported strong strength of evidence for both written and narrative exposure therapies for PTSD. The American Psychological Association conditionally recommended narrative exposure therapy for PTSD but did not mention written exposure therapy.

Present-Centered Therapy

PCT is a supportive, nondirective therapy originally developed as a control condition to isolate the effects of CBT from nonspecific therapeutic factors. The treatment is not trauma focused; rather, the content of treatment is oriented toward facilitating problem solving for current life challenges. As described earlier (see "Prolonged Exposure Therapy"), one RCT comparing this treatment to PE in active-duty military personnel found equivalent outcomes on PTSD symptoms (Foa et al. 2018), and another clinical trial in veterans found no differences between these approaches at 6-month follow-up, although PE outperformed PCT at posttreatment (Schnurr et al. 2007). Another trial found that group CPT was equivalent to PCT on clinician-rated PTSD symptoms in active-duty military personnel (Resick et al. 2015). In a meta-analysis of five studies, PCT was not statistically different from other evidence-based treatments in terms of PTSD and secondary outcomes but had significantly lower dropout rates (Frost et al. 2014) and had a large effect size ($d=0.88$) compared to no treatment.

The VA/DoD reported that the available evidence in support of PCT for PTSD is weak. The American Psychological Association guideline did not include PCT.

Innovations in PTSD Treatment

Nightmare Interventions

Several innovations in the treatment of PTSD have been developed since the early 2000s and are reviewed in more detail in Table 32–3. Imagery rehearsal therapy, developed in 2001, is a CBT program that combines sleep hygiene and cognitive restructuring with imaginal exposure to the content of a nightmare (Krakow et al. 2001). However, during the exposure practice, the content of the nightmare is intentionally altered in some way. As described in the table, imagery rehearsal therapy and imaginal confrontation with nightmare contents have a growing evidence base as treatments for PTSD, but as for many studies on CBT, evidence is not sufficient to suggest that these treatments outperform active comparison conditions. The VA/DoD's clinical practice guidelines (Department of Veterans Affairs and Department of Defense 2017) no longer include the prior recommendation in support of imagery rehearsal therapy. Although a 2004 American Psychiatric Association guideline recommended the use of imagery rehearsal therapy, the 2017 American Psychological Association guidelines did not make a recommendation for or against the therapy.

Yoga and Mindfulness-Based Interventions

Yoga and mindfulness-based interventions have been explored for PTSD, as reviewed in Table 32–3. A few studies have revealed small to medium effect sizes for either yoga or mindfulness-based interventions, whereas others have found no benefit for these interventions. In addition, some reviews have criticized the quality of available published studies on the topic. Therefore, the evidence for yoga and mindfulness-based interventions for PTSD is tentative at best.

Technology-Assisted Interventions

Several innovations in technology-assisted interventions have been developed, ranging from telehealth to independently operated internet treatments, reviewed in Table 32–4. In general, studies found strong evidence in support of telehealth interventions for PTSD, although some evidence suggests that they might be inferior to in-person PTSD interventions (with some recent exceptions that were not included in these

TABLE 32–3.   **Innovative treatments for PTSD**

	Study	Articles reviewed	Summary
Nightmare interventions	Hansen et al. 2013	20	This meta-analysis found that imaginal confrontation with nightmare contents was associated with significant reduction in nightmares, but both imagery rehearsal therapy and imaginal confrontation were associated with large reductions in nightmare frequency ($g=1.04$), number of nights per week with nightmares ($g=0.99$), and PTSD severity ($g=0.92$).
Yoga and mindfulness-based interventions	Hopwood and Schutte 2017	18	This meta-analysis revealed small to medium effects on PTSD symptoms for mindfulness-based interventions compared to active control ($d=0.44$) or waitlist conditions ($d=0.59$).

meta-analyses; Sloan et al. 2011). Internet-delivered CBT interventions have demonstrated medium to large effect sizes compared to treatment as usual or passive control comparisons but smaller effect sizes compared to active interventions (Kuester et al. 2016).

Virtual reality exposure (VRE) therapy for PTSD interventions has received empirical support since 2010, as reviewed in Table 32–4. Several RCTs have demonstrated that VRE therapy is a promising intervention compared to waitlist. VRE performed similarly to PE in two studies (Difede et al. 2019; Reger et al. 2016), although PE performed better at follow-up assessments in one study with active-duty service members (Reger et al. 2016).

Special Samples, Comorbidities, and Practical Considerations

CBT has been used successfully in controlled studies to relieve the symptoms of PTSD in several special populations, including adult victims of rape, physical assault, domestic violence, natural disasters, terrorism, or torture, and in adolescents and refugees (see Foa et al. 2013a; Resick et al. 2002). In addition, as discussed earlier, CBT has a robust body of evidence for efficacy among veterans and active-duty military personnel. As is consistent with the larger literature on CBT for PTSD, no evidence has been published supporting recommendations for particular variants of CBT based on the sample under consideration.

However, clinicians frequently report concerns about using CBT for PTSD in patients with complex comorbidities. In general, PTSD has high rates of comorbidity with psychiatric and physical diagnoses, and therefore it is essential to understand the efficacy of treatments in samples with comorbid diagnoses.

TABLE 32–4.   Technology-assisted interventions for PTSD

Citation	Articles reviewed	Summary
Internet or telehealth interventions		
Kuester et al. 2016	20	This meta-analysis found medium to large effect sizes for internet-delivered CBT compared to passive control conditions for PTSD (g range = 0.66–0.83), although CBT and expressive writing were not superior to active control conditions.
Sloan et al. 2011	13	This meta-analysis found that telehealth treatment was associated with large reductions in PTSD symptoms ($d = 0.99$) and in large effect sizes when telehealth treatments were compared to waitlist ($d = 1.01$). However, telehealth was inferior to in-person treatments for PTSD ($d = -0.68$).
Virtual reality interventions		
Reger et al. 2016	1	This RCT compared PE to VRE in active-duty military personnel and found that PE outperformed VRE at 3- and 6-month follow-up assessments ($d = 0.88, 0.83$).
Rothbaum et al. 2014	1	This RCT found that VRE augmented with DCS performed comparably to VRE augmented with placebo when assessed from pretreatment to follow-up (mean reduction on CAPS for DCS 37.3 points, for placebo 34.2 points). Similarly, VRE augmented with alprazolam performed comparably to VRE augmented with placebo on a clinician-rated severity scale from pretreatment to follow-up (mean reduction on CAPS for alprazolam 30.8, placebo 34.2). The alprazolam group had significantly higher CAPS scores than the placebo group at posttreatment, and more participants given alprazolam met criteria for PTSD at 3-month follow-up.
Gonçalves et al. 2012	10	This systematic review of virtual reality studies for PTSD found that several studies demonstrated a benefit of VRE compared to waitlist, although no differences emerged when VRE was compared to in exposure therapy.

Note.   CAPS = Clinician-Administered PTSD Scale; CBT = cognitive-behavioral therapy; DCS = D-cycloserine; PE = prolonged exposure; RCT = randomized controlled trial; VRE = virtual reality exposure.

Substance Use

Substance use disorders are prevalent among individuals with a diagnosis of PTSD. Fortunately, a growing literature supports the efficacy of PTSD treatments for individuals with comorbid substance use disorders. For example, one study of veterans ($N=536$) who received CPT found that the presence of an alcohol use disorder did not alter PTSD or depression outcomes (Kaysen et al. 2014). An RCT of PE and naltrexone for PTSD and alcohol use disorder found less relapse in the follow-up period among participants assigned to exposure compared to participants assigned to supportive counseling (Foa et al. 2013b). However, the vast majority of RCTs for PTSD explicitly excluded participants on the basis of their substance use status. No studies to date have reported significant increases in substance use throughout the course of PTSD treatment.

Much of the recent research on PTSD and substance use disorder treatment outcomes has focused on integrated treatments. A meta-analysis of 14 CBT studies found that integration of CBT plus substance use treatment was associated with significantly greater improvements in PTSD symptoms compared to a waitlist or treatment as usual (SMD=−0.41; Roberts et al. 2016). CBT was associated with significant reductions in substance use, but these reductions were not maintained at follow-up, and CBT completion rates were lower than completion rates for treatment as usual. Across all aspects of this study, the available evidence was classified as ranging from very low to low quality, suggesting that more research is needed in this area.

Sleep Disturbance

Sleep disturbance is the most common PTSD symptom endorsed before and after CPT or PCT treatment for PTSD (Pruiksma et al. 2016). Even among service members who experienced remission from PTSD, 57% continued to report insomnia (Pruiksma et al. 2016). One study comparing CPT to PE for female rape survivors found that although both treatments outperformed the minimal attention condition on sleep symptoms, neither resulted in remission of sleep disturbance (Gutner et al. 2013). Therefore, more research is needed on strategies to reduce sleep disruption among individuals with PTSD.

Perhaps in light of these findings, some researchers have attempted to examine the impact of sleep-focused interventions on PTSD symptoms. One meta-analysis of 11 studies found that sleep-specific CBT was associated with significant medium-effect-size reductions in PTSD symptoms and insomnia compared to waitlist control groups ($g=0.41$; Ho et al. 2016). In addition, attrition from sleep-specific CBT was low (12.8%). Therefore, directly addressing sleep disorder symptoms, either independently or as an augmentation to evidence-based treatments, may have some benefit for PTSD. Future research should directly explore an integration of sleep- and PTSD-focused treatment effects on both sleep and PTSD outcomes.

Depression and Suicide

A large body of literature supports the efficacy of evidence-based PTSD treatments for depression. For instance, a meta-analysis of 116 treatment comparisons across 93 publications found that evidence-based PTSD treatments are as effective for reducing symptoms of depression as they are for PTSD (Ronconi et al. 2015). In addition, a recent study of three RCTs examining PE for PTSD found strong evidence for bidirectional change between PTSD and depression in treatment (Brown et al. 2018b).

Less evidence is available on the impact of PTSD treatments on suicide risk reduction. One explanation for this gap in the literature is that most RCTs for PTSD explicitly exclude patients at risk for death from suicide. Therefore, the conclusions that can be drawn from the available literature are limited. Nevertheless, some studies have explored change in suicidal ideation over time in response to PE or CPT. The first such study found significant reductions in suicidal ideation for female survivors of sexual assault (Gradus et al. 2013). Although this study found steeper declines in suicidal ideation with CPT than with PE, this finding was confounded by a significantly higher baseline severity of suicidal ideation in the CPT group. Furthermore, the degree of reduction in PTSD symptom severity was correlated with the degree of reduction in suicidal ideation. In a naturalistic sample of veterans in the VA health system who received PE, a significant reduction in suicidal ideation was observed, and as in the study by Gradus et al. (2013), the degree of reduction in PTSD symptoms correlated with the degree of reduction in suicidal ideation (Cox et al. 2016). A naturalistic study of civilians with an anxiety-related disorder, including PTSD, demonstrated significant reductions in response to CBT from pre- to posttreatment (Brown et al. 2018a). Finally, an RCT comparing CPT to PCT for PTSD in active-duty service members found significant reductions in suicidal ideation that were comparable in both treatment conditions (Bryan et al. 2016). Collectively, the available studies suggest that PTSD treatments are safe and efficacious for individuals at relatively lower risk for suicide; however, given that most of these studies formally excluded individuals at higher risk, more research is needed on the efficacy and safety of PTSD treatments in patients at high risk for suicide.

Psychosis

One meta-analysis of 12 studies exploring the efficacy of evidence-based PTSD treatments among individuals with comorbid psychosis symptoms demonstrated that trauma-focused treatments were associated with small reductions in positive symptoms of psychosis ($g=0.31$) and PTSD ($g=0.21$), and effects were not observed for negative symptoms of psychosis ($g=0.28$) (Brand et al. 2018). This pattern of findings suggests that evidence-based treatments for PTSD may be less effective among individuals with psychosis, although these treatments may be worth pursuing even if they are associated with only a small benefit.

Conclusion

It has been widely recognized that traumatic events can lead to psychological disturbances and chronic distress. CBT significantly reduces symptoms of PTSD from a wide variety of traumas, including combat, natural disasters, sexual assault, nonsexual physical assault, childhood abuse, and a combination of traumas. PE and CPT are currently the best-supported approaches to treatment, with large effect sizes consistently reported. They are relatively short-term treatments that can be administered effectively by clinicians who have limited experience with CBT. Narrative and written exposure therapies have also gained empirical support. Finally, several important developments have occurred in the treatment of PTSD with comorbid substance use, sleep disorders, depression, suicidal behavior, and psychosis.

Key Points

- Chronic psychological disturbances following traumatic experiences are common, but most of these symptoms remit with time. Some individuals, however, develop chronic symptoms that require therapeutic intervention.

- Cognitive-behavioral techniques significantly reduce symptoms of chronic PTSD and may promote more rapid recovery following trauma.

- Prolonged exposure and cognitive processing therapy are highly effective cognitive-behavioral therapy–based methods of reducing PTSD symptoms.

References

American Psychiatric Association: Diagnostic and Statistical Manual of Mental Disorders, 5th Edition. Arlington, VA, American Psychiatric Association, 2013

American Psychological Association: Clinical Practice Guideline for the Treatment of PTSD. Guideline Development Panel for the Treatment of PTSD in Adults. Washington, DC, American Psychological Association, 2017. Available at: https://www.apa.org/ptsd-guideline/ptsd.pdf. Accessed July 18, 2019.

Brand RM, McEnery C, Rossell S, et al: Do trauma-focused psychological interventions have an effect on psychotic symptoms? A systematic review and meta-analysis. Schizophr Res 195:13–22, 2018 28844432

Brown LA, Gallagher T, Petersen J, et al: Does CBT for anxiety-related disorders alter suicidal ideation? Findings from a naturalistic sample. J Anxiety Disord 59:10–16, 2018a 30107264

Brown LA, Jerud A, Asnaani A, et al: Changes in posttraumatic stress disorder (PTSD) and depressive symptoms over the course of prolonged exposure. J Consult Clin Psychol 86(5):452–463, 2018b 29683702

Bryan CJ, Clemans TA, Hernandez AM, et al: Evaluating potential iatrogenic suicide risk in trauma-focused group cognitive behavioral therapy for the treatment of PTSD in active duty military personnel. Depress Anxiety 33(6):549–557, 2016 26636426

Cox KS, Mouilso ER, Venners MR, et al: Reducing suicidal ideation through evidence-based treatment for posttraumatic stress disorder. J Psychiatr Res 80:59–63, 2016 27295122

Cusack K, Jonas DE, Forneris CA, et al: Psychological treatments for adults with posttraumatic stress disorder: a systematic review and meta-analysis. Clin Psychol Rev 43:128–141, 2016 26574151

Department of Veterans Affairs, Department of Defense: VA/DoD Clinical Practice Guideline for the Management of Posttraumatic Stress Disorder and Acute Stress Disorder. Washington, DC, Department of Veterans Affairs, 2017. Available at: https://www.healthquality.va.gov/guidelines/MH/ptsd/VADoDPTSDCPGFinal012418.pdf. Accessed July 18, 2019.

Difede J, Rothbaum B, Rizzo A, et al: Enhancing exposure therapy for posttraumatic stress disorder (PTSD): virtual reality and imaginal exposure with a cognitive enhancer. New York, Weill Medical College of Cornell University, 2019. Available at: https://clinicaltrials.gov/ct2/show/NCT01352637. Accessed July 18, 2019.

Ehlers A, Clark DM: A cognitive model of posttraumatic stress disorder. Behav Res Ther 38(4):319–345, 2000 10761279

Foa EB, Hembree EA, Rothbaum BO: Prolonged Exposure Therapy for PTSD. New York, Oxford University Press, 2007

Foa EB, McLean CP, Capaldi S, et al: Prolonged exposure vs supportive counseling for sexual abuse-related PTSD in adolescent girls: a randomized clinical trial. JAMA 310(24):2650–2657, 2013a 24368465

Foa EB, Yusko DA, McLean CP, et al: Concurrent naltrexone and prolonged exposure therapy for patients with comorbid alcohol dependence and PTSD: a randomized clinical trial. JAMA 310(5):488–495, 2013b 23925619

Foa EB, McLean CP, Zang Y, et al: Effect of prolonged exposure therapy delivered over 2 weeks vs 8 weeks vs present-centered therapy on PTSD symptom severity in military personnel: a randomized clinical trial. JAMA 319(4):354–364, 2018 29362795

Forman-Hoffman V, Middleton JC, Feltner C, et al: Psychological and Pharmacological Treatments for Adults With Posttraumatic Stress Disorder: A Systematic Review Update (AHRQ Comparative Effectiveness Review No 207). Rockville, MD, Agency for Healthcare Research and Quality, 2018

Frost ND, Laska KM, Wampold BE: The evidence for present-centered therapy as a treatment for posttraumatic stress disorder. J Trauma Stress 27(1):1–8, 2014 24515534

Gonçalves R, Pedrozo AL, Coutinho ESF, et al: Efficacy of virtual reality exposure therapy in the treatment of PTSD: a systematic review. PLoS One 7(12):e48469, 2012 23300515

Gradus JL, Suvak MK, Wisco BE, et al: Treatment of posttraumatic stress disorder reduces suicidal ideation. Depress Anxiety 30(10):1046–1053, 2013 23636925

Gutner CA, Casement MD, Stavitsky Gilbert K, et al: Change in sleep symptoms across cognitive processing therapy and prolonged exposure: a longitudinal perspective. Behav Res Ther 51(12):817–822, 2013 24184428

Haagen JF, Smid GE, Knipscheer JW, et al: The efficacy of recommended treatments for veterans with PTSD: a metaregression analysis. Clin Psychol Rev 40:184–194, 2015 26164548

Hansen K, Höfling V, Kröner-Borowik T, et al: Efficacy of psychological interventions aiming to reduce chronic nightmares: a meta-analysis. Clin Psychol Rev 33(1):146–155, 2013 23186732

Ho FY, Chan CS, Tang KN: Cognitive-behavioral therapy for sleep disturbances in treating posttraumatic stress disorder symptoms: a meta-analysis of randomized controlled trials. Clin Psychol Rev 43:90–102, 2016

Hopwood TL, Schutte NS: A meta-analytic investigation of the impact of mindfulness-based interventions on post traumatic stress. Clin Psychol Rev 57:12–20, 2017

Kaysen D, Schumm J, Pedersen ER, et al: Cognitive processing therapy for veterans with comorbid PTSD and alcohol use disorders. Addict Behav 39(2):420–427, 2014 24035644

Kline AC, Cooper AA, Rytwinksi NK, et al: Long-term efficacy of psychotherapy for posttraumatic stress disorder: a meta-analysis of randomized controlled trials. Clin Psychol Rev 59:30–40, 2018 29169664

Krakow B, Hollifield M, Johnston L, et al: Imagery rehearsal therapy for chronic nightmares in sexual assault survivors with posttraumatic stress disorder: a randomized controlled trial. JAMA 286(5):537–545, 2001 11476655

Kuester A, Niemeyer H, Knaevelsrud C: Internet-based interventions for posttraumatic stress: a meta-analysis of randomized controlled trials. Clin Psychol Rev 43:1–16, 2016 26655959

Montero-Marin J, Garcia-Campayo J, López-Montoyo A, et al: Is cognitive-behavioural therapy more effective than relaxation therapy in the treatment of anxiety disorders? A meta-analysis. Psychol Med 48(9):1427–1436, 2018 29037266

Morland LA, Mackintosh MA, Rosen CS, et al: Telemedicine versus in-person delivery of cognitive processing therapy for women with posttraumatic stress disorder: a randomized noninferiority trial. Depress Anxiety 32(11):811–820, 2015 26243685

Otte C: Cognitive behavioral therapy in anxiety disorders: current state of the evidence. Dialogues Clin Neurosci 13(4):413–421, 2011 22275847

Pruiksma KE, Taylor DJ, Wachen JS, et al: Residual sleep disturbances following PTSD treatment in active duty military personnel. Psychol Trauma 8(6):697–701, 2016 27243567

Reger GM, Koenen-Woods P, Zetocha K, et al: Randomized controlled trial of prolonged exposure using imaginal exposure vs. virtual reality exposure in active duty soldiers with deployment-related posttraumatic stress disorder (PTSD). J Consult Clin Psychol 84(11):946–959, 2016 27606699

Resick PA, Nishith P, Weaver TL, et al: A comparison of cognitive-processing therapy with prolonged exposure and a waiting condition for the treatment of chronic posttraumatic stress disorder in female rape victims. J Consult Clin Psychol 70(4):867–879, 2002 12182270

Resick PA, Galovski TE, Uhlmansiek MO, et al: A randomized clinical trial to dismantle components of cognitive processing therapy for posttraumatic stress disorder in female victims of interpersonal violence. J Consult Clin Psychol 76(2):243–258, 2008 18377121

Resick PA, Wachen JS, Mintz J, et al: A randomized clinical trial of group cognitive processing therapy compared with group present-centered therapy for PTSD among active duty military personnel. J Consult Clin Psychol 83(6):1058–1068, 2015 25939018

Resick PA, Monson CM, Chard KM: Cognitive Processing Therapy for PTSD: A Comprehensive Manual. New York, Guilford, 2016

Resick PA, Wachen JS, Dondanville KA, et al: Effect of group vs individual cognitive processing therapy in active-duty military seeking treatment for posttraumatic stress disorder: a randomized clinical trial. JAMA Psychiatry 74(1):28–36, 2017 27893032

Roberts NP, Roberts PA, Jones N, et al: Psychological therapies for post-traumatic stress disorder and comorbid substance use disorder. Cochrane Database Syst Rev 4:CD010204, 2016 27040448

Ronconi JM, Shiner B, Watts BV: A meta-analysis of depressive symptom outcomes in randomized, controlled trials for PTSD. J Nerv Ment Dis 203(7):522–529, 2015 26075838

Rothbaum BO, Price M, Jovanovic T, et al: A randomized, double-blind evaluation of d-cycloserine or alprazolam combined with virtual reality exposure therapy for posttraumatic stress disorder in Iraq and Afghanistan War veterans. Am J Psychiatry 171(6):640–648, 2014 24743802

Schauer M, Neuner F, Elbert T: Narrative Exposure Therapy: A Short-Term Treatment for Traumatic Stress Disorders, 2nd Edition. Cambridge, MA, Hogrefe, 2011

Schnurr PP, Friedman MJ, Engel CC, et al: Cognitive behavioral therapy for posttraumatic stress disorder in women: a randomized controlled trial. JAMA 297(8):820–830, 2007 17327524

Shapiro F: Efficacy of eye movement desensitization procedure in the treatment of traumatic memories. J Trauma Stress 2(2):199–223, 1989

Shapiro F: Eye Movement Desensitization and Reprocessing: Basic Principles, Protocols, and Procedures. New York, Guilford, 1995

Sloan DM, Gallagher MW, Feinstein BA, et al: Efficacy of telehealth treatments for posttraumatic stress-related symptoms: a meta-analysis. Cogn Behav Ther 40(2):111–125, 2011 21547778

Sloan DM, Lee DJ, Litwack SD, et al: Written exposure therapy for veterans diagnosed with PTSD: a pilot study. J Trauma Stress 26(6):776–779, 2013 24203914

Sloan DM, Marx BP, Lee DJ, Resick PA: A brief exposure-based treatment vs cognitive processing therapy for posttraumatic stress disorder: a randomized noninferiority clinical trial. JAMA Psychiatry 75(3):233–239, 2018 29344631

Spates CR, Koch E, Pagoto S: Eye movement desensitization and reprocessing, in Effective Treatments for PTSD: Practice Guidelines From the International Society for Traumatic Stress Studies, 2nd Edition. Edited by Foa EB, Keane TM, Friedman MJ, et al. New York, Guilford, 2008, pp 279–305

Surís A, Link-Malcolm J, Chard K, et al: A randomized clinical trial of cognitive processing therapy for veterans with PTSD related to military sexual trauma. J Trauma Stress 26(1):28–37, 2013 23325750

Tran US, Gregor B: The relative efficacy of bona fide psychotherapies for post-traumatic stress disorder: a meta-analytical evaluation of randomized controlled trials. BMC Psychiatry 16:266, 2016 27460057

van Emmerik AA, Reijntjes A, Kamphuis JH: Writing therapy for posttraumatic stress: a meta-analysis. Psychother Psychosom 82(2):82–88, 2013 23295550

Watts BV, Schnurr PP, Mayo L, et al: Meta-analysis of the efficacy of treatments for posttraumatic stress disorder. J Clin Psychiatry 74(6):e541–e550, 2013 23842024

Recommended Readings

Brown LA, Belli G, Asnaani A, et al: A review of the role of negative cognitions about oneself, others, and the world in the treatment of PTSD. Cogn Ther Res 43(1):13–22, 2018

Cusack K, Jonas DE, Forneris CA, et al: Psychological treatments for adults with posttraumatic stress disorder: a systematic review and meta-analysis. Clin Psychol Rev 43:128–141, 2016 26574151

Foa EB, Hembree EA, Rothbaum BO: Prolonged Exposure Therapy for PTSD. New York, Oxford University Press, 2007

Resick PA, Monson CM, Chard KM: Cognitive Processing Therapy for PTSD: A Comprehensive Manual. New York, Guilford, 2016

CHAPTER 33

Phenomenology of Acute and Persistent Grief

Sidney Zisook, M.D.

Naomi Simon, M.D., M.Sc.

Charles Reynolds, M.D.

Ilanit R. Tal, Ph.D.

Barry Lebowitz, Ph.D.

Stephen J. Cozza, M.D.

M. Katherine Shear, M.D.

"The risk of love is loss, and the price of loss is grief. But the pain of grief is only a shadow when compared with the pain of never risking love.

Hilary Stanton Zunin

Grief describes the emotional, cognitive, functional, and behavioral responses to a meaningful loss. Throughout life, individuals face many losses capable of triggering grief. In this chapter we focus on grief after *bereavement*—the death of someone close. Bereavement is a nearly universal phenomenon that may be experienced many times by those living long enough to lose loved ones. Of all the life events and stresses of ordinary life, bereavement may have the greatest impact. Bereavement usually triggers an *acute grief* response of intense emotional pain and disruption of normal activities, both expectable and socially sanctioned. Although not unique in all respects, some aspects of grief after bereavement are distinctive. Grief after the death of someone close is especially stressful because of the permanence of the loss and the central importance of close relationships in our lives.

Although grief is often painful and impairing, with emotional and somatic distress, most people adapt to their loss, get through the acute grief period, and ultimately get on with their lives without professional assistance. *Mourning* is the process of adapting to loss, transforming acute grief to *integrated grief*. Adaptation entails accepting the finality and consequences of the loss, including a changed relationship to the deceased, and re-envisioning the future with the possibility for happiness in a world without the deceased. Cultural and religious rituals are a part of the mourning process, and these vary worldwide. When mourning is successful, the painful and disruptive experience of acute grief transforms into a form of integrated grief that is bittersweet and in the background: the bereaved recognize what the loss of the person means to them and how the person continues to be a part of their life; they are able to shift from focusing on their loss to living a meaningful life in a world without the deceased (Shear et al. 2016; Zisook and Shear 2009).

For a minority of bereaved individuals, mourning is not successful. Instead, maladaptive thoughts, feelings, or behaviors interfere with adapting to the loss, and the agony of the loss and yearning for and preoccupation with the deceased remain intense and debilitating. This condition, referred to in this chapter as *complicated grief* (see the section on "Complicated Grief" for a more complete discussion of the name and criteria), is a unique and recognizable disorder that responds to specific treatment (Shear and Bloom 2017; Shear et al. 2016). In this chapter, we describe the features, phenomenology, and course of acute and integrated grief and discuss the epidemiology, clinical features, evaluation, and pathophysiology of complicated grief.

Acute Grief

Clinical Characteristics

The hallmark of acute grief is intense focus on thoughts and memories of the deceased person, with sadness and yearning. Grief is not a linear process with concrete stages or boundaries but rather is a composite of overlapping and fluid cognitions, emotions, and behaviors, varying across individuals and differing in the same person after different losses and over time. Social, religious, and cultural norms influence the experience of grief, as do age, health, religious and ethnic identity, coping style, attachment style, available social support and material resources, situation and circumstances of the death, and experience of prior losses. Yet despite the variation and individual nuances, there are some common features of acute grief (Shear et al. 2017b; Zisook and Shear 2009).

A Sense of Disbelief

Most pronounced in the first hours to day to weeks, varying degrees of disbelief and denial are common. Statements such as "it can't be" or "I don't believe it" are ubiquitous, and the accompanying feeling of numbness pervades much of the initial period. Feeling numb and paralyzed, the bereaved may not believe the death is real. Mourning rituals and the gathering of family and friends support acceptance of death's reality.

Frequent Strong Feelings of Yearning and Sorrow

As the reality of the death is confronted, powerful feeling states settle in, generally occurring in waves of intense emotional arousal. Sometimes described as painful eruptions of autonomic responses, these feelings may include a wrenching of the gut, shortness of breath, chest pain, lightheadedness, weakness, rapid welling up of tears, and uncontrollable crying. During the early days and weeks, these responses tend to erupt often, suddenly, and unexpectedly in connection with a thought or reminder of the deceased. Over time, their frequency and intensity diminish.

Feelings of Insecurity, Emptiness, and Loss

The survivor experiences an increasing feeling of loss—not simply for the person who has died but also for that part of the survivor that was "connected" to the deceased. Additionally, many aspects of the survivor's daily life change because the person is no longer present. Hopes and plans for the future with the person who has died are lost. These feelings of loss, after a period of great intensity, gradually lessen as the person adapts to the changes.

A Mixture of Other Feelings

Several other feelings and thoughts, both positive and negative, are also common. *Anger* may be experienced as irritability, hatred, resentment, envy, or unfairness. It may be directed at the deceased, the deceased's physician, the hospital, God, fate, the world in general, or even the bereaved person him- or herself. *Guilt* may be experienced as caregiver self-blame or survivor guilt. Bereaved persons may believe they contributed to the death or suffering of the deceased, blaming themselves for many "transgressions," including improper feeding, inadequate support, failing to prevent unhealthy behavior or lifestyle, or not pushing the physician hard enough to detect or treat the disorder. The survivor may dwell on missed opportunities to do or say something that might have helped with suffering or completed some unfinished business. No matter how many exigencies one can anticipate and provide for, and how loving the relationship may have been, when someone close dies, there are always regrets. However, self-blame and survival guilt can be especially strong if the survivor has an element of responsibility for the death (e.g., if the bereaved person was the driver in a fatal vehicle accident). Other common feelings include *anxiety, fearfulness, mental disorganization, feeling overwhelmed,* and *loneliness.* Often, loneliness becomes more severe or may even initially manifest after the first several months of bereavement.

Thoughts of a loved one typically engender positive as well as painful emotions. Even during acute grief, painful experiences are intermingled with *positive feelings.* For example, bereaved people may experience *warmth, amusement,* or *pride* when thinking about the loved one. Sometimes they may feel a sense of *relief* at the ending of suffering. Depending on beliefs about death and the afterlife, *joy, peace,* and *happiness* may be present. Positive emotions can also be experienced during periods of distraction from the reality of the loss. Although positive thoughts and emotions may sometimes elicit a sense of disloyalty and survivor guilt, positive feelings are important for resilience and healthy long-term outcomes.

Insistent Thoughts and Images Focused on the Deceased

During acute grief, bereaved people may have recurring and often preoccupying, unshakable thoughts, memories, and images of the deceased. They may ruminate about things related to the deceased, looking at pictures or admiring prized possessions or other memorabilia. Especially after a traumatic loss, intrusive images may occur in the form of "instant replays" of the circumstances of the death or visions of the dying person in scenes of deterioration or suffering. Particularly in the early weeks or months of bereavement, these intrusive images can cause overwhelming distress.

Loss of Interest in Ongoing Life

With attention initially focused on loss, little energy may be left for other roles, responsibilities, and relationships. Most cultures acknowledge and facilitate the mourner's need for respite from life's demands by providing bereavement leave, help with child care, meals and "condolence baskets," and other such supports. Progress adapting to loss is typically erratic but ultimately allows for increasing reengagement in ongoing life and the renewed capacity for joy and meaning to unfold.

Course

Acute grief is usually time limited. Although cultures vary in expectations for the time-frame of acute grief, the process of adapting to the loss is generally believed to begin soon after the loss, and restoration of ongoing life is often achieved within 6–12 months (Shear 2015). As a person adapts, grief becomes more subdued, and thoughts and memories of the deceased recede into the background and are no longer insistent. Grief becomes integrated as the finality and consequences of the death and the changed relationship to the deceased are understood and accepted. However, the response to the loss of a loved one does not end. Rather, acute grief is transformed into an abiding form, *integrated grief* (Shear et al. 2017b).

Transition to Integrated Grief

Support from family and friends and cultural traditions assist adaptation to loss, transforming acute grief to integrated grief. Every culture has its own beliefs, customs, and behaviors related to bereavement. These include rituals for mourning (e.g., wakes, shiva), for disposing of the body, for religious ceremonies, and for periodic official remembrances. These rituals facilitate a focus on thoughts and feelings related to the deceased, particularly in the earliest period after the loss and periodically thereafter. The funeral is the prevailing public display of bereavement in contemporary North America. The funeral and burial service underscore the real and final nature of the death, garner support for the bereaved, encourage tribute to the dead, unite families, and empower community expressions of sorrow. Visits, prayers, and other ceremonies allow for support, coming to terms with reality, remembering, emotional expression, and concluding unfinished business with the deceased. Several cultural and religious rituals provide purpose and meaning, protect the survivors from isolation and vulnerability, and set limits on grieving. Over time, eruptions of autonomic distress give way to bittersweet remembrance, which is often brought on by holidays, birthdays, anniversaries, and other special events that remind the living of the dead and are experienced as comforting.

Unlike acute grief, integrated grief is permanent. As bereaved people adapt to the many changes that accompany the death of a loved one, their wounds begin to heal, and they find their way back to a fulfilling life. The reality and meaning of the death are assimilated, and the relationship with the deceased has a new place in the life of the bereaved, who can engage once again in pleasurable and satisfying relationships

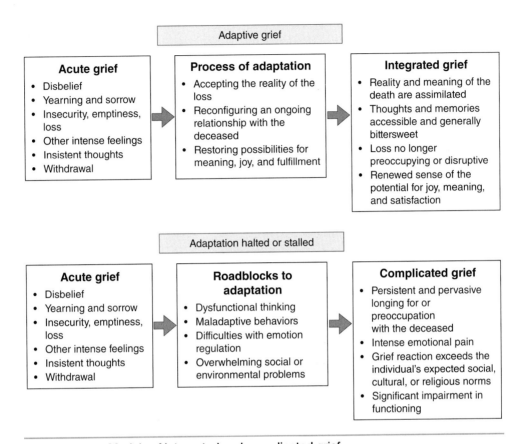

FIGURE 33–1. Models of integrated and complicated grief.

and activities. The bereaved do not forget or stop missing lost ones or relinquish their sadness, and intense grief may reawaken around the time of significant events, another loss, or other particularly meaningful or stressful times; however, these feelings do not interfere with the ongoing experience of a renewed sense of joy and satisfaction.

Complicated Grief

For a significant minority, adaptation to loss is impeded by dysfunctional thinking, maladaptive behaviors, difficulties with emotion regulation, and social or environmental problems (Figure 33–1). The result is that acute grief persists, continuing to invade the person's life. The reality of the death is not integrated into autobiographical memory, nor are satisfying activities restored to the bereaved's life (Shear 2015; Shear et al. 2017a). An array of terms have been used to describe persistent grief—*abnormal, atypical, chronic, complicated, delayed, distorted, morbid, pathological, prolonged, traumatic,* and *unresolved,* to name a few. DSM-5 calls it *persistent complex bereavement disorder* (American Psychiatric Association 2013), and ICD-11 names the condition *prolonged grief disorder* (Augsburger and Maercker 2018; Mauro et al. 2019). Here we use the term *complicated grief* because it appears in the literature most commonly. This syndrome is characterized by intense and persistent sadness, longing, and yearning that last longer than expected according to social norms and that cause impairment in major roles (Reynolds et al. 2017).

Epidemiology

No consensus has yet been reached on specific diagnostic criteria for complicated grief, and studies regarding its prevalence and risk factors are sparse and preliminary. Furthermore, the currently available studies are characterized by considerable methodological diversity in study design, participant characteristics (e.g., age, sex, relationship to the deceased), time since loss, instruments used, and cutoff points applied. Thus, the variation of prevalence rates across studies (e.g., 1.8%–25.4%; Lundorff et al. 2017) is not surprising. The best data thus far estimate a worldwide rate of 2%–4% in the general adult population and 10% among persons bereaved by natural causes (Lundorff et al. 2017).

Complicated grief can follow the loss of any close relationship, but prevalence rates appear to be higher after the death of a romantic partner and higher still among parents who have lost children, compared with the loss of a parent, grandparent, sibling, or close friend (Meert et al. 2011). Furthermore, complicated grief is more likely when a death is sudden or violent (e.g., by suicide, homicide, or accident) than after natural or anticipated deaths (Kristensen et al. 2012; Tal et al. 2017). It also appears elevated in clinical settings, with high rates among patients with mood disorders (Simon et al. 2005; Sung et al. 2011), PTSD (Charney et al. 2018; Simon et al. 2018), and anxiety disorders (Marques et al. 2013). Other risk factors include female sex, older age, past or co-occurring mood or anxiety disorder, low socioeconomic status, nonwhite race, severe medical illness, insecure attachment style (anxious/avoidant), childhood separation anxiety, and an especially close relationship with the deceased. Emerging evidence also points to neurobiological and genetic vulnerabilities (Shear et al. 2017a). Whatever the causes or unique triggering conditions, clinical experience suggests that without treatment, symptoms of complicated grief commonly diminish slowly and incompletely, resulting in chronic impairments in quality of life and function (Shear et al. 2011).

Clinical Features

Key Features

Complicated grief is characterized by an accentuation of the intensity, pervasiveness, and persistence of acute grief, along with specific thoughts, feelings, behaviors, and situations that impede adaptation and lead to its persistence (Table 33–1). One study found the most frequent symptoms to be yearning for the deceased (88%), feeling upset by memories of the deceased (82%), loneliness (81%), emptiness (80%), disbelief (76%), and inability to accept the death (70%) (Simon et al. 2011). Thus, individuals with complicated grief find themselves caught up in seemingly endless yearning for, longing for, or preoccupation with the deceased, unable to see possibilities for happiness. They may perceive their grief as frightening, shameful, and strange, believing that life is over and that their intense pain will never cease. Some people with complicated grief do not want the grief to end, believing it is all that is

TABLE 33–1.	Features of complicated grief

Accentuation of intensity, pervasiveness, and persistence of acute grief symptoms

Disbelief

Yearning and sorrow

Emptiness and loss

Insecurity

Thinking focused on the deceased

Loss of interest in ongoing life

Mixture of other feelings (positive and negative): anger, guilt, anxiety, loneliness, mental disorganization; feeling overwhelmed, relieved, proud, at peace

Complications

Maladaptive thoughts: second-guessing, grief judging, self-blaming, catastrophizing

Maladaptive feelings: overly intense negative emotions, low positive emotions, low self-compassion

Maladaptive behaviors: excessive avoidance, social withdrawal, substance use, negative health behaviors

Maladaptive social/environmental problems: lack of any supportive companion, feeling blamed by or blaming others for the death, homelessness, poverty, loss of employment

left of the relationship with their loved one or that enjoying their life would be a betrayal. They frequently feel estranged from others, including people with whom they used to be close (Zisook and Shear 2009).

Diagnosis

Diagnostic criteria for complicated grief are now available; although some questions remain about the optimal way to diagnose this condition (Cozza et al. 2016; Mauro et al. 2017, 2019; Prigerson and Maciejewski 2017; Reynolds et al. 2017), the core clinical features are not under debate. Table 33–2 compares the four leading proposed criteria sets for this condition. Of these, the ICD-11 criteria (World Health Organization 2018) are the simplest and briefest and accurately identify bereaved individuals with prolonged, persistent, and impairing grief who respond to targeted treatment (Mauro et al. 2019). Thus, the ICD-11 guideline is well suited for clinical settings. ICD-11 defines the new condition of prolonged grief disorder as

> a disturbance in which, following the death of a partner, parent, child, or other person close to the bereaved, there is persistent and pervasive grief response characterized by longing for the deceased or persistent preoccupation with the deceased accompanied by intense emotional pain (e.g., sadness, guilt, anger, denial, blame, difficulty accepting the death, feeling one has lost a part of one's self, an inability to experience positive mood, emotional numbness, difficulty in engaging with social or other activities). The grief response has persisted for an atypically long period of time following the loss (more than 6 months at a minimum) and clearly exceeds expected social, cultural or religious norms for the individual's culture and context…. The disturbance causes significant impairment in personal, family, social, educational, occupational or other important areas of functioning. (World Health Organization 2018)

TABLE 33–2.   Proposed diagnostic criteria for persistent and impairing grief

	Persistent complex bereavement disorder (DSM-5)	Prolonged grief disorder (ICD-11)	Prolonged grief disorder (Prigerson et al. 2009)	Complicated grief disorder (Mauro et al. 2019)
Criterion A	Loss > 12 months	Loss > 6 months	Loss > 6 months	Loss > 6 months
Criterion B	At least 1 of 4: Yearning Preoccupation with the deceased Intense sorrow Preoccupation with the death	At least 1 of 2: Longing for the deceased Persistent preoccupation with the deceased	1 of 1: Yearning	At least 1 of 4: Yearning Insistent thoughts of the deceased Life is unbearable Intense loneliness
Criterion C	At least 6 of 12: Difficulty accepting the death Feeling disbelief/numbness Difficulty with positive reminiscing Bitterness/Anger Self-blame Avoidance of reminders Desire to die Difficulty trusting others Alone/Detached Life is meaningless Confusion about role/diminished identity Difficulty pursuing interests/making plans	At least 1 of 10 (intense emotional pain): Anger Denial Emotional numbness Difficulty accepting the death Difficulty engaging with social or other activities Guilt Sadness Blame Feeling one has lost a part of oneself Inability to experience positive mood	At least 5 of 9: Avoiding reminders Mistrustful of others Bitterness/Anger Numbness Feel stunned or shocked Role confusion Difficulty accepting the death Difficulty moving on Life is unfulfilling	At least 2 of 8: Avoiding reminders or seeking to feel close Mistrustful of others Bitterness/Anger Disbelief Shocked or numb Troubling thoughts Hearing/Seeing deceased Strong reactivity to reminders

Associated Features

People with complicated grief may spend excessive time seeking proximity to the lost person (e.g., frequent visits to the grave or other memorials, spending long periods daydreaming about being with the person) or avoiding reminders of the loss. Difficulty imagining a promising future without the deceased contributes to feelings of emptiness and futility and reduces the sense of purpose and meaning in ongoing life (Shear et al. 2017a). Complicated grief is associated with an elevated risk for suicide, including indirect suicidal behavior (Szanto et al. 2006). Thus, suicide risk should be assessed in all patients (Latham and Prigerson 2004; Szanto et al. 2006; Tal et al. 2017).

Differential Diagnosis

Complicated grief must be differentiated from the three most similar conditions: uncomplicated (i.e., acute and integrated) grief, major depressive disorder (MDD), and PTSD. It differs from uncomplicated grief primarily by the prominence of counterfactual thoughts, avoidance behavior, and persistent intense emotions, as well as persistent interference with functioning lasting more than a year after the death (6 months in ICD-11). Complicated grief has many symptoms in common with MDD, such as intense sadness, crying, sleep disturbance, and withdrawal from customary activities; however, depressive symptoms are centered on loss rather than the more pervasive depressed mood seen in MDD. Similarly, guilt is specifically related to letting the deceased down in some way and not the pervasive sense of guilt seen in MDD. Suicidal ideation is focused on not wanting to live without the deceased or on wishes to be reunited with the lost loved one; in MDD, suicidal thoughts more often reflect feelings of being unworthy to live. Features of complicated grief not seen in MDD include intense yearning for the deceased, behaviors enacted to feel close to the deceased, intrusive or preoccupying thoughts of the deceased, intense emotions activated by reminders of the loss, and efforts to avoid these reminders (Zisook et al. 2012).

Complicated grief also shares features with PTSD. Experiencing the death of a loved one is a life event that meets the trauma criterion of observing or learning of death. People with complicated grief describe intrusive images of the deceased, avoid reminders of the loss, feel estranged from others, and report sleep disturbances or difficulty concentrating. However, because being confronted with physical danger is fundamentally different from losing a sustaining relationship, many grief symptoms differ correspondingly from those of PTSD. The hallmarks of complicated grief are sadness and yearning, whereas the hallmark of PTSD is fear. Symptoms of complicated grief focus on the loved one, and intrusive images of the deceased may be pleasurable or bittersweet; intense yearning or searching for the deceased, behaviors enacted to feel close to the deceased, and insistent thoughts or daydreams of the deceased that may be pleasurable are common. These are not seen in PTSD, which entails frightening reexperiencing of thoughts and images of the traumatic event, excessive startle response, and nightmares (Shear et al. 2011). Avoidance in complicated grief helps avert painful thoughts or feelings related to the loss; avoidance in PTSD is generally aimed at preventing thoughts and feelings related to fear or the recurrence of danger.

Comorbidity

Complicated grief may be accompanied by comorbid psychopathology, most commonly MDD, PTSD, generalized anxiety disorder, panic disorder, and substance use disorders (Shear et al. 2017a). Severity of grief symptoms and functional impairment are greater in individuals with comorbid psychopathology (Simon et al. 2007).

Other Consequences

Complicated grief has been associated with an elevated risk of MDD, suicidal ideation, cancer, hypertension, and cardiac events; functional impairments (social, family, and occupational dysfunction); adverse health behaviors (e.g., alcohol abuse, increased use of tobacco); and hospitalization as well as reduced quality of life and increased mortality due to general medical conditions, suicidal behaviors (Latham and Prigerson 2004; Shear et al. 2017a; Szanto et al. 2006), and cognitive impairment (Hall et al. 2014).

Course

Adequate long-term studies of complicated grief are not yet available to determine course, but the best available evidence suggests that once features persist beyond about 6 months, symptoms and impairment tend to last for years, if not a lifetime, absent focused treatment interventions. In several studies that identified patients currently experiencing complicated grief, the average elapsed time since the loss ranged from 10 to 16 years (Shear et al. 2017a).

Evaluation

Questions about important losses should be part of a standard diagnostic evaluation, especially in older patients, for whom loss is common, and in patients with mood, anxiety, or trauma-related disorders and bereavement who may have unrecognized complicated grief—potentially a hidden factor in treatment resistance. The presence of thoughts and behaviors that are indicative of complicated grief should be assessed with the use of a clinical interview.

The Brief Grief Questionnaire (Ito et al. 2012) is a five-item self-report questionnaire that can be used to screen patients for complicated grief; a score of 5 or higher indicates a positive screen (Patel et al. 2018; Shear et al. 2006). The Structured Clinical Interview for Complicated Grief is a validated semistructured interview (Bui et al. 2015) that can be used to systematically assess complicated grief; a short form of this instrument is available (Shear 2015). The Inventory of Complicated Grief (Prigerson et al. 1995) is a 19-item self-report questionnaire that can be used to monitor treatment response; a score greater than 25 identifies clinically significant symptoms that predict negative health outcomes (Meert et al. 2011; Prigerson et al. 1995). Other psychiatric conditions (e.g., substance use disorders) should also be assessed.

Pathophysiology of Complicated Grief

Preliminary neurobiological research has suggested the potential for smaller brain volumes in complicated grief (Saavedra Pérez et al. 2015). Specific brain areas involved in emotion regulation and reward, which may be a component of the attachment-related distress that is key to this diagnosis, have been identified in neuroimaging research (Arizmendi et al. 2016; O'Connor et al. 2008). Alterations in cortisol, with flatter slopes across the day, have been reported (O'Connor et al. 2012), but much more work is needed to understand the biological causes and consequences of and biomarkers for the condition. Finally, a growing literature identifies differences in information processing and memory in complicated grief, including attention biases toward loss-related events (Maccallum and Bryant 2010) and reduced imagining of the future (Boelen et al. 2010; Golden et al. 2007; Maccallum and Bryant 2011; Robinaugh and McNally 2013).

Conclusion

Each individual's grief process is unique, and most bereaved individuals demonstrate great resilience. Mourning rituals, which may vary by culture and religion, and the love and support of friends and relatives help most bereaved individuals adapt to their loss without need of professional assistance. However, for a meaningful minority of bereaved persons, mourning is not successful, adaptation stalls, and the condition known as complicated grief develops. Complicated grief is painful; interferes with health, relationships, function, and quality of life; and, in the absence of targeted interventions, may last indefinitely. Potentially life-altering, life-saving, evidence-based interventions for this serious condition are discussed in Chapter 34, "Treatment of Acute and Persistent Grief."

Key Points

- Acute grief is a natural, often painful and disruptive, but generally time-limited response to bereavement.

- In the absence of complications, acute grief is usually transformed and integrated as a person adapts to the loss; integrated grief is an enduring form of grief that is minimally disruptive, often associated with personal growth, and compatible with well-being.

- Dysfunctional thinking, maladaptive behaviors, difficulties with emotion regulation, and social or environmental problems can disrupt adaptation to bereavement, leaving grief persistent and pervasive and producing the syndrome of complicated grief.

- Complicated grief can be reliably diagnosed and differentiated from its nearest neighbors: normal (uncomplicated, adaptive) grief, major depressive disorder, and PTSD.

- Complicated grief is painful, impairing, and associated with various general medical and psychiatric sequelae. If untreated, it can last for years or even decades.

References

American Psychiatric Association: Diagnostic and Statistical Manual of Mental Disorders, 5th Edition. Arlington, VA, American Psychiatric Association, 2013

Arizmendi B, Kaszniak AW, O'Connor MF: Disrupted prefrontal activity during emotion processing in complicated grief: an fMRI investigation. Neuroimage 124(pt A):968–976, 2016 26434802

Augsburger M, Maercker A: Mental disorders specifically associated with stress in the upcoming ICD-11: an overview [in German]. Fortschr Neurol Psychiatr 86(3):156–162, 2018 29621820

Boelen PA, Huntjens RJC, van Deursen DS, et al: Autobiographical memory specificity and symptoms of complicated grief, depression, and posttraumatic stress disorder following loss. J Behav Ther Exp Psychiatry 41(4):331–337, 2010 20394916

Bui E, Mauro C, Robinaugh DJ, et al: The structured clinical interview for complicated grief: reliability, validity, and exploratory factor analysis. Depress Anxiety 32(7):485–492, 2015 26061724

Charney ME, Bui E, Sager JC, et al: Complicated grief among military service members and veterans who served after September 11, 2001. J Trauma Stress 31(1):157–162, 2018 29384232

Cozza SJ, Fisher JE, Mauro C, et al: Performance of DSM-5 persistent complex bereavement disorder criteria in a community sample of bereaved military family members. Am J Psychiatry 173(9):919–929, 2016 27216262

Golden AM, Dalgleish T, Mackintosh B: Levels of specificity of autobiographical memories and of biographical memories of the deceased in bereaved individuals with and without complicated grief. J Abnorm Psychol 116(4):786–795, 2007 18020724

Hall CA, Reynolds CF 3rd, Butters M, et al: Cognitive functioning in complicated grief. J Psychiatr Res 58:20–25, 2014 25088285

Ito M, Nakajima S, Fujisawa D, et al: Brief measure for screening complicated grief: reliability and discriminant validity. PLoS One 7(2):e31209, 2012 22348057

Kristensen P, Weisæth L, Heir T: Bereavement and mental health after sudden and violent losses: a review. Psychiatry 75(1):76–97, 2012 22397543

Latham AE, Prigerson HG: Suicidality and bereavement: complicated grief as psychiatric disorder presenting greatest risk for suicidality. Suicide Life Threat Behav 34(4):350–362, 2004 15585457

Lundorff M, Holmgren H, Zachariae R, et al: Prevalence of prolonged grief disorder in adult bereavement: a systematic review and meta-analysis. J Affect Disord 212:138–149, 2017 28167398

Maccallum F, Bryant RA: Attentional bias in complicated grief. J Affect Disord 125(1–3):316–322, 2010

Maccallum F, Bryant RA: Imagining the future in complicated grief. Depress Anxiety 28(8):658–665, 2011 21796741

Marques L, Bui E, LeBlanc N, et al: Complicated grief symptoms in anxiety disorders: prevalence and associated impairment. Depress Anxiety 30(12):1211–1216, 2013 23495105

Mauro C, Shear MK, Reynolds CF, et al: Performance characteristics and clinical utility of diagnostic criteria proposals in bereaved treatment-seeking patients. Psychol Med 47(4):608–615, 2017 27821201

Mauro C, Reynolds CF, Maercker A, et al: Prolonged grief disorder: clinical utility of ICD-11 diagnostic guidelines. Psychol Med 49(5):861–867, 2019 29909789

Meert KL, Shear K, Newth CJ, et al: Follow-up study of complicated grief among parents eighteen months after a child's death in the pediatric intensive care unit. J Palliat Med 14(2):207–214, 2011 21281122

O'Connor MF, Wellisch DK, Stanton AL, et al: Craving love? Enduring grief activates brain's reward center. Neuroimage 42(2):969–972, 2008 18559294

O'Connor MF, Wellisch DK, Stanton AL, et al: Diurnal cortisol in complicated and non-complicated grief: slope differences across the day. Psychoneuroendocrinology 37(5):725–728, 2012 21925795

Patel SR, Cole A, Little V, et al: Acceptability, feasibility and outcome of a screening programme for complicated grief in integrated primary and behavioural health care clinics. Family Pract 36(2):125–131, 2018

Prigerson HG, Maciejewski PK: Rebuilding consensus on valid criteria for disordered grief. JAMA Psychiatry 74(5):435–436, 2017 28355449

Prigerson HG, Maciejewski PK, Reynolds CF, et al: Inventory of Complicated Grief: a scale to measure maladaptive symptoms of loss. Psychiatry Res 59(1):65–79, 1995 8771222

Prigerson HG, Horowitz MJ, Jacobs SC, et al: Prolonged grief disorder: psychometric validation of criteria proposed for DSM-V and ICD-11. PLoS Med 6(8):e1000121, 2009 19652695

Reynolds CF, Cozza SJ, Shear MK: Clinically relevant diagnostic criteria for a persistent impairing grief disorder: putting patients first. JAMA Psychiatry 74(5):433–434, 2017 28355457

Robinaugh DJ, McNally RJ: Remembering the past and envisioning the future in bereaved adults with and without complicated grief. Clin Psychol Sci 1(3):290–300, 2013

Saavedra Pérez HC, Ikram MA, Direk N, et al: Cognition, structural brain changes and complicated grief: a population-based study. Psychol Med 45(7):1389–1399, 2015 25363662

Shear MK: Clinical practice: complicated grief. N Engl J Med 372(2):153–160, 2015 25564898

Shear MK, Bloom CG: Complicated grief treatment: an evidence-based approach to grief therapy. J Ration Emot Cogn Behav Ther35(1):6–25, 2017

Shear KM, Jackson CT, Essock SM, et al: Screening for complicated grief among Project Liberty service recipients 18 months after September 11, 2001. Psychiatr Serv 57(9):1291–1297, 2006 16968758

Shear MK, Simon N, Wall M, et al: Complicated grief and related bereavement issues for DSM-5. Depress Anxiety 28(2):103–117, 2011 21284063

Shear MK, Reynolds CF 3rd, Simon NM, et al: Optimizing treatment of complicated grief: a randomized clinical trial. JAMA Psychiatry 73(7):685–694, 2016 27276373

Shear MK, Reynolds CF 3rd, Simon NM, et al: Complicated Grief in Adults: Epidemiology, Clinical Features, Assessment, and Diagnosis. Waltham, MA, Uptodate, 2017a

Shear MK, Reynolds CF 3rd, Simon NM, et al: Grief and Bereavement in Adults: Clinical Features. Waltham, MA, Uptodate, 2017b

Simon NM, Pollack MH, Fischmann D, et al: Complicated grief and its correlates in patients with bipolar disorder. J Clin Psychiatry 66(9):1105–1110, 2005 16187766

Simon NM, Shear KM, Thompson EH, et al: The prevalence and correlates of psychiatric comorbidity in individuals with complicated grief. Compr Psychiatry 48(5):395–399, 2007 17707245

Simon NM, Wall MM, Keshaviah A, et al: Informing the symptom profile of complicated grief. Depress Anxiety 28(2):118–126, 2011 21284064

Simon NM, O'Day EB, Hellberg SN, et al: The loss of a fellow service member: complicated grief in post-9/11 service members and veterans with combat-related posttraumatic stress disorder. J Neurosci Res 96(1):5–15, 2018

Sung SC, Dryman MT, Marks E, et al: Complicated grief among individuals with major depression: prevalence, comorbidity, and associated features. J Affect Disord 134(1–3):453–458, 2011 21621849

Szanto K, Shear MK, Houck PR, et al: Indirect self-destructive behavior and overt suicidality in patients with complicated grief. J Clin Psychiatry 67(2):233–239, 2006

Tal I, Mauro C, Reynolds CF III, et al: Complicated grief after suicide bereavement and other causes of death. Death Stud 41(5):267–275, 2017 27892842

World Health Organization: International Statistical Classification of Diseases and Related Health Problems, 11th Revision (advance preview). Geneva, World Health Organization, 2018

Zisook S, Shear K: Grief and bereavement: what psychiatrists need to know. World Psychiatry 8(2):67–74, 2009 19516922

Zisook S, Corruble E, Duan N, et al: The bereavement exclusion and DSM-5. Depress Anxiety 29(5):425–443, 2012 22495967

Recommended Readings

Bui E: Grief: from normal to pathological reactions, in Clinical Handbook of Bereavement and Grief Reactions. Cham, Switzerland, Humana, 2018, pp 85–101

Shear MK: Clinical practice: complicated grief. N Engl J Med 372(2):153–160, 2015 25564898

Shear MK, Reynolds CF 3rd, Simon NM, et al: Optimizing treatment of complicated grief: a randomized clinical trial. JAMA Psychiatry 73(7):685–694, 2016 27276373

Zisook S, Shear K: Grief and bereavement: what psychiatrists need to know. World Psychiatry 8(2):67–74, 2009 19516922

CHAPTER 34

Treatment of Acute and Persistent Grief

M. Katherine Shear, M.D.

Natalia Skritskaya, Ph.D.

Colleen Gribbin Bloom, M.S.W.

People we love are important to our well-being. We provide each other with a safe haven when we are stressed or troubled and a secure base from which we explore the world, learn new things, and take risks to achieve things that matter to us. As if that were not enough, we contribute to each other's psychological and physiological regulation—both in and out of awareness. Our close relationships mediate feelings of belonging in our community and of mattering to others. No wonder that the loss of a loved one is considered the most stressful of life events.

Bereavement, defined as the state of having lost someone close, triggers acute grief. A meaningful loss further initiates natural processes to facilitate ways to adapt to the absence of the person as well as the host of changes that accompany the loss. Grief is complex and multifaceted, containing both painful and pleasant emotions, troubling and comforting thoughts, and grief-related behaviors. Acute grief can be intensely painful, and it can take over a bereaved person's life. As we adapt to the loss, grief settles down and finds a place in our lives. We gradually learn to accept the finality and consequence of the loss, including the changed—although not ended—relationship with the person who died. We discover how to live fully in a world filled with reminders of absence and to see the future as having purpose and possibilities for happiness. Adapting is not easy, and it is not linear. Sometimes people continue to grapple with the effects of a terrible loss for decades, even as they also reengage in meaningful ways in their ongoing lives. Often, those who have lost a cherished companion continue to feel that person's comforting presence, keeping him or her close for years, decades, or even the rest of their lives. Overall and in varying ways, most people adjust to even the most difficult loss without requiring mental health treatment. Moreover, a painful loss often leads to personal growth. Death of a loved one can open our hearts to the suffering of others, engender a deeper sense of spirituality, or foster a greater appreciation of other people and of our own lives. It is a testament to human resilience that we find so many ways to flourish after adversity.

Grief, as the response to bereavement, is complex, with variable and changing cognitive, emotional, behavioral, and physiological features. Everyone grieves in their own way. We also adapt in our own way. Adaptation to loss progresses in fits and starts, and at times it may feel as though gains have been lost. Grief tags along behind our efforts to adapt, waxing and waning in intensity as we struggle to accept the reality and make sense of our lives in a new way. We do not emerge unscathed or unchanged, but we can still thrive. Heartbreaking and unwelcome though it may be, the devastation of loss creates fertile ground for new growth. Gradually, painfully, we find our way forward, granting grief a permanent place in our lives. It's not surprising that this journey sometimes goes off course.

A persistent impairing grief disorder is now part of the psychiatric nomenclature, provisionally included in DSM-5 as *persistent complex bereavement disorder* (American Psychiatric Association 2013) and in ICD-11 as *prolonged grief disorder*. However, the term *complicated grief* is the most commonly used designation in the clinical and research literature. At the writing of this chapter, we still await consensus about the name, so in the meantime we use *complicated grief*. Untreated, this is a life-draining experience that can last for decades or even indefinitely. Happily, the introduction of the provisional diagnoses in ICD-11 and DSM-5 was accompanied by a solid body of treatment research to guide clinicians. In this chapter, we provide an overview of the growing body of evidence-informed and efficacy-tested treatment approaches for complicated grief. We include a brief overview of treatment-relevant phenomenology and a model of pathogenesis to guide intervention.

What a Clinician Should Look For: Treatment-Relevant Phenomenology

In Chapter 33, "Phenomenology of Acute and Persistent Grief," Zisook and colleagues provide a detailed description of the ICD-11 diagnostic guideline for prolonged grief disorder, including the differential diagnosis, clinical features, and course of this condition. Here, we want to emphasize the importance of a focus on the framework for adapting to loss. Grief emerges with recognition of a loss and is transformed as we adapt. The persistence of intense and impairing grief is a marker for problems in adaptation. Grief itself is not the problem. This is important to recognize, because efforts to directly reduce grief intensity can backfire. Clinicians can be misled because the name of the disorder and the symptoms in the criteria describe grief. This is somewhat analogous to the difference between treating a fever with aspirin as opposed to treating an underlying infection. Still, just as a fever indicates an infection, so is grief a cardinal indicator of inadequate adaptation. Clinicians need to recognize and differentiate acute, integrated, and complicated grief.

> Grace is a bereaved 40-year-old woman. Her story is typical for people dealing with complicated grief. Since her sister Jane died, it is as though Grace is frozen in time, unable to see a way forward. She is caught up in maladaptive thoughts and dysfunctional

behaviors that hamper her ability to adapt. Ruminating about reasons Jane didn't have to die distracts Grace from coming to terms with the reality of the loss and from attempting to envision an inviting future without her sister. She is unable to adapt, and acute grief symptoms persist, pervasive and unabating. Grace has persistent pervasive yearning and longing, preoccupation with thoughts and images of her sister, and other evidence of emotional pain and thoughts and behaviors that hamper adaptation.

Persistent pervasive yearning and longing: Four years after Jane died, Grace is still experiencing intense grief. She knows her grief is excessive, but she thinks less grief means forgetting Jane or leaving her behind. Sometimes her yearning is so strong she thinks it will surely bring Jane back.

Preoccupation with thoughts, images, or memories: Grace often daydreams about being with her sister, gossiping, sharing secrets, trying on clothes, or hiking in the woods.

Evidence of emotional pain: The feeling of her sister's absence invades the most ordinary places and fills Grace with guilt, anxiety, sadness, and anger.

Thoughts and behaviors that hamper adaptation: Grace does not want to look at pictures of her sister or do anything that reminds her that Jane is gone. Her thoughts often focus on why Jane did not have to die. She can think of so many ways it could have been different. She does not see how she can live in a world without her sister. She and Jane had so many plans, and now the future looks bleak and empty.

Clinicians need to be clear about similarities and differences between complicated grief and other DSM diagnoses, attending to both differential diagnosis and comorbidity (Table 34–1). These are well described in Chapter 33. We draw attention to the frequent occurrence with complicated grief of suicidal thinking and behavior, including lethal attempts. Bereaved individuals may believe they want to join their deceased loved one, that they do not want to live in a world without their loved one, or that they do not deserve to live because their loved one can no longer live. Those bereaved by a suicide death may be especially prone to active suicidal thinking (Young 2017).

Using a Model of Pathogenesis to Guide Intervention

Because grief is the response to loss of a loved one, understanding love is important in understanding grief. Considerable data document the myriad ways close relationships contribute to self-regulation, cognitive functioning, and physiological regulation both in and out of awareness. Hence, bereavement heralds a period of regulatory dysfunction (see Shear and Shair 2005). Additionally, a loss triggers activation of the attachment system, proximity seeking, separation anxiety, separation guilt, and inhibition of exploration. Taken together, these effects describe acute grief (Figure 34–1).

Fortunately, grief does not usually remain acute and disruptive. Why not? Bowlby (1982) provided an answer. He posited that adaptation is an instinctive process, triggered naturally by a loss. In order to adapt, we must accept the painful reality that a loved one has died. The death of a loved one does not end our relationship with that person, but it does move him or her off center stage. This change must be acknowledged for proximity seeking to abate and for the bereaved to envision a promising future. Reciprocally, capacity to see an inviting future facilitates acceptance of the reality of the death. Thus, adaptation requires both accepting the reality of the death and finding a way to envision the future as holding possibilities for happiness. Grief is transformed as the new reality is integrated into attachment-related mental processes.

TABLE 34–1.   **Key differences between complicated grief and other conditions**

Symptoms	Complicated grief	Acute grief	Integrated grief	MDD	PTSD
Yearning or longing	+++	++	+	–	–
Preoccupying thoughts or memories of the deceased	+++	++	–	–	–
Other evidence of emotional pain	+++	++	–	+	+
Counterfactual or judgmental grief-related thoughts	+++	+	–	–	–
Grief-related behaviors	+++	+	–	–	–
Persist ≥1 year after the death	+++	–	+++	++	++

Note.   MDD=major depressive disorder.
–=rarely or not present; +=sometimes present; ++=often present; +++=always or almost always present.

Clinicians can assume that natural instinctive processes for adaptation are still present in people with complicated grief, although these processes have been derailed by dysregulated emotions, maladaptive thoughts, and dysfunctional behaviors. These impediments subvert acknowledgment of the reality of the death and block adaptation. Treatment needs to resolve the impediments and reengage adaptive processes along with their natural facilitators.

Persistent intense emotions fuel avoidance of reminders of the loss, which limits freedom to move about and restricts possibilities for positive experiences. Avoidance also undercuts reward extinction, leaving intact powerful urges for proximity seeking—the intense yearning and longing for the deceased that is a hallmark of complicated grief (Robinaugh et al. 2016). Put another way, the unchallenged expectation of rewarding interactions with the deceased prevents necessary transformation of the attachment working model. Unrevised, the working model remains activated, meaning it is in searching, seeking mode. An activated attachment system hijacks mental resources in a futile search for reunion with no feasible end point. Treatment thus needs to include a focus on avoidance and on facilitating recognition of the changed relationship with the deceased.

Social support is an important facilitator of adaptation; however, persistent intense grief often leads to estrangement from others. Real and growing social isolation makes the future look bleak. Moreover, the strong orientation toward seeking proximity leaves few remaining resources for imagining new pathways to joy and satisfaction. Clinicians need to help patients generate some enthusiasm for the future.

In summary, the overall objective of intervention for complicated grief is to promote adaptation. Clinicians need to help patients understand and accept grief; identify and manage maladaptive thoughts, feelings, and behaviors; confront the reality of the death; and envision an inviting future. A clinician can address these goals in many ways. In the remainder of this chapter, we outline some of them. Beginning with loss assessment, we provide an overview of evidence-based approaches to psychotherapy, such as complicated grief treatment (CGT), which is supported by three randomized controlled trials (RCTs), and other promising approaches and provide information about when and how to use pharmacotherapy to optimize treatment.

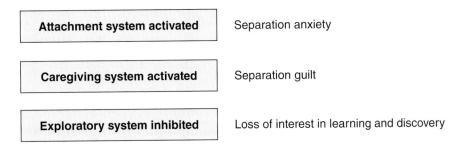

Attachment system activated	Separation anxiety
Caregiving system activated	Separation guilt
Exploratory system inhibited	Loss of interest in learning and discovery

FIGURE 34–1. The effects of loss on attachment, caregiving, and exploration explaining acute grief.

Role of Loss Assessment in Treatment Planning

Assessment of important losses is a part of a standard clinical evaluation. Persistent impairing grief may be a clinical concern either as the chief complaint that brings a patient to treatment or as an emerging problem for a patient already in treatment. Either way, a brief psychiatric history and mental status examination should accompany or precede the assessment of loss and grief. Evaluating clinicians should keep in mind that loss of a loved one is a major stressor that can trigger the onset of a wide range of clinically significant problems (Keyes et al. 2014). Assessment of a bereaved patient includes a brief discussion of the relationship with the deceased and the circumstances of the death, a review of grief symptoms and impairment since the loss, and appraisal of progress adapting to the loss. Assessment of typical maladaptive thoughts, behaviors, and emotion regulation strategies is done to alert clinicians to possible complications. Examples include counterfactual ruminations; assignment of blame; judging or questioning grief; persistent intense guilt, anger, or anxiety; excessive avoidance; negative health behaviors; or excessive risk-taking behavior. Grief assessment can be done as a clinical interview with or without a semistructured interview guide (Bui et al. 2015; Shear 2015) or with validated self-report questionnaires such as the Inventory of Complicated Grief (Prigerson et al. 1995) or Brief Grief Questionnaire (Shear et al. 2006). Assessment of a bereaved patient includes questions about suicidal thoughts and behaviors (e.g., Columbia Suicide Scale; Posner et al. 2011). The occurrence of PTSD or major depressive disorder in the first 3–6 months after a loss is a risk factor for complicated grief (Guldin et al. 2012) and should be treated.

Treatment Approaches

Psychotherapy

A large number of psychotherapy approaches have been proposed, with case studies to support their usefulness. Others have been studied in small pilot samples, and a handful have shown efficacy in single RCTs. In this section we briefly describe CGT, a hybrid of cognitive-behavioral, interpersonal, motivational interviewing, and psychodynamic methods. In three studies funded by the National Institutes of Health, among a total of 641 participants randomly assigned to different treatments, CGT significantly outperformed proven efficacious treatments for depression (number needed to treat, 2.6–4.6; Shear et al. 2005, 2014, 2016), providing replicated, clinically significant evidence of efficacy and strong evidence that grief and depression are not the same (Shear 2012). CGT is the most extensively studied approach to date. However, several other investigators have studied similar treatments that are described as purely cognitive-behavioral approaches (Boelen et al. 2007; Bryant et al. 2014). In the section that follows we provide information about these and other, more eclectic and creative approaches that have not been studied in RCTs.

Complicated Grief Treatment

Treatment Model. CGT is based on a simple model of bereavement, grief, and adaptation to loss described previously (Figure 34–2). According to Bowlby (1982) and supported by empirical studies of adaptive implicit cognitive processes (Wilson and Gilbert 2006), loss of a close relationship triggers an intense psychological response (acute grief) and processes that support adaptation to the loss. The latter achieve two main goals: accepting the reality of the loss and restoring a meaningful future. Understanding and accepting the reality revises the working model of the deceased person and frees the ability to envision a promising future. Seeing possibilities for future happiness, in turn, enables acceptance of the unwanted reality. Thus, it makes sense to address both facets of adaptation in tandem. CGT was designed to achieve resolution of these impediments and to facilitate or reactivate natural adaptive processes.

Treatment Approach. CGT is delivered in a structured, weekly, 16-session model with four phases: 1) getting started (sessions 1–3); 2) revisiting sequence (4–9); 3) midcourse review (10); and 4) closing sequence (11–16). Each session is also structured, beginning with a review of the previous week, moving to a loss focus and then a restoration focus, and ending with a review of the session and plan for the upcoming week. Sessions include a small number of specific, well-defined procedures as listed in Table 34–2. The structured framework and well-specified procedures provide a scaffold to help the clinician guide the patient in a highly individualized way.

The clinician helps each patient understand and accept grief as a natural response to loss. Patients are invited to tell the story of a loved one's death, repeating this as many times as necessary to make this "unthinkable" event "thinkable." Patients are guided to think about the future even as they grapple with the reality of the loss and learn to live with reminders of the loss. The strategy is to guide people to find their intrinsic motivation (Ryan and Deci 2000) and identify a meaningful and specific long-term goal. CGT also helps with emotion regulation, rebuilding social relationships, and connecting with memories. These supportive processes use specific procedures throughout the treatment.

CGT was developed on the basis of principles derived from relevant empirical science and uses a range of strategies and procedures from different successful psychotherapies. The structure and framework are rooted in findings from cognitive, behavioral, and biological science. The techniques are modified from interpersonal psychotherapy (IPT; Markowitz and Weissman 2004), cognitive-behavioral therapy (CBT), motivational interviewing (Miller and Rollnick 2002), and psychodynamic

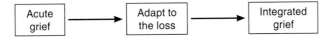

Bereavement evokes acute grief and triggers adaptive processes

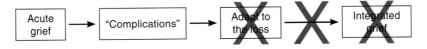

Grief complications interfere with adaptation

FIGURE 34–2. The complicated grief treatment model.

Loss of a loved one evokes acute grief and also stimulates implicit and explicit processes that mediate adaptation. Grief is diminished and integrated as adaptation progresses. Grief complications (maladaptive thoughts, dysfunctional behaviors, ineffective emotion regulation) interfere with adaptation and prolong the period of acute grief. Complicated grief treatment addresses the grief complications and facilitates natural adaptive processes.

psychotherapy. Therapists from any persuasion have been able to make use of the treatment framework, goals, and well-described procedures and to work in the interstices in the way they prefer. Clinicians can use the principles and procedures in whatever way fits with their own work.

CGT has been directly compared with IPT, which targets interpersonal problem areas, including grief, with the goal of improving mood. IPT focuses on strengthening relationships, helping patients move the relationship with the deceased loved one off center stage, and resolving grief. CGT includes daily grief monitoring, an aspirational goals procedure, a ritualized way of telling the story of the death, a behavioral approach to reminders of the loss, and an imaginal conversation with the deceased (Shear and Gribbin Bloom 2017). In two trials comparing CGT to IPT (Shear et al. 2005, 2014), response rates were significantly better among patients randomly assigned to CGT (70% vs. 32%). Pilot studies of this treatment have been conducted in diverse samples (Cruz et al. 2007), among people with substance abuse problems (Zuckoff et al. 2006), and across cultures (Asukai et al. 2011; Nam 2016). Group CGT has also been examined in a small study of older adults (Supiano and Luptak 2014).

Cognitive-Behavioral Treatment

Several smaller RCTs have tested different forms of CBT administered individually (Boelen et al. 2007; Rosner et al. 2014), in groups (Bryant et al. 2014), or over the internet (Eisma et al. 2015; Kersting et al. 2013; Wagner et al. 2006). Control conditions for these studies have included supportive counseling (Boelen et al. 2007) or a waitlist (Eisma et al. 2015; Kersting et al. 2013; Rosner et al. 2014; Wagner et al. 2006). The main CBT strategies are similar to CGT and include addressing maladaptive thoughts and avoidance of thoughts of the death as well as activities and places that are reminders of the loss. Two small studies (Litz et al. 2014; Papa et al. 2013) have suggested that interventions focused on behavioral activation alone (i.e., increasing enjoyable activities) are effective, although these methods also encourage patients to do things even when these activities are reminders of the loss.

TABLE 34–2.   **Specific complicated grief treatment procedures**

Procedure	Session number	Within session	Between sessions	Purpose
Psychoeducation	2 and as needed	Therapist presentation	Review handout on complicated grief and its treatment	To learn about the condition of complicated grief
Grief monitoring diary	1–15	Therapist review and guidance	Patient completes diary	Understand grief; support emotion regulation
Aspirational goals work	2–16	Therapist review and guidance	Activities planned by patient	Reactivate sense of purpose and meaning; generate enthusiasm
Meet with significant other	3 or later	Provide psychoeducation and elicit support	Planned social interactions	Strengthen relationships
Tell the story of the death	4–9	Imaginal revisiting exercise	Listen to recording from session at home daily	Develop a narrative; accept the reality of the death
Situational revisiting	5–16	Set up and plan revisiting exercise	Do planned exercise	Learn to live with reminders of the loss
Work with memories and imaginal conversation	6–11	Introduce and review memories forms; conduct imaginal conversation with the deceased	Complete memories forms	Connect with memories and foster sense of continuing bonds

Other Approaches

A number of more eclectic treatment approaches are available, some targeting specific kinds of loss and some more generic. Examples include Rynearson's (1994) restorative retelling of violent death and Jordan's (2017) postvention for individuals bereaving a loss due to suicide. Palmer (1973) reported successful use of psychodrama in which burial rites are reenacted. Melges and DeMaso (1980) reported on helping patients relive, revise, and revisit scenes of loss in present-day imagery as a way to remove obstacles to grieving; Ingram et al. (1985) used this approach in pastoral counseling. Essa (1986) described an effective grief therapy for the elderly. In a series of studies, Piper et al. (2007) successfully used a psychodynamic grief therapy to treat complicated grief. Neimeyer and Wogrin (2008) advocated for a meaning-oriented approach to psychotherapy for complicated grief. Botella et al. (2008) reported on the use of a virtual reality environment to facilitate grief therapy. Barbosa et al. (2014) conducted a small randomized trial of a cognitive narrative intervention in older widowed adults. Horowitz (2014) advocated a focus on the importance of self-reorganization in grieving. Smid et al. (2015) created a brief eclectic psychotherapy for complicated grief after a violent death. Iliya (2015) developed grief-specific music therapy based on CGT imaginal conversation and a method of vocal psychotherapy; this treatment received preliminary support in a small pilot study. Spuij et al. (2015) developed and successfully used a nine-session grief help intervention for children and adolescents with five accompanying parental sessions. Barlé et al. (2017) proposed an approach to loss under traumatic circumstances that entails building resources, processing trauma, and facilitating mourning. Kosminsky and Jordan (2016) suggested an approach to clearing cognitive obstacles to healing from loss. Rubin et al. (2017) suggested the clinical use of a two-track model targeting biopsychosocial functioning of the bereaved and the ongoing relational bond to the deceased. Any of these techniques might be of interest to clinicians.

Pharmacotherapy

Data from randomized trials of pharmacotherapy for complicated grief are fairly sparse. However, some have indicated that antidepressant medication may be of use. Our recent multicenter study failed to find a statistical or clinical difference in grief symptoms for citalopram compared to placebo (Shear et al. 2016). This was true when the citalopram or placebo was used with supportive clinical management alone or in combination with CGT. In the combination treatment arm, however, citalopram was significantly better than placebo in treating co-occurring depression symptoms. Moreover, use of citalopram or placebo with supportive management did result in a moderate response, so this may be a reasonable approach if grief-targeted psychotherapy is not available. This possibility is supported by five open-label trials involving a total of 50 patients that also suggested improvement in patients who received antidepressants but not benzodiazepines (Bui et al. 2012; Simon 2013). Also of interest, in an early study (Simon et al. 2008), rates of response to both CGT (61%) and IPT (40%) were higher in patients who also received antidepressants than in those who did not (CGT 42%, IPT 19%).

Conclusion

Complicated grief is a prevalent condition that has been reported in bereaved individuals worldwide. ICD-11 includes a diagnostic guideline for prolonged grief disorder that should help clinicians know how to identify bereaved people in need of treatment. Good evidence indicates that complicated grief causes substantial distress and impairment, and therefore it is important for clinicians to recognize and treat this condition. Working with bereaved people can seem sad and hopeless, and clinicians might fear burnout and shy away from work with grief. However, effective short-term treatment is available. Knowing how to administer a short-term treatment that had an average 70% response rate across three separate National Institute of Mental Health–funded trials is a powerful antidote to burnout and, by contrast, is very gratifying. Therapists using CGT often tell us that this work has been the most rewarding experience of their career.

CGT is outlined in this chapter; more detailed instructions and training are available from the Center for Complicated Grief (www.complicatedgrief.columbia.edu). The evidence base continues to grow for other grief-targeted approaches that clinicians may find helpful. Medication treatment might also be helpful in some situations, particularly in the setting of depression or when therapy is not available or accepted by the patient. Overall, clinicians must be optimistic about the possibility of helping people with this highly distressing and impairing condition.

Key Points

- Loss triggers a natural response of grief and activation of adaptive processes; grief quiets as the bereaved accepts the new reality and restores a sense of meaning and purpose and possibilities for happiness; complicated grief occurs when impediments to adaptation arise.

- Complicated grief requires treatment. However, grief is not the problem; rather, treatment needs to facilitate adaptation and resolve impediments to adaptive processes.

- Complicated grief does not respond well to efficacious treatment for depression, but it can be effectively treated with a short-term targeted intervention.

- Effective treatment includes helping patients 1) understand and accept grief, 2) tell a coherent story of the death, 3) live in a world of reminders, and 4) envision a promising future. Therapists also support effective emotion regulation, work to strengthen relationships, and provide opportunities for the patient to connect with memories of the deceased person.

- A wide range of strategies can be used to treat complicated grief, but only a few are evidence tested, and complicated grief treatment currently has the most data supporting its efficacy.

References

American Psychiatric Association: Diagnostic and Statistical Manual of Mental Disorders, 5th Edition. Arlington, VA, American Psychiatric Association, 2013

Asukai N, Tsuruta N, Saito A: Pilot study on traumatic grief treatment program for Japanese women bereaved by violent death. J Trauma Stress 24(4):470–473, 2011 21780192

Barbosa V, Sá M, Carlos Rocha J: Randomised controlled trial of a cognitive narrative intervention for complicated grief in widowhood. Aging Ment Health 18(3):354–362, 2014 24073815

Barlé N, Wortman CB, Latack JA: Traumatic bereavement: basic research and clinical implications. J Psychother Integration 27(2):127–139, 2017

Barlow DH: Promises to keep. Behav Ther 28(4):589–596, 1997

Boelen PA, de Keijser J, van den Hout MA, et al: Treatment of complicated grief: a comparison between cognitive-behavioral therapy and supportive counseling. J Consult Clin Psychol 75(2):277–284, 2007 17469885

Botella C, Osma J, Palacios AG, et al: Treatment of complicated grief using virtual reality: a case report. Death Stud 32(7):674–692, 2008 18924294

Bowlby J: Attachment and loss: retrospect and prospect. Am J Orthopsychiatry 52(4):664–678, 1982 7148988

Bryant RA, Kenny L, Joscelyne A, et al: Treating prolonged grief disorder: a randomized clinical trial. JAMA Psychiatry 71(12):1332–1339, 2014 25338187

Bui E, Nadal-Vicens M, Simon NM: Pharmacological approaches to the treatment of complicated grief: rationale and a brief review of the literature. Dialogues Clin Neurosci 14(2):149–157, 2012 22754287

Bui E, Mauro C, Robinaugh DJ, et al: The Structured Clinical Interview for Complicated Grief: reliability, validity, and exploratory factor analysis. Depress Anxiety 32(7):485–492, 2015 26061724

Cruz M, Scott J, Houck P, et al: Clinical presentation and treatment outcome of African Americans with complicated grief. Psychiatr Serv 58(5):700–702, 2007 17463353

Eisma MC, Boelen PA, van den Bout J, et al: Internet-based exposure and behavioral activation for complicated grief and rumination: a randomized controlled trial. Behav Ther 46(6):729–748, 2015 26520217

Essa M: Grief as a crisis: psychotherapeutic interventions with elderly bereaved. Am J Psychother 40(2):243–251, 1986 3728751

Guldin M-B, Vedsted P, Zachariae R, et al: Complicated grief and need for professional support in family caregivers of cancer patients in palliative care: a longitudinal cohort study. Support Care Cancer 20(8):1679–1685, 2012 21892795

Horowitz M: Grieving: the role of self-reorganization. Psychodyn Psychiatry 42(1):89–97, 2014 24555462

Iliya YA: Music therapy as grief therapy for adults with mental illness and complicated grief: a pilot study. Death Stud 39(1–5):173–184, 2015 25730407

Ingram TL, Hurley EC, Riley MT: Grief-resolution therapy in a pastoral context. J Pastoral Care 39(1):69–72, 1985 10270365

Jordan JR: Postvention is prevention: the case for suicide postvention. Death Stud 41(10):614–621, 2017 28557579

Kersting A, Dölemeyer R, Steinig J, et al: Brief internet-based intervention reduces posttraumatic stress and prolonged grief in parents after the loss of a child during pregnancy: a randomized controlled trial. Psychother Psychosom 82(6):372–381, 2013 24061387

Keyes KM, Pratt C, Galea S, et al: The burden of loss: unexpected death of a loved one and psychiatric disorders across the life course in a national study. Am J Psychiatry 171(8):864–871, 2014 24832609

Kosminsky P, Jordan JR: Attachment-Informed Grief Therapy: The Clinician's Guide to Foundations and Applications. New York, Routledge, 2016

Litz BT, Schorr Y, Delaney E, et al: A randomized controlled trial of an internet-based therapist-assisted indicated preventive intervention for prolonged grief disorder. Behav Res Ther 61:23–34, 2014 25113524

Markowitz JC, Weissman MM: Interpersonal psychotherapy: principles and applications. World Psychiatry 3(3):136–139, 2004 16633477

Melges FT, DeMaso DR: Grief-resolution therapy: reliving, revising, and revisiting. Am J Psychother 34(1):51–61, 1980 7369431

Miller WR, Rollnick S: Motivational Interviewing: Preparing People for Change, 2nd Edition. New York, Guilford, 2002

Nam I: Complicated grief treatment for older adults: the critical role of a supportive person. Psychiatry Res 244:97–102, 2016 27479098

Neimeyer RA, Wogrin C: Psychotherapy for complicated bereavement: a meaning-oriented approach. Illness, Crisis and Loss 16(1):1–20, 2008

Palmer J: Treating prolonged mourning in Spanish-speaking psychiatric patients. Hosp Community Psychiatry 24(5):337–338, 1973 4705608

Papa A, Sewell MT, Garrison-Diehn C, et al: A randomized open trial assessing the feasibility of behavioral activation for pathological grief responding. Behav Ther 44(4):639–650, 2013 24094789

Piper WE, Ogrodniczuk JS, Joyce AS, et al: Group composition and group therapy for complicated grief. J Consult Clin Psychol 75(1):116–125, 2007 17295570

Posner K, Brown GK, Stanley B, et al: The Columbia-Suicide Severity Rating Scale: initial validity and internal consistency findings from three multisite studies with adolescents and adults. Am J Psychiatry 168(12):1266–1277, 2011 22193671

Prigerson HG, Maciejewski PK, Reynolds CF 3rd, et al: Inventory of Complicated Grief: a scale to measure maladaptive symptoms of loss. Psychiatry Res 59(1–2):65–79, 1995 8771222

Robinaugh DJ, Mauro C, Bui E, et al: Yearning and its measurement in complicated grief. J Loss Trauma 21(5):410–420, 2016

Rosner R, Pfoh G, Kotoučová M, et al: Efficacy of an outpatient treatment for prolonged grief disorder: a randomized controlled clinical trial. J Affect Disord 167:56–63, 2014 25082115

Rubin SS, Witztum E, Malkinson R: Bereavement and traumatic bereavement: working with the two-track model of bereavement. J Ration Emot Cogn Behav Ther 35(1):78–87, 2017

Ryan RM, Deci EL: Self-determination theory and the facilitation of intrinsic motivation, social development, and well-being. Am Psychol 55(1):68–78, 2000 11392867

Rynearson T: Psychotherapy of bereavement after homicide. J Psychother Pract Res 3(4):341–347, 1994 22700202

Shear MK: Getting straight about grief. Depress Anxiety 29(6):461–464, 2012 22730310

Shear MK: Clinical practice: complicated grief. N Engl J Med 372(2):153–160, 2015 25564898

Shear MK, Gribbin Bloom C: Complicated grief treatment: an evidence-based approach to grief therapy. J Ration-Emot Cogn-Behav Ther 35(1):6–25, 2017

Shear MK, Shair H: Attachment, loss, and complicated grief. Dev Psychobiol 47(3):253–267, 2005 16252293

Shear MK, Frank E, Houck PR, et al: Treatment of complicated grief: a randomized controlled trial. JAMA 293(21):2601–2608, 2005 15928281

Shear MK, Jackson CT, Essock SM, et al: Screening for complicated grief among Project Liberty service recipients 18 months after September 11, 2001. Psychiatr Serv 57(9):1291–1297, 2006 16968758

Shear MK, Wang Y, Skritskaya N, et al: Treatment of complicated grief in elderly persons: a randomized clinical trial. JAMA Psychiatry 71(11):1287–1295, 2014 25250737

Shear MK, Reynolds CF 3rd, Simon NM, et al: Optimizing treatment of complicated grief: a randomized clinical trial. JAMA Psychiatry 73(7):685–694, 2016 27276373

Simon NM: Treating complicated grief. JAMA 310(4):416–423, 2013 23917292

Simon NM, Shear MK, Fagiolini A, et al: Impact of concurrent naturalistic pharmacotherapy on psychotherapy of complicated grief. Psychiatry Res 159(1–2):31–36, 2008 18336918

Smid GE, Kleber RJ, de la Rie SM, et al: Brief Eclectic Psychotherapy for Traumatic Grief (BEP-TG): toward integrated treatment of symptoms related to traumatic loss. Eur J Psychotraumatol 6(1):27324, 2015 26154434

Spuij M, Dekovic M, Boelen PA: An open trial of 'grief-help': a cognitive-behavioural treatment for prolonged grief in children and adolescents. Clin Psychol Psychother 22(2):185–192, 2015 24227661

Supiano KP, Luptak M: Complicated grief in older adults: a randomized controlled trial of complicated grief group therapy. Gerontologist 54(5):840–856, 2014 23887932

Wagner B, Knaevelsrud C, Maercker A: Internet-based cognitive-behavioral therapy for complicated grief: a randomized controlled trial. Death Stud 30(5):429–453, 2006 16610157

Wilson T, Gilbert D: Miswanting: some problems in the forecasting of future affective states, in Feeling and Thinking: The Role of Affect in Social Cognition Studies in Emotion and Social Interaction, 2nd Series. New York, Cambridge University Press, 2006, pp 178–197

Young H: Overcoming barriers to grief: supporting bereaved people with profound intellectual and multiple disabilities. Int J Dev Disabil 63(3):131–137, 2017

Zuckoff A, Shear K, Frank E, et al: Treating complicated grief and substance use disorders: a pilot study. J Subst Abuse Treat 30(3):205–211, 2006 16616164

Recommended Readings

Bowlby J: Attachment and loss: retrospect and prospect. Am J Orthopsychiatry 52(4):664–678, 1982 7148988

Horowitz M: Grieving: the role of self-reorganization. Psychodyn Psychiatry 42(1):89–97, 2014 24555462

Keyes KM, Pratt C, Galea S, et al: The burden of loss: unexpected death of a loved one and psychiatric disorders across the life course in a national study. Am J Psychiatry 171(8):864–871, 2014 24832609

Ryan RM, Deci EL: Self-determination theory and the facilitation of intrinsic motivation, social development, and well-being. Am Psychol 55(1):68–78, 2000 11392867

Shear MK: Getting straight about grief. Depress Anxiety 29(6):461–464, 2012 22730310

Shear MK: Clinical practice: complicated grief. N Engl J Med 372(2):153–160, 2015 25564898

Shear MK, Shair H: Attachment, loss, and complicated grief. Dev Psychobiol 47(3):253–267, 2005 16252293

Wilson T, Gilbert D: Miswanting: some problems in the forecasting of future affective states, in Feeling and Thinking: The Role of Affect in Social Cognition Studies in Emotion and Social Interaction, 2nd Series. New York, Cambridge University Press, 2006, pp 178–197

PART IX

Anxiety Disorders and Comorbidity

CHAPTER 35

Mixed Anxiety-Depressive Disorder

Jan Fawcett, M.D.

Rebecca P. Cameron, Ph.D.

Alan F. Schatzberg, M.D.

Mixed anxiety-depressive disorder, a diagnostic category proposed in DSM-IV (American Psychiatric Association 1994) for further study, is characterized by dysphoria combined with other depressive and anxiety symptoms that are subthreshold for a diagnosis of a primary affective or anxiety disorder (Box 35–1). This diagnosis followed the lead of the World Health Organization, which included a similar subsyndromal diagnosis with anxious and depressed features—mixed anxiety-depressive disorder—in ICD-10 (World Health Organization 1992c). It reflected a fresh attempt to address several clinical phenomena that had been underrecognized in recent versions of DSM: anxiety and depression frequently co-occur; patients' disorders do not always fit neatly into the primary diagnostic categories, such as major depressive disorder (MDD) and generalized anxiety disorder (GAD); and subsyndromal symptoms may be clinically significant. Unfortunately, few data were available to support the reliability of the diagnosis, and it was dropped from DSM-5 (American Psychiatric Association 2013).

Box 35–1. DSM-IV research criteria for mixed anxiety-depressive disorder

A. Persistent or recurrent dysphoric mood lasting at least 1 month.
B. The dysphoric mood is accompanied by at least 1 month of four (or more) of the following symptoms:

 1. Difficulty concentrating or mind going blank
 2. Sleep disturbance (difficulty falling or staying asleep, or restless unsatisfying sleep)
 3. Fatigue or low energy
 4. Irritability

5. Worry
6. Being easily moved to tears
7. Hypervigilance
8. Anticipating the worst
9. Hopelessness (pervasive pessimism about the future)
10. Low self-esteem or feelings of worthlessness

C. The symptoms cause clinically significant distress or impairment in social, occupational, or other important areas of functioning.

D. The symptoms are not due to the direct physiological effects of a substance (e.g., a drug of abuse, a medication) or a general medical condition.

E. All of the following:

1. Criteria have never been met for Major Depressive Disorder, Dysthymic Disorder, Panic Disorder, or Generalized Anxiety Disorder.
2. Criteria are not currently met for any other Anxiety or Mood Disorder (including an Anxiety or Mood Disorder, In Partial Remission).
3. The symptoms are not better accounted for by any other mental disorder.

Source.   Reprinted from American Psychiatric Association: *Diagnostic and Statistical Manual of Mental Disorders,* 4th Edition. Washington, DC, American Psychiatric Association, 1994. Copyright © 1994 American Psychiatric Association. Used with permission.

A more prominent mixed anxiety-depression has long been recognized in the literature (Clayton et al. 1991; Fava et al. 2008). This has taken the form of full-criteria major depression with a high level of anxiety—usually accompanied by diagnoses of one or more comorbid anxiety disorders—that predicts a poorer treatment outcome and a higher risk of suicidal thoughts and behaviors. In this chapter, we review this form of anxious depression, along with the subsyndromal mixed disorder and studies of the common co-occurrence of GAD with MDD that have led to suggestions that GAD be classified in the mood disorders section of DSM-5.

Prior to DSM-III (American Psychiatric Association 1980), the concept of mixed anxiety-depressive disorders had been widely accepted, as evidenced in diagnostic labels such as anxiety-depressive neurosis (Shammas 1977), psychoneurotic depressive illness with associated anxiety or anxiety-depressive syndromes (Houck 1970), and anxiety masquerading as depression or depression with prominent features of anxiety (Verner 1969). The use of earlier psychopharmacological agents (benzodiazepines and tricyclic antidepressants [TCAs]) with seemingly more specific effects for anxious or depressive symptoms and the emphasis in DSM-III on differential categorical classification encouraged an exaggerated dichotomy between the two broad diagnostic categories that has persisted.

Despite somewhat successful attempts to separate various anxiety and depressive syndromes, the distinction between GAD and MDD has never been clear cut, and genetic evidence suggests that these two disorders are outcomes of the same underlying diathesis (Kendler 1996; Kendler et al. 1992). In 1983, Fawcett and Kravitz found that among patients diagnosed with major depression, 29% had co-occurring panic attacks, and more than 60% scored at least moderate psychic anxiety, as measured by the Schedule for Affective Disorders and Schizophrenia–Change (SADS-C) ratings. Although, as characterized in DSM-IV, mixed anxiety-depressive disorder reflected symptomatology below diagnostic thresholds for existing anxiety and mood diagnoses (except the residual categories of anxiety disorder not otherwise specified [NOS] and depressive disorder NOS), the syndrome appeared to have potentially clinically important implications for patients' distress and disability and for the treatability of their illnesses. However, the inclusion of a subsyndromal mixed anxiety-depressive disorder did not resolve the issue of overlap between anxiety and depression (in particular, GAD and MDD). Rather, it described a syndrome with milder symptoms of this overlapping construct. See Box 35–1 for proposed DSM-IV criteria (First 2011; Möller et al. 2016).

History of Combined Anxiety-Depressive Syndromes

1960s–1970s: Development of Specific Psychopharmacological Agents

Anxiety and Depression as Overlapping Constructs

Anxiety and depression were not as stringently differentiated in the era prior to DSM-III, when it was widely accepted that many patients presented for treatment with symptoms of both disorders. For example, Roth et al. (1972) noted that "a wide range of workers drawn from many schools of thought have (explicitly or implicitly) upheld the view that anxiety states and depressive disorders merge insensibly with one another or belong to different parts of a single continuum of affective disturbance" (pp. 147–148).

Dichotomization of Anxiety and Depression

The concept of two separate classes of disorders was increasingly accepted by clinicians during the 1960s and 1970s. In a seminal study, Roth et al. (1972) investigated the difficulty of differentiating between depressed and anxious patients and found that they could be distinguished despite areas of overlap. Factor analysis of symptoms suggested that two factors appeared to describe patients with either panic disorder or major depression with melancholia, and a third, residual factor corresponded to GAD and depression. Historical data and social functioning indicated that individuals in the anxious group were more disturbed by their symptoms and experienced greater disability. These findings led to incorporation of the distinction between panic disorder and major depression in DSM-III. However, the study results did not help to resolve the debate regarding the existence of a mixed anxiety-depressive disorder.

The development of pharmacological agents with relatively specific antidepressant or anxiolytic effects, particularly TCAs and benzodiazepines, supported the dichotomization of depression and anxiety. Initial confusion over whether benzodiazepines should be considered an antidepressant class of drugs gave way over time to evidence that they were primarily and specifically useful for anxiety symptoms. In contrast, TCAs were found to be useful primarily for depressive symptoms and for endogenous or severe depression, although data did emerge regarding their effectiveness in panic disorder as well.

Rickels and Downing (1972) and Rickels et al. (1970) found that outpatients with depression who were classified with different degrees of depression and anxiety differed in their treatment responses to a TCA, a minor tranquilizer, a combination, or placebo. Patients with high levels of depression and high levels of anxiety responded best to a combined regimen of amitriptyline and chlordiazepoxide, whereas amitriptyline alone was indicated for patients with high depression and low anxiety, and chlordiazepoxide was most effective for patients with low depression and high anxiety. Patients with low depression and low anxiety showed no difference in response among the three active treatments and placebo (Rickels et al. 1970).

In the late 1970s, we reviewed the efficacy of benzodiazepines and TCAs in the treatment of depressive disorders (Schatzberg 1978; Schatzberg and Cole 1978) and suggested the need to differentiate endogenous from nonendogenous depression, noting that nonendogenous depressive syndromes resembled neurotic anxiety disorders. *Endogenous depression* was defined as depression with symptoms (e.g., diurnal variation). *Nonendogenous depression* was considered more heterogeneous, but it could include histrionic behavior, anxiety, or early insomnia. This latter syndrome is less easily distinguishable from anxiety states, which also are frequently accompanied by mild depressive symptoms. We suggested a continuum ranging from anxiety states to endogenous depression, with nonendogenous depression being intermediate between the two.

Advent of DSM-III and Changes in DSM-III-R: Categorical Classification

Multiple Models of the Possible Relationship Between Generalized Anxiety and Depression

Several models of the relationship between anxiety and depression have been proposed (Stahl 1993; Stavrakaki and Vargo 1986). The unitary position suggests that anxiety and depression are aspects of the same disorder but differ quantitatively or temporally. In the pluralistic model, anxiety and depression are viewed as distinct disorders. A third position maintains that mixed anxiety and depression is distinct from both primary anxiety and primary depression. A fourth position, put forward by Clayton et al. (1991) and Fava et al. (2006), suggests a type of full-criteria major depression accompanied by significant levels of anxiety that could meet criteria for the full range of anxiety disorders. This combination results in a poorer treatment outcome. In fact, N.M. Simon et al. (2007) reported that five epidemiological studies, two clinical studies of unipolar major depression, and two clinical studies of bipolar disorders have shown a higher risk of suicidal behaviors and, in one study, a higher rate of suicide in patients with comorbid anxiety or anxiety disorders (Table 35–1).

A major issue in developing such models is the frequent comorbidity among anxiety disorders and between anxiety and depression. Anxiety and depression can be comorbid in various ways: comorbidity of full-syndrome disorders; one full-syndrome condition with significant subsyndromal overlay from the other; or a residual category of mixed, subsyndromal symptoms. Excluding residual symptom cases greatly decreases the prevalence rates.

TABLE 35–1. Studies linking severe psychic anxiety or anxiety disorders to suicidal behavior and poor response to treatment in patients with depression and probands

Study	Finding
Fawcett et al. 1990	Severe psychic anxiety (>5) on the SADS-C psychic anxiety scale was significantly associated with suicide in MDD over 1 year.
Clayton et al. 1991	Subjects with MDD who had higher ratings for anxiety took longer to recover.
Hall et al. 1999	90% of patients interviewed after admission for severe suicide attempt had expressed severe anxiety during the month before the attempt.
Busch et al. 2003	76% of inpatients who died from suicide had had at least 3 days of severe anxiety or agitation within 7 days prior to the suicide.
Wunderlich et al. 1998	Comorbidity, especially anxiety disorders, increases risk of suicide attempts more than any DSM-IV diagnosis.
Sareen et al. 2005	Data clearly indicate that comorbid anxiety disorders amplify the risk of suicide in mood disorders.
Foley et al. 2006	Suicidal risk was greatest in association with current MDD plus GAD (OR 468.5).
Boden et al. 2007	Any anxiety disorder increased the risk of suicide attempts by 5.65 times. Rates of suicidal behavior increased with the number of anxiety disorders present.
Bolton et al. 2008	Presence of one or more anxiety disorders at baseline was significantly associated with subsequent onset of suicide attempts (OR 2.2).
Fava et al. 2004	46% met criteria for anxious MDD on HAM-D subscale (score ≥7). These patients had more severe MDD and increased rates of suicidal ideation.
Fava et al. 2006	Individuals with anxious MDD were more likely to endorse IDS-C30 items concerning melancholic endogenous features, both before and after adjusting for baseline severity of MDD.
N.M. Simon et al. 2007	In patients with bipolar disorder, a lifetime anxiety disorder doubled the odds of a past suicide attempt and current anxiety. Comorbidity more than doubled the odds of current suicide ideation.
G.E. Simon et al. 2007	Comorbid anxiety disorder was associated with significantly higher risk of suicide attempt (HR 1.4) and suicide death (HR 1.81).
Fava et al. 2008	In levels 1 and 2 of STAR*D, patients with anxious MDD had significantly lower remission rates than did nonanxious patients.
Saveanu et al. 2015	In the iSPOT-D study, patients with anxious MDD demonstrated significantly lower remission rates than did nonanxious patients with MDD.
Arnow et al. 2015	In iSPOT-D, anxiety syndromes were nonpredictive of response.

Note. GAD=generalized anxiety disorder; HAM-D=Hamilton Rating Scale for Depression; IDS-C30=Inventory of Depressive Symptomatology–Clinician–Rated; iSPOT-D= International Study to Predict Optimised Treatment in Depression; MDD=major depressive disorder; SADS-C=Schedule for Affective Disorders and Schizophrenia– Change; STAR*D=Sequenced Treatment Alternatives to Relieve Depression.

In a study of comorbidity, Wetzler and Katz (1989) discussed the problems of differentiating anxiety and depression. They distinguished two conceptual stances: a dimensional approach and a categorical approach. In the dimensional approach, anxiety and depression are considered separate, continuous constructs, whereas in the categorical approach, anxiety and depression are viewed as syndromes that characterize different groups of patients.

DSM-III, DSM-III-R, and Comorbidity

Changes in classifications from DSM-II (American Psychiatric Association 1968) through DSM-IV have reflected then-current views and further influenced our conceptualizations of anxiety, depression, and their overlap. DSM-III contained a more elaborate system for classifying anxiety and depressive disorders than did DSM-II, with more subtypes under each broad syndrome and more specific criteria for each diagnostic category. DSM-III also implemented exclusion criteria that prioritized diagnoses of depression over diagnoses of anxiety. DSM-III-R (American Psychiatric Association 1987) eliminated this hierarchy for anxiety disorders, thereby making it easier for comorbid anxiety and mood disorders to be diagnosed as such. Despite such efforts, debate has remained about the differentiation of GAD and MDD, and this debate is only heightened by their somewhat arbitrary criteria. For example, the difference in duration of symptoms required for diagnosis of the two disorders (6 months for GAD vs. 2 weeks for MDD) still makes it difficult to assess the true extent of overlap in symptom presentation. In fact, except for the distinction in duration of symptoms, GAD and MDD, as defined in DSM-IV, could easily be applied to the same clinical presentation if both dysphoria and worry were present.

Generalized Anxiety Disorder Differentiation

In his review of GAD and comorbidity, Maser (1998) noted the shifting diagnostic criteria for GAD over time, with respect to both the duration of symptoms (1 month in DSM-III, yielding a 45% prevalence of GAD in a probability sample; 6 months in DSM-III-R and DSM-IV, yielding a 9% prevalence) and the hierarchical rules disallowing GAD from being diagnosed as a comorbid disorder with other anxiety and depressive disorders (present in DSM-III but gradually eliminated in subsequent versions of DSM).

Maser (1998) further noted that obtaining comorbidity data from clinical samples confounds questions about the nature and frequency of comorbidity with the fact that treatment-seeking populations are more likely to be experiencing comorbidity and are more likely to be relatively severe cases. With these limitations in mind, he reviewed studies that found that 91% of clinic patients with GAD had at least one comorbid condition. In this sample, 41% of clinic patients with GAD had a mood disorder (usually dysthymia). In other clinical samples, rates of comorbid mood disorders ranged from 9% to 45% for major depression and from 29% to 69% for mood disorders defined more broadly (e.g., including dysthymia).

Alternative Conceptualizations

Evidence From Psychometric Studies of Self-Report Instruments: Affect Dimensions

Increasing evidence indicates that depression and anxiety have common dimensional features or risk factors (e.g., genetics), although discriminating characteristics may also exist. Clark and Watson (1991) and Watson et al. (1988) investigated a tripartite model in which measures of negative affect, positive affect, and hyperarousal were used to differentiate depression and anxiety. Low-state positive affect is a specific feature of depression, whereas positive affect is largely unrelated to anxiety. Hyperarousal or autonomic arousal corresponds to the physiological symptoms of anxiety, such as pounding heart, feelings of constriction, and lightheadedness. It is highly relevant to panic disorder and is less clearly temperamental. Negative affect is a common risk factor for both depression and anxiety, and it may reflect, in part, the overlap in phenomenological distress between these two disorders.

Findings From Genetic and Familial Studies

Kendler (1996; Kendler et al. 1992) examined genetic and environmental contributions to the frequent comorbidity of GAD and major depression. Lifetime diagnosis was used for the first study, and 1-year follow-up prevalence was used for the second. In a sample of approximately 1,000 female twin pairs, Kendler et al. (1992) found that GAD (diagnosed according to modified DSM-III-R criteria) and MDD (as defined by DSM-III-R criteria) share a common genetic diathesis. Furthermore, shared environmental experiences, such as aspects of family environment, played no role in the etiology of MDD or GAD. Instead, individual-specific experiences were responsible for whether the genetic diathesis was expressed as MDD or GAD. Kendler (1996) replicated these findings and suggested that different stressful life events might be responsible for the occurrence of these disorders.

Generalized Anxiety Disorder as Anxious Temperament Type

Akiskal (1998) suggested that GAD could be reconceptualized as the extreme manifestation of an anxious temperament type, called *generalized anxious temperament*. This constellation of traits represents a vigilant stance focused on harm avoidance and is considered narrower in scope than either neuroticism or negative affectivity. It may be associated with increased risk for depression and other disorders (e.g., phobias, substance use disorders). Evidence in support of this view includes the finding that GAD symptoms (e.g., worry, nausea) are lifelong and trait-like, rather than acute, for many individuals. Acute life events may thus provoke a more severe episode (GAD) in the context of longstanding symptoms (generalized anxious temperament).

In 1990, Fawcett et al. found that severe psychic anxiety, panic attacks, and severe (global) insomnia, measured prospectively by SADS-C ratings, were associated with

TABLE 35–2.   **Prevalence of mixed anxiety-depressive disorder in specific settings**

Reference	Sample type	N	Prevalence, %
Wittchen and Essau 1993	Epidemiological	1,366	0.8
Roy-Byrne et al. 1994	Primary care	267	5.1
Sartorius and Üstün 1995	Primary care	25,916	1.3
Stein et al. 1995	Primary care	501	2.0
Spijker et al. 2010	Epidemiological survey	4,796	0.6

Note.   Definitions of mixed anxiety-depressive disorder vary; see text.

the occurrence of suicide over a follow-up period of 12 months, whereas standard predictors of suicide such as recent or prior suicide attempts, suicidal ideation, and severe hopelessness did not show a correlation with suicide over the 1-year period but did demonstrate a correlation with suicide as an outcome during a 2- to 10-year follow-up period. This work suggested a change in focus from the presence of comorbid anxiety disorders to the severity of the anxiety symptoms. See Table 35–2 for a summary of studies.

Anxiety as a Premonitor of Major Depression

Kessler's group as well as ours and others reported that anxiety disorders in adolescence (particularly social phobia) were frequently premonitory of depression in adulthood (Kessler et al. 2015; Ohayon and Schatzberg 2010; Regier et al. 1998). Most recently, Kessler et al. (2015) reported on a World Health Organization study of more than 300,000 subjects that clearly indicated that this sequence is common. Although one might want to conclude that this is a common comorbidity, it is more likely that we are looking at a biological process in which the initial presentation in adolescence is anxiety, which progresses to major depression in adulthood (Schatzberg 2015). In adults we have reported that GAD and MDD do show a common biology, with secondary differences explaining specific symptoms (Etkin and Schatzberg 2011).

Advent of Selective Serotonin Reuptake Inhibitors

The development of selective serotonin reuptake inhibitors (SSRIs) and other new compounds provided clinicians with access to treatments that are safer and better tolerated than older categories of antidepressants. Over time, evidence has accumulated that these drugs are effective in treating depression, panic disorder, and, more recently, GAD. The ability of these drugs to address a range of symptoms facilitates their use in primary care settings, where clinicians may not have the time to clarify complex differential diagnoses. The broad applicability of newer pharmacological agents may raise questions about distinctions in the underlying biochemical dysregulation of anxiety and depression, but it also highlights a need to understand how to best treat patients with MDD and comorbid anxiety who are poorly responsive to SSRIs alone.

Major Depression With Pronounced Anxiety: Clinical Course and Treatment

As indicated in Table 35–1, results from both the Sequenced Treatment Alternatives to Relieve Depression (STAR*D) and the International Study to Predict Optimised Treatment in Depression (iSPOT-D) showed that patients with MDD and marked anxiety symptoms respond significantly more poorly to antidepressants (SSRIs or serotonin-norepinephrine reuptake inhibitors) alone than do patients without significant anxiety symptoms (Fava et al. 2008; Saveanu et al. 2015). Of particular note in both studies is the observation that the poorer response relates to anxiety but not to fully comorbid anxiety disorders (Arnow et al. 2015; Fava et al. 2008). Thus, pronounced anxiety in the context of major depression—but not a full comorbid anxiety disorder—predicts poor response to first-line agents. This may help explain the odd contrast that in non-comorbid anxiety disorders, these same agents are effective as monotherapy in treating, for example, GAD or panic. For the more severe forms of mixed anxiety-depression, evidence has shown that augmentation of antidepressants or mood stabilizers with clonazepam (Londborg et al. 2000; Papakostas et al. 2010; Smith et al. 1998, 2002) or, in more recent findings, with atypical antipsychotic agents such as quetiapine and olanzapine (Hirschfeld et al. 2006; Houston et al. 2006; McIntyre et al. 2007; Papakostas et al. 2015) may significantly reduce severe anxiety symptoms with ruminations as well as agitation. We have reported that mirtazapine was more effective for reducing anxiety and insomnia in geriatric patients with depression than was paroxetine (Schatzberg et al. 2002).

Development of DSM-IV and the Introduction of Mixed Anxiety-Depressive Disorder

Changes Prior to DSM-IV

Two earlier changes to DSM reshaped the conceptualization of the relation between generalized anxiety and depression (Stahl 1993). First, GAD was redefined from its former status as a residual anxiety diagnosis (i.e., diagnosed only in the absence of any other anxiety disorder) to a generalized anxiety syndrome with symptoms of mild depression that are less severe than the symptoms of anxiety. Thus, GAD became more explicitly a mixed disorder. In addition, from DSM-III-R onward, GAD has been defined as a chronic disorder, with a minimum of 6 months' duration required to warrant the diagnosis. Second, mixed anxiety-depressive disorder was introduced and defined as a stable core of subsyndromal symptoms that do not reach the threshold for a diagnosis of GAD, MDD, or any other full-syndrome disorder. It was always unclear whether this syndrome was in fact a stable disorder or whether, under stress, it could be exacerbated, leading to an overt anxiety or depressive disorder.

Changes in DSM-IV

DSM-IV (American Psychiatric Association 1994) criteria for mixed anxiety-depressive disorder were somewhat different from ICD-10 criteria. ICD-10 defined the disorder as comprising symptoms of both anxiety and depression, with neither more salient than the other and neither at a level that would warrant a separate diagnosis (World Health Organization 1992c). The ICD-10 clinical descriptions (World Health Organization 1992a) offered further specificity by requiring that autonomic symptoms be present and that a significant life change not be associated with the onset of symptoms (in which case the diagnosis should be adjustment disorder). Finally, the ICD-10 research criteria suggested that researchers develop their own criteria within the guidelines described (World Health Organization 1992b).

Effect of Subsyndromal States on Functioning

Many researchers have documented the effect of subsyndromal states on disability. Johnson et al. (1992) carried out an epidemiological survey and found that threshold diagnoses of MDD or dysthymia resulted in increased service use and social morbidity (medication use, impaired physical and emotional health, time lost from work, and attempted suicide). However, the presence of subthreshold depressive symptoms resulted in higher levels of service use and social morbidity as well, and on a population basis, subthreshold symptomatology resulted in greater social impairment and service cost than did diagnosable disorders.

Preparations for DSM-IV

The recognition of high levels of comorbidity of full-syndrome anxiety and depressive disorders, as well as the ICD-10 inclusion of a subsyndromal mixed disorder, prompted the developers of DSM-IV to consider several questions related to revising existing diagnoses or adding new ones. The work group charged with considering the possibility of including a mixed anxiety-depression diagnosis in DSM-IV delineated two relevant issues (Moras 1989, as cited in Moras et al. 1996). The first was whether to include a diagnosis that would correspond to the ICD-10 diagnosis of mixed anxiety-depressive disorder. The second was whether DSM-IV diagnoses should be altered to better reflect the overlap between anxiety and depression or whether a new diagnosis should be included to reflect empirical knowledge about comorbid anxiety and depressive disorders. Literature reviews were undertaken to answer these questions.

Evidence for a Subsyndromal Category

Katon and Roy-Byrne (1991) examined literature based on community, primary care, and psychiatric samples to determine whether a patient population with clinically important symptoms of anxiety and depression that fell below the thresholds for specific DSM-III-R diagnoses (consistent with the ICD-10 description of mixed anxiety-depressive disorder) could be identified. With respect to community samples, their review found that diagnosable mood disorders occurred in 3%–8% of the population (based on Epidemiologic Catchment Area data), that subsyndromal depression occurred in 13%–20% of the population, and that community members who experienced depressive symptoms were more likely to have mixed anxious-depressive profiles than more purely depressive profiles. In their review, they found higher rates of distress (40%) than of diagnosable disorder (25%), suggesting a 15% prevalence of subsyndromal distressed patients in these settings. Furthermore, patients with mixed-symptom profiles in this setting did have deficits in functioning.

A Possible Comorbid Diagnostic Category

In his review of the literature on comorbidity, Moras (1989, as cited in Moras et al. 1996) focused on concurrent comorbidity rather than lifetime comorbidity. He selected MDD and dysthymia from the mood disorders and included a range of anxiety disorders, such as agoraphobia, panic disorder, GAD, OCD, social phobia, simple phobia, and PTSD. He found that comorbidity rates varied but that, generally, patients with anxiety disorders were more likely to have a concomitant depressive diagnosis than patients with depression were to have an anxiety disorder. He concluded that the data did not support the creation of mixed diagnoses that would reflect current understandings of comorbidity.

The work group concluded that field trials should be conducted for the proposed mixed-symptom, subsyndromal disorder; that existing diagnoses should not be changed to reflect comorbidity; and that research should be conducted on the Clark and Watson (1991) tripartite model of depression and anxiety to prepare for DSM-IV revisions.

Field Trial for Mixed Anxiety-Depressive Disorder

The DSM-IV field trial for mixed anxiety-depression (Zinbarg et al. 1994) was designed to answer four questions: 1) Do patients with subsyndromal symptoms and functional impairment exist? 2) Does medical pathology, rather than psychopathology, account for their functional deficits? 3) What is the breakdown of this population with respect to anxiety symptoms, depressive symptoms, or mixed symptoms? 4) What is the best way to operationalize the criteria for any subsyndromal diagnosis?

Patients ($N=666$) were studied at five primary care medical sites and two mental health sites, chosen to yield a sample with a range of demographic characteristics. Patients presenting to primary care clinics were screened for subjective distress with the General Health Questionnaire and the Medical Outcomes Study/RAND Short-Form General Health Survey. Those whose scores were at or above the cutoff and half as many patients whose scores were below the cutoff were interviewed in depth. Every patient presenting to the psychiatry clinics was interviewed. In-depth evaluations used included the Anxiety Disorders Interview Schedule—Revised, the Mixed Anxiety-Depression Field Trial Revision of the Hamilton Anxiety Scale and the Hamilton Rating Scale for Depression, and the Chronic Disease Score.

In addition to DSM-III-R diagnoses with previously established criteria sets, diagnoses of anxiety disorder NOS and depressive disorder NOS (i.e., patient is sufficiently distressed or impaired to be considered a probable or definite "case" but not better fitting another diagnostic category) were identified. Patients with NOS diagnoses constituted 11.7% of the patients surveyed, making that group the third-largest diagnostic group after those with panic disorder (29.1%) and GAD (20.2%) and just ahead of the group with MDD (11.6%). These patients were characterized by high levels of impairment or distress (80% met criteria for definite caseness).

A principal component analysis of the Hamilton symptom ratings (anxiety and depression) of all patients yielded three factors, which the investigators labeled *anxiety* (e.g., tension, apprehension), *physiological arousal* (e.g., tachycardia, choking), and *depression* (e.g., helplessness, diminished libido). These components were used to define symptom scales. A fourth symptom scale was constructed of items loading on both the anxiety and the depression components. This scale was labeled *negative affect* and included such items as irritability and fatigue.

Patients in the largest diagnostic groups (anxiety or depression NOS, panic disorder with agoraphobia, GAD, MDD, and no diagnosis) were analyzed according to the symptom scales described earlier. Patients with anxiety or depression NOS could be identified with the negative affect scale. Profile analyses suggested that this negative affect scale characterized the subsyndromal group and differentiated it from the other groups of more established disorders. Although altering the criteria for GAD or MDD would be an alternative that would include many of these patients in existing categories, mixed anxiety-depressive disorder was seen as a more accurate and useful category for these patients. Investigators concluded that at least as many patients had subsyndromal affective symptoms (defined as meeting criteria for anxiety disorder NOS or depressive disorder NOS) as had symptoms meeting criteria for certain well-delineated diagnostic categories; that these patients had meaningful levels of functional impairment; that nonspecific mixed-symptom profiles were the most common pattern of subsyndromal disorder; and that these patients could be distinguished from patients with GAD, MDD, and panic disorder with agoraphobia.

What Do We Know About Subsyndromal Mixed Anxiety-Depressive Disorder?

Given the decision to include mixed anxiety-depressive disorder as a proposed category in DSM-IV, and given the ongoing debate over how to account for comorbidity and overlap between anxiety and depression, epidemiological data and data on clinical course are needed. Although defining a subsyndromal diagnosis of mixed anxiety-depressive disorder did not resolve many of the big questions about continuity between risk factors, symptoms, and syndromes, it did afford an opportunity to characterize a distressed and impaired group that is not currently a focus of attention. Little had been established about patients with mixed anxiety-depressive disorder in terms of gender, sex, age at onset, and so on. We do have some information on the prevalence of mixed anxiety-depressive disorder (based on different criteria sets) in various settings (see Table 35–2).

Wittchen and Essau (1993) reported results of the Munich 15-Year Follow-Up Study, including data from a general population sample. They assessed depression and dysthymia as well as panic disorder, agoraphobia, and simple and social phobias, but not GAD. The prevalence of mixed anxiety-depressive disorder, on the basis of the ICD-10 definition (i.e., the presence of subsyndromal anxiety and subsyndromal depression), was 0.8% in their epidemiological sample, less than that of pure subsyndromal categories (21.9% subsyndromal anxiety and 2.4% subsyndromal depression). Comorbid depression and anxiety, whether above or below diagnostic thresholds, was associated with higher levels of subjective suffering, functional impairment, and health service use than were pure disorders.

Roy-Byrne et al. (1994) used data from a field trial to describe a sample of 267 primary care patients. A brief screen, followed by a structured interview, revealed that

5.1% of the patients had subsyndromal symptoms of anxiety and depression (defined as depression NOS or anxiety NOS based on DSM-III-R criteria) accompanied by functional impairment. This prevalence rate was comparable with the prevalence of mood disorders in this sample and was about one-fourth the prevalence of anxiety disorders. In addition, the patients with subsyndromal symptoms demonstrated functional impairments comparable with those of patients in the anxiety and mood disorder groups.

Stein et al. (1995) studied 501 primary care patients who denied having a current psychiatric diagnosis or receiving current psychiatric treatment. Of these, 78 (15.6%) were systematically interviewed after screening positive for distress on the Beck Depression Inventory or the Beck Anxiety Inventory. Of the patients interviewed, 12.8% met the authors' criteria for mixed anxiety-depressive disorder (2.0% of the larger sample).

Sartorius and Üstün (1995) studied depression and anxiety, as defined in ICD-10, using a large data set of 25,916 patients in general health care facilities in 14 countries. A sample of 5,379 patients, including those who scored high and low on the General Health Questionnaire, received in-depth evaluations. The rate of depressive disorders was 11.8%, and the rate of anxiety disorders was 10.2%. The prevalence rates of subthreshold depression and subthreshold anxiety were 6.5% and 5.0%, respectively. Although some variability was found from country to country, the overall rate of mixed anxiety-depressive disorder was 1.3%.

In their review of the literature, Boulenger et al. (1997) estimated that the prevalence of mixed anxiety-depressive disorder ranged from 0.8% to 2.5% in epidemiological studies and from 5% to 15% in primary care settings. Furthermore, they concluded that longitudinal evidence supported the conceptualization of mixed anxiety-depressive disorder as a risk factor for full-syndrome depressive and anxiety disorders. An epidemiological study in the Netherlands of nearly 5,000 subjects reported a 1-year prevalence rate of 0.6% in individuals who did not meet criteria for a previous anxiety or depressive disorder (Spijker et al. 2010).

Controversy About Adding a Mixed Anxiety-Depressive Disorder Category

Several authors have addressed the need for and potential problems with adding a new category of mixed anxiety-depressive disorder (Boulenger et al. 1997; Katon and Roy-Byrne 1991; Möller et al. 2016; Roy-Byrne 1996; Wittchen and Essau 1993). Beyond providing for compatibility with ICD-10, several arguments for adding mixed anxiety-depressive disorder to the DSM classification have been offered. Unfortunately, some of these authors confuse the notion of fully comorbid disorders with mixed subsyndromal anxiety and depression, which is characterized by the following:

- Mixed subsyndromal anxiety-depressive disorder is seen in primary care settings, particularly because anxious and depressed patients tend to present to their physicians with somatic symptoms. Distinguishing this group of patients may help physicians identify patients in need of intervention and may reduce excessive or inappropriate medical visits. Providing appropriate treatment is particularly important because subthreshold symptomatology can have a marked effect on distress and disability.

- Mixed subsyndromal anxiety-depressive disorder may represent a prodromal or residual phase of a more severe disorder, so identifying this at-risk group may facilitate development of secondary preventive interventions.
- Mixed subsyndromal anxiety-depressive disorder may be a more appropriate diagnosis than adjustment disorder for some patients who do not identify a precipitating stressor or who may be particularly reactive to stress (Liebowitz 1993).
- Mixed anxiety-depressive disorder may comprise a spectrum ranging from subsyndromal anxiety-depression to full-syndrome major depression with severe anxiety or comorbid anxiety disorders, representing a disorder that is important to recognize and requires special treatment to avoid poor response or even suicide.

Potential problems with the subsyndromal diagnosis of mixed anxiety-depressive disorder were also raised. The diagnostic category of mixed anxiety-depressive disorder may increase the risk of trivializing distress that is severe enough to affect functioning (Stahl 1993), overlap too much with adjustment disorder or other DSM diagnoses (Liebowitz 1993), or become a "wastebasket" category and thus discourage more careful diagnosis. These problems could ultimately impede research and reduce identification of major depression and other diagnoses requiring prompt, serious, and specific intervention (Liebowitz 1993; Preskorn and Fast 1993). In addition, mixed anxiety-depressive disorder may be an unstable diagnosis leading to episodes of traditional affective or anxiety disorders. Minor depression may provide a subsyndromal diagnostic category adequate to meet clinical needs (Liebowitz 1993). Other authors argued that more effort should be put into distinguishing patients with anxiety from those with depression (rather than combining them into one category) and offered strategies for making the appropriate primary diagnosis (Clayton 1990; Preskorn and Fast 1993). The deliberations over whether to incorporate mixed anxiety-depressive order into DSM or ICD have been nicely reviewed by Möller et al. (2016).

Implications of an Anxiety-Depression Spectrum Diagnosis for DSM-5

The DSM-5 workgroup proposed a new set of criteria to better delineate the subsyndromal aspects of both the anxiety and the depressive disorders (First 2011; Möller et al. 2016; see Table 35–1). They then included these newer criteria in the field trials for DSM-5, but the kappa coefficients for reliability were extremely low for both sites in the trial (Regier et al. 2013). In addition, the prevalence rates were modest. For these reasons, it was decided to not elevate the syndrome into the nomenclature. Moreover, because the progress made for developing a reliable construct for the disorder over time has been modest at best, it was decided to not include it in the DSM-5 system nor to carry it again in the appendix.

A concept of mixed anxiety-depressive disorder may well recognize a syndrome associated with significant suffering and disability. However, given the evidence that full-syndrome MDD with comorbid anxiety is associated with poor treatment outcome and increased risk of suicidal behavior, it should be asked whether the introduction into DSM-5 of a new diagnosis implying a less severe, but treatment-worthy, anxiety-depressive syndrome would inappropriately reduce the perceived risk associated with full-syndrome MDD with severe comorbid anxiety. One solution would be to establish a category for mixed anxiety-depression with agreed-on dimensions of severity, which would imply different treatment approaches. Such an approach would present the advantage of introducing the concept of symptom severity (as opposed to only identifying the number of symptoms) back into the DSM diagnostic system as a meaningful dimension to guide treatment decisions, while still recognizing the presence of a mixed anxiety-depression category. This would require agreement on and use of an accepted dimensional measure of the severity of anxiety and depression for patients classified in this category. ICD-10 has continued to include mixed anxiety-depression, and more specific criteria for making the diagnosis have been proposed for ICD-11 (Möller et al. 2016).

Conclusion

Mixed anxiety-depression is a subsyndromal combination of depression and anxiety, which, left untreated, has been thought to result in significant disability. In addition, numerous studies have demonstrated the clinical significance of a full-syndrome MDD with comorbid severe anxiety symptoms or anxiety disorders, resulting in a more difficult course, higher relapse rates, and increased risk of suicide attempts and death from suicide.

Following the lead of ICD-10, a mixed-symptom, subsyndromal diagnostic category of mixed anxiety-depressive disorder was included in DSM-IV for further study. This reflected the increasing recognition of the potentially disabling effect of subsyndromal states as well as the consistent observations of co-occurring symptoms. However, the low reliability in making the diagnosis and low prevalence of subjects who had not previously met criteria for MDD or an anxiety disorder (i.e., residual syndromes) in the field trials led to the category being abandoned in DSM-5. Routine application of dimensional measures of anxiety and depression may help bring DSM closer to understanding comorbid anxiety and depression.

Key Points

- In its subsyndromal form, mixed anxiety-depression has been thought to be a significant cause of impairment, but this has been controversial. Severe anxiety accompanying a full-syndrome major depression has been associated with clearly poorer treatment response and outcome, as well as a heightened risk for suicidal behavior and suicide.

- The reliability of diagnosing subsyndromal mixed anxiety-depression was low in the DSM-5 field trials, and the syndrome was dropped from the appendix in DSM-5.

- Distinguishing between mild and full-syndrome forms of anxiety is potentially important. The frequency of the full-syndrome form is about 50%, as indicated in reports from the STAR*D study (Fava et al. 2008), but full-syndrome comorbidity—in contrast to significant anxiety—does not predict poor response (Arnow et al. 2015; Fava et al. 2008; Saveanu et al. 2015).

- Use of dimensional severity ratings for this diagnostic designation may also focus attention on more effective treatments for comorbid anxiety associated with depression.

References

Akiskal HS: Toward a definition of generalized anxiety disorder as an anxious temperament type. Acta Psychiatr Scand Suppl 393(suppl):66–73, 1998 9777050

American Psychiatric Association: Diagnostic and Statistical Manual of Mental Disorders, 2nd Edition. Washington, DC, American Psychiatric Association, 1968

American Psychiatric Association: Diagnostic and Statistical Manual of Mental Disorders, 3rd Edition. Washington, DC, American Psychiatric Association, 1980

American Psychiatric Association: Diagnostic and Statistical Manual of Mental Disorders, 3rd Edition, Revised. Washington, DC, American Psychiatric Association, 1987

American Psychiatric Association: Diagnostic and Statistical Manual of Mental Disorders, 4th Edition. Washington, DC, American Psychiatric Association, 1994

American Psychiatric Association: Diagnostic and Statistical Manual of Mental Disorders, 5th Edition. Arlington, VA, American Psychiatric Association, 2013

Arnow BA, Blasey C, Williams LM, et al: Depression subtypes in predicting antidepressant response: a report from the iSPOT-D trial. Am J Psychiatry 172(8):743–750, 2015 25815419

Boden JM, Fergusson DM, Horwood LJ: Anxiety disorders and suicidal behaviours in adolescence and young adulthood: findings from a longitudinal study. Psychol Med 37(3):431–440, 2007 17109776

Bolton JM, Cox BJ, Afifi TO, et al: Anxiety disorders and risk for suicide attempts: findings from the Baltimore Epidemiologic Catchment Area follow-up study. Depress Anxiety 25(6):477–481, 2008 17541978

Boulenger J-P, Fournier M, Rosales D, et al: Mixed anxiety and depression: from theory to practice. J Clin Psychiatry 58(suppl 8):27–34, 1997 9236733

Busch KA, Fawcett J, Jacobs DG: Clinical correlates of inpatient suicide. J Clin Psychiatry 64(1):14–19, 2003 12590618

Clark LA, Watson D: Tripartite model of anxiety and depression: psychometric evidence and taxonomic implications. J Abnorm Psychol 100(3):316–336, 1991 1918611

Clayton PJ: The comorbidity factor: establishing the primary diagnosis in patients with mixed symptoms of anxiety and depression. J Clin Psychiatry 51(suppl):35–39, 1990 2228992

Clayton PJ, Grove WM, Coryell W, et al: Follow-up and family study of anxious depression. Am J Psychiatry 148(11):1512–1517, 1991 1928465

Etkin A, Schatzberg AF: Common abnormalities and disorder-specific compensation during implicit regulation of emotional processing in generalized anxiety and major depressive disorders. Am J Psychiatry 168(9):968–978, 2011 21632648

Fava M, Alpert JE, Carmin CN, et al: Clinical correlates and symptom patterns of anxious depression among patients with major depressive disorder in STAR*D. Psychol Med 34(7):1299–1308, 2004 15697056

Fava M, Rush AJ, Alpert JE, et al: What clinical and symptom features and comorbid disorders characterize outpatients with anxious major depressive disorder: a replication and extension. Can J Psychiatry 51(13):823–835, 2006 17195602

Fava M, Rush AJ, Alpert JE, et al: Difference in treatment outcome in outpatients with anxious versus nonanxious depression: a STAR*D report. Am J Psychiatry 165(3):342–351, 2008 18172020

Fawcett J, Kravitz HM: Anxiety syndromes and their relationship to depressive illness. J Clin Psychiatry 44:8–11, 1983 6874657

Fawcett J, Scheftner WA, Fogg L, et al: Time-related predictors of suicide in major affective disorder. Am J Psychiatry 147(9):1189–1194, 1990 2104515

First MB: DSM-5 proposals for mood disorders: a cost-benefit analysis. Curr Opin Psychiatry 24(1):1–9, 2011 21042219

Foley DL, Goldston DB, Costello EJ, et al: Proximal psychiatric risk factors for suicidality in youth: the Great Smoky Mountains Study. Arch Gen Psychiatry 63(9):1017–1024, 2006 16953004

Hall RC, Platt DE, Hall RC: Suicide risk assessment: a review of risk factors for suicide in 100 patients who made severe suicide attempts. Evaluation of suicide risk in a time of managed care. Psychosomatics 40(1):18–27, 1999 9989117

Hirschfeld RM, Weisler RH, Raines SR, et al: Quetiapine in the treatment of anxiety in patients with bipolar I or II depression: a secondary analysis from a randomized, double-blind, placebo-controlled study. J Clin Psychiatry 67(3):355–362, 2006 16649820

Houck J: Combined therapy in anxiety-depressive syndromes. II. Comparative effects of amitriptyline and limbitrol (chlordiazepoxide-amitriptyline). Dis Nerv Syst 31(6):421–426, 1970 4917419

Houston JP, Ahl J, Meyers AL, et al: Reduced suicidal ideation in bipolar I disorder mixed-episode patients in a placebo-controlled trial of olanzapine combined with lithium or divalproex. J Clin Psychiatry 67(8):1246–1252, 2006 16965203

Johnson J, Weissman MM, Klerman GL: Service utilization and social morbidity associated with depressive symptoms in the community. JAMA 267(11):1478–1483, 1992 1538538

Katon W, Roy-Byrne PP: Mixed anxiety and depression. J Abnorm Psychol 100(3):337–345, 1991 1918612

Kendler KS: Major depression and generalized anxiety disorder: same genes, (partly) different environments—revisited. Br J Psychiatry 168(suppl):68–75, 1996

Kendler KS, Neale MC, Kessler RC, et al: Major depression and generalized anxiety disorder. Same genes, (partly) different environments? Arch Gen Psychiatry 49(9):716–722, 1992 1514877

Kessler RC, Sampson NA, Berglund P, et al: Anxious and non-anxious major depressive disorder in the World Health Organization World Mental Health Surveys. Epidemiol Psychiatr Sci 24(3):210–226, 2015 25720357

Liebowitz MR: Mixed anxiety and depression: should it be included in DSM-IV? J Clin Psychiatry 54(suppl):4–7, discussion 17–20, 1993 8509357

Londborg PD, Smith WT, Glaudin V, et al: Short-term cotherapy with clonazepam and fluoxetine: anxiety, sleep disturbance and core symptoms of depression. J Affect Disord 61(1–2):73–79, 2000 11099743

Maser JD: Generalized anxiety disorder and its comorbidities: disputes at the boundaries. Acta Psychiatr Scand Suppl 393:12–22, 1998 9777042

McIntyre A, Gendron A, McIntyre A: Quetiapine adjunct to selective serotonin reuptake inhibitors or venlafaxine in patients with major depression, comorbid anxiety, and residual depressive symptoms: a randomized, placebo-controlled pilot study. Depress Anxiety 24(7):487–494, 2007 17177199

Möller HJ, Bandelow B, Volz HP, et al: The relevance of "mixed anxiety and depression" as a diagnostic category in clinical practice. Eur Arch Psychiatry Clin Neurosci 266:725–736, 2016 27002521

Moras K: Diagnostic comorbidity in the DSM-III and DSM-III-R anxiety and mood disorder: implications for the DSM-IV. Review paper for the DSM-IV Generalized Anxiety Disorder and Mixed Anxiety Depression Work Group. Albany, NY, Center for Stress and Anxiety Disorders, University at Albany, State University of New York, 1989

Moras K, Telfer LA, Barlow DH: Efficacy and specific effects data on new treatments: a case study strategy with mixed anxiety-depression. J Consult Clin Psychol 61(3):412–420, 1993 8326041

Moras K, Clark LA, Katon W, et al: Mixed anxiety-depression, in DSM-IV Sourcebook, Vol 2. Edited by Widiger TA, Frances AJ, Pincus HA, et al. Washington, DC, American Psychiatric Association, 1996, pp 623–643

Ohayon MM, Schatzberg AF: Social phobia and depression: prevalence and comorbidity. J Psychosom Res 68(3):235–243, 2010 20159208

Papakostas GI, Clain A, Ameral VE, et al: Fluoxetine-clonazepam cotherapy for anxious depression: an exploratory, post-hoc analysis of a randomized, double blind study. Int Clin Psychopharmacol 25(1):17–21, 2010 19898245

Papakostas GI, Fava M, Baer L, et al: Ziprasidone augmentation of escitalopram for major depressive disorder: efficacy results from a randomized, double-blind, placebo-controlled study. Am J Psychiatry 172(12):1251–1258, 2015 26085041

Preskorn SH, Fast GA: Beyond signs and symptoms: the case against a mixed anxiety and depression category. J Clin Psychiatry 54(suppl):24–32, 1993 8425872

Regier DA, Rae DS, Narrow WE, et al: Prevalence of anxiety disorders and their comorbidity with mood and addictive disorders. Br J Psychiatry Suppl 173(34):24–28, 1998 9829013

Regier DA, Narrow WE, Clarke DE, et al: DSM-5 field trials in the United States and Canada, part II: test-retest reliability of selected categorical diagnoses. Am J Psychiatry 170(1):59–70, 2013 23111466

Rickels K, Downing RW: Methodological aspects in the testing of antidepressant drugs, in Depressive Illness: Diagnosis, Assessment, Treatment, International Symposium, St. Moritz. Edited by Kielholz P. Stuttgart, Germany, Huber Berne, 1972, pp 84–99

Rickels K, Hesbacher P, Downing RW: Differential drug effects in neurotic depression. Dis Nerv Syst 31(7):468–475, 1970 4918448

Roth M, Gurney C, Garside RF, et al: Studies in the classification of affective disorders: the relationship between anxiety states and depressive illnesses. I. Br J Psychiatry 121(561):147–161, 1972 5072240

Roy-Byrne P: Generalized anxiety and mixed anxiety-depression: association with disability and health care utilization. J Clin Psychiatry 57(suppl 7):86–91, 1996 8690701

Roy-Byrne P, Katon W, Broadhead WE, et al: Subsyndromal ("mixed") anxiety-depression in primary care. J Gen Intern Med 9(9):507–512, 1994 7996294

Sareen J, Cox BJ, Afifi TO, et al: Anxiety disorders and risk for suicidal ideation and suicide attempts: a population-based longitudinal study of adults. Arch Gen Psychiatry 62(11):1249–1257, 2005 16275812

Sartorius N, Üstün TB: Mixed anxiety and depressive disorder. Psychopathology 28(suppl 1):21–25, 1995 8903888

Saveanu R, Etkin A, Duchemin AM, et al: The International Study to Predict Optimized Treatment in Depression (iSPOT-D): outcomes from the acute phase of antidepressant treatment. J Psychiatr Res 61:1–12, 2015 25586212

Schatzberg AF: Benzodiazepines in depressive disorders: a clinical guide. South Med J 71(suppl 2):18–23, 1978 28570

Schatzberg AF: The chicken and egg of anxiety and depression. Epidemiol Psychiatr Sci 24(3):227–229, 2015 25997897

Schatzberg AF, Cole JO: Benzodiazepines in depressive disorders. Arch Gen Psychiatry 35(11):1359–1365, 1978 30428

Schatzberg AF, Kremer C, Rodrigues HE, et al: Double-blind, randomized comparison of mirtazapine and paroxetine in elderly depressed patients. Am J Geriatr Psychiatry 10(5):541–550, 2002 12213688

Shammas E: Controlled comparison of bromazepam, amitriptyline, and placebo in anxiety-depressive neurosis. Dis Nerv Syst 38(3):201–207, 1977 13969

Simon GE, Hunkeler E, Fireman B, et al: Risk of suicide attempt and suicide death in patients treated for bipolar disorder. Bipolar Disord 9(5):526–530, 2007 17680924

Simon NM, Zalta AK, Otto MW, et al: The association of comorbid anxiety disorders with suicide attempts and suicidal ideation in outpatients with bipolar disorder. J Psychiatr Res 41(3–4):255–264, 2007 17052730

Smith WT, Londborg PD, Glaudin V, et al: Short-term augmentation of fluoxetine with clonazepam in the treatment of depression: a double-blind study. Am J Psychiatry 155(10):1339–1345, 1998 9766764

Smith WT, Londborg PD, Glaudin V, et al: Is extended clonazepam cotherapy of fluoxetine effective for outpatients with major depression? J Affect Disord 70(3):251–259, 2002 12128237

Spijker J, Batelaan N, de Graaf R, et al: Who is MADD? Mixed anxiety depressive disorder in the general population. J Affect Disord 121(1–2):180–183, 2010 19577307

Stahl SM: Mixed anxiety and depression: clinical implications. J Clin Psychiatry 54(suppl):33–38, 1993 8425874

Stavrakaki C, Vargo B: The relationship of anxiety and depression: a review of the literature. Br J Psychiatry 149:7–16, 1986 3535981

Stein MB, Kirk P, Prabhu V, et al: Mixed anxiety-depression in a primary-care clinic. J Affect Disord 34(2):79–84, 1995 7665808

Verner JV Jr: Comparison of imipramine and chlordiazepoxide in the treatment of the depressed and anxious patient. J Fla Med Assoc 56(1):15–21, 1969 4883339

Watson D, Clark LA, Carey G: Positive and negative affectivity and their relation to anxiety and depressive disorders. J Abnorm Psychol 97(3):346–353, 1988 3192830

Wetzler S, Katz MM: Problems with the differentiation of anxiety and depression. J Psychiatr Res 23(1):1–12, 1989 2666646

Wittchen H-U, Essau CA: Comorbidity and mixed anxiety-depressive disorders: is there epidemiologic evidence? J Clin Psychiatry 54(suppl):9–15, 1993 8425875

World Health Organization: The ICD-10 Classification of Mental and Behavioural Disorders: Clinical Descriptions and Diagnostic Guidelines. Geneva, World Health Organization, 1992a

World Health Organization: The ICD-10 Classification of Mental and Behavioural Disorders: Diagnostic Criteria for Research. Geneva, World Health Organization, 1992b

World Health Organization: International Statistical Classification of Diseases and Related Health Problems, 10th Revision, Vol 1. Geneva, World Health Organization, 1992c

Wunderlich U, Bronisch T, Wittchen HU: Comorbidity patterns in adolescents and young adults with suicide attempts. Eur Arch Psychiatry Clin Neurosci 248(2):87–95, 1998 9684918

Zinbarg RE, Barlow DH, Liebowitz M, et al: The DSM-IV field trial for mixed anxiety-depression. Am J Psychiatry 151(8):1153–1162, 1994 8037250

Recommended Readings

Kessler RC, Sampson NA, Berglund P, et al: Anxious and non-anxious major depressive disorder in the World Health Organization World Mental Health Surveys. Epidemiol Psychiatr Sci 24(3):210–226, 2015 25720357

Möller HJ, Bandelow B, Volz HP, et al: The relevance of "mixed anxiety and depression" as a diagnostic category in clinical practice. Eur Arch Psychiatry Clin Neurosci 266:725–736, 2016 27002521

Ohayon MM, Schatzberg AF: Social phobia and depression: prevalence and comorbidity. J Psychosom Res 68(3):235–243, 2010 20159208

Schatzberg AF: The chicken and egg of anxiety and depression. Epidemiol Psychiatr Sci 24(3):227–229, 2015 25997897

Spijker J, Batelaan N, de Graaf R, et al: Who is MADD? Mixed anxiety depressive disorder in the general population. J Affect Disord 121(1–2):180–183, 2010 19577307

CHAPTER 36

Anxiety in the Context of Substance Use Disorders

Sudie E. Back, Ph.D.

Kathleen T. Brady, M.D., Ph.D.

The relationship between anxiety disorders and substance use disorders (SUDs) is complex and bidirectional. Studies of treatment-seeking individuals and epidemiological surveys indicate that anxiety disorders, symptoms of anxiety, and SUDs commonly co-occur and that the interaction is multifaceted and variable. Anxiety disorders may be a risk factor for the development of an SUD. Furthermore, anxiety disorders are likely to modify the presentation and outcome of SUDs, just as substance use and SUDs modify the presentation and outcome of anxiety disorders. In addition, anxiety symptoms may emerge during the course of chronic intoxication and withdrawal from alcohol or drugs. In this chapter, we review the epidemiology, etiological relationships, and diagnostic considerations of co-occurring anxiety disorders and SUDs.

Epidemiology

General Population

Several epidemiological studies conducted in the United States since the 1990s have concluded that anxiety disorders and SUDs co-occur more commonly than would be expected by chance alone (Kessler et al. 1994, 1997; Lai et al. 2015; Regier et al. 1990). Table 36–1 presents prevalence rates for SUDs and anxiety disorders. The National Epidemiological Survey on Alcohol and Related Conditions (NESARC) is the most recent and largest comorbidity study to date, involving more than 43,000 adults. It was designed to distinguish between independent mood and anxiety disorders (i.e., those that cannot be attributed to withdrawal or intoxication) and substance-induced

TABLE 36–1.   **Prevalence of substance use and anxiety disorders per 100 people in the United States**

	ECA (lifetime prevalence)	NCS-R (lifetime prevalence)	NESARC (12-month prevalence)
Alcohol abuse	5.6	13.2	4.7
Alcohol dependence	7.9	5.4	3.8
Drug abuse	2.6	7.9	1.4
Drug dependence	3.5	3.0	0.6
Generalized anxiety disorder	—	5.7	2.1
Social phobia	2.8	12.1	2.8
OCD	2.5	1.6	—
PTSD	—	6.8	—
Panic disorder			
with agoraphobia	0.5	1.1	0.6
without agoraphobia	—	3.7	1.6

Note. ECA=Epidemiologic Catchment Area (Regier et al. 1990); NCS-R=National Comorbidity Survey–Replication (Kessler et al. 2006); NESARC=National Epidemiologic Survey on Alcohol and Related Conditions (Grant et al. 2004).

mood and anxiety disorders. Over 17.7% of respondents with an SUD in the prior 12 months met criteria for an independent anxiety disorder. Among respondents with any anxiety disorder in the prior 12 months, approximately 15% had at least one co-occurring SUD (Grant et al. 2004). The relationship between anxiety and drug use disorders (OR 2.8) was stronger than for anxiety and alcohol use disorders (OR 1.7). Associations between SUDs and specific anxiety disorders were virtually all significantly positive ($P<0.05$), with the odds ratios for women more positive than for men. Among individuals with anxiety disorders, marijuana use disorders were the most common drug use disorder (15.1%), followed by cocaine (5.4%), amphetamine (4.8%), hallucinogen (3.7%), and sedative (2.6%) use disorder (Conway et al. 2006).

A secondary analysis of six international epidemiological data sets, including the National Comorbidity Survey (NCS), examined co-occurring anxiety disorders and SUDs among 14- to 64-year-olds (Merikangas et al. 1998). Across sites, 32% of individuals with lifetime alcohol dependence and 45% of individuals with lifetime drug dependence also met criteria for a lifetime anxiety disorder.

Neurobiology: Anxiety Disorders and Substance Use Disorders

A growing body of evidence implicates abnormalities in the common neurobiological pathways involved in anxiety and addictions. One bridging construct involves the role of stress. Corticotropin-releasing factor (CRF), a key hormone involved in the stress response, has been implicated in the pathophysiology of anxiety, affective, and addictive disorders (Brady and Sinha 2005; Koob and Kreek 2007). Preclinical evidence suggests that CRF and noradrenergic pathways are involved in stress-induced reinstatement of drug-seeking behavior in drug-dependent laboratory animals (Piazza and Le Moal 1998). Similarly, emotional stress and negative affect states increase drug craving in drug-dependent humans (Sinha 2008). In animal models, early life stress and chronic stress result in long-term changes in stress response, altering the sensitivity of the dopamine system to stress and increasing susceptibility to drug self-administration (Meaney et al. 2002). Current models of addiction and anxiety posit that aberrant functioning and remodeling of neuronal circuits involving brain systems mediating fear and reward underlie the pathological behavior. As such, a disease-defining experience (i.e., drug reward or stress) triggers specific forms of synaptic plasticity that can become persistent in susceptible individuals and lead to disease. These circuits involve diverse brain structures, such as the amygdala, ventral tegmental area, nucleus accumbens, and prefrontal cortices and have functionally diverse neurons including glutamatergic/GABAergic, endogenous opiate, noradrenergic, neuropeptide Y, nociceptin, and oxytocin (Lüthi and Lüscher 2014). New techniques, such as optogenetics, allow more precise exploration of this circuitry and will hopefully lead to new treatment strategies in the future.

Diagnostic Considerations

Accurate diagnosis and differentiation between drug-induced states and primary anxiety diagnoses are critical. Use of some substances (e.g., marijuana, stimulants) is associated with anxiety symptoms, and withdrawal from others (e.g., opiates, benzodiazepines) is marked by anxiety. Chronic use of substances of abuse, which have powerful effects on neurotransmitter systems involved in anxiety, may also unmask vulnerability or to lead to neurobiological changes that manifest as anxiety disorders. The best way to differentiate transient, substance-induced symptoms from true anxiety symptoms is through observation during a period of abstinence. A key issue is the duration of abstinence necessary for accurate diagnosis; this will vary by diagnosis and substance. For drugs with long half-lives (e.g., some benzodiazepines, methadone), withdrawal symptoms may be protracted, and several weeks of abstinence may be essential for accurate diagnoses. For shorter-acting substances (e.g., cocaine, short-half-life benzodiazepines), both the acute intoxication and withdrawal durations are likely to be briefer, and it may be possible to make diagnoses after shorter abstinence. When the diagnosis remains unclear, the following factors favor the diagnosis of an anxiety disorder: onset of anxiety symptoms before SUD onset, positive family history of anxiety disorders, and sustained anxiety symptoms during lengthy periods of abstinence.

Because anxiety is common in SUDs, patients presenting with anxiety should be screened for alcohol and drug use. Useful brief screening tools for SUDs in the psychiatric setting include the Alcohol Use Disorders Identification Test (Bohn et al. 1995), Michigan Alcohol Screening Test (Teitelbaum and Carey 2000), Drug and Alcohol Screening Test (Maisto et al. 2000), and CAGE questions (Ewing 1984). Caffeine and some over-the-counter medications (e.g., pseudoephedrine, diet pills) can also cause substantial anxiety (Kendler et al. 2006), and although their use might not constitute substance abuse, decreasing use may be of enormous benefit in decreasing anxiety.

We have divided the remainder of this chapter into sections addressing individual anxiety disorders. For each disorder, we discuss comorbidity prevalence as well as diagnostic and treatment considerations. For many disorders, few data exist. In areas where data are lacking, we cite relevant studies and review general principles guiding appropriate clinical management of comorbidity.

Psychosocial Treatments

Among psychosocial treatments, cognitive-behavioral therapy (CBT) has been shown to decrease both anxiety symptoms in anxiety disorders and relapse in individuals with SUDs. Techniques such as relaxation, coping skills, behavioral activation, problem solving, and sleep hygiene can assist patients with both disorders (McKeehan and Martin 2002). Nutritional counseling and regular exercise may also be useful in helping individuals learn alternative strategies for coping with anxiety, but empirical trials are lacking. Associative learning and classical conditioning are involved in the association of drug craving in SUDs or fearful responses in anxiety disorders with cues and contextual stimuli (Weinstein et al. 2015). Extinction learning is an active process that reduces the value or salience of these conditioned cues and contexts and can be effective in reducing cue- and context-induced symptoms in addiction and anxiety, improving outcomes (Kaplan et al. 2011). Convergent neurobiological evidence documents the central role of the prefrontal cortex in extinction of conditioned fear and drug reward behaviors. Extinction training targeting both disorders and the use of pharmacotherapeutic agents in facilitating extinction training warrant further investigation.

Anxiety Disorders

Generalized Anxiety Disorder

Epidemiology

Second to major depression, SUDs are the most common comorbid psychiatric disorder with generalized anxiety disorder (GAD) (Wittchen et al. 1994). Data from the NESARC showed a strong association between 12-month GAD prevalence and both alcohol (OR 2.0) and drug use disorders (OR 4.5) (Grant et al. 2005). Comorbid GAD is associated with an accelerated progression from first use to the onset of dependence (Sartor et al. 2007). Furthermore, comorbid SUDs significantly decrease the likelihood of recovery from GAD (Bruce et al. 2005).

Differential Diagnosis

GAD is particularly difficult to diagnose in the face of SUDs because every GAD symptom can be mimicked by substance use or withdrawal. For accurate diagnosis, the definitive diagnosis of GAD should be delayed until intoxication or withdrawal has terminated.

Pharmacological Treatment

Although benzodiazepines are effective for GAD, their use in individuals with current or previous SUDs is controversial because of abuse liability. Some authors (Posternak and Mueller 2001) have posited that the empirical evidence of danger in SUDs is insufficient and that benzodiazepines may be safely used in some SUD patients. In several studies, buspirone, a partial serotonin 1A (5-HT$_{1A}$) agonist with low abuse potential, has been shown to be efficacious in patients with alcoholism and anxiety (Kranzler et al. 1994; Malec et al. 1996; McKeehan and Martin 2002). In contrast, Malcolm et al. (1992) found no between-group differences in anxiety or alcohol use severity in patients treated with buspirone or placebo. Another randomized trial of buspirone among opiate-dependent individuals with anxiety found a trend toward improvement in depressive symptomatology and a slower return to substance use in the buspirone group but no significant improvement in anxiety symptoms (McRae et al. 2004). Selective serotonin reuptake inhibitors (SSRIs) are efficacious in GAD (Lydiard et al. 1988); however, no clinical trials of SSRIs in individuals with comorbid GAD and SUDs have been conducted.

Social Anxiety Disorder

Epidemiology

Individuals with social anxiety disorder are two to three times more likely than those without social phobia to develop an alcohol use disorder (Kushner et al. 1990). Alcohol is the most common substance of abuse among patients with social anxiety. Social anxiety disorder is also associated with illicit drug use, with odds ratios ranging from 1.6 to 2.3 (Sareen et al. 2006). Consistent with the self-medication model as well as the early age of onset of social anxiety disorder, SUDs generally follow the onset of social anxiety (Carrigan and Randall 2003; Myrick and Brady 1997; Terra et al. 2006). In the NCS data, 16.4% of individuals with social phobia endorsed self-medicating with alcohol and drugs (Bolton et al. 2006).

Differential Diagnosis

Compared with other anxiety disorders, less abstinence may be needed to establish a diagnosis of social anxiety disorder. Because the average onset of the disorder occurs before adolescence, symptoms are often present before alcohol or drug use (Bakken et al. 2005). Also, the cardinal symptom, fear of public scrutiny, is specific and not mimicked by substance use and withdrawal. Social anxiety symptoms that arise only during acute intoxication or withdrawal are not sufficient to meet disorder criteria.

Pharmacological Treatment

Randall et al. (2001a) examined paroxetine, an SSRI, in 15 outpatients with alcohol dependence and social phobia in a double-blind, placebo-controlled trial. The paroxetine-treated group had significantly lower social anxiety symptoms at endpoint but no significant differences in alcohol-use outcomes. Gabapentin, an anticonvulsant agent, has demonstrated efficacy for social anxiety disorder in a placebo-controlled, double-blind trial (Pande et al. 1999) and for the treatment of alcohol withdrawal in other trials (Malcolm et al. 2001; Voris et al. 2003), and although some reports of gabapentin misuse have been made, it has considerably less abuse potential than benzodiazepines. Further exploration of anxiolytic anticonvulsants in individuals with SUDs and social anxiety disorder is needed.

Psychosocial Treatment

Several controlled trials examined psychosocial treatment for co-occurring social anxiety and SUDs. Randall et al. (2001b) compared 12 weeks of CBT for alcohol dependence alone with an integrated CBT approach for both disorders and found that the alcohol-dependence-only treatment group evidenced better outcomes. The authors hypothesized that exposure to feared social situations during early recovery may have led to increases in alcohol use to cope. Schadé et al. (2004) conducted a randomized trial in individuals with alcohol dependence and comorbid social anxiety disorder with or without agoraphobia. Groups were assigned to relapse prevention alone or relapse prevention plus CBT for social anxiety. Both groups were offered concomitant SSRI pharmacotherapy (fluvoxamine), but more than half (53%) refused it. Combined treatment led to significantly greater improvement in anxiety symptoms than relapse prevention alone, but no significant between-group differences in alcohol use severity were found. The use of fluvoxamine did not predict improved anxiety or alcohol use severity.

Obsessive-Compulsive Disorder

Epidemiology

The association between OCD and SUDs is less robust than other anxiety disorders (Kessler et al. 2005). In a clinical sample of 254 individuals, approximately 4% of patients with OCD met criteria for a lifetime SUD (Sbrana et al. 2005). Schuckit et al. (1997) estimated lifetime rates of OCD at 1.3% for individuals with alcohol dependence and 0.9% for control subjects. Individuals with OCD are not prone to impulsive behaviors, often have high harm avoidance, and do not enjoy the loss of control that drugs and alcohol often produce. The most commonly used illicit drug among individuals with OCD is marijuana (Sbrana et al. 2005).

Differential Diagnosis

SUDs contain elements of obsessions and compulsions (Modell et al. 1992); individuals with SUDs have recurrent intrusive thoughts about using alcohol or drugs, often feel compelled to use, and may realistically believe that if they use, their distressing thoughts or cravings will be quelled. For people with SUDs, however, the content of the cognitions and compulsions is restricted to alcohol or drug use.

Substances of abuse, such as alcohol or stimulants, have been associated with the occurrence of compulsive behaviors (McKeehan and Martin 2002). Case reports have also described the emergence of obsessive-compulsive symptoms during acute intoxication with cocaine and other stimulants (Satel and McDougle 1991). However, the differential diagnosis of OCD with SUDs is not difficult because obsessions and compulsions focused solely on procuring and using drugs or that occur only during intoxication do not meet diagnostic criteria for OCD.

Pharmacological Treatment

Little research has been done on the treatment of comorbid OCD and SUDs. A case report (Chatterjee and Ringold 1999) of gabapentin augmentation of paroxetine in OCD and alcohol dependence found a significant decrease in craving and alcohol consumption but a mixed impact on OCD symptoms. SSRIs are efficacious for OCD (Greist et al. 1995) but have not been systematically tested with comorbid SUDs.

Psychosocial Treatment

Literature regarding the psychosocial treatment of comorbid OCD and SUDs is also limited. Fals-Stewart and Schafer (1992) randomly assigned patients with OCD and SUDs to integrated psychotherapy for both disorders, therapy for SUDs only, or a progressive muscle relaxation–attention control condition. The integrated-treatment group evidenced significantly greater reductions in OCD symptoms, alcohol abstinence rates, and treatment retention.

Posttraumatic Stress Disorder

Epidemiology

The NCS showed adults with PTSD were two to four times more likely to have co-morbid SUDs than adults without PTSD (Kessler et al. 1995). Similarly, data from the Australian National Survey of Mental Health and Well-Being (*N*=10,000) found that 34.4% of respondents with PTSD had at least one SUD, with alcohol use disorders being most common (Mills et al. 2006). Among treatment-seeking substance abusers, the prevalence of lifetime PTSD has been reported as high as 50% (Roberts et al. 2015; Seal et al. 2011). In most cases, the development of PTSD precedes the development of the SUD (Back et al. 2005, 2006b; Jacobsen et al. 2001).

Differential Diagnosis

A characteristic unique to PTSD is that the diagnosis requires a traumatic event. Thus, less abstinence is needed to establish the diagnosis of PTSD among patients with SUD. Intrusive symptoms (e.g., recurrent trauma related thoughts or images, psychological or physiological reactivity to trauma reminders, nightmares) are characteristic of PTSD and unlikely to be mimicked by substance use or withdrawal. Other symptoms (e.g., irritability, sleep impairment, difficulty concentrating, exaggerated startle response, negative cognitions) could be exacerbated by intoxication or withdrawal from alcohol and drugs and should be carefully assessed.

Pharmacological Treatment

Relatively more empirical research is available on the pharmacological treatment of comorbid PTSD and SUDs (Ralevski et al. 2014; Sofuoglu et al. 2014). Petrakis and Simpson (2017) reviewed nine pharmacological trials focused on agents that 1) targeted alcohol use disorder, 2) targeted PTSD, or 3) targeted both alcohol use disorders and PTSD by addressing shared neuropathology. Studies targeting alcohol use disorder (e.g., with naltrexone, disulfiram) found that medications improved alcohol-related outcomes regardless of comorbid PTSD. The studies that focused on medications targeting PTSD examined SSRIs; in a 12-week double-blind, placebo-controlled trial, Brady et al. (2005) investigated sertraline, which is FDA approved for PTSD, in individuals with alcohol dependence and PTSD. Those with less severe alcohol dependence and early onset PTSD demonstrated greater improvement in alcohol use severity when treated with sertraline versus placebo. In contrast, individuals with more severe alcohol dependence and later-onset PTSD demonstrated better alcohol use outcomes with placebo than with sertraline. The sertraline-treated group showed a trend toward greater PTSD improvement. No other studies examining medications for PTSD found group differences in alcohol use disorder or PTSD outcomes. Finally, several studies investigating medications hypothesized to address both alcohol use disorder and PTSD (e.g., prazosin, aprepitant) found no clear benefit on alcohol-related or PTSD outcomes. However, Batki et al. (2014) examined topiramate versus placebo in military veterans with alcohol use disorder and PTSD and found that topiramate was associated with significant reductions in alcohol use and craving and a trend toward reduced PTSD symptoms. A double-blind, randomized controlled pilot study in veterans with SUDs and PTSD found that *N*-acetylcysteine, an antioxidant with glutamatergic modulation properties, resulted in significantly lower PTSD symptoms, substance craving, and depressive symptoms (Back et al. 2016). Substance use was significantly reduced in both groups, and there no were retention or tolerability differences. In summary, although topiramate and *N*-acetylcysteine show promise, no single pharmacological agent has yet demonstrated clear evidence of efficacy for use in treating co-occurring alcohol use disorder and PTSD. However, patients with comorbid alcohol use disorder and PTSD can be safely prescribed pharmacotherapies used in non-comorbid populations.

Psychosocial Treatment

Several reviews and meta-analyses have evaluated psychosocial interventions for the treatment of comorbid SUDs and PTSD (Ralevski et al. 2014; Roberts et al. 2015; Simpson et al. 2017). Simpson et al. (2017) evaluated 24 studies categorized as either 1) exposure-based interventions, 2) coping-based interventions, or 3) addiction-focused interventions. Exposure-based treatments were the most effective in reducing PTSD severity and yielded significant and comparable improvements in SUDs. Although most treatments led to some reduction in SUD and PTSD severity, treatments integrating exposure-based PTSD treatment were recommended. Despite concerns that trauma-focused or exposure-based therapy might worsen SUDs (Norman and Hamblen 2017), data from numerous studies clearly demonstrate that integrated treatments are safe, feasible, and effective. Furthermore, a large percentage of patients with SUDs and PTSD indicate that they prefer to receive integrated treatments that address both disorders (Back et al. 2006a, 2014b).

The most widely studied integrated psychosocial treatment to date is Seeking Safety, a 25-session manualized treatment (Najavits 2002) that is designed to bolster stabilization and safety with psychoeducation and coping skills and does not include discussion of the trauma memories or events. A review by Simpson et al. (2017) included six studies evaluating Seeking Safety, three of which controlled for time and attention, and found reductions in PTSD symptoms, with no differences in PTSD for Seeking Safety and control groups at any time point. SUD outcomes were mixed. Two studies that compared Seeking Safety to conditions that were not controlled for time and attention found better SUD outcomes on some, but not all, parameters.

Another integrated psychosocial treatment, Concurrent Treatment of PTSD and Substance Use Disorders Using Prolonged Exposure (COPE), is a 12-session individual treatment integrating prolonged exposure with CBT for SUDs (Back et al. 2014a). Randomized controlled trials of COPE in the United States and Australia have demonstrated significantly greater reductions in PTSD and significant and comparable reductions in SUD severity (Back et al. 2019; Mills et al. 2012; Norman et al. 2019; Ruglass et al. 2017). In a recent study of COPE versus relapse prevention among military veterans, COPE resulted in significantly greater PTSD symptom reduction and significantly higher rates of PTSD diagnostic remission (OR 5.3). Both groups evidenced significant reductions in SUDs during treatment and at 6-month follow-up; COPE participants evidenced significantly fewer drinks per drinking day than the control group (Back et al. 2019). Taken together, these studies indicate that exposure-based integrated treatment is effective among civilians and veterans and can result in significant improvements in both PTSD and SUDs.

Panic Attacks, Panic Disorder, and Agoraphobia

Epidemiology

In the NESARC study, panic disorder with agoraphobia was the anxiety disorder with the strongest association with SUDs. The 12-month odds ratio of individuals experiencing panic disorder with agoraphobia were 1.4 with alcohol abuse, 3.6 with alcohol dependence, 3.5 with drug abuse, and 10.5 with drug dependence (Grant et al. 2004). The 12-month odds ratio of having panic disorder without agoraphobia were 0.8 with alcohol abuse, 3.4 with alcohol dependence, 1.6 with drug abuse, and 7.6 with drug dependence (Grant et al. 2004). In the NCS replication study (Kessler et al. 2006), of respondents with panic disorder only, agoraphobia only, or their combination, 35.3% had comorbid alcohol use disorder and 20.6% had an illicit drug use disorder.

Differential Diagnosis

The ubiquitous nature of panic attacks in many psychiatric disorders and the ability of some substances to evoke panic-like symptoms indicate the need for careful differential diagnosis. Heavy alcohol use increases sensitivity to carbon dioxide, thereby increasing the possibility of a panic attack in heavy drinkers (Cosci et al. 2007). Because of noradrenergic stimulation, stimulant drugs can induce panic attacks that may develop into full-blown panic disorder over time (Louie et al. 1996). MDMA (3,4-methylenedioxymethamphetamine; "Ecstasy") has also been associated with the development of panic disorder in case studies (Pallanti and Mazzi 1992). Whether the panic attacks are ever untriggered or unexpected is important to consider. Alcohol and opioid withdrawal also are associated with noradrenergic overdrive that can result in a panic attack. However, panic disorder requires persistent worry about having an attack and symptoms that cause significant distress or impairment in at least one area (American Psychiatric Association 2013).

Pharmacological Treatment

Clinical trials generally exclude participants with active SUDs. To date, no pharmacotherapy trials of co-occurring panic disorder and SUDs have been published. SSRIs, however, are FDA approved for panic disorder.

Psychosocial Treatment

Two studies investigated psychosocial treatments for panic disorder with comorbid SUDs. Among inpatients with alcohol dependence and panic disorder (with or without agoraphobia), one study compared treatment as usual for alcohol dependence to an empirically supported (e.g., Craske et al. 1991) CBT-oriented group for panic disorder plus treatment as usual. Although the combined treatment group received an additional 12 hours of treatment, no significant differences were found in anxiety or drinking (Bowen et al. 2000). Moreover, both groups improved on anxiety and alcohol abstinence up to 1 year after treatment with no significant between-group differences. Hypothesized reasons for these findings included limited cognitive skills and motivation for engagement among patients and the severity of inpatient populations.

An integrated group cognitive-behavioral intervention for co-occurring panic and alcohol dependence was developed and tested in addition to a partial hospitalization program for addictions (Kushner et al. 2006). The treatment contained three modules—psychoeducation, cognitive restructuring, and exposure—and explicitly addressed links between alcohol use, panic symptoms, and agoraphobia. Participants who completed the treatment were significantly less likely to meet criteria for panic disorder at 4-month follow-up. Relapse rates did not differ, but patients who participated in the integrated treatment had less severe relapses (i.e., fewer drinks, fewer binges).

Anxiety and Opioid Use Disorders

The United States is currently in the midst of an opioid epidemic. The rate of deaths from opioid overdose quadrupled between 1999 and 2008 and continues to rise every year; more than 72,000 lives were lost to overdose in 2017. As such, the relationship of anxiety to opioid use disorders is of particular interest. Both basic science and clinical studies demonstrate that the endogenous opioid system plays a critical role in the neural modulation of anxiety and that activation of the opioid system leads to anxiolytic responses in healthy subjects and those with anxiety disorders (Colasanti et al. 2011). In the NESARC study, anxiety disorders were identified in approximately 61% of subjects with opioid dependence (Conway et al. 2006), and all associations between opioid use disorders and specific anxiety disorders were significant and strong. Of interest, opioid withdrawal states are characterized by noradrenergic overactivity and anxiety, and panic attacks are not infrequent. These aversive symptoms of opioid withdrawal may be exaggerated in individuals with anxiety disorders and could contribute to escalation to compulsive drug use. It is particularly important to screen individuals with opioid use disorders for anxiety disorders and to aggressively treat the anxiety, because this may be critical to successful recovery.

Conclusions and Future Directions

Interest in the co-occurrence of anxiety disorders and SUDs has grown tremendously in recent years. Co-occurrence of these disorders is common and has a significant impact on prognosis and treatment. Furthermore, treatment of anxiety disorders may be associated with decreased substance use. Increasing evidence concerning the common neurobiology of anxiety and SUDs, combined with the development of new methodologies that allow investigation of specific neural circuitry, may lead to new therapeutic approaches. Although promising developments in both pharmacotherapeutic and psychotherapeutic treatments provide cause for considerable optimism, much work remains to be done.

Key Points

- Because substance intoxication and withdrawal are often associated with anxiety, diagnostic clarity in the face of active use or during early abstinence is challenging. For generalized anxiety disorder in particular, symptom overlap is substantial, and the diagnosis must be carefully assessed and reassessed as individuals attain more time in recovery.

- Use of over-the-counter medications and excessive use of caffeine should be carefully assessed in anyone with significant anxiety.

- Advances in the pharmacotherapy of anxiety disorders have led to the development of newer agents with less toxicity, fewer side effects, and fewer interactions with substances of abuse. Research on pharmacotherapeutic treatments in individuals with co-occurring disorders indicate that similar pharmacotherapeutic agents work well for anxiety disorders with or without substance use disorders (SUDs).

- In the absence of specific data about the treatment of co-occurring disorders, the use of agents with known efficacy in the treatment of the anxiety disorder is recommended once the diagnosis has been established. However, special considerations include toxic interactions with drugs and alcohol should relapse occur, medical conditions that are particularly common in individuals with SUDs, and the abuse potential of the agent being used.

- Poor medication adherence is a problem in patients with SUDs as a result of their complex and conflicting attitudes about medications. It is important to address the need for adherence to medications proactively and directly early in treatment and to follow up closely to monitor adherence and response.

- The pharmacotherapy of SUDs is rapidly developing, and a number of studies have investigated the pharmacological treatment of SUDs and comorbid anxiety disorders, in particular PTSD. Available data suggest that agents that target SUDs, such as naltrexone or disulfiram, can be safely used among patients with anxiety comorbidities and may be beneficial.

- It is important to maximize the use of nonpharmacological treatments. The ability to self-regulate emotional states can be extremely helpful to patients in recovery. Learning strategies to self-regulate anxiety symptoms may help them break out of the mindset of using external agents to combat distressing subjective states and acquire healthy alternative coping strategies.

- Several studies have demonstrated that cognitive-behavioral therapies are among the most effective treatments for anxiety disorders and SUDs, and integrated approaches to the treatment of several anxiety disorders have shown promise. However, findings are mixed, and further investigation is needed.

References

American Psychiatric Association: Diagnostic and Statistical Manual of Mental Disorders, 5th Edition. Arlington, VA, American Psychiatric Association, 2013

Back SE, Jackson JL, Sonne S, et al: Alcohol dependence and posttraumatic stress disorder: differences in clinical presentation and response to cognitive-behavioral therapy by order of onset. J Subst Abuse Treat 29(1):29–37, 2005 15979529

Back SE, Brady KT, Jaanimägi U, et al: Cocaine dependence and PTSD: a pilot study of symptom interplay and treatment preferences. Addict Behav 31(2):351–354, 2006a 15951125

Back SE, Brady KT, Sonne SC, et al: Symptom improvement in co-occurring PTSD and alcohol dependence. J Nerv Ment Dis 194(9):690–696, 2006b 16971821

Back SE, Foa E, Killeen T, et al: Concurrent Treatment of PTSD and Substance Use Disorders Using Prolonged Exposure (COPE) Therapist Manual. New York, Oxford University Press, 2014a

Back SE, Killeen TK, Teer AP, et al: Substance use disorders and PTSD: an exploratory study of treatment preferences among military veterans. Addict Behav 39(2):369–373, 2014b 24199930

Back SE, McCauley JL, Korte KJ, et al: A double-blind, randomized, controlled pilot trial of N-acetylcysteine in veterans with posttraumatic stress disorder and substance use disorders. J Clin Psychiatry 77(11):e1439–e1446, 2016 27736051

Back SE, Killeen T, Badour CL, et al: Concurrent treatment of PTSD and substance use disorders using prolonged exposure: a randomized clinical trial in military veterans. Addict Behav 90:369–377, 2019 6488423

Bakken K, Landheim AS, Vaglum P: Substance-dependent patients with and without social anxiety disorder: occurrence and clinical differences. A study of a consecutive sample of alcohol-dependent and poly substance-dependent patients treated in two counties in Norway. Drug Alcohol Depend 80(3):321–328, 2005 15964156

Batki SL, Pennington DL, Lasher B, et al: Topiramate treatment of alcohol use disorder in veterans with posttraumatic stress disorder: a randomized controlled pilot trial. Alcohol Clin Exp Res 38(8):2169–2177, 2014 25092377

Bohn MJ, Babor TF, Kranzler HR: The Alcohol Use Disorders Identification Test (AUDIT): validation of a screening instrument for use in medical settings. J Stud Alcohol 56(4):423–432, 1995 7674678

Bolton J, Cox B, Clara I, Sareen J: Use of alcohol and drugs to self-medicate anxiety disorders in a nationally representative sample. J Nerv Ment Dis 194(11):818–825, 2006 17102705

Bowen RC, D'Arcy C, Keegan D, et al: A controlled trial of cognitive behavioral treatment of panic in alcoholic inpatients with comorbid panic disorder. Addict Behav 25(4):593–597, 2000 10972451

Brady KT, Sinha R: Co-occurring mental and substance use disorders: the neurobiological effects of chronic stress. Am J Psychiatry 162(8):1483–1493, 2005 16055769

Brady KT, Sonne S, Anton RF, et al: Sertraline in the treatment of co-occurring alcohol dependence and posttraumatic stress disorder. Alcohol Clin Exp Res 29(3):395–401, 2005 15770115

Bruce SE, Yonkers KA, Otto MW, et al: Influence of psychiatric comorbidity on recovery and recurrence in generalized anxiety disorder, social phobia, and panic disorder: a 12-year prospective study. Am J Psychiatry 162(6):1179–1187, 2005 15930067

Carrigan MH, Randall CL: Self-medication in social phobia: a review of the alcohol literature. Addict Behav 28(2):269–284, 2003 12573678

Chatterjee CR, Ringold AL: A case report of reduction in alcohol craving and protection against alcohol withdrawal by gabapentin. J Clin Psychiatry 60(9):617, 1999 10520981

Colasanti A, Rabiner EA, Lingford-Hughes A, et al: Opioids and anxiety. J Psychopharmacol 25(11):1415–1433, 2011 20530588

Conway KP, Compton W, Stinson FS, et al: Lifetime comorbidity of DSM-IV mood and anxiety disorders and specific drug use disorders: results from the National Epidemiologic Survey on Alcohol and Related Conditions. J Clin Psychiatry 67(2):247–257, 2006 16566620

Cosci F, Schruers KR, Abrams K, et al: Alcohol use disorders and panic disorder: a review of the evidence of a direct relationship. J Clin Psychiatry 68(6):874–880, 2007

Craske MG, Brown TA, Barlow DH: Behavioral treatment of panic disorder: a two-year follow-up. Behav Ther 22:289–304, 1991

Ewing JA: Detecting alcoholism. The CAGE questionnaire. JAMA 252(14):1905–1907, 1984 6471323

Fals-Stewart W, Schafer J: The treatment of substance abusers diagnosed with obsessive-compulsive disorder: an outcome study. J Subst Abuse Treat 9(4):365–370, 1992 1479631

Grant BF, Stinson FS, Dawson DA, et al: Prevalence and co-occurrence of substance use disorders and independent mood and anxiety disorders: results from the National Epidemiologic Survey on Alcohol and Related Conditions. Arch Gen Psychiatry 61(8):807–816, 2004 15289279

Grant BF, Hasin DS, Stinson FS, et al: Co-occurrence of 12-month mood and anxiety disorders and personality disorders in the US: results from the National Epidemiologic Survey on Alcohol and Related Conditions. J Psychiatr Res 39(1):1–9, 2005 15504418

Greist J, Chouinard G, DuBoff E, et al: Double-blind parallel comparison of three dosages of sertraline and placebo in outpatients with obsessive-compulsive disorder. Arch Gen Psychiatry 52(4):289–295, 1995 7702445

Jacobsen LK, Southwick SM, Kosten TR: Substance use disorders in patients with posttraumatic stress disorder: a review of the literature. Am J Psychiatry 158(8):1184–1190, 2001 11481147

Kaplan GB, Heinrichs SC, Carey RJ: Treatment of addiction and anxiety using extinction approaches: neural mechanisms and their treatment implications. Pharmacol Biochem Behav 97(3):619–625, 2011 20723558

Kendler KS, Myers J, O Gardner C: Caffeine intake, toxicity and dependence and lifetime risk for psychiatric and substance use disorders: an epidemiologic and co-twin control analysis. Psychol Med 36(12):1717–1725, 2006 16893482

Kessler RC, McGonagle KA, Zhao S, et al: Lifetime and 12-month prevalence of DSM-III-R psychiatric disorders in the United States. Results from the National Comorbidity Survey. Arch Gen Psychiatry 51(1):8–19, 1994 8279933

Kessler RC, Sonnega A, Bromet E, et al: Posttraumatic stress disorder in the National Comorbidity Survey. Arch Gen Psychiatry 52(12):1048–1060, 1995 7492257

Kessler RC, Crum RM, Warner LA, et al: Lifetime co-occurrence of DSM-III-R alcohol abuse and dependence with other psychiatric disorders in the National Comorbidity Survey. Arch Gen Psychiatry 54(4):313–321, 1997 9107147

Kessler RC, Chiu WT, Demler O, et al: Prevalence, severity, and comorbidity of 12-month DSM-IV disorders in the National Comorbidity Survey Replication. Arch Gen Psychiatry 62(6):617–627, 2005 15939839

Kessler RC, Chiu WT, Jin R, et al: The epidemiology of panic attacks, panic disorder, and agoraphobia in the National Comorbidity Survey Replication. Arch Gen Psychiatry 63(4):415–424, 2006 16585471

Koob G, Kreek MJ: Stress, dysregulation of drug reward pathways, and the transition to drug dependence. Am J Psychiatry 164(8):1149–1159, 2007 17671276

Kranzler HR, Burleson JA, Del Boca FK, et al: Buspirone treatment of anxious alcoholics: a placebo-controlled trial. Arch Gen Psychiatry 51(9):720–731, 1994 8080349

Kushner MG, Sher KJ, Beitman BD: The relation between alcohol problems and the anxiety disorders. Am J Psychiatry 147(6):685–695, 1990 2188513

Kushner MG, Donahue C, Sletten S, et al: Cognitive behavioral treatment of comorbid anxiety disorder in alcoholism treatment patients: presentation of a prototype program and future directions. J Ment Health 15:697–707, 2006

Lai HMX, Cleary M, Sitharthan T, et al: Prevalence of comorbid substance use, anxiety and mood disorders in epidemiological surveys, 1990–2014: a systematic review and meta-analysis. Drug Alcohol Depend 154:1–13, 2015 26072219

Louie AK, Lannon RA, Rutzick EA, et al: Clinical features of cocaine-induced panic. Biol Psychiatry 40(9):938–940, 1996 8896786

Lüthi A, Lüscher C: Pathological circuit function underlying addiction and anxiety disorders. Nat Neurosci 17(12):1635–1643, 2014 25402855

Lydiard RB, Roy-Byrne PP, Ballenger JC: Recent advances in the psychopharmacological treatment of anxiety disorders. Hosp Community Psychiatry 39(11):1157–1165, 1988 2906319

Maisto SA, Carey MP, Carey KB, et al: Use of the AUDIT and the DAST-10 to identify alcohol and drug use disorders among adults with a severe and persistent mental illness. Psychol Assess 12(2):186–192, 2000 10887764

Malcolm R, Anton RF, Randall CL, et al: A placebo-controlled trial of buspirone in anxious inpatient alcoholics. Alcohol Clin Exp Res 16(6):1007–1013, 1992 1335217

Malcolm R, Myrick H, Brady KT, et al: Update on anticonvulsants for the treatment of alcohol withdrawal. Am J Addict 10(suppl):s16–s23, 2001 11268817

Malec E, Malec T, Gagné MA, et al: Buspirone in the treatment of alcohol dependence: a placebo-controlled trial. Alcohol Clin Exp Res 20(2):307–312, 1996 8730222

McKeehan MB, Martin D: Assessment and treatment of anxiety disorders and co-morbid alcohol/other drug dependency. Alcohol Treat Q 20:45–59, 2002

McRae AL, Sonne SC, Brady KT, et al: A randomized, placebo-controlled trial of buspirone for the treatment of anxiety in opioid-dependent individuals. Am J Addict 13(1):53–63, 2004 14766438

Meaney MJ, Brake W, Gratton A: Environmental regulation of the development of mesolimbic dopamine systems: a neurobiological mechanism for vulnerability to drug abuse? Psychoneuroendocrinology 27(1–2):127–138, 2002 11750774

Merikangas KR, Mehta RL, Molnar BE, et al: Comorbidity of substance use disorders with mood and anxiety disorders: results of the International Consortium in Psychiatric Epidemiology. Addict Behav 23(6):893–907, 1998 9801724

Mills KL, Teesson M, Ross J, et al: Trauma, PTSD, and substance use disorders: findings from the Australian National Survey of Mental Health and Well-Being. Am J Psychiatry 163(4):652–658, 2006 16585440

Mills KL, Teesson M, Back SE, et al: Integrated exposure-based therapy for co-occurring post-traumatic stress disorder and substance dependence: a randomized controlled trial. JAMA 308(7):690–699, 2012 22893166

Modell JG, Glaser FB, Cyr L, et al: Obsessive and compulsive characteristics of craving for alcohol in alcohol abuse and dependence. Alcohol Clin Exp Res 16(2):272–274, 1992 1590549

Myrick H, Brady KT: Social phobia in cocaine-dependent individuals. Am J Addict 6(2):99–104, 1997 9134071

Najavits LM: Seeking Safety: A Treatment Manual for PTSD and Substance Abuse. New York, Guilford, 2002

Norman SB, Hamblen JL: Promising directions for treating comorbid PTSD and substance use disorder. Alcohol Clin Exp Res 41(4):708–710, 2017 28181264

Norman SB, Trim R, Haller M, et al: Efficacy of integrated exposure therapy vs integrated coping skills therapy for comorbid posttraumatic stress disorder and alcohol use disorder: a randomized clinical trial. JAMA Psychiatry 2019 Epub ahead of print

Pallanti S, Mazzi D: MDMA (Ecstasy) precipitation of panic disorder. Biol Psychiatry 32(1):91–95, 1992 1356491

Pande AC, Davidson JR, Jefferson JW, et al: Treatment of social phobia with gabapentin: a placebo-controlled study. J Clin Psychopharmacol 19(4):341–348, 1999 10440462

Petrakis IL, Simpson TL: Posttraumatic stress disorder and alcohol use disorder: a critical review of pharmacologic treatments. Alcohol Clin Exp Res 41(2):226–237, 2017 28102573

Piazza PV, Le Moal M: The role of stress in drug self-administration. Trends Pharmacol Sci 19(2):67–74, 1998 9550944

Posternak MA, Mueller TI: Assessing the risks and benefits of benzodiazepines for anxiety disorders in patients with a history of substance abuse or dependence. Am J Addict 10(1):48–68, 2001 11268828

Ralevski E, Olivera-Figueroa LA, Petrakis I: PTSD and comorbid AUD: a review of pharmacological and alternative treatment options. Subst Abuse Rehabil 5:25–36, 2014 24648794

Randall CL, Johnson MR, Thevos AK, et al: Paroxetine for social anxiety and alcohol use in dual-diagnosed patients. Depress Anxiety 14(4):255–262, 2001a 11754136

Randall CL, Thomas S, Thevos AK: Concurrent alcoholism and social anxiety disorder: a first step toward developing effective treatments. Alcohol Clin Exp Res 25(2):210–220, 2001b 11236835

Regier DA, Farmer ME, Rae DS, et al: Comorbidity of mental disorders with alcohol and other drug abuse. Results from the Epidemiologic Catchment Area (ECA) Study. JAMA 264(19):2511–2518, 1990 2232018

Roberts NP, Roberts PA, Jones N, et al: Psychological interventions for post-traumatic stress disorder and comorbid substance use disorder: a systematic review and meta-analysis. Clin Psychol Rev 38:25–38, 2015 25792193

Ruglass LM, Lopez-Castro T, Papini S, et al: Concurrent treatment with prolonged exposure for co-occurring full or subthreshold posttraumatic stress disorder and substance use disorders: a randomized clinical trial. Psychother Psychosom 86(3):150–161, 2017 28490022

Sareen J, Chartier M, Paulus MP, et al: Illicit drug use and anxiety disorders: findings from two community surveys. Psychiatry Res 142(1):11–17, 2006 16712953

Sartor CE, Lynskey MT, Heath AC, et al: The role of childhood risk factors in initiation of alcohol use and progression to alcohol dependence. Addiction 102(2):216–225, 2007 17222275

Satel SL, McDougle CJ: Obsessions and compulsions associated with cocaine abuse. Am J Psychiatry 148(7):947, 1991 2053637

Sbrana A, Bizzarri JV, Rucci P, et al: The spectrum of substance use in mood and anxiety disorders. Compr Psychiatry 46(1):6–13, 2005 15714188

Schadé A, Marquenie LA, Van Balkom AJ, et al: Alcohol-dependent patients with comorbid phobic disorders: a comparison between comorbid patients, pure alcohol-dependent and pure phobic patients. Alcohol Alcohol 39(3):241–246, 2004 15082462

Schuckit MA, Tipp JE, Bergman M, et al: Comparison of induced and independent major depressive disorders in 2,945 alcoholics. Am J Psychiatry 154(7):948–957, 1997 9210745

Seal KH, Cohen G, Waldrop A, et al: Substance use disorders in Iraq and Afghanistan veterans in VA healthcare, 2001–2010: implications for screening, diagnosis and treatment. Drug Alcohol Depend 116(1–3):93–101, 2011 21277712

Simpson TL, Lehavot K, Petrakis IL: No wrong doors: findings from a critical review of behavioral randomized clinical trials for individuals with co-occurring alcohol/drug problems and posttraumatic stress disorder. Alcohol Clin Exp Res 41(4):681–702, 2017 28055143

Sinha R: Chronic stress, drug use, and vulnerability to addiction. Ann N Y Acad Sci 1141:105–130, 2008 18991954

Sofuoglu M, Rosenheck R, Petrakis I: Pharmacological treatment of comorbid PTSD and substance use disorder: recent progress. Addict Behav 39(2):428–433, 2014 24035645

Teitelbaum LM, Carey KB: Temporal stability of alcohol screening measures in a psychiatric setting. Psychol Addict Behav 14(4):401–404, 2000 11130159

Terra MB, Barros HM, Stein AT, et al: Social anxiety disorder in 300 patients hospitalized for alcoholism in Brazil: high prevalence and undertreatment. Compr Psychiatry 47(6):463–467, 2006

Voris J, Smith NL, Rao SM, et al: Gabapentin for the treatment of ethanol withdrawal. Subst Abus 24(2):129–132, 2003 12766380

Weinstein A, Maayan G, Weinstein Y: A study on the relationship between compulsive exercise, depression and anxiety. J Behav Addict 4(4):315–318, 2015 26690627

Wittchen H-U, Zhao S, Kessler RC, et al: DSM-III-R generalized anxiety disorder in the National Comorbidity Survey. Arch Gen Psychiatry 51(5):355–364, 1994 8179459

Recommended Readings

Bolton J, Cox B, Clara I, et al: Use of alcohol and drugs to self-medicate anxiety disorders in a nationally representative sample. J Nerv Ment Dis 194:818–825, 2006

Compton WM, Cottler LB, Jacobs JL, et al: The role of psychiatric disorders in predicting drug dependence treatment outcome. Am J Psychiatry 160:890–895, 2003

Dunner DL: Management of anxiety disorders: the added challenge of comorbidity. Depress Anxiety 13:57–71, 2001

Merikangas KR, Mehta RL, Molnar BE, et al: Comorbidity of substance use disorders with mood and anxiety disorders: results of the International Consortium in Psychiatric Epidemiology. Addict Behav 23:893–907, 1998

Posternak MA, Mueller TI: Assessing the risks and benefits of benzodiazepines for anxiety disorders in patients with a history of substance abuse or dependence. Am J Addict 10:48–68, 2001

Tiet QQ, Mausbach B: Treatments for patients with dual diagnosis: a review. Alcohol Clin Exp Res 31:513–536, 2007

Websites of Interest

National Institute on Drug Abuse: www.nida.nih.gov
Substance Abuse and Mental Health Services Administration: www.samhsa.gov
Teen Drug Abuse: www.teendrugabuse.us

CHAPTER 37

Anxiety and Anxiety Disorders in Medical Settings

Rushi H. Vyas, M.D.

Antolin Trinidad, M.D., Ph.D.

Thomas N. Wise, M.D.

Health-related concerns and primary anxiety disorders often present as comorbid conditions. Sherbourne et al. (1996) estimated rates of 15%–18% of primary care patients having a concurrent comorbid primary anxiety disorder, with lifetime rates of anxiety of 26%–28%. Specific phobias and generalized anxiety disorder (GAD) are the anxiety disorders most commonly seen in medically ill patients, with panic disorder showing greater prevalence in medically ill patients with comorbid depression (Sherbourne et al. 1996). With lifetime prevalence of anxiety disorders in the United States at 18% (Kessler et al. 2012), and higher rates in those with comorbid medical illnesses, clinicians should consider anxiety disorders in the differential diagnoses.

It remains helpful to consider McHugh and Slavney's (1998) argument that psychiatry should be viewed from multiple perspectives. Each perspective has a specific internal grammar of its own, possessing both strengths and weaknesses (McHugh and Slavney 1998; Schwartz and Wiggins 1988). This multifaceted approach remains very useful for the clinician working in the medical setting. Two perspectives discussed here are the life history perspective and the more common disease approach.

Life History Perspective

In the *life history perspective*, each patient's developmental vicissitudes create a personal biography with a variety of special meanings (Engel 1997; Slavney and McHugh

1984). Understanding such meaningful connections is the essence of dynamic psychiatry. Medical illness evokes personal meanings that can create or worsen anxieties in patients and their families. The life history perspective facilitates understanding of how patients will react to a specific diagnosis. They may resort to catastrophic thinking with new diagnoses; unrealistic fears about medications are also common. Clinicians ideally use their own empathic abilities to better understand how patients are reacting to their conditions.

Disease Approach

The *disease approach* is based on the medical model, in which a syndromic category is defined based on signs and symptoms that allow a categorical designation to be developed and investigated for pathophysiological causes (McHugh and Slavney 1982). These categorical distinctions are the essence of DSM-5 and ICD-11 (American Psychiatric Association 2013; Gureje 2018).

DSM-5 catalogs various syndromes in which anxiety is the main symptom. Goldenberg et al. (1996) showed that "pure culture," or defining symptom clusters presenting in one patient, is rare because comorbidity is common. DSM-5 differs from previous iterations because it has a separate section on "Somatic Symptom and Related Disorders" that includes multiple varying somatic diagnoses. Anxiety can be present in many of the somatic diagnoses such as illness anxiety disorder, somatic symptom disorder, and psychological factors affecting other medical conditions (Hüsing et al. 2018).

Another confounder is the demarcation between benign and pathological anxiety. Clinicians often underdiagnose anxiety disorders because they rationalize it is "normal" to be anxious about health issues (Jackson et al. 2007). Time limitations in a busy practice often hinder accurate assessments. This underrecognition could benefit from the use of effective structured screening instruments. For example, the seven-item Generalized Anxiety Disorder Scale (GAD-7; Kroenke et al. 2007) has been demonstrated to be well accepted by primary care patients and easy to score.

One category of anxiety results from a diagnosable medical/physical disorder (Table 37–1). Medical conditions, such as congestive heart failure, hyperthyroid disease, and metabolic disorders, often present with anxiety as part of the plethora of symptoms of the disorder (Hall 1980). Thus, appropriate endocrine, laboratory, and imaging studies should be considered if they have not already been performed. Various drugs (e.g., caffeine or exogenous, or even illicit, steroids) also have the potential to cause anxiety in some patients.

Common DSM-5 Anxiety Disorder Categories Often Presenting in the Medical Setting

Panic disorder presents acutely with frightening physical symptoms; patients with panic disorder have higher utilization rates of medical care as a consequence of misinterpretation and misattribution of their symptomatology (Katon 1996). Apart from accurate diagnosis and treatment, a critical step is educating patients that their symp-

TABLE 37–1.   Drug–drug interactions

Antianxiety medication	Enzyme	Inhibition/Induction	Interactions
Benzodiazepines			
Lorazepam, temazepam, oxazepam	No liver metabolism-glucuronidation	None	Decreased by ritonavir, nelfinavir
Alprazolam, triazolam, estazolam	3A4	None	Increased by carbamazepine, phenytoin, rifampin, barbiturates, ritonavir, delavirdine, macrolides, calcium channel blockers, fluvoxamine, erythromycin, nefazodone, fluoxetine, sertraline, midazolam
Midazolam	3A4	Inhibits 3A4	Increased by the same medications as alprazolam, triazolam, estazolam
β-Blockers			
Atenolol	Minimal metabolism		Additive effects with other hypertensive medications Exaggerated clonidine withdrawal Hypotension with trazodone, thioridazine, chlorpromazine, olanzapine, risperidone, quetiapine, TCAs
Metoprolol	2D6		
Propranolol	2D6, 2C19		
Selective serotonin reuptake inhibitors			
Fluvoxamine	Unknown	Inhibits 1A2, 3A4 Less inhibition of 2C19, 2C9, 3A4	Increases warfarin levels/INR, amiodarone, quinidine, simvastatin, calcium channel blockers
Fluoxetine, paroxetine	2D6	Inhibit 2D6	Increased by β-blockers, ritonavir, protease inhibitors, many antiarrhythmics

TABLE 37–1. Drug–drug interactions (continued)

Antianxiety medication	Enzyme	Inhibition/Induction	Interactions
Antipsychotics			
Haloperidol, perphenazine	2D6		Increased by fluoxetine, paroxetine, fluvoxamine Perphenazine substrate increased by carbamazepine Haloperidol substrate decreased by carbamazepine
Clozapine	1A2 (primary) 2D6 (secondary)		Increased by fluoxetine, paroxetine, fluvoxamine, sertraline Decreased by carbamazepine
Risperidone	2D6		Altered by same medications as haloperidol and perphenazine
Olanzapine	1A2		Altered by same medications as clozapine
Quetiapine, ziprasidone	3A4		Altered by same medications as alprazolam, triazolam, and estazolam
Other			
Buspirone	3A4	Inhibits	Altered by the same medications as alprazolam, triazolam, and estazolam
Venlafaxine	2D6	Inhibits	May elevate blood pressure Risk of increase in bleeding disorders HRV may be reduced when used with mirtazapine or quetiapine
Duloxetine	2D6	Inhibits	Should not be coadministered with MAOI
Vortioxetine	2D6	Inhibits	Reduce bupropion dose by half if used concurrently

Note. HRV=heart rate variability; INR=international normalized ratio; MAOI=monoamine oxidase inhibitor; TCA=tricyclic antidepressant.
Source. Data from Crone and Gabriel 2004; DeVane and Markowitz 2000; Dresser et al. 2000; Markowitz et al. 1995; Prior and Baker 2003; Tanaka and Hisawa 1999.

toms are a part of panic disorder rather than of another serious illness (Hocking and Koenig 1995). This is a good opportunity to educate patients and lessen stigmatization while showing their interpretation of panic symptoms from a psychological perspective rather than just as physical symptoms due to sympathetic overdrive from anxiety.

Adjustment disorder with anxiety is one of the more common psychiatric diagnoses seen in medically ill patients (Wilson-Barnett 1992). In this diagnosis, a stressor, such as a physical illness, is clearly defined, and the individual exhibits marked distress or functional impairment in excess of what would be expected from exposure to that particular stressor.

Acute stress disorder is characterized by exposure to a traumatic event and nine symptoms from five categories of symptoms (i.e., intrusions, negative mood, dissociation, avoidance, and arousal), which differentiates it from adjustment disorder. The exact incidence of acute stress disorder within medical settings is not known. However, this entity, as well as PTSD, may be found in both patients and their supportive caregivers. Notably, radical surgeries and medical procedures along with prolonged, life-threatening hospitalizations may be causative factors in acute stress disorder or PTSD (Bienvenu et al. 2013; Tully et al. 2015).

Illness anxiety disorder is a new category in DSM-5 similar to older DSM categories of hypochondriasis, wherein the individual fears having or acquiring an illness. It is usually comorbid with the personality dimension of neuroticism and can be seen in individuals who meet DSM-5 criteria for psychological factors affecting other medical conditions. The difference between the two is that those with illness anxiety are often perseverating and anxious about developing an illness, whereas those with psychological factors affecting other medical conditions already have a known medical diagnosis.

GAD involves a chronic anxiety state with both psychological and physical symptomatology; patients may also seek medical care excessively, including medical evaluations and interventions.

Pharmacotherapy

A medication's side effect profile, drug–drug interactions (Table 37–2), and impact on ongoing clinical issues must be considered in the medical setting. First-line treatments often include faster-acting agents (e.g., benzodiazepines) and then consideration of longer-acting anxiolytics such as antidepressants or buspirone. Alternative agents are considered for more chronic forms of anxiety. Considerations by class are further discussed in the following sections.

Benzodiazepines

For acute, rapid treatment, benzodiazepines are often the first option prescribed in the medical setting, but this choice is not without considerations. These agents have a variety of half-lives, metabolic routes, and dosages that allow the physician to tailor the regimen to a patient's acute episode of anxiety; however, long-term use carries a risk of increased side effects, tolerance, and dependency. Common issues that complicate benzodiazepine administration in medically ill patients are impaired pulmonary function, liver disease, pregnancy considerations, diminished cognitive capacity, and

TABLE 37–2.   **Common medical conditions that may cause anxiety**

Cardiovascular	Metabolic	Neurological
Anemia	Acidosis	Cerebral anoxia
Arrhythmia	Hyperthermia	Cerebral vascular disease
Congestive heart failure	Hypocalcemia	Encephalopathy (i.e.,
Coronary artery disease	Hypokalemia	delirium)
Hypovolemic states	Hypophosphatemia	Huntington's chorea
Mitral valve prolapse	Acute intermittent porphyria	Mass lesion of the brain*
	Vitamin B_{12} deficiency	Multiple sclerosis
		Myasthenia gravis
Respiratory	**Substance intoxication**	Pain
Asthma and COPD	Alcohol	Parkinson's disease
Hyperventilation	Amphetamines	Polyneuritis
Hypoxia	Caffeine	Postconcussion syndrome
Oat cell carcinoma	Cannabis	Postencephalitic disorders
Pneumonia	Cocaine	Posterolateral sclerosis
Pneumothorax	Hallucinogens	Simple or complex partial
Pulmonary embolism	Inhalants	seizure
	Phencyclidine	Vestibular dysfunction–
		related vertigo
Endocrinological	**Substance withdrawal**	**Toxicological**
Adrenal gland dysfunction	Medications	Carbon dioxide
Hypoglycemia	Anxiolytics	Carbon monoxide
Menopause and ovarian	Clonidine	Gasoline
dysfunction	Hypnotics and sedatives	Heavy metals
Parathyroid disease	SSRIs and TCAs	Insecticides and
Pheochromocytoma	Other substances	organophosphates
Pituitary disorders	Alcohol	Paint
Premenstrual syndrome	Cocaine	
Thyroid dysfunction	Nicotine	
	Opiates	

Note.   COPD=chronic obstructive pulmonary disease; SSRIs=selective serotonin reuptake inhibitors; TCAs=tricyclic antidepressants.
*Especially third ventricle.

encephalopathy or delirium. Central respiratory suppression should be closely monitored and can affect vulnerable patients with compromised pulmonary function. Lorazepam, oxazepam, and temazepam should be considered in patients with liver impairment because these agents do not undergo hepatic oxidation but are primarily excreted via the kidney after glucuronidation (Trevor and Way 2007). Previous concerns that benzodiazepine use may have associations with birth defects such as cleft palate are being overturned by newer studies that show this association is less likely (Ban et al. 2014). The American College of Obstetricians and Gynecologists and American Family Physician note that the use of benzodiazepines in women does not appear to carry a significant teratogenic risk but acknowledged the association between oral cleft and prenatal benzodiazepine exposure primarily increased the absolute risk by 0.01%. Disadvantages of benzodiazepines include crossing the placental barrier and the attendant effects on neonate health; cognitive impairments in the elderly; and worsening confusion in delirious patients. In addition, the geriatric population often have an increased risk of falls and oversedation, regardless of inpatient or outpatient status. Thus, benzodiazepines are not an ideal choice to start with in this population.

Antipsychotics

Low-dose antipsychotics can be used to treat severe and persistent anxiety when benzodiazepine treatment fails, although this is considered an off-label use (Kreys and Phan 2015). Their use in the medical setting includes an adjunctive role in delirious or agitated patients, particularly because antipsychotics generally have fewer respiratory concerns than benzodiazepines. For steroid-induced anxiety and anxiety secondary to organic causes, especially delirium, low-dose antipsychotics such as haloperidol or quetiapine are effective.

The second-generation antipsychotics have become the most widely used antipsychotic agents in many settings, and awareness of their metabolism is essential when patients may have medical comorbidities. Low initial dosages and frequent monitoring are recommended, as well as monitoring for extrapyramidal side effects and the possibility of neuroleptic malignant syndrome.

Beta-Blockers

By directly blocking β-adrenergic stimulation, β-blockers can be effective in treating anxiety symptoms secondary to specific medical illnesses such as hyperthyroidism. Also occasionally used for situational anxiety, they can be useful to reduce physiological signs of general hyperarousal (e.g., sweating, tremors, hypertension, tachycardia). Patients with asthma, chronic obstructive pulmonary disease, diabetes, or bradycardia should avoid β-blockers. Concurrent use of amiodarone and β-blockers may result in hypotension, bradycardia, or cardiac arrest. The use of clonidine with a β-blocker should be avoided because an exaggerated clonidine withdrawal response (rebound hypertension) may occur (Kaplan 2007). Additional caution is warranted in patients with type 1 diabetes because the anxiolytic mechanisms of β-blockers can also mask the sympathetic response caused by hypoglycemia, and patients then may not easily recognize their hypoglycemic states (Kaplan 2007).

Antidepressants

Selective serotonin reuptake inhibitors (SSRIs) are the most commonly prescribed antidepressants and are ideal medications for long-term treatment of anxiety, with adjunctive medications such as a limited course of benzodiazepines used for acute treatment over the first month while the SSRI takes time to reach full therapeutic efficacy. This is an ideal regimen in the average adult outpatient population, and one that should be considered first line for populations with primary anxiety disorders without any comorbidities. (However, this is not often the case in medical and elderly populations, often leading to use of the antidepressant without the benzodiazepine). Careful titration is the rule; start with low dosages, monitoring for drug–drug interactions and side effects.

The side effects of tricyclic antidepressants (TCAs) and monoamine oxidase inhibitors, as well as the risk of toxicity and drug–drug interactions, make them more difficult to use in medically ill patients. TCAs are eliminated by cytochrome P450 isoenzymes, and they interact with sympathomimetics, such that arrhythmia, hypertension, and tachycardia may result (Huyse et al. 2006). Caution is also advised when combining TCAs with other sedative medications, medications that lower the seizure threshold, or hypotensive agents.

Buspirone

Buspirone is a well-tolerated partial agonist that preferentially binds to serotonin 1A (5-HT$_{1A}$) receptors, with fewer effects on cognition or seizure risk and less concern for tolerance, dependence, or withdrawal. However, it has a slow time of onset (3–4 weeks). Buspirone has the advantage of not causing sedation or respiratory depression and may improve pulmonary ventilation (Lee et al. 2005). It is thus useful for patients who are on mechanical ventilators or who have poor respiratory drive (Craven and Sutherland 1991; Mendelson et al. 1991). In addition, because it does not bind to GABA receptors, it has lower liability to be abused and no cross-reaction with alcohol. It is metabolized primarily by CYP3A4. The clinician should be aware of drug–drug interactions because levels of buspirone are increased by enzyme inhibitors including itraconazole, verapamil, diltiazem, nefazodone, and erythromycin (Dresser et al. 2000; Mahmood and Sahajwalla 1999) and decreased by rifampin (Lamberg et al. 1998).

Antihistamines

If respiratory function is a major concern or benzodiazepine abuse is present, antihistamines can be used acutely, because they are less likely than benzodiazepines to cause pulmonary depression. Hydroxyzine is recommended because it causes fewer anticholinergic side effects while still maintaining the anxiolytic, sedative, and analgesic effects, and it may be used effectively in treatment not only of acute anxiety but also possibly of GAD (Guaiana et al. 2010). Antihistamines have side effects such as dizziness, confusion, and anticholinergic effects; lower the seizure threshold; and are not as potent as benzodiazepines in reducing anxiety. Caution should again be used in the elderly and those predisposed to delirium.

Others

Anticonvulsants such as pregabalin, gabapentin, and valproic acid are used anecdotally in medical settings to assist with the management of anxiety and delirium. They can be useful treatments for anxious, agitated patients, especially those predisposed to CNS insults such as traumatic brain injuries, seizure disorders, or neurocognitive disorders. Valproic acid is used in the management of delirium and also is sedating, which assists with reducing aggression and anxiety. Gabapentin and pregabalin can help with anxiety, especially in patients with neuropathy or anxiety secondary to pain, as well as alcohol withdrawal–related anxiety (Generoso et al. 2017; Lavigne et al. 2012).

Another compound commonly encountered in the clinical setting is marijuana and its various active ingredients, compounds, and derivatives. Although many states are increasing legalization of recreational marijuana use, the American Psychiatric Association (APA) supports the view that no clear scientific evidence has shown marijuana useful for the treatment of anxiety (or any psychiatric disorder).

Despite the increasing number of patients using marijuana for management of pain, seizure control, or other varied medical reasons, neither the FDA nor the APA support its use in treating psychiatric disorders (Zaman et al. 2013).

Psychotherapy

Physician–Patient Relationship

The physician must establish a working therapeutic alliance with any patient (Wise 1990). In a potential crisis emanating from a new diagnosis of cancer or heart disease or when faced with a major surgery, patients uniquely view the physician as the individual who can save their life. This role demands supportive and empathic care in both imparting information and offering hope, regardless of how serious the situation is. A study found that placebo was as effective as alprazolam in reducing anxiety in cancer patients (Wald et al. 1993), and this underscores the idea that nondrug factors may alleviate anxiety. It is then conceivable that physician empathy and understanding belong to the category of nondrug agents that can alleviate anxiety. Other nonphysician members of the treatment team also are well poised to ease the patient's burden. Physicians must include their staff in planning for the emotional care of the patient because often support staff have more interaction with the patient outside of the physician appointment.

Supportive and Other Forms of Psychotherapy

Something in the human brain responds to, and potentially heals from, narratives, which are the main and common tool for the different forms of psychotherapies. *Narratives* are the recitation of the patients' unique story of their illness, and they require active listening. They allow patients to experience the passage of time and to glean meaning from difficult life events, such as medical illness, that involve suffering.

Listening to patients' fears may be a uniquely supportive activity. Viederman and Perry (1980) outlined an assessment of the individual's life trajectory in which the consultant attempts to understand where patients are in their lives and how their illness has modified their hopes and dreams. Understanding patients' marital relationships and how their spouses are coping with the crisis of a serious disease further elucidates the social systems in which the patients reside (Spiegel 1997). It is also essential for psychiatric consultants to pay attention to patients' wider support systems such as friends and employers. Group support has shown promise of benefit. Studies show that supportive group therapy is associated with longer survival in patients with breast cancer (Spiegel and Kato 1996). Other forms of psychotherapy have been demonstrated to improve the affective status (often anxiety as well as depression) in patients with late-stage cancer. As examples of this narrative approach, dignity therapy and meaning-oriented therapies have empirical evidence of benefit (Breitbart et al. 2018; Dose et al. 2018).

Bedside psychotherapy can be one of the most powerful psychotherapies in effecting positive change in patients and catalyzing good medical outcomes for medical inpatients. Daily rounds can provide opportunities to develop rapport, build therapeutic relationships, and educate patients about their own conditions as well as continuously assess how they are adaptively coping. James Griffith (Griffith and Gaby 2005) described helping demoralized medical patients by fostering the treatment alliance between physician and patient while addressing demoralization at the bedside.

Cognitive-behavioral therapy (CBT) approaches to anxiety disorders in general have been shown to be effective (Hedman et al. 2016; Roberge et al. 2018). The centering themes of these approaches include the cognitive (reframing and reconfiguring distorted interpretations of events and symptoms) along with the behavioral, which includes specific strategies to effect dialing-down the sympathetic overdrive caused by mental constructs of danger. In other words, the automatic, instinctive fight-or-flight response may be modulated downward by behavioral techniques such as breathing exercises, mental imagery, and distraction. Fundamentally based on principles of classical and operant learning theories, behavioral medicine has broadened its concept of psychological life to include not only behaviors but also cognitions, emotions, and psychosocial environments. Along with this conceptual shift, many behavioral techniques have been developed, ranging from relaxation, hypnosis, and biofeedback training to environmental modification, CBT, and group education. These techniques have been applied to various medically ill populations to successfully reduce anxiety and its effect on the outcome of disease processes. Meditation and mindfulness have been demonstrated in various studies to diminish anxiety in chronic neurological diseases (Chan et al. 2015). Stress reduction diminishes the risk of cardiac mortality and reinfarction (Frasure-Smith 1991). Mindfulness meditation has been demonstrated to both subjectively improve sense of well-being and to improve salient cardiac physiology in patients with cardiac disease (Younge et al. 2015). The marriage of the cognitive and the behavioral into what we now know as CBT has proven to be a very robust hybrid that has helped many anxiety syndromes in the medically ill, such as patients with inflammatory bowel disease (Bennebroek Evertsz et al. 2017), primary care patients with panic disorder (Roy-Byrne et al. 2005), and diabetic patients with both depression and anxiety (Tovote et al. 2014).

Acceptance and commitment therapy (ACT; Hayes et al. 2016) is a relatively recent systematization of an adage from Linehan (1993), who came up with the notion in her book on the treatment of borderline personality disorder. She said that one of the options people have when faced with any problem is "radical acceptance." Paired with mindfulness principles, ACT has risen as a useful alternative in treating syndromes such as borderline personality disorder. In irreversible medical conditions, the idea of acceptance circumvents the stress and anxiety inherent in the longing for improvement or cure. Such circumvention evokes a mindfulness-based striving toward serenity in the face of something that cannot be changed. In radical acceptance therapy, patients are encouraged to accept life on its own terms, to condition themselves so that higher grades of stress and anxiety will not ensue, and to focus on the practical things that they can change versus those they cannot. This idea is therefore poised to be very useful to patients with chronic or terminal medical illnesses.

Evidence for the efficacy of ACT has been shown in several studies. It was tried for patients with anxiety and obsessive-compulsive spectrum disorders and shown to be as effective as CBT (Bluett et al. 2014), and ACT also has been shown to improve pain intensity and catastrophizing measures in patients with chronic pain as compared to control subjects (Trompetter et al. 2015). What is common between CBT and ACT modalities is the conscious readjustment of patients' attitudes and perspectives regarding their conditions while challenging their assumptions that contribute to magnification of their distress. These modalities nod to accepting that medical illnesses are often chronic, if not lifelong, and sometimes terminal. Anxiety can be modulated, if not eliminated, through these psychotherapeutic methods.

Conclusion

Anxiety disorders remain an important issue for many patients presenting for treatment of general medical illnesses. Even in an age when assessment and treatments have been conceptualized using outcomes-based algorithms and structured rating scales, a clinician's empathy, interview skills, and sensitivity to developmental and personal psychosocial perspectives are crucial components of care. Preexisting anxiety disorders may present as comorbidities, or anxiety may result from the medical illness itself. More and more of these disorders will be treated in embedded-care settings in the future. Relevant pharmacokinetic and pharmacodynamic principles must be considered in the treatment, along with newer forms of psychotherapy.

Key Points

- Anxiety is common in patients experiencing a medical illness and may occur in various forms, such as panic disorder or generalized anxiety disorder. Medical causes for anxiety, which can include endocrine, neurological, and cardiac diseases, must be identified before making the assumption that the patient's distress is solely due to psychiatric factors.

- It is important for the clinician to diagnose the form of the anxiety disorder and to understand which elements of the patient's fears are realistic and which are not. It is also essential to understand the patient's basic personality dimensions and whether they include a propensity for worry and fear.

- Treatment includes a supportive physician–patient relationship, use of supportive help to modify factors that foster anxiety, and use of rational psychopharmacology that is effective, safe, and tolerable.

References

American Psychiatric Association: Diagnostic and Statistical Manual of Mental Disorders, 5th Edition. Arlington, VA, American Psychiatric Association, 2013

Ban L, West J, Gibson JE, et al: First trimester exposure to anxiolytic and hypnotic drugs and the risks of major congenital anomalies: a United Kingdom population-based cohort study. PLoS One 9(6):e100996, 2014

Beitman BD, Basha I, Flaker G, et al: Atypical or nonanginal chest pain: panic disorder or coronary artery disease? Arch Intern Med 147(9):1548–1552, 1987 3632161

Bennebroek Evertsz' F, Sprangers MAG, Sitnikova K, et al: Effectiveness of cognitive-behavioral therapy on quality of life, anxiety, and depressive symptoms among patients with inflammatory bowel disease: a multicenter randomized controlled trial. J Consult Clin Psychol 85(9):918–925, 2017 28857595

Bienvenu OJ, Gellar J, Althouse BM, et al: Post-traumatic stress disorder symptoms after acute lung injury: a 2-year prospective longitudinal study. Psychol Med 43(12):2657–2671, 2013 23438256

Bluett EJ, Homan KJ, Morrison KL, et al: Acceptance and commitment therapy for anxiety and OCD spectrum disorders: an empirical review. J Anxiety Disord 28(6):612–624, 2014 25041735

Breitbart W, Pessin H, Rosenfeld B, et al: Individual meaning-centered psychotherapy for the treatment of psychological and existential distress: a randomized controlled trial in patients with advanced cancer. Cancer 124(15):3231–3239, 2018 29757459

Chan RR, Larson JL: Meditation interventions for chronic disease populations: a systematic review. J Holist Nurs 33(4):351–356, 2015

Craven J, Sutherland A: Buspirone for anxiety disorders in patients with severe lung disease (letter). Lancet 338(8761):249, 1991 1676794

Crone CC, Gabriel GM: Treatment of anxiety and depression in transplant patients: pharmacokinetic considerations. Clin Pharmacokinet 43:361–394, 2004

DeVane CL, Markowitz JS: Avoiding psychotropic drug interactions in the cardiovascular patient. Bull Menninger Clin 64:49–59, 2000

Dose AM, McCabe PJ, Krecke CA, et al: Outcomes of a dignity therapy/life plan intervention for patients with advanced cancer undergoing chemotherapy. J Hosp Palliat Nurs 20(4):400–406, 2018 30063634

Dresser GK, Spence JD, Bailey DG: Pharmacokinetic-pharmacodynamic consequences and clinical relevance of cytochrome P450 3A4 inhibition. Clin Pharmacokinet 38(1):41–57, 2000 10668858

Engel GL: From biomedical to biopsychosocial. Being scientific in the human domain. Psychosomatics 38(6):521–528, 1997 9427848

Frasure-Smith N: In-hospital symptoms of psychological stress as predictors of long-term outcome after acute myocardial infarction in men. Am J Cardiol 67(2):121–127, 1991 1987712

Generoso MB, Tevizol AP, Kasper S, et al: Pregabalin for generalized anxiety disorder: an updated systematic review and meta-analysis. Int Clin Psychopharmacol 32(1):49–55, 2017

Goldenberg IM, White K, Yonkers K, et al: The infrequency of "pure culture" diagnoses among the anxiety disorders. J Clin Psychiatry 57(11):528–533, 1996 8968302

Griffith JL, Gaby L: Brief psychotherapy at the bedside: countering demoralization from medical illness. Psychosomatics 46(2):109–116, 2005 15774948

Guaiana G, Barbui C, Cipriani A: Hydroxyzine for generalized anxiety disorder. Cochrane Database Syst Rev (12):DC006815, 2010 21154375

Gureje O: ICD-11 chapter on mental and behavioural disorders: heralding new ways of seeing old problems. Epidemiol Psychiatr Sci 27(3):209–211, 2018 29697046

Hall RCW: Anxiety, in Psychiatric Presentations of Medical Illness: Somatopsychic Disorders. Edited by Hall RCW. New York, Spectrum, 1980, pp 180–210

Hayes SC, Strohsal KD, Wilson KG: Acceptance and Commitment Therapy: The Process and Practice of Mindful Change, 2nd Edition. New York, Guilford, 2016

Hedman E, Axelsson E, Andersson E, et al: Exposure-based cognitive-behavioural therapy via the internet and as bibliotherapy for somatic symptom disorder and illness anxiety disorder: randomised controlled trial. Br J Psychiatry 209(5):407–413, 2016 27491531

Hocking LB, Koenig HG: Anxiety in medically ill older patients: a review and update (review). Int J Psychiatry Med 25(3):221–238, 1995 8567190

Hüsing P, Löwe B, Toussaint A: Comparing the diagnostic concepts of ICD-10 somatoform disorders and DSM-5 somatic symptom disorders in patients from a psychosomatic outpatient clinic. J Psychosom Res 113:74–80, 2018 30190052

Huyse FJ, Touw DJ, van Schijndel RS, et al: Psychotropic drugs and the perioperative period: a proposal for a guideline in elective surgery. Psychosomatics 47(1):8–22, 2006 16384803

Jackson JL, Passamonti M, Kroenke K: Outcome and impact of mental disorders in primary care at 5 years. Psychosom Med 69(3):270–276, 2007 17401055

Kaplan N: Systemic hypertension therapy, in Braunwald's Heart Disease: A Textbook of Cardiovascular Medicine, 8th Edition. Edited by Libby P, Bonow RO, Mann DL, et al. Philadelphia, PA, WB Saunders, 2007, pp 1049–1068

Katon W: Panic disorder: relationship to high medical utilization, unexplained physical symptoms, and medical costs. J Clin Psychiatry 57(suppl 10):11–18, discussion 19–22, 1996 8917128

Kessler RC, Petukhova M, Sampson NA, et al: Twelve-month and lifetime prevalence and life-time morbid risk of anxiety and mood disorders in the United States. Int J Methods Psychiatr Res 21(3):169–184, 2012 22865617

Kreys TJ, Phan SV: A literature review of quetiapine for generalized anxiety disorder. Pharmacotherapy 35(2):175–188, 2015 25689246

Kroenke K, Spitzer RL, Williams JB, et al: Anxiety disorders in primary care: prevalence, impairment, comorbidity, and detection. Ann Intern Med 146(5):317–325, 2007 17339617

Lamberg TS, Kivistö KT, Neuvonen PJ: Concentrations and effects of buspirone are considerably reduced by rifampicin. Br J Clin Pharmacol 45(4):381–385, 1998 9578186

Lavigne JE, Heckler C, Mathews JL, et al: A randomized, controlled, double-blinded clinical trial of gabapentin 300 versus 900 mg versus placebo for anxiety symptoms in breast cancer survivors. Breast Cancer Res Treat 136(2):479–486, 2012

Lee ST, Park JH, Kim M: Efficacy of the 5HT1A agonist, buspirone hydrochloride, in migraines with anxiety: a randomized, prospective, parallel group, double-blind, placebo-controlled study. Headache 45(8):1004–1011, 2005 16109114

Linehan M: Cognitive-Behavioral Therapy of Borderline Personality Disorder. New York, Guilford, 1993

Mahmood I, Sahajwalla C: Clinical pharmacokinetics and pharmacodynamics of buspirone, an anxiolytic drug. Clin Pharmacokinet 36(4):277–287, 1999 10320950

Markowitz JS, Wells BG, Carson WH: Interactions between antipsychotic and antihypertensive drugs. Ann Pharmacother 29:603–609, 1995

McHugh PR, Slavney PR: Methods of reasoning in psychopathology: conflict and resolution. Compr Psychiatry 23(3):197–215, 1982 7083848

McHugh PR, Slavney PR: The Perspectives of Psychiatry, 2nd Edition. Baltimore, MD, Johns Hopkins University Press, 1998

Mendelson WB, Maczaj M, Holt J: Buspirone administration to sleep apnea patients. J Clin Psychopharmacol 11(1):71–72, 1991 2040719

Prior TI, Baker GB: Interactions between the cytochrome P450 system and the second-generation antipsychotics. J Psychiatry Neurosci 28:99–112, 2003

Roberge P, Provencher MD, Gosselin P, et al: A pragmatic randomized controlled trial of group transdiagnostic cognitive-behaviour therapy for anxiety disorders in primary care: study protocol. BMC Psychiatry 18(1):320, 2018 30285672

Roy-Byrne P, Stein MB, Russo J: Medical illness and response to treatment in primary care panic disorder. Gen Hosp Psychiatry 27:237–243, 2005

Schwartz MA, Wiggins OP: Perspectivism and the methods of psychiatry. Compr Psychiatry 29(3):237–251, 1988 3378413

Sherbourne CD, Jackson CA, Meredith LS, et al: Prevalence of comorbid anxiety disorders in primary care outpatients. Arch Fam Med 5(1):27–34, discussion 35, 1996 8542051

Slavney PR, McHugh PR: Life stories and meaningful connections: reflections on a clinical method in psychiatry and medicine. Perspect Biol Med 27:279–288, 1984

Spiegel D: Psychosocial aspects of breast cancer treatment (review). Semin Oncol 24(1 suppl):S1-36–S1-47, 1997 9045314

Spiegel D, Kato PM: Psychosocial influences on cancer incidence and progression (review). Harv Rev Psychiatry 4(1):10–26, 1996 9384968

Tanaka E, Hisawa S: Clinically significant pharmacokinetic drug interactions with psychoactive drugs: antidepressants and antipsychotics and the cytochrome P450 system. J Clin Pharmacol Ther 24:7–16, 1999

Tovote KA, Fleer J, Snippe E, et al: Individual mindfulness-based cognitive therapy and cognitive behavior therapy for treating depressive symptoms in patients with diabetes: results of a randomized controlled trial. Diabetes Care 37(9):2427–2434, 2014 24898301

Trevor AJ, Way WL: Sedative-hypnotic drugs, in Basic and Clinical Pharmacology, 10th Edition. Edited by Katzung BG. New York, McGraw-Hill, 2007, pp 347–362

Trompetter HR, Bohlmeijer ET, Veehof MM, et al: Internet-based guided self-help intervention for chronic pain based on acceptance and commitment therapy: a randomized controlled trial. J Behav Med 38(1):66–80, 2015 24923259

Tully PJ, Winefield HR, Baker RA, et al: Depression, anxiety and major adverse cardiovascular and cerebrovascular events in patients following coronary artery bypass graft surgery: a five year longitudinal cohort study. Biopsychosoc Med 9:14, 2015 26019721

Viederman M, Perry SW 3rd: Use of a psychodynamic life narrative in the treatment of depression in the physically ill. Gen Hosp Psychiatry 2(3):177–185, 1980 7429146

Wald TG, Kathol RG, Noyes R Jr, et al: Rapid relief of anxiety in cancer patients with both alprazolam and placebo. Psychosomatics 34(4):324–332, 1993 8351307

Wilson-Barnett J: Psychological reactions to medical procedures. Psychother Psychosom 57(3):118–127, 1992 1518919

Wise TN: The physician–patient relationship, in Behavioral Science. Edited by Wiener J. Media, PA, Harwal, 1990, pp 193–202

Younge JO, Gotink RA, Baena CP, et al: Mind-body practices for patients with cardiac disease: a systematic review and meta-analysis. Eur J Prev Cardiol 22(11):1385–1398, 2015

Zaman T, Rosenthal R, Renner J Jr, et al: Resource Document on Marijuana as Medicine. Arlington, VA, American Psychiatric Association, 2013. Available at: https://www.psychiatry.org/File%20Library/Psychiatrists/Directories/Library-and-Archive/resource_documents/rd2013_MarijuanaMedicine.pdf. Accessed July 25, 2019.

Recommended Readings

Levinson JL, Ferrando SJ: Clinical Manual of Psychopharmacology in the Medically Ill, 2nd Edition, Revised. Washington, DC, American Psychiatric Association Publishing, 2017

Taylor S, Asmundson GJG: Treating Health Anxiety: A Cognitive Behavioral Approach, 1st Edition. New York, Guilford, 2004

Wyszynski B, Ambrosino A: Manual of Psychiatric Care for the Medically Ill (Concise Guides). Washington, DC, American Psychiatric Publishing, 2005

CHAPTER 38

Anxiety and Insomnia

Thomas W. Uhde, M.D.

Nicole A. Short, Ph.D.

Bernadette M. Cortese, Ph.D.

The high comorbidity of anxiety and sleep complaints, including insomnia, is widely recognized. Among the anxiety disorders, DSM-5 (American Psychiatric Association 2013) lists sleep disturbances as a core feature of generalized anxiety disorder (GAD), and among the trauma- and stressor-related disorders, it lists them as a core feature of PTSD. Despite not being listed as a specific symptom in other anxiety disorders, sleep disturbance is prevalent in those disorders as well, with rates of sleep disturbances as high as 68% for panic disorder (Stein et al. 1993) and 30%–50% for social anxiety disorder (Zalta et al. 2013). Moreover, panic disorder is characterized by a high prevalence of sleep panic attacks, which often produce conditioned fear of sleep and resultant avoidance of sleep and the sleep environment (Uhde 2000). Interestingly, patients with primary insomnia also experience coexistent anxiety (Spira et al. 2008), and patients with insomnia may be at greater risk for developing anxiety later in life (Batterham et al. 2012; Breslau et al. 1996; Jansson-Fröjmark and Lindblom 2008; Morphy et al. 2007; Neckelmann et al. 2007; Weissman et al. 1997). Thus, the prevalence of comorbid insomnia in anxiety disorders and comorbid anxiety in insomnia suggests an important underlying relationship. Although the directionality and exact nature of this relationship remain unclear, it is prudent for the clinician to either develop separate treatments for each symptom cluster (i.e., anxiety and insomnia) or select a single treatment that produces a complete and full therapeutic response for the comorbid syndrome. In the latter case, this theoretically would take place when the anxiety and sleep disorders are the manifestations of a common underlying pathological abnormality (Uhde and Cortese 2008).

The purpose of this chapter is to provide an overview of the neurobiology and treatment of insomnia in GAD, social anxiety disorder, panic disorder, and PTSD and in related anxiety conditions that manifest sleep disturbances as key features of their phenomenology. In addition, we conclude with suggestions for future research.

Neurobiology: Arousal, Alarm, Vigilance, and Wake-Sleep Systems

Although a single neurotransmitter system does not alone mediate anxiety or sleep-wake states, several systems (GABAergic, serotonergic, noradrenergic, hypocretinergic [orexinergic], and histaminergic) are implicated in the neurobiology of arousal, alarm, vigilance, and wakefulness (i.e., systems reasonably thought to mediate hyperarousal). We focus on these systems because *states of hyperarousal* often are observed in many anxiety disorders and insomnia (Kalmbach et al. 2018; Nofzinger 2004; Riemann et al. 2010). We acknowledge that an exclusive focus on neurotransmitter-receptor systems involved in arousal-hyperarousal functions has limitations. No scientific consensus has been reached on what actually constitutes hyperarousal (i.e., different biological, cognitive, and behavioral manifestations). Moreover, no single operational or biological definition of hyperarousal is consistently used across all anxiety disorders or insomnia.

GABAergic System

As the brain's major inhibitory neurotransmitter system, crucial to regulation of brain excitability, the GABAergic system is the neurotransmitter pathway most widely implicated in both anxiety and insomnia, with the ionotropic $GABA_A$-benzodiazepine-chloride receptor complex that regulates chloride channels being particularly relevant for the biological functions of alarm, arousal, and sedation. Several lines of evidence in rodents and humans suggest that the $GABA_A$ receptors, perhaps particularly the α_1, α_2, α_3, and β_3 subunits, may play a partial role in the pathophysiology and treatment of insomnia and comorbid anxiety symptoms (Möhler et al. 2005; Rowlett et al. 2005).

Serotonergic System

The reticular formation has long been associated with functions of wakefulness. Moruzzi and Magoun (1949) conducted studies demonstrating that the transection of the reticular formation above the pons in the face of intact sensory inputs to higher brain regions is associated with behavior and electroencephalographic patterns consistent with sleep, whereas lesions of the reticular formation below the pons are associated with a reduction in sleep. These classic studies and subsequent research indicate that different neural networks within and impinging on the reticular formation mediate wakefulness and arousal functions, including serotonergic projections and activation of serotonin 2A ($5\text{-}HT_{2A}$) receptors at the level of the cerebral cortex and, possibly, the hypothalamus. The serotonergic receptor system is also strongly implicated in fearful animal behaviors and human anxiety disorders, particularly panic and obsessive-compulsive disorders. Knockouts of $5\text{-}HT_{1A}$ receptors are associated with increased fear behaviors in animal models, including, but not limited to, performance on elevated-plus maze and foot-shock, forced-swim, and open-field tests.

Noradrenergic System

Within the noradrenergic system, the pontine nucleus locus coeruleus plays a key role in arousal and vigilance in animals, and disturbances in this nucleus or its neuronal projections to the amygdala and related limbic substrates, hypothalamus, and nucleus accumbens have been implicated in panic disorder, GAD, PTSD, and insomnia (Alttoa et al. 2007; Aston-Jones et al. 1991; Charney et al. 1990, 1995; DeViva et al. 2004). Preclinical studies in rodents and monkeys have demonstrated that noradrenergic effects associated with fear and stress are in part mediated through activation of the locus coeruleus and subsequent increase of norepinephrine in the brain regions associated with anxiety (Aston-Jones and Cohen 2005; Korf et al. 1973; Redmond 1981). The locus coeruleus likely mediates its wakefulness-promoting effects, and presumably insomnia, via a number of actions, including direct activation of the cortex and pedunculopontine tegmental nucleus and inhibitory inputs to the ventral lateral preoptic nucleus, a galanin-related structure implicated in insomnia associated with aging (Gaus et al. 2002).

Emerging evidence indicates important interactions between the noradrenergic locus coeruleus and hypocretinergic (orexinergic) systems in the neurobiology of arousal and sleep.

Hypocretinergic (Orexinergic) System

Hypocretins (also known as orexins) are neuropeptides synthesized in the hypothalamus that play important roles in the neurobiology of arousal states such vigilance, alertness, anxiety, and wakefulness (for review, see James et al. 2017). The hypocretin (orexin) neurons (i.e., hypocretin 1 [orexin A] and hypocretin 2 [orexin B]) are located in the lateral hypothalamus, with projections to brain areas regulating arousal and anxiety. The hypocretins (orexins) mediate their effects via two receptor subtypes: hypocretin-orexin-1 and hypocretin-orexin-2 receptors. The hypocretin 1 (orexin A) endogenous ligand binds to both receptor subtypes, whereas the hypocretin 2 (orexin B) neuropeptide acts preferentially at the hypocretin-orexin-2 receptor subtype. Some overlapping, as well as regional specificity, occurs in the distribution of these brain receptor subtypes. For example, the rodent locus coeruleus exclusively expresses hypocretin-orexin-1 receptors. The differential brain distribution, as well as differences in the biological functions, of hypocretin-orexin receptor subtypes suggests that one could, in theory, develop hypocretinergic (orexinergic) antagonists with specific and nonspecific therapeutic profiles (Gozzi et al. 2011; for review see Kumar et al. 2016). For example, given the dense expression of hypocretin-orexin-1 receptors that activate firing of neurons from the locus coeruleus and the pathophysiological association between noradrenergic hyperactivity and panic disorder (Charney and Heninger 1986; Charney et al. 1990, 1995; Uhde et al. 1984), it is reasonable to hypothesize that hypocretin-orexin-1 receptor blockade might be effective in treating sleep-related disturbances in panic disorder, particularly in the subgroup of patients with panic disorder who experience panic attacks while sleeping. In contrast, hypocretin (orexin) antagonists with dual antagonism at both receptor subtypes might possess a broader spectrum of action in states of generalized anxiety or hyperarousal and primary insomnia.

Histaminergic System

Histamine and the histaminergic system have long been known to regulate arousal and wakefulness. Histaminergic neurons are located within and around the tuberomammillary nucleus (TMN) in humans and, similar to the noradrenergic locus coeruleus and serotonergic raphe, are excitatory neurotransmitters in terms of inducing and maintaining arousal. Histamine mediates its effects by binding to four histamine receptors (H_1, H_2, H_3, H_4), with the H_1 and H_3 receptors being most relevant to the neurobiology of anxiety and insomnia. H_1 agonists produce arousal/wakefulness, and H_1 antagonists induce sleep. The histamine H_3 receptor is an autoreceptor. H_3 agonists decrease and H_3 antagonists increase the release of histamine, which, as expected, induces sleep and wakefulness, respectively. The dose-dependent increase in wakefulness induced by H_3 antagonists (Parmentier et al. 2007) is absent in H_1 knockout mice (Huang et al. 2006). Together, these observations suggest functional interactions between the H_3 and H_1 receptors in the regulation of arousal and sleep-to-wakefulness transitions (Atkin et al. 2018).

Interestingly, the hypocretinergic-orexinergic system likely mediates much of the arousal-wakefulness properties via activation of histamine. Both local TMN and central administration of hypocretin-1 (orexin A) produce histamine release and wakefulness, which is absent in H_1 knockout mice (Huang et al. 2006). These findings indicate that downstream histamine actions may mediate a component of the wakefulness-promoting effects of hypocretin-orexin. Moreover, H_1 receptor agonists increase firing of neurons from the locus coeruleus, a system strongly linked to arousal, alarm, and anxiety.

Taken together, these findings indicate that the histaminergic system has important functional interactions with two other systems strongly linked to the neurobiology of arousal and wakefulness-sleep regulation. The histaminergic system, perhaps particularly H_1 receptor antagonists, should not be forgotten as a potential therapeutic target for mixed anxiety-insomnia conditions.

Melatoninergic System

Melatonin is primarily synthesized by the pituitary gland, and its effects are mediated via two G-protein coupled receptors (MT_1 and MT_2). Melatonin rises about 2 hours before the onset of sleep (Lewy and Sack 1989), remains elevated during sleep (unless subject is exposed to bright light), and then, under normal sleep-wake conditions, stays low throughout the day. Both of these factors (onset/offset of melatonin secretion and light exposure) influence the timing of the sleep-wake cycle.

Melatonin is suppressed by light, particularly short-wavelength or blue light, via the retinohypothalamic tract, which sends light signals from the retina to the master clock (i.e., the suprachiasmatic nucleus located in the anterior hypothalamus). The timing of melatonin and bright light exposure, respectively, can delay or advance the sleep-wake cycle. Light has greater phase-shifting potency than melatonin; thus, light exposure in the evening induces a phase delay (i.e., the individual goes to sleep much later), whereas light exposure in the morning causes a phase advance (waking up earlier in the morning). Melatonin has the opposite effect; melatonin taken in the early evening induces phase advance, whereas morning administration results in phase delay. These fundamental principles have resulted in the development of various therapeutic strategies using melatonin, melatonin agonists, and bright light exposure, alone or in combination, to treat insomnia and circadian rhythm sleep disorders.

Pharmacological Treatments

Although a neurotransmitter receptor–based model of pathophysiology and therapeutic drug selection has some practical utility for decision making, it is also overly simplistic because 1) anxiolytic medications influence, directly or indirectly, more than one neurotransmitter-receptor system and 2) the neurobiology of anxiety and insomnia, although often linked to physiological hyperarousal, is not identical. To the extent that the underlying anxiety state and its associated sleep disturbance (e.g., insomnia) are mediated by the same hyperarousal system(s), a medication that "normalizes" the arousal system(s) should, in theory, demonstrate convergent improvements in both anxiety and insomnia.

Tables 38–1 and 38–2, respectively, list FDA-approved drugs for the treatment of anxiety and the known effects of these drugs on sleep. These agents are generally used as first-line medications in the treatment of anxiety disorders. Table 38–3 presents a partial listing of medications that may be used off-label for treatment of anxiety or sleep disturbances; these drugs should be considered backup options for treating anxiety that is refractory or only partially responsive to first-line antianxiety medications. The sleep effects of the agents presented in Tables 38–2 and 38–3 represent best estimates based on a range of evidence, from low-quality and unvalidated observations (e.g., case reports) to high-quality evidence based on meta-analyses and placebo-controlled, randomized clinical trials; the quality of evidence should be considered and is available in the citations. Finally, any dosages or observations regarding effects on sleep are based upon findings in adults and should not be extrapolated to children.

GABAergic, Benzodiazepines, Z-Drugs

Although some benzodiazepine hypnotics and sleep-promoting Z-drugs may have transient antianxiety effects, traditional hypnotics such as flurazepam, estazolam, temazepam, triazolam, and quazepam are generally considered impractical for the off-label treatment of daytime anxiety because of their short half-life pharmacokinetics.

Serotonergic Medications

Selective serotonin reuptake inhibitors (SSRIs) are widely used by clinicians to treat most of the anxiety disorders, whereas trazodone, a tetracyclic SSRI with 5-HT$_2$ antagonist effects, may be the most frequently prescribed medication for the treatment of insomnia by psychiatrists and primary care physicians. Data are limited regarding secondary improvement in insomnia following targeted treatment of anxiety (or vice

TABLE 38–1.   **List of FDA-approved anxiolytics and indications**

Drugs and sites of action	Trade name	Indication
GABAergic		
Alprazolam	Xanax	Anxiety disorders, GAD, PD
Chlordiazepoxide	Librium	Anxiety disorders
Clonazepam	Klonopin	PD
Clorazepate dipotassium	Tranxene	Anxiety disorders
Diazepam	Valium	Anxiety disorders
Lorazepam	Ativan	Anxiety disorders
Meprobamate	Equanil	Anxiety disorders
Oxazepam	Serepax	Anxiety disorders
Serotonergic		
Escitalopram	Lexapro	GAD
Fluoxetine	Prozac	OCD, PD
Fluvoxamine maleate	Luvox	OCD
Paroxetine	Paxil	GAD, PD, PTSD, SAD, OCD
Paroxetine mesylate	Pexeva	GAD, PD, PTSD, SAD, OCD
Sertraline	Zoloft	PD, PTSD, SAD, OCD
Noradrenergic/Serotonergic		
Buspirone	BuSpar	Anxiety disorders
Duloxetine	Cymbalta	GAD
Venlafaxine	Effexor	GAD, PD, SAD
Histaminergic and mixed targets		
Amitriptyline-chlordiazepoxide	Limbitrol	Mixed depression/anxiety
Amitriptyline-perphenazine	Triavil	Mixed depression/anxiety
Amoxapine	Asendin	Mixed depression/anxiety
Clomipramine	Anafranil	OCD
Doxepin	Sinequan (Silenor)	Depression and/or anxiety
Hydroxyzine dihydrochloride	Atarax	Psychoneurotic anxiety
Hydroxyzine pamoate	Vistaril	Psychoneurotic anxiety
Prochlorperazine dimaleate	Compazine	Generalized nonpsychotic anxiety
Trifluoperazine dihydrochloride	Stelazine	Generalized nonpsychotic anxiety

Note.   GAD=generalized anxiety disorder; PD=panic disorder; SAD=social anxiety disorder.

versa). Older patients with anxiety disorders show improved sleep quality (e.g., age 60 years, with mainly GAD; Blank et al. 2006). However, not all individuals with anxiety disorder show parallel improvements in anxiety and insomnia when treated with SSRIs. Moreover, some SSRIs may be ineffective or may actually induce insomnia (Winokur et al. 2001). Thus, although SSRIs play a crucial role in the treatment of anxiety disorders, including those in which sleep problems are a core feature, the effects on insomnia are less predictable (Everitt et al. 2018).

TABLE 38–2.   FDA-approved anxiolytics: subjective and objective effects on sleep

Drug (trade name)	Subjective effects	Objective effects	References
GABAergic			
Alprazolam (Xanax), chlordiazepoxide (Librium)	↑ Sleep quality in panic disorder ↓ Insomnia in PTSD	↑ Sleep efficiency in panic disorder	Saletu-Zyhlarz et al. 2000 Braun et al. 1990
Clonazepam (Klonopin), clorazepate (Tranxene)	↑ Symptoms in chronic insomniacs	—	Schenck and Mahowald 1996
	—	↓ Total wake time in primary insomnia	Kales et al. 1991
	No change in PTSD	—	Cates et al. 2004
Diazepam (Valium)	↑ Sleep soundness/quality in primary insomnia	↓ Total wake time/sleep latency, ↑ stage 2/REM in primary insomnia	Kales et al. 1988
Lorazepam (Ativan)	↑ Sleep quality in GAD	↓ Awakenings/Time awake in GAD	Saletu et al. 1997
Meprobamate (Equanil)	—	↑ Stage 2, ↓ REM in healthy subjects	Freemon et al. 1965
Oxazepam (Serepax)	—	↑ Sleep duration, ↓ awakenings for insomnia	Gallais et al. 1983
Serotonergic			
Escitalopram (Lexapro)	Trend-level ↑ in sleep disturbance in PTSD	—	Robert et al. 2006
Fluoxetine (Prozac)	Some ↑ in sleep disturbance in MDD with insomnia	↓ Sleep efficiency/REM sleep, ↑ awakenings in MDD with insomnia	Gillin et al. 1997
Fluvoxamine (Luvox)	↑ HAM-D sleep items score in MDD ↑ Sleep quality in PTSD	↑ REM latency, ↓ REM sleep in MDD	Wilson et al. 2000 Neylan et al. 2001
Paroxetine (Paxil), paroxetine mesylate (Pexeva)	↑ Sleep quality in primary insomnia	No significant change in objective measures in primary insomnia	Nowell et al. 1999
Sertraline (Zoloft)	↓ Sleep disturbance in PTSD No change in sleep in MDD Insomnia most common adverse event in PTSD	↑ Sleep latency, ↓ REM sleep in MDD	Stein et al. 2003 Jindal et al. 2003 Davidson et al. 2001

TABLE 38–2. FDA-approved anxiolytics: subjective and objective effects on sleep *(continued)*

Drug (trade name)	Subjective effects	Objective effects	References
Noradrenergic/Serotonergic			
Buspirone (BuSpar)	No significant change in sleep in primary insomnia	↑ Time awake in primary insomnia	Manfredi et al. 1991
Duloxetine (Cymbalta)	Gradually ↑ insomnia symptoms in MDD	—	Hirschfeld et al. 2005
		↑ REM latency, ↓ REM sleep in MDD	Kluge et al. 2007
Venlafaxine (Effexor)	Gradually ↑ insomnia symptoms in GAD	—	Stahl et al. 2007
Mixed targets			
Amitriptyline-chlordiazepoxide (Limbitrol), amitriptyline-perphenazine (Triavil), amoxapine (Asendin)	↑ HAM-D, GAS, POMS, SAS in MDD with insomnia	↑ Sleep efficiency, ↓ awakenings/REM sleep in MDD with insomnia	Scharf et al. 1986
Clomipramine (Anafranil)	—	↓ REM sleep, sleep efficiency, maintenance, ↑ wakefulness in MDD	Kupfer et al. 1989
Doxepin (Sinequan)	↑ Sleep quality and working ability in primary insomnia	↑ Sleep efficiency in primary insomnia	Hajak et al. 2001
	↑ Sleep quality	↑ Sleep efficiency in primary insomnia	Roth et al. 2007
Hydroxyzine (Atarax, Vistaril), compazine, stelazine	↑ Sleep duration and sleep quality, ↓ nightmares and sleep latency in PTSD	—	Ahmadpanah et al. 2014

Note. Drugs grouped by primary neurotransmitter target.
GAD=generalized anxiety disorder; GAS=Global Assessment Scale; HAM-D=Hamilton Rating Scale for Depression; MDD=major depressive disorder; POMS=Profile of Mood State; REM=rapid eye movement; SAS=State Anxiety Scale.

TABLE 38–3. Off-label anxiolytics[a]: mechanisms of action and effects on sleep

Drug (trade name)	Off-label use		Mechanisms of action[b]		References
	Anxiety	**Sleep**	**Anxiety**	**Sleep**	
Amitriptyline (Elavil)	Pain-related anxiety Social anxiety disorder EMA (half life, 12–24 hours)	Insomnia ↓ Sleep latency ↓ REM ↑ Slow wave sleep ↑ Sleep efficiency	↑ NE, 5-HT via reuptake blocker	H₁, H₂ antagonists 5-HT₂A/5-HT₂C antagonists	Atkin et al. 2018; Wilson et al. 2010
Carbamazepine (Tegretol) Oxcarbazepine (Trileptal)	*100–200 mg/day* PTSD Panic disorder/PTSD *Carbamazepine 400 mg/ day*	*25–50 mg at bedtime* Healthy control subjects: ↓ Sleep latency ↓ REM ↑ Slow wave sleep ↑ Total sleep time Secondary insomnia[c]: ↑ Slow wave sleep *Carbamazepine 400–700 mg/day*	↑ GABA inhibition ↑ EAAT3 activity	↑ GABA inhibition ↑ EAAT3 activity	Ketter et al. 1999; Lee et al. 2005; Mula et al. 2007
Clonidine (Catapres)	Preoperative anxiety *0.1 mg* Withdrawal related anxiety (opiate, nicotine) Panic disorder (short-term prescription) *0.1–0.2 mg every 6–8 hours*	PTSD-related nightmares Nightmare disorder *Low dose (0.025 mg)* Presynaptic α₂ agonist ↓ NE release ↑ REM *Higher dose (0.15–2.0 mg)* Postsynaptic α₂ agonist ↓ REM	α₂ agonist ↓ NE release	Nonspecific binding to α₂A, α₂B, α₂C receptor subtypes	Belkin and Schwartz 2015; Detweiler et al. 2016; Henry et al. 2018; Uhde et al. 1989

TABLE 38–3. Off-label anxiolytics[a]: mechanisms of action and effects on sleep *(continued)*

Drug (trade name)	Off-label use — Anxiety	Off-label use — Sleep	Mechanisms of action[b] — Anxiety	Mechanisms of action[b] — Sleep	References
Gabapentin (Neurontin)	Panic disorder Social anxiety disorder PTSD *300–3,600 mg/day*	Primary insomnia: ↑ Slow wave sleep ↓ Wake after sleep onset ↑ Sleep efficiency ↑ Sleep quality *200–1,800 mg/day*	$\alpha_2\delta$-1 subunit of VGCC ↓ Release of glutamate	↑ GABA synthesis	Foldvary-Schaefer et al. 2002; Lo et al. 2010; Mula et al. 2007
Imipramine (Tofranil)	Panic disorder GAD PTSD *100–300 mg/day*	Cataplexy *10–100 mg/day*	↑ NE, 5-HT via reuptake blocker	↑ NE, 5-HT via reuptake blocker	Roth et al. 2007
Lamotrigine (Lamictal)	PTSD *500 mg/day*	Secondary insomnia[c]: ↑ REM ?↑ Slow wave sleep *200 mg/day*	Glutamate inhibitor		Foldvary et al. 2001; Mula et al. 2007; Placidi et al. 2000
Mirtazapine/Remeron	Cancer-related anxiety Pathological excoriation *15–45 mg/day*	Secondary insomnia: − Sleep latency ↑ Slow wave sleep ↑ Sleep efficiency *15 mg/day*	Presynaptic α_2 antagonist produces ↑ NE ↑ 5-HT release 5-HT$_2$/5-HT$_3$ receptor antagonists	H$_1$ antagonist	Atkin et al. 2018
Prazosin (Minipress)	PTSD *3–15 mg/day*	Trauma-related nightmares ↑ Sleep quality ↓ Severity of nightmares ↓ Frequency of nightmares *3–15 mg/day*	α_1 antagonist	α_1 antagonist	Ahmadpanah et al. 2014; Germain et al. 2012; Raskind et al. 2003, 2007, 2018

TABLE 38–3. Off-label anxiolytics[a]: mechanisms of action and effects on sleep *(continued)*

Drug (trade name)	Off-label use		Mechanisms of action[b]		References
	Anxiety	**Sleep**	**Anxiety**	**Sleep**	
Pregabalin (Lyrica)[d]	GAD Social anxiety disorder *300–600 mg/day*	↓Sleep latency ↑Slow wave sleep ↓Sleep maintenance insomnia ↓Early morning awakening *300–600 mg/day*	↓Release glutamate $\alpha_2\delta$-1 subunit of VGCC	$\alpha_2\delta$-1 subunit of VGCC	Boschen 2011; Frampton 2014; Holsboer-Trachsler and Prieto 2013; Houghton et al. 2017
Quetiapine (Seroquel)	GAD *IR 50–200 mg/day* *XR 50–150 mg/day* PTSD *50–400 mg/day*	Healthy control subjects: ↑Total sleep time ↑Sleep efficiency Secondary insomnia[c]: ↑Total sleep time ↑Sleep efficiency *25–100 mg/day*	5-HTα_2 5-HT$_{2C}$ D$_2$ antagonists	H$_1$ antagonist	Anderson and Vande Griend 2014; Atkin et al. 2018; Katzman et al. 2011; Khan et al. 2013
Tiagabine (Gabitril)	GAD *4–16 mg/day* PTSD	↑Sleep quality ↑Total sleep time Slow wave sleep ±↑REM	GABA receptor inhibitor	GABA receptor inhibitor	Mathias et al. 2001; Rosenthal 2003
Trazodone (Desyrel)	Panic disorder GAD (not typically prescribed even for major depression at higher dosage levels) *100–400 mg/day*	Secondary insomnia[c]: ↓Sleep latency ↓Sleep maintenance insomnia ↑Slow wave sleep ↓REM –Sleep efficiency *25–100 mg/day*	5-HT reuptake blocker 5-HT$_2$ receptor antagonist	H$_1$ antagonist	Atkin et al. 2018

TABLE 38–3.   Off-label anxiolytics[a]: mechanisms of action and effects on sleep (*continued*)

| Drug (trade name) | Off-label use | | Mechanisms of action[b] | | References |
	Anxiety	Sleep	Anxiety	Sleep	
Valproate (Depakote)	Panic disorder PTSD Social anxiety disorder *750–1,500 mg/day*	Secondary insomnia[c]: ↓ Sleep latency ↓ REM ↓ Wake after sleep onset *750–1,500 mg/day*	VGNC	↑ GABA transmission	Ketter et al. 1999; Mula et al. 2007

Note. ↑=increase; ↓=decrease; –=no change or not effective; ?=possible; 5-HT=serotonin; EAAT3=glutamate excitatory amino acid transporter subtype 3; GAD=generalized anxiety disorder; H=histamine receptor; IR=immediate release; NE=norepinephrine; REM=rapid eye movement; VGCC=voltage-gated calcium channel; VGNC=voltage-gated sodium channel; XR=extended release.

[a]Drugs sometimes used by clinicians to treat anxiety symptoms.

[b]Although most of these drugs have effects at multiple different receptor targets, those listed are believed to be the main targets or mechanisms involved in the anxiolytic and sedative-hypnotic properties.

[c]Insomnia attributed to a medical and/or mental health disorder (e.g., cancer, epilepsy, Alzheimer's, Parkinson's disease, major depression, schizophrenia).

[d]United Kingdom: GAD.

Noradrenergic Medications

Clonidine, an α_2-adrenergic agonist, has short-term but not long-term antianxiety effects in humans (Uhde et al. 1989). Theoretically, this effect parallels the initial inhibition of, followed by later tolerance to, the direct application of clonidine via iontophoresis onto the locus coeruleus in animals (Aghajanian and VanderMaelen 1982). Inhibition of the locus coeruleus also likely mediates the sedating and antianxiety effects of other α_2-adrenergic agonists such as dexmedetomidine and lofexidine. Similarly, the α_1-adrenergic antagonist prazosin has become a widely used medication for the treatment of anxiety, hyperarousal, and related PTSD symptoms, especially insomnia and nightmares (Raskind et al. 2003, 2007). A recent negative study in military veterans by the same researchers (Raskind et al. 2018), however, suggested the need for additional research to identify personalized as well as biological and genetic predictors of response (Ressler 2018). Peskind et al. (2003) also reported that nightmares strongly reappeared in older men (67–83 years of age) with PTSD when prazosin was discontinued.

Hypocretinergic (Orexinergic) Medications

Given that hypocretin (orexin)–locus coeruleus pathways interact to maintain wakefulness, that blockade of hypocretin-orexin receptors produces sleep in animals (Brisbare-Roch et al. 2007; Winrow et al. 2011), and that deficiencies in cerebrospinal fluid hypocretin-1 are associated with pathological hypersomnia (excessive daytime sleepiness) in narcolepsy (Mignot et al. 2002), it was inevitable that the pharmaceutical industry would develop and investigate hypocretin (orexin) antagonists as potential sleep-promoting agents (for review, see Scammell and Winrow 2011). This line of drug discovery proved fruitful; most, but not all, orexin antagonist compounds, especially those with greater binding to the hypocretinergic-orexinergic-2 receptor, were found to promote sleep in animals (see Janto et al. 2018; Kumar et al. 2016). These preclinical studies affirmed the concept that antagonism of hypocretin-orexin receptors can promote sleep, which has led to several hypocretin-orexin antagonists being investigated as sleep-promoting agents. At this point, only Suvorexant, which blocks hypocretin (orexin) neuropeptides at both hypocretin-orexin-1 and hypocretin-orexin-2 receptors (and thus is classified as a dual orexin receptor antagonist), is FDA approved for the treatment of insomnia in humans.

A word of caution regarding the use of orexin antagonists: sleep paralysis and frightening hypnopompic hallucinations may occur with Suvorexant. In a prior survey, we found that 50% of psychiatrists misdiagnose recurrent sleep paralysis and associated sleep-related hallucinations as psychotic disorders. Use of Suvorexant is contraindicated in people with prior histories of sleep paralysis or narcolepsy, but these untoward experiences may also occur in individuals without prior experiences of sleep paralysis, cataplexy, or hypnopompic/hypnagogic hallucinations.

Histaminergic Medications

Antihistamine drugs are not first-line medications for treatment of the anxiety and stress-related disorders that are the focus of this chapter (i.e., GAD, social anxiety disorder, panic disorder, and PTSD). However, antihistamine compounds such as hydroxyzine (in its various preparations: oral solutions, intramuscular injection, oral tablets) are often used by nonpsychiatric physicians to manage anxiety and distress associated with certain dermatological conditions (e.g., chronic idiopathic urticaria, contact dermatitis) and pre- or postoperative procedures. At the standard daily antidepressant dosage of 100–300 mg/day, doxepin likely mediates its therapeutic effects via blockade of the serotonin transporter (K_i [nM] 66.7 [Lexi-Drugs, Antidepressant Receptor Profile]) and norepinephrine transporter (K_i [nM] 29.4 [Lexi-Drugs, Antidepressant Receptor Profile]). At the dosage range approved by the FDA for insomnia (3–6 mg), doxepin most likely exerts its hypnotic effects via H_1 receptor blockade (K_i [nM] 0.24 [Lexi-Drugs, Antidepressant Receptor Profile]). Thus, doxepin has strong effects as a histamine receptor inhibitor. Interestingly, the lower dosage of doxepin (i.e., Silenor) was approved by the FDA for maintenance insomnia (i.e., insomnia characterized by awakenings after sleep onset with difficulty returning to sleep) but not for sleep-onset insomnia. However, a small study directly comparing doxepin with citalopram (non–placebo controlled) found doxepin to have similar positive effects on sleep latency (Wu et al. 2015). Like doxepin (Goforth 2009), amitriptyline at lower dosages (10–50 mg [Wilson et al. 2010]) probably induces sedative-hypnotic effects via blockade of H_1 receptors (K_i [nM] 1.1 [Lexi-Drugs, Antidepressant Receptor Profile]) rather than inhibition of serotonin and norepinephrine transporters at the dosages used to achieve an antidepressant response (100–300 mg/day).

Dermatological problems such as chronic and sleep-related pathological excoriations are sometimes observed in patients with panic disorder and GAD. Mirtazapine, another drug with FDA-approved indications for treatment of depression, is used off-label to treat anxiety associated with these dermatological problems; other anxiolytics with antihistaminergic effects also may be considered. Similar to doxepin and amitriptyline, the sedative-hypnotic effects of mirtazapine are attributable to blockade of H_1 receptors.

Melatoninergic Medications

Melatonin is relevant to the timing of sleep and therefore plays a role in the neurobiology and treatment of circadian rhythm sleep disorders and sleep-onset insomnia. Several different circadian rhythm sleep disorders exist (American Academy of Sleep Medicine 2014; American Psychiatric Association 2013), but the subtype most relevant to anxiety disorders is delayed sleep-phase disorder (DSPD). People with DSPD have a natural tendency to go to sleep much later in the evening (often 2–4 A.M.), and when they attempt to go to sleep at a conventionally normal time, they have great difficulty doing so (i.e., they experience sleep-onset insomnia). They also have difficulty waking up at the appropriate time to meet external expectations (e.g., going to school or work) and frequently experience sleep inertia (grogginess and confusion upon awakening).

In our clinical experience, DSPD is not uncommon in patients with anxiety disorders (i.e., GAD, panic disorder), but this clinical impression has not been confirmed by research. When DSPD is coexistent with pathological anxiety in adults, our recommended treatment approach includes a combination of patient-specific cognitive-behavioral therapy (CBT) for insomnia (see discussion later) and melatonin (2–5 mg, given 2–3 hours before desired bedtime). To achieve desired sleep-wake times in

DSPD, melatonin and light exposure can be combined with gradual (e.g., 1-hour) advances in the person's wake up time.

Nonpharmacological Interventions

CBT is the most commonly used nonpharmacological intervention for both anxiety and insomnia. Although CBT-targeted interventions for GAD or worry appear to reduce insomnia, additional research is required to establish the clinical significance of these effects (Bélanger et al. 2004; Bootzin 1972; McGowan and Behar 2013). With regard to social anxiety disorder, evidence is quite mixed; the effectiveness of CBT for social anxiety may be reduced in the presence of insomnia and may have no impact on co-occurring sleep problems (Kushnir et al. 2014; Tang 2010; Zalta et al. 2013). From a practical perspective, symptoms of social anxiety and insomnia should be independently evaluated on a case-by-case basis both during and after treatment with CBT.

CBT has also been assessed for comorbid PTSD and insomnia. Although PTSD, along with some symptoms of sleep disturbance such as nightmares (Keane et al. 1989), improves with treatment, insomnia may not respond well to CBT for PTSD. Specifically, insomnia symptoms may decrease following CBT for PTSD (Belleville et al. 2011; Galovski et al. 2009; Gutner et al. 2013), but they do not fully remit, and many participants continue to exhibit clinically significant symptoms of insomnia even after treatment. For complete symptom resolution, it may be necessary for patients to undergo additional CBT specifically targeting insomnia (DeViva et al. 2005).

A typical component of CBT for insomnia is *sleep restriction*, with the goal of maximizing sleep efficiency, or the amount of time in bed spent sleeping (>85%), and improving sleep latency and wake after sleep onset. Basically, sleep restriction limits the amount of time patients spend in bed (usually no less than 4–5 hours) to the amount of real time that they spend sleeping while in bed. The actual time patients sleep while in bed is obtained via self-report, actigraphy, or polysomnography and takes into account sleep latency and wake after sleep onset (Perlis et al. 2000).

Sleep restriction is generally well tolerated (despite initial "resistance" when patients whose experience is that they get "too little" sleep are instructed to decrease their time in bed) (Perlis et al. 2000; Smith et al. 2005). Sleep restriction should be avoided in sleep apnea.

Limitations of the Evidence

From a *theoretical* perspective, it makes sense to treat the disorder (e.g., anxiety disorder or insomnia) that heralded the onset of illness. However, from a *practical* perspective, it will often be necessary to treat the anxiety and insomnia symptoms separately.

Future Research

Although highly speculative, the possibility exists that the hypocretinergic (orexinergic) system emerged during evolution as a specialized system to monitor threat during sleep, a period of maximum vulnerability to threats in the wild. Such a system might be relevant to patients who experience nonrestorative sleep and those who are intolerant to the muscle-relaxant properties of benzodiazepine hypnotic compounds. Orexin antagonists have been shown to improve sleep while at the same time allowing animals to awaken to external stimuli more easily than traditional hypnotic compounds. Given that the hypocretinergic/orexinergic system increases firing of neurons from the locus coeruleus via hypocretin-A/orexin-1 receptors, the possible role of selective hypocretin-A/orexin-1 antagonists in the treatment of anxiety-insomnia disorders, especially those syndromes characterized by noradrenergic hyperactivity and hyperarousal, is a particularly appealing area for research.

Key Points

- The high prevalence of comorbid insomnia in primary anxiety disorder and comorbid anxiety symptoms in primary insomnia suggests an important underlying relationship between these entities.

- Several neurotransmitter systems (noradrenergic, GABAergic, serotonergic, histaminergic, and hypocretinergic-orexinergic) are involved in the pathophysiology of anxiety-insomnia.

- Anxiety and insomnia sometimes respond favorably to similar pharmacological treatments (e.g., benzodiazepines, selective serotonin reuptake inhibitors) and nonpharmacological interventions (e.g., cognitive-behavioral therapy).

- In all likelihood, many patients with comorbid anxiety and insomnia will fail to achieve full remission after successful treatment of one disorder, making separate treatment necessary.

References

Aghajanian GK, VanderMaelen CP: Alpha 2-adrenoceptor-mediated hyperpolarization of locus coeruleus neurons: intracellular studies in vivo. Science 215(4538):1394–1396, 1982 6278591

Ahmadpanah M, Sabzeiee P, Hosseini SM, et al: Comparing the effect of prazosin and hydroxyzine on sleep quality in patients suffering from posttraumatic stress disorder. Neuropsychobiology 69(4):235–242, 2014 24993832

Alttoa A, Eller M, Herm L, et al: Amphetamine-induced locomotion, behavioral sensitization to amphetamine, and striatal D2 receptor function in rats with high or low spontaneous exploratory activity: differences in the role of locus coeruleus. Brain Res 1131(1):138–148, 2007 17156751

American Academy of Sleep Medicine: International Classification of Sleep Disorders, 3rd Edition: Diagnostic and Coding Manual. Darien, IL, American Academy of Sleep Medicine, 2014

American Psychiatric Association: Diagnostic and Statistical Manual of Mental Disorders, 5th Edition. Arlington, VA, American Psychiatric Association, 2013

Anderson SL, Vande Griend JP: Quetiapine for insomnia: a review of the literature. Am J Health Syst Pharm 71(5):394–402, 2014 24534594

Aston-Jones G, Cohen JD: Adaptive gain and the role of the locus coeruleus-norepinephrine system in optimal performance. J Comp Neurol 493(1):99–110, 2005 16254995

Aston-Jones G, Chiang C, Alexinsky T: Discharge of noradrenergic locus coeruleus neurons in behaving rats and monkeys suggests a role in vigilance. Prog Brain Res 88:501–520, 1991 1813931

Atkin T, Comai S, Gobbi G: Drugs for insomnia beyond benzodiazepines: pharmacology, clinical applications, and Discovery. Pharmacol Rev 70(2):197–245, 2018 29487083

Batterham PJ, Glozier N, Christensen H: Sleep disturbance, personality and the onset of depression and anxiety: prospective cohort study. Aust N Z J Psychiatry 46(11):1089–1098, 2012 22899700

Bélanger L, Morin CM, Langlois F, et al: Insomnia and generalized anxiety disorder: effects of cognitive behavior therapy for GAD on insomnia symptoms. J Anxiety Disord 18(4):561–571, 2004 15149714

Belkin MR, Schwartz TL: Alpha-2 receptor agonists for the treatment of posttraumatic stress disorder. Drugs Context 4:212286, 2015 26322115

Belleville G, Guay S, Marchand A: Persistence of sleep disturbances following cognitive-behavior therapy for posttraumatic stress disorder. J Psychosom Res 70(4):318–327, 2011 21414451

Blank S, Lenze EJ, Mulsant BH, et al: Outcomes of late-life anxiety disorders during 32 weeks of citalopram treatment. J Clin Psychiatry 67(3):468–472, 2006 16649835

Bootzin RR: Stimulus control treatment for insomnia. Proceedings of the American Psychological Association 7:395–396, 1972

Boschen MJ: A meta-analysis of the efficacy of pregabalin in the treatment of generalized anxiety disorder. Can J Psychiatry 56(9):558–566, 2011 21959031

Braun P, Greenberg D, Dasberg H, et al: Core symptoms of posttraumatic stress disorder unimproved by alprazolam treatment. J Clin Psychiatry 51(6):236–238, 1990 2189869

Breslau N, Roth T, Rosenthal L, et al: Sleep disturbance and psychiatric disorders: a longitudinal epidemiological study of young adults. Biol Psychiatry 39(6):411–418, 1996 8679786

Brisbare-Roch C, Dingemanse J, Koberstein R, et al: Promotion of sleep by targeting the orexin system in rats, dogs and humans. Nat Med 13(2):150–155, 2007 17259994

Cates ME, Bishop MH, Davis LL, et al: Clonazepam for treatment of sleep disturbances associated with combat-related posttraumatic stress disorder. Ann Pharmacother 38(9):1395–1399, 2004 15252193

Charney DS, Heninger GR: Abnormal regulation of noradrenergic function in panic disorders: effects of clonidine in healthy subjects and patients with agoraphobia and panic disorder. Arch Gen Psychiatry 43(11):1042–1052, 1986 3021083

Charney DS, Woods SW, Nagy LM, et al: Noradrenergic function in panic disorder. J Clin Psychiatry 51(suppl A):5–11, 1990 2258377

Charney DS, Deutch AY, Southwick SM, et al: Neural circuits and mechanisms of post-traumatic stress disorder, in Neurobiological and Clinical Consequences of Stress: From Normal Adaptation to Post Traumatic Stress Disorder. Edited by Friedman MJ, Charney DS, Deutch AY. Philadelphia, PA, Lippincott-Raven, 1995, pp 271–287

Davidson JR, Rothbaum BO, van der Kolk BA, et al: Multicenter, double-blind comparison of sertraline and placebo in the treatment of posttraumatic stress disorder. Arch Gen Psychiatry 58(5):485–492, 2001 11343529

Detweiler MB, Pagdala B, Candelario J, et al: Treatment of post-traumatic stress disorder nightmares at a Veterans Affairs medical center. J Clin Med 5(12):117, 2016 27999253

DeViva JC, Zayfert C, Mellman TA: Factors associated with insomnia among civilians seeking treatment for PTSD: an exploratory study. Behav Sleep Med 2(3):162–176, 2004 15600231

DeViva JC, Zayfert C, Pigeon WR, et al: Treatment of residual insomnia after CBT for PTSD: case studies. J Trauma Stress 18(2):155–159, 2005 16281208

Everitt H, Baldwin DS, Stuart B, et al: Antidepressants for insomnia in adults. Cochrane Database Syst Rev 5:CD010753, 2018 29761479

Foldvary N, Perry M, Lee J, et al: The effects of lamotrigine on sleep in patients with epilepsy. Epilepsia 42(12):1569–1573, 2001 11879368

Foldvary-Schaefer N, De Leon Sanchez I, Karafa M, et al: Gabapentin increases slow-wave sleep in normal adults. Epilepsia 43(12):1493–1497, 2002 12460250

Frampton JE: Pregabalin: a review of its use in adults with generalized anxiety disorder. CNS Drugs 28(9):835–854, 2014 25149863

Freemon FR, Agnew HW Jr, Williams RL: An electroencephalographic study of the effects of meprobamate on human sleep. Clin Pharmacol Ther 6(2):172–176, 1965 14288186

Gallais H, Casanova P, Fabregat H: Midazolam and oxazepam in the treatment of insomnia in hospitalized patients. Br J Clin Pharmacol 16(suppl 1):145S–149S, 1983 6138068

Galovski TE, Monson C, Bruce SE, et al: Does cognitive-behavioral therapy for PTSD improve perceived health and sleep impairment? J Trauma Stress 22(3):197–204, 2009 19466746

Gaus SE, Strecker RE, Tate BA, et al: Ventrolateral preoptic nucleus contains sleep-active, galaninergic neurons in multiple mammalian species. Neuroscience 115(1):285–294, 2002 12401341

Germain A, Richardson R, Moul DE, et al: Placebo-controlled comparison of prazosin and cognitive-behavioral treatments for sleep disturbances in US Military Veterans. J Psychosom Res 72(2):89–96, 2012 22281448

Gillin JC, Rapaport M, Erman MK, et al: A comparison of nefazodone and fluoxetine on mood and on objective, subjective, and clinician-rated measures of sleep in depressed patients: a double-blind, 8-week clinical trial. J Clin Psychiatry 58(5):185–192, 1997 9184611

Goforth HW: Low-dose doxepin for the treatment of insomnia: emerging data. Expert Opin Pharmacother 10(10):1649–1655, 2009 19496739

Gozzi A, Turrini G, Piccoli L et al: Functional magnetic resonance imaging reveals different neural substrates for the effects of orexin-1 and orexin-2 receptor antagonists. PLoS One 6(1):e16406, 2011 21307957

Gutner CA, Casement MD, Stavitsky Gilbert K, et al: Change in sleep symptoms across cognitive processing therapy and prolonged exposure: a longitudinal perspective. Behav Res Ther 51(12):817–822, 2013 24184428

Hajak G, Rodenbeck A, Voderholzer U, et al: Doxepin in the treatment of primary insomnia: a placebo-controlled, double-blind, polysomnographic study. J Clin Psychiatry 62(6):453–463, 2001 11465523

Henry RG, Raybould TP, Romond K, et al: Clonidine as a preoperative sedative. Spec Care Dentist 38(2):80–88, 2018 24184428

Hirschfeld RM, Mallinckrodt C, Lee TC, et al: Time course of depression-symptom improvement during treatment with duloxetine. Depress Anxiety 21(4):170–177, 2005 16035056

Holsboer-Trachsler E, Prieto R: Effects of pregabalin on sleep in generalized anxiety disorder. Int J Neuropsychopharmacol 16(4):925–936, 2013 23009881

Houghton KT, Forrest A, Awad A, et al: Biological rationale and potential clinical use of gabapentin and pregabalin in bipolar disorder, insomnia and anxiety: protocol for a systematic review and meta-analysis. BMJ Open 7(3):e013433, 2017 28348186

Huang Z-L, Mochizuki T, Qu W-M, et al: Altered sleep-wake characteristics and lack of arousal response to H3 receptor antagonist in histamine H1 receptor knockout mice. Proc Natl Acad Sci USA 103(12):4687–4692, 2006 16537376

James MH, Campbell EJ, Dayas CV: Role of the orexin/hypocretin system in stress-related psychiatric disorders. Curr Top Behav Neurosci 33:197–219, 2017 28083790

Jansson-Fröjmark M, Lindblom K: A bidirectional relationship between anxiety and depression, and insomnia? A prospective study in the general population. J Psychosom Res 64(4):443–449, 2008 18374745

Janto K, Prichard JR, Pusalavidyasagar S: An update on dual orexin receptor antagonists and their potential role in insomnia therapeutics. J Clin Sleep Med 14(8):1399–1408, 2018 30092886

Jindal RD, Friedman ES, Berman SR, et al: Effects of sertraline on sleep architecture in patients with depression. J Clin Psychopharmacol 23(6):540–548, 2003 14624183

Kales A, Soldatos CR, Bixler EO, et al: Diazepam: effects on sleep and withdrawal phenomena. J Clin Psychopharmacol 8(5):340–346, 1988 3183072

Kales A, Manfredi RL, Vgontzas AN, et al: Clonazepam: sleep laboratory study of efficacy and withdrawal. J Clin Psychopharmacol 11(3):189–193, 1991 2066457

Kalmbach DA, Cuamatzi-Castelan AS, Tonnu CV, et al: Hyperarousal and sleep reactivity in insomnia: current insights. Nat Sci Sleep 10:193–201, 2018 30046255

Katzman MA, Brawman-Mintzer O, Reyes EB, et al: Extended release quetiapine fumarate (quetiapine XR) monotherapy as maintenance treatment for generalized anxiety disorder: a long-term, randomized, placebo-controlled trial. Int Clin Psychopharmacol 26(1):11–24, 2011 20881846

Keane TM, Fairbank JA, Caddell JM, et al: Implosive (flooding) therapy reduces symptoms of PTSD in Vietnam combat veterans. Behav Ther 20:245–260, 1989

Ketter TA, Post RM, Theodore WH: Positive and negative psychiatric effects of antiepileptic drugs in patients with seizure disorders. Neurology 53(5 suppl 2):S53–S67, 1999 10496235

Khan A, Atkinson S, Mezhebovsky I, et al: Extended-release quetiapine fumarate (quetiapine XR) as adjunctive therapy in patients with generalized anxiety disorder and a history of inadequate treatment response: a randomized, double-blind study. Ann Clin Psychiatry 25(4):E7–E22, 2013 24199224

Kluge M, Schüssler P, Steiger A: Duloxetine increases stage 3 sleep and suppresses rapid eye movement (REM) sleep in patients with major depression. Eur Neuropsychopharmacol 17(8):527–531, 2007 17337164

Korf J, Aghajanian GK, Roth RH: Increased turnover of norepinephrine in the rat cerebral cortex during stress: role of the locus coeruleus. Neuropharmacology 12(10):933–938, 1973 4750561

Kumar A, Chanana P, Choudhary S: Emerging role of orexin antagonists in insomnia therapeutics: an update on SORAs and DORAs. Pharmacol Rep 68(2):231–242, 2016 26922522

Kupfer DJ, Ehlers CL, Pollock BG, et al: Clomipramine and EEG sleep in depression. Psychiatry Res 30(2):165–180, 1989 2694201

Kushnir J, Marom S, Mazar M, et al: The link between social anxiety disorder, treatment outcome, and sleep difficulties among patients receiving cognitive behavioral group therapy. Sleep Med 15(5):515–521, 2014 24767722

Lee G, Huang Y, Washington JM, et al: Carbamazepine enhances the activity of glutamate transporter type 3 via phosphatidylinositol 3-kinase. Epilepsy Res 66(1–3):145–153, 2005 16150575

Lewy AJ, Sack RL: The dim light melatonin onset as a marker for circadian phase position. Chronobiol Int 6(1):93–102, 1989 2706705

Lo HS, Yang CM, Lo HG, et al: Treatment effects of gabapentin for primary insomnia. Clin Neuropharmacol 33(2):84–90, 2010 20124884

Manfredi RL, Kales A, Vgontzas AN, et al: Buspirone: sedative or stimulant effect? Am J Psychiatry 148(9):1213–1217, 1991 1883000

Mathias S, Wetter TC, Steiger A, et al: The GABA uptake inhibitor tiagabine promotes slow wave sleep in normal elderly subjects. Neurobiol Aging 22(2):247–253, 2001 11182474

McGowan SK, Behar E: A preliminary investigation of stimulus control training for worry: effects on anxiety and insomnia. Behav Modif 37(1):90–112, 2013 22977265

Mignot E, Lammers GJ, Ripley B, et al: The role of cerebrospinal fluid hypocretin measurement in the diagnosis of narcolepsy and other hypersomnias. Arch Neurol 59(10):1553–1562, 2002 12374492

Möhler H, Fritschy JM, Vogt K, et al: Pathophysiology and pharmacology of GABA(A) receptors. Handb Exp Pharmacol (169):225–247, 2005 16594261

Morphy H, Dunn KM, Lewis M, et al: Epidemiology of insomnia: a longitudinal study in a UK population. Sleep 30(3):274–280, 2007 17425223

Moruzzi G, Magoun HW: Brain stem reticular formation and activation of the EEG. Electroencephalogr Clin Neurophysiol 1(4):455–473, 1949 18421835

Mula M, Pini S, Cassano GB: The role of anticonvulsant drugs in anxiety disorders: a critical review of the evidence. J Clin Psychopharmacol 27(3):263–272, 2007 17502773

Neckelmann D, Mykletun A, Dahl AA: Chronic insomnia as a risk factor for developing anxiety and depression. Sleep 30(7):873–880, 2007 17682658

Neylan TC, Metzler TJ, Schoenfeld FB, et al: Fluvoxamine and sleep disturbances in posttraumatic stress disorder. J Trauma Stress 14(3):461–467, 2001 11534878

Nofzinger EA: What can neuroimaging findings tell us about sleep disorders? Sleep Med 5(suppl 1):S16–S22, 2004 15301993

Nowell PD, Reynolds CF 3rd, Buysse DJ, et al: Paroxetine in the treatment of primary insomnia: preliminary clinical and electroencephalogram sleep data. J Clin Psychiatry 60(2):89–95, 1999 10084634

Parmentier R, Anaclet C, Guhennec C, et al: The brain H3-receptor as a novel therapeutic target for vigilance and sleep-wake disorders. Biochem Pharmacol 73(8):1157–1171, 2007 17288995

Perlis M, Aloia M, Milliken A, et al: Behavioral treatment of insomnia: a clinical case series study. J Behav Med 23(2):149–161, 2000 17288995

Peskind ER, Bonner LT, Hoff DJ, et al: Prazosin reduces trauma-related nightmares in older men with chronic posttraumatic stress disorder. J Geriatr Psychiatry Neurol 16(3):165–171, 2003 12967060

Placidi F, Marciani MG, Diomedi M, et al: Effects of lamotrigine on nocturnal sleep, daytime somnolence and cognitive functions in focal epilepsy. Acta Neurol Scand 102(2):81–86, 2000 10949523

Raskind MA, Peskind ER, Kanter ED, et al: Reduction of nightmares and other PTSD symptoms in combat veterans by prazosin: a placebo-controlled study. Am J Psychiatry 160(2):371–373, 2003 12562588

Raskind MA, Peskind ER, Hoff DJ, et al: A parallel group placebo controlled study of prazosin for trauma nightmares and sleep disturbance in combat veterans with post-traumatic stress disorder. Biol Psychiatry 61(8):928–934, 2007 17069768

Raskind MA, Peskind B, Chow C, et al: Trial of prazosin for post-traumatic stress disorder in military veterans. N Engl J Med 378(6):507–517, 2018 29414272

Redmond DE Jr: Clonidine and the primate locus coeruleus: evidence suggesting anxiolytic and anti-withdrawal effects. Prog Clin Biol Res 71:147–163, 1981 6276892

Ressler KJ: Alpha-adrenergic receptors in PTSD—failure or time for precision medicine? N Engl J Med 378(6):575–576, 2018 29414268

Riemann D, Spiegelhalder K, Feige B, et al: The hyperarousal model of insomnia: a review of the concept and its evidence. Sleep Med Rev 14(1):19–31, 2010 19481481

Robert S, Hamner MB, Ulmer HG, et al: Open-label trial of escitalopram in the treatment of posttraumatic stress disorder. J Clin Psychiatry 67(10):1522–1526, 2006 17107242

Rosenthal M: Tiagabine for the treatment of generalized anxiety disorder: a randomized, open-label, clinical trial with paroxetine as a positive control. J Clin Psychiatry 64(10):1245–1249, 2003 14658975

Roth T, Rogowski R, Hull S, et al: Efficacy and safety of doxepin 1 mg, 3 mg, and 6 mg in adults with primary insomnia. Sleep 30(11):1555–1561, 2007 18041488

Rowlett JK, Cook JM, Duke AN, et al: Selective antagonism of GABAA receptor subtypes: an in vivo approach to exploring the therapeutic and side effects of benzodiazepine-type drugs. CNS Spectr 10(1):40–48, 2005 15618946

Saletu B, Saletu-Zyhlarz G, Anderer P, et al: Nonorganic insomnia in generalized anxiety disorder. 2. Comparative studies on sleep, awakening, daytime vigilance and anxiety under lorazepam plus diphenhydramine (Somnium) versus lorazepam alone, utilizing clinical, polysomnographic and EEG mapping methods. Neuropsychobiology 36(3):130–152, 1997 9313245

Saletu-Zyhlarz GM, Anderer P, Berger P, et al: Nonorganic insomnia in panic disorder: comparative sleep laboratory studies with normal controls and placebo-controlled trials with alprazolam. Hum Psychopharmacol 15(4):241–254, 2000 12404319

Scammell TE, Winrow CJ: Orexin receptors: pharmacology and therapeutic opportunities. Annu Rev Pharmacol Toxicol 51:243–266, 2011 21034217

Scharf MB, Hirschowitz J, Zemlan FP, et al: Comparative effects of limbitrol and amitriptyline on sleep efficiency and architecture. J Clin Psychiatry 47(12):587–591, 1986 3536890

Schenck CH, Mahowald MW: Long-term, nightly benzodiazepine treatment of injurious parasomnias and other disorders of disrupted nocturnal sleep in 170 adults. Am J Med 100(3):333–337, 1996 8629680

Smith MT, Huang MI, Manber R: Cognitive behavior therapy for chronic insomnia occurring within the context of medical and psychiatric disorders. Clin Psychol Rev 25(5):559–592, 2005 15970367

Spira AP, Friedman L, Aulakh JS, et al: Subclinical anxiety symptoms, sleep, and daytime dysfunction in older adults with primary insomnia. J Geriatr Psychiatry Neurol 21(2):149–153, 2008 18474724

Stahl SM, Ahmed S, Haudiquet V: Analysis of the rate of improvement of specific psychic and somatic symptoms of general anxiety disorder during long-term treatment with venlafaxine ER. CNS Spectr 12(9):703–711, 2007 17805217

Stein DJ, Davidson J, Seedat S, et al: Paroxetine in the treatment of post-traumatic stress disorder: pooled analysis of placebo-controlled studies. Expert Opin Pharmacother 4(10):1829–1838, 2003 14521492

Stein MB, Kroft CD, Walker JR: Sleep impairment in patients with social phobia. Psychiatry Res 49(3):251–256, 1993 8177919

Tang NK: Brief CBT-I for insomnia comorbid with social phobia: a case study. Behav Cogn Psychother 38(1):113–122, 2010 19852878

Uhde T: The anxiety disorders, in Principles and Practice in Sleep Medicine, 3rd Edition. Edited by Kryger MH, Roth T, Dement W. Philadelphia, PA, WB Saunders, 2000, pp 1123–1139

Uhde T, Cortese BM: Anxiety and insomnia: theoretical relationship and future research, in Anxiety in Health Behaviors and Physical Illness. Edited by Zvolensky MJ, Smits JA. New York, Springer, 2008, pp 105–127

Uhde TW, Boulenger JP, Post RM, et al: Fear and anxiety: relationship to noradrenergic function. Psychopathology 17(suppl 3):8–23, 1984 6505121

Uhde TW, Stein MB, Vittone BJ, et al: Behavioral and physiologic effects of short-term and long-term administration of clonidine in panic disorder. Arch Gen Psychiatry 46(2):170–177, 1989 2643934

Weissman MM, Greenwald S, Niño-Murcia G, et al: The morbidity of insomnia uncomplicated by psychiatric disorders. Gen Hosp Psychiatry 19(4):245–250, 1997 9327253

Wilson SJ, Bell C, Coupland NJ, et al: Sleep changes during long-term treatment of depression with fluvoxamine—a home-based study. Psychopharmacology (Berl) 149(4):360–365, 2000 10867963

Wilson SJ, Nutt DJ, Alford C, et al: British Association for Psychopharmacology consensus statement on evidence-based treatment of insomnia, parasomnia and circadian rhythm disorders. J Psychopharmacol 24(11):1577–1601, 2010 20813762

Winokur A, Gary KA, Rodner S, et al: Depression, sleep physiology, and antidepressant drugs. Depress Anxiety 14(1):19–28, 2001 11568979

Winrow CJ, Gotter AL, Cox CD, et al: Promotion of sleep by suvorexant—a novel dual orexin receptor antagonist. J Neurogenet 25(1–2):52–61, 2011 21473737

Wu J, Chang F, Zu H: Efficacy and safety evaluation of citalopram and doxepin on sleep quality in comorbid insomnia and anxiety disorders. Exp Ther Med 10(4):1303–1308, 2015 26622482

Zalta AK, Dowd S, Rosenfield D, et al: Sleep quality predicts treatment outcome in CBT for social anxiety disorder. Depress Anxiety 30(11):1114–1120, 2013 24038728

Recommended Readings

Everitt H, Baldwin DS, Stuart B, et al: Antidepressants for insomnia in adults (review). Cochrane Database Syst Rev 5:CD010753, 2018

Kryger MH, Roth T (eds): Principles and Practice of Sleep Medicine, 6th Edition. Philadelphia, PA, Elsevier, 2017

Perlis MJ, Jungquist C, Smith MT, et al: Cognitive Behavioral Treatment of Insomnia. New York, Springer Science+Business Media, 2008

Short NA, Allan NP, Schmidt NB: Sleep disturbance as a predictor of affective functioning and symptom severity among individuals with PTSD: an ecological momentary assessment study. Behav Res Ther 97:146–153, 2017

Tobias T, Comai S, Gobbi G: Drugs for insomnia beyond benzodiazepines: pharmacology, clinical applications, and discovery. Pharmacol Rev 70(2):197–245, 2018

PART X

Anxiety Disorders in Special Populations

CHAPTER 39

Childhood Anxiety Disorders

Sandra S. Pimentel, Ph.D.

Carolyn Spiro-Levitt, Ph.D.

Anne Marie Albano, Ph.D., ABPP

This chapter provides an overview of child- and adolescent-onset anxiety disorders, including separation anxiety disorder, generalized anxiety disorder (GAD), social anxiety disorder, panic disorder, selective mutism, and specific phobias. Anxiety is a normative emotion, and fears experienced by children and adolescents are generally developmentally appropriate. Anxiety serves a neurobiologically based protective function that alerts the individual to potential threat, motivates preparatory behaviors, and is instructive during childhood for developing and refining adaptive skills.

Phenomenology

When anxiety becomes excessive, prolonged, uncontrollable, and interfering, it can become pathological, disrupting developmental functioning. Youth anxiety disorders are the most common class of psychiatric disorders, with a lifetime prevalence of almost 32% (Merikangas et al. 2010). Regardless of epidemiological methodology (Costello et al. 2004), anxiety disorders in youth are a significant public health concern. Even subclinical presentations may be associated with impairments (Angold et al. 1999), which may functionally impact youth trajectories into adulthood (Swan and Kendall 2016).

Anxiety disorders in youth are highly comorbid and can co-occur with other disorders, most frequently other anxiety disorders and OCD (Kendall et al. 2010). Although they may also co-occur with depression (Costello et al. 2004), they often precede mood disorders and indicate heightened risk for depression and suicide (Beesdo et al. 2007; Gould et al. 1998). Youth with both anxiety and depression have a significantly worse long-term prognosis than those with anxiety alone (Pine et al. 1998). Social anxiety disorder and panic disorder also indicate risk for substance abuse disorders (Clark and Neighbors 1996). Anxiety disorders are also comorbid with ADHD, disruptive behavior disorders, and externalizing conditions, and comorbidity likely reflects increased impairment (Costello et al. 2004; Curry et al. 2004). Age and developmental stage are relevant as well. Children may have difficulty expressing the specific nature of anxiety, further complicating diagnostic clarification. Multiple fears (e.g., safety, dark, illness) can overlap across anxiety disorders; excessive worry can be difficult to disentangle from intrusive obsessions and depressogenic rumination; inattention may emerge from apprehensive preoccupation in GAD as well as an attention deficit in ADHD.

Experiencing distress upon separating from a primary caregiver is developmentally appropriate and normatively transient for most young children. However, youth with separation anxiety disorder express anxiety that is excessive and beyond developmental appropriateness (American Psychiatric Association 2013). Diagnostic criteria can include distress in anticipation of or during times of separation, refusals to separate, excessive fears about harm befalling themselves or their parent, difficulty sleeping independently, nightmares, and somatic symptoms (American Psychiatric Association 2013). Youth with separation anxiety disorder may exhibit tearfulness, tantrums, reassurance-seeking, and extreme clinginess and must exhibit associated functional impairment for at least 4 weeks. They may ask their parents repeated questions about separations, demand a parent stay with them at bedtime, and have difficulty staying at school.

Worry, characterized in DSM-5 as "apprehensive expectation" (American Psychiatric Association 2013), is the central feature of GAD when it becomes excessive and uncontrollable. Evidence suggests that youth can normatively worry about topics including school, friends, health, and safety (Muris et al. 1998); what distinguishes clinical from nonclinical worry is the intensity and number of worries (Weems et al. 2000). To be diagnosed, youth must experience at least one of the following as a result of their worry: restlessness, excessive fatigue, difficulty concentrating, irritability, and trouble sleeping (American Psychiatric Association 2013). Adult diagnosis requires three of these symptoms. Worry must cause significant academic, interpersonal, and developmental impairment, and evidence suggests youth diagnosed with GAD are more functionally impaired than their nonanxious counterparts (Alfano 2012). These youth may experience disruptive somatic distress and engage in anxious behaviors such as avoidance (e.g., homework procrastination) or excessive reassurance-seeking from others or external sources (e.g., online).

Social anxiety disorder in youth involves experiencing significant anxiety in social situations in which they are interacting with others or perceive they are being observed, with fears of negative evaluation, scrutiny, or embarrassment (American Psychiatric Association 2013). To be diagnosed in youth, the social situations must involve same-age peers, and the youth must nearly always experience anxiety in these social situations, trying to avoid them or enduring with distress. In social situations, youth likely are overestimating the threat posed, may display physical symptoms, and experience functional impairments in school (e.g., avoiding participation), interpersonal relationships (e.g., conversations), and everyday activities (e.g., ordering food). Diagnostically, it is important to consider normative and transient environmental factors (e.g., starting a new school), and diagnosis can only be applied if youth experience these symptoms for at least 6 months (American Psychiatric Association 2013).

Unexpected, intense, and recurrent panic attacks are the central feature of panic disorder. Panic attacks include a surge of physiological symptoms that peak in several minutes and can include heart palpitations, dizziness, chest discomfort, shortness of breath, derealization, depersonalization, and fears of losing control, going crazy, or dying (American Psychiatric Association 2013). Youth must experience excessive worry about the recurrence of a panic attack within 1 month of the initial attack and engage in maladaptive behaviors in efforts to avoid future panic attacks. Panic disorder can be comorbid with agoraphobia because youth may avoid various situations (e.g., crowded spaces) fearing onset of an attack, lack of controllability, or inability to escape. It is important to differentiate, considering developmental age, the language youth may use to describe fear responses that are connected to other anxiety states (e.g., intense worry) from a true panic attack and to establish anticipatory anxiety about recurrence of panic attacks.

New to DSM-5 as an anxiety disorder, selective mutism is diagnosed in youth who exhibit failure to speak in situations where they are expected to do so (e.g., school) despite being able to speak in other situations (e.g., home) and who experience academic and social impairments as a result (American Psychiatric Association 2013). Important for diagnosis is to consider any communication- or language-based conditions and onset and duration of symptoms beyond 1 month. For example, is the failure to speak associated with the start of the school year? Diagnosis also must consider youth familiarity with the dominant language.

Specific phobias are characterized by intense, excessive fear associated with particular phobic domains including animals (e.g., snakes), natural environment (e.g., thunderstorms), blood-injection-injury (e.g., needles), and situations (e.g., transportation), among others (e.g., vomit) (American Psychiatric Association 2013). When encountering a phobic stimulus, youth must almost always experience significant distress, and the phobic reaction must be present for at least 6 months. Youth (and now adults) need not acknowledge that their response is not proportionate to actual threat. Different phobias may overlap, and attention must be paid to developmental and transient factors (American Psychiatric Association 2013). Please see Table 39–1.

Pathogenesis

The pathogenesis of anxiety disorders is not yet clearly understood. Many complex and dynamic biological, psychosocial, and psychological factors appear to be involved in the development of anxiety.

Biological Factors

Genetics

Substantial evidence supports the familial and heritable nature of anxiety disorders. Genetic epidemiological studies report moderate levels of family aggregation (OR 4–6),

TABLE 39–1.   **Summary of youth anxiety disorders, prevalence, onset and gender difference**

	Core clinical feature	Prevalence rates	Age correlates/onset	Gender
Separation anxiety disorder	Extreme distress when separating from primary caregivers/attachment figures	1%–8%	Cannot be diagnosed in those younger than 6 years; most are diagnosed by age 12	1:1 in clinically referred; more females in the community
Generalized anxiety disorder	Excessive, uncontrollable worry across multiple domains	1%–3%		1:1 for younger children; greater in adolescent females
Social anxiety disorder	Fears of negative evaluation in various social situations	1%–9%	Between 8 and 15 years of age	1:1 for younger children; greater in adolescent females
Panic disorder	Unexpected, intense physiological arousal and anxious anticipation of future panic "attacks"	<1%–4%	More likely to onset in adolescence	Higher prevalence in females
Selective mutism	Persistent failure to speak when expected to do so	<1%	Onsets in younger children < age 5 and with school entry	Some research suggests 1:1; some suggests slightly higher prevalence in females
Specific phobias	Impairing fear and distress associated with specific objects or situations	1%–19%	More common in adolescents	Higher prevalence in females

and the familial risk is believed to be largely genetic, with heritability estimates of 30%–50% (Shimada-Sugimoto et al. 2015) across a range of disorders.

Neurocircuitry

Cortico-amygdala circuitry has been implicated in anxiety disorders (LeDoux 2000). Research from animal and human models shows that fear extinction in early development is heavily dependent on the amygdala, whereas at later ages, the amygdala, ventromedial prefrontal cortex, and hippocampus all are implicated (Shechner et al. 2014). Findings in pediatric samples have found that anxious youth demonstrated thicker cortex in the ventromedial prefrontal cortex than did healthy youth (Gold et al. 2017).

Psychosocial and Psychological Factors

Childhood/Developmental Factors

Many behavioral systems have been implicated in the cross-generational influences of childhood anxiety disorders, including vicarious learning, social referencing, modeling of anxious behaviors by parents, and parent accommodation to anxious behaviors (Lebowitz et al. 2016). *Family accommodation* describes how family members change their behavior to reduce their child's anxious distress; parental accommodation is common among youth with anxiety disorders and is related to severity (Lebowitz et al. 2013).

Temperament

Temperament, specifically *behavioral inhibition*—a pattern of withdrawal, hypervigilance, and avoidance in response to novel stimuli and social situations—is a risk factor for anxiety disorders. High levels of behavioral inhibition in early childhood have been linked to the development of later anxiety disorders (Bufferd et al. 2018). Behavioral inhibition may have conceptual similarities to several of the anxiety disorders, particularly social anxiety disorder, but data suggest it is an independent construct and does not overlap completely with any single disorder. Although the relationship between behavioral inhibition and anxiety has been well established in adults, their connection in pediatric anxiety disorders remains unclear.

Fear Learning and Threat Appraisal

Abnormal fear-safety learning during childhood may lead to the development of threat-related biases, which may contribute to the development of anxiety disorders (Britton et al. 2011). Moderate evidence suggests that anxious individuals demonstrate elevated fear in response to danger/safety cues (Shechner et al. 2014) and are more likely to classify ambiguous stimuli as threatening (Britton et al. 2011). Anxiety also is associated with attention biases; anxious individuals are quicker to engage with threatening stimuli and show greater difficulty disengaging from threats (Bar-Haim et al. 2007).

Life Events

Childhood maltreatment, including physical and sexual abuse and neglect, has been associated with increased risk of anxiety disorders. One meta-analysis demonstrated an odds ratio of 2.70 between any type of maltreatment and development of anxiety (Li et al. 2016). Additionally, stressful life events have been longitudinally associated with increases in anxiety sensitivity, and certain stressors (e.g., health-related events, family discord) were predictive of increases in anxiety sensitivity (McLaughlin and Hatzenbuehler 2009).

Assessment

Assessment tools for pediatric anxiety have been refined (Silverman and Ollendick 2005), with newer measures taking developmental considerations into account, including the unique differences in the daily environments and lives of youth versus adults (i.e., focus on school). The progression of normative fear development in youth has been well documented; for example, fear of separation increases in infancy and early childhood, fears of the dark in middle childhood, and fears of social evaluation in adolescence and later years (Ollendick et al. 1989). As such, youth assessment tools must take these developmentally normative fears into account.

The past several decades have seen a growing number of self-report instruments and structured clinical interviews developed specifically for youth. However, although measures of observed behavior such as the Behavioral Approach Test (BAT; Ollendick et al. 2011) are increasingly used, they have not yet been standardized. Spence (2017) provided an in-depth review of evidence-based assessment of anxiety disorders in youth and offered specific recommendations for selecting developmentally appropriate instruments.

Questionnaires and Rating Scales

Although some anxiety symptoms are easily observable by others (e.g., phobic refusal to go near a dog), other symptoms are experienced internally. For this reason, self-report anxiety questionnaires are important because they provide youth an opportunity to reveal their internal experience. Additionally, questionnaires have been developed for parents and teachers to provide information from multiple perspectives. Some questionnaires assess the symptoms of one disorder, whereas others are broadband and assess multidimensional constructs of anxiety.

Multidimensional measures of youth anxiety provide a total anxiety score and subscales meant to reflect specific anxiety disorders. The strongest evidence-based multidimensional measures for youth are the Multidimensional Anxiety Scale for Children (March et al. 1997), the Screen for Child Anxiety-Related Emotional Disorders (Birmaher et al. 1997), and the Spence Children's Anxiety Scale (Spence 1998, 2017), which was refined to include a depression subscale. This revision led to the development of the Revised Child Anxiety and Depression Scale (Chorpita et al. 2000). Each measure listed has child and parent versions and has shown good test-retest reliability over periods of about 4 weeks as well as solid convergent validity with other anxiety measures and divergent validity with measures of externalizing problems. Notably, each of these scales was originally developed for DSM-IV (American Psychiatric Association 1994), and data on their diagnostic validity for DSM-5 are limited. A newer measure correlating with existing measures, the Youth Anxiety Measure for DSM-5 (Muris et al. 2017), was developed to align with DSM-5 criteria.

Useful narrowband measures are worth highlighting, including the Liebowitz Social Anxiety Scale for Children and Adolescents (Masia-Warner et al. 2003), Children's Yale-Brown Obsessive-Compulsive Scale (Goodman et al. 1991), and the youth-adapted Penn State Worry Questionnaire (Chorpita et al. 1997).

Diagnostic Interviews

Dimensional self-report measures can highlight the severity of clinically relevant symptoms; however, they are not sufficient to establish a DSM-5 diagnosis and should be used in conjunction with an evidence-based clinical interview. Structured and semistructured interviews allow quantification of clinical data, reduce possible interviewer bias, and increase diagnostic reliability (Silverman 1987). Given the high comorbidity of anxiety disorders in youth, these interviews allow for thorough symptom assessment to inform diagnostic clarity and treatment planning. Interviews generally are designed for youth ages 7–17 years. Semistructured interviews allow the interviewer flexibility to elaborate and ask questions in a developmentally appropriate way.

Many diagnostic interviews for youth require that both the parent and child be interviewed with complementary versions of the assessment, because multi-informant methods allow evaluators to better understand symptoms from multiple perspectives. The most commonly used and well-established interviews for youth are the Schedule for Affective Disorders and Schizophrenia for School-Age Children (Kaufman et al. 1997); National Institute of Mental Health Diagnostic Interview Schedule for Children–IV (Shaffer et al. 2000); and Anxiety Disorders Interview Schedule for DSM-5 Child/Parent Version (Albano and Silverman, in press), which is known as the gold standard assessment of youth anxiety because it assesses the range of anxiety disorders, mood disorders, and related behavioral symptoms in 7- to 17-year-olds, with developmentally tailored descriptors. Parents and children are interviewed separately, typically by the same evaluator.

Behavioral Observation

Although self-report, checklist, and interview measures can provide useful information in the assessment of anxiety disorders in youth, disagreement often arises between informants (e.g., parents, children, teachers) that can lead to a confusing diagnostic picture and unclear treatment targets (Becker-Haimes et al. 2018). Therefore, including behavioral observation of the child in anxiety-provoking situations can provide invaluable clinical information. For example, the BAT requires the child to take several increasingly difficult steps in approach toward a feared stimulus, with the option to terminate at any time (Ollendick et al. 2011). This assesses the level of approach and avoidance behaviors as well as distress experienced when facing an anxiety-provoking situation in real time. Clinical interviewers can obtain samples of anxious behaviors through home and school observation or the use of in-session behavioral approach tests. Additionally, including parents in this behavioral observation can provide useful information about possible parental accommodation.

In summary, multi-method and multi-informant evaluation is critical for generating an accurate diagnostic picture and cognitive-behavioral treatment plan (March et al. 1995).

Treatment

Decades of randomized clinical trials (RCTs) and treatment studies have demonstrated that cognitive-behavioral therapy (CBT), medication, and their combination are the most effective therapeutic modalities for anxiety disorders in children and adolescents (see Palitz et al. 2019). The largest RCT to date, the Child/Adolescent Anxiety Multimodal Study (CAMS), randomly assigned 488 youths (ages 7–17 years) with separation anxiety disorder, social anxiety disorder, and GAD to receive CBT, sertraline, their combination, or pill placebo (Compton et al. 2010). Independent evaluators found an 81% response rate for youth randomized to combination treatment as compared to the monotherapies and pill placebo at 12 weeks, with CBT and medication alone being relatively equally effective (60% and 55%, respectively) and superior to placebo (24%; Walkup et al. 2008). Although gains were maintained for treatment responders at a 6-month follow-up maintenance session (Piacentini et al. 2014), further uncontrolled follow-up over a 4-year period was more sobering. CAMS responder status was associated with an increased likelihood of remission, but only 22% of youths retained their response over the long term (Ginsburg et al. 2018). Moreover, investigators found that 30% of youths were chronically ill and that 48% had relapsed. Type of treatment (selective serotonin reuptake inhibitor [SSRI]) was not associated with remission status at any point during the follow-up. Positive response to acute treatment may reduce the risk for chronic anxiety disorder and disability, but overall results emphasize the need to address ways to improve identification of youth at risk and provide access to early intervention. CBT and medication remain the only treatments to date with solid empirical support for the treatment of anxiety disorders in children.

Cognitive-Behavioral Therapy

CBT espouses a theoretical framework of social learning theory, steeped in classical and operant conditioning, that asserts that person–environment interactions are mediated by cognitive processes and solidified by the principles of reinforcement (Pimentel and Albano 2017). CBT is often short term and administered in individual, group, or family format. Treatment goals are to assist patients in recognizing and changing the interaction of thoughts, feelings, and behavior that serves to decrease their adaptive behaviors and to replace unhealthy habits with coping-focused healthy thinking and actions (Kendall 1994). CBT adapts flexibly to age and cognitive ability while staying true to its empirical foundation.

CBT is comprehensive and includes a set of interventions (Table 39–2; Moore et al. 2010). All CBT interventions involve *education* for youth and parents about anxiety, avoidance conditioning (escape provides immediate relief but leads to long-term, sustained anxiety through negative reinforcement), role of parents/safety persons, and the change process. *Goal setting* is critical, because youth and parents must understand why the child is in therapy, what is realistic to attain during treatment, and how

TABLE 39–2. Techniques used in cognitive-behavioral therapy for pediatric anxiety disorders

Term	Definition	Examples
Cognitive restructuring	Active altering of maladaptive thought patterns; replacing negative thoughts with more constructive adaptive cognitions and beliefs	Challenging aberrant risk appraisal in patient with panic disorder
Differential reinforcement of appropriate behavior	Attending to and positively rewarding appropriate behavior, especially when incompatible with inappropriate behavior	Praising child with social phobia for answering the telephone in therapist's office or at home when a responsible adult is not present
Exposure	Prolonged contact with the phobic stimulus in the absence of real threat to decrease anxiety; contact and interaction with a phobic stimulus or in a phobic situation with a focus on managing real threat (e.g., a needle stick will cause momentary discomfort) to decrease avoidance; may be contrived (sought-out contact with feared stimuli) or not contrived (unavoidable contact with feared stimuli)	Patient with fear of heights goes up a ladder: the first time, it is scary, the tenth time, it is boring
Extinction	Conventionally defined as the elimination of problem behaviors through removal of parental positive reinforcement; technically defined as removing the negative reinforcement effect of the problem behavior so that it no longer persists	Refusal to reassure anxious patient; refusal by mother to cave in to anxious oppositional child's tantrums by withdrawing a command
Generalization training	Moving the methods and success of problem-focused interventions to targets not specifically addressed in treatment	Exposure and response prevention in imagination for developmentally appropriate fears, even if not particularly bothersome or not specifically addressed in treatment
Negative reinforcement	Self-reinforcing purposeful removal of an aversive stimulus; stated differently, the termination of an aversive stimulus, which, when stopped, increases or stamps in the behavior that removed the aversive stimulus	Reassurance from parent provides short-term relief of anxiety in child; eliminating reassurance, which also blocks negative reinforcement for parent when child's distress and difficult behavior decrease, is prime goal of treatment

TABLE 39–2.   Techniques used in cognitive-behavioral therapy for pediatric anxiety disorders (continued)

Term	Definition	Examples
Positive reinforcement	Imposing a pleasurable stimulus to increase a desirable behavior	Praising selectively mute youngster who talks to the teacher
Prompting, guiding, and shaping	External commands and suggestions that increasingly direct the child toward more adaptive behavior that is then reinforced; typically, shaping procedures rapidly fade in preference to generalization training	Gradually encouraging and helping youngster with social phobia to talk in class and with other children
Punishment	Imposing an aversive stimulus to decrease an undesirable behavior	"Time-out" because of unacceptable behavior or overcorrection (as in extra chores to make restitution for aggressive behavior) Typically, punishment worsens anxiety disorders
Relapse prevention	Interventions designed to anticipate triggers for reemergence of symptoms; practicing skillful coping in advance	Imaginal exposure to a possible new fear followed by use of cognitive therapy and response prevention to successfully resist the incursion of anxiety-driven operant reinforcers
Response cost	Removal of positive reinforcer as a consequence of undesirable behavior	Loss of points in a token economy
Response prevention	Assisting patient to resist completing an anxiety-maintaining behavior	Typically used to treat OCD, in which response prevention means not performing rituals Also applies in other situations, such as eliminating an avoidance or escape withdrawal behavior in patients with social anxiety or agoraphobia
Restructuring the environment	Changes in setting or stimuli that decrease problem behaviors or facilitate adaptive behavior	Intervening to protect anxious child from punishment by teacher or teasing by peers

TABLE 39–2. Techniques used in cognitive-behavioral therapy for pediatric anxiety disorders *(continued)*

Term	Definition	Examples
Somatic management	Interventions used to target the physiological symptoms associated with anxiety (e.g., muscle tension, shortness of breath, gastrointestinal distress)	Teaching progressive muscle relaxation to individuals with generalized anxiety disorder who experience pain in their shoulders; teaching paced diaphragmatic breathing for individuals with panic disorder Monitor use as safety behaviors/avoidance from feared stimuli Can be used in conjunction with exposure therapy to facilitate engagement with feared stimuli
Stimulus hierarchy	A list of phobic stimuli ranked from least to most difficult to resist, with fear thermometer rating scores	Unique list of exposure targets ranked by fear thermometer score Individual patient may have one or more hierarchies, depending on complexity of symptoms (e.g., particular patient may have separate hierarchies for social fears and for separation anxiety)

to facilitate meeting goals. *Skills training* is employed to teach problem solving, cognitive restructuring, assertiveness training, emotion regulation, and other behavioral targets. Adapted for age, these skills can be taught through therapist modeling, role playing, and home-based practice and are found in programs such as "The Coping Cat" (Kendall and Hedtke 2006) and "Stand-Up, Speak-Out" (Albano and DiBartolo 2007), among others. Central to CBT for anxiety is *therapeutic exposure,* a process used to address avoidance behavior, such as behavioral refusal to engage with anxiety-provoking situations (e.g., sleeping in own bed; giving oral reports); more subtle "safety" accommodations, such as a parent allowing the child to stay home on the day of a field trip; and other means of escape or attenuation of anxiety that result in solidifying the anxiety response and preventing the experience of natural consequences that can shape adaptive functioning (Albano and Pepper 2013). Key is for anxious youth to be exposed to feared stimuli while processing realistic information that disputes their anxious ideas and helps them learn to cope with any less-than-ideal circumstances. Hence, *parent involvement* is often critical, given empirical findings that parents often inadvertently maintain anxious avoidance by completing tasks that the youth should do for him- or herself in order to relieve the child's distress (Albano and Pepper 2013; Wei and Kendall 2014). Hence, models for involving parents in the active treatment process are being developed (e.g., Lebowitz et al. 2019).

Advances in technology have allowed for the development of computer- and web-based treatments such as Khanna and Kendall's (2010) Camp Cope-A-Lot and Spence et al.'s (2011) Brave Online. A significant literature documents that internet-delivered CBT is effective, cost-effective, acceptable, and adaptable to various settings (Hill et al. 2018).

Pharmacotherapy

Whereas CBT is the recommended first-line treatment for youth with mild to moderate anxiety, a multimodal treatment approach is most effective for youth overall and recommended for youth who either do not respond to CBT or who have moderate to severe anxiety (Rapp et al. 2013). Practice parameters are based on primarily acute, short-term clinical efficacy trials with relatively brief follow-up periods (Patel et al. 2018). RCTs for the child anxiety triad (GAD, separation anxiety disorder, social anxiety disorder) support the efficacy and safety of SSRIs and serotonin-norepinephrine reuptake inhibitors for children with anxiety (Rapp et al. 2013). The CAMS (Walkup et al. 2008) compared the relative efficacy of CBT, medication (sertraline, 25–200 mg/day), combination treatment, and pill placebo for the child anxiety triad and yielded excellent acute treatment response for medication alone or combined with CBT. To date, however, no randomized trials have addressed the critical question of "what to start with first, for whom, and for how long" (Hussain et al. 2016), nor have evaluating algorithms been developed for discontinuing treatments or managing comorbidity. The SSRIs (Table 39–3) are effective and safe in youth with anxiety disorders and are the recommended first-line medication either as a monotherapy or in combination with CBT (American Academy of Child and Adolescent Psychiatry 2007). The safety and efficacy of other medications in this population have not been fully evaluated.

Patient-centered practice begins with a comprehensive baseline evaluation, including administration of rating scales (self, parent, teacher), clinical interview, and if

TABLE 39–3. **Commonly prescribed selective serotonin reuptake inhibitor and serotonin-norepinephrine reuptake inhibitor medications for anxiety in children and adolescents**

Drug (trade name)	Initial and maximum dosage, *mg/day*	Half-life	FDA indications
Citalopram (Celexa)	Initial: 10 Maximum: 60	24–48 hours	Off-label indication for OCD
Escitalopram (Lexapro)	Initial: 5 Maximum: 30	27–32 hours	
Fluoxetine (Prozac)	Initial: 10 Maximum: 20–30 (lower weight); 20–60 (higher weight)	4–6 days	OCD
Fluvoxamine IR (Luvox)	Initial: 25 Maximum: 200 (8–11 years); 300 (≥ 12 years)	14–16 hours	OCD
Paroxetine (Paxil)	Initial: 10 Maximum: 50–60	21 hours	Off-label indications for OCD and social anxiety disorder
Sertraline (Zoloft)	Initial: 25 (6–12 years); 50 (≥13 years) Maximum: 200	14–16 hours	OCD
Venlafaxine ER (Effexor)	Initial: 37.5 Maximum: 112.5 (25–39 kg); 225 (≥ 0 kg)	3–7 hours	
Duloxetine (Cymbalta)	Initial: 30 Maximum: 120	12 hours	Generalized anxiety disorder
Mirtazapine (Remeron)	Initial: 15 Maximum: 45	20–40 hours	

Note. ER=extended release; IR=immediate release.

appropriate, laboratory measures (Moore et al. 2010), along with a review of the child's physical health history. Additional therapeutics for physical health disorders (e.g., antiepileptics) should be carefully examined, as well as the family's use of homeopathic and alternative remedies, to avoid potential adverse interactions. After examining risk/benefit ratios for each agent under consideration and obtaining informed consent and child assent to initiate a medication trial, starting with the least-complicated and least-risky dosing strategy is recommended (Moore et al. 2010). Collaboration with the child's individual CBT therapist is advised; adopting concise communication strategies for tracking key symptoms and outcome indicators will assist the prescribing clinician with titration and maintenance decisions (Freidl et al. 2018). Prescribers are cautioned to use only one medication at a time, if possible, and to track target symptoms in a systematic manner. Dose-response (intensity) and time-response (temporal) characteristics of the medication in relation to the child's disorder should be considered.

Typically, children do not seek treatment, and adolescents may reject intervention. Pressures from school or outside agents may prompt parents to seek treatment for their child even as they have uncertain investment in the intervention. Prescribers should assess the child's and caretakers' understanding of the pros and cons of "leaving well enough alone" with regard to anxiety disorders as well as the risks and benefits of medication treatment with or without psychotherapy. Adolescents also should be encouraged to collaborate with the provider by assuming appropriate increasing responsibility for aspects of their care, including discussing response and side effects, independently taking medications, and refilling prescriptions.

For patients whose illness does not respond to pharmacotherapy or CBT, or only partially responds, careful monitoring of treatment targets and engagement of the parents and youth are necessary to examine if the goals of treatment were appropriately identified and whether treatment was appropriately implemented. Self- and parent-monitoring of symptoms and response will assist prescribers and psychotherapists in tracking progress. For the prescribing clinician, increasing the dosage, switching to a different medication, augmenting with another agent, or referring for additional evidence-based therapies may be necessary for achieving the desired treatment response.

Key Points

- Anxiety disorders in children and adolescents are common, result in clinical distress and significant impairment in role functioning, and may result in chronic disability for many youth over the long term.

- Although anxiety and fear are normal emotions and vary over the course of development, the severity and persistence of the anxiety, as well as the level of impairment, require careful evaluation to determine the need for treatment.

- Although the pathogenesis of anxiety disorders is not yet clearly understood, research supports a dynamic and complex interaction of both biological (i.e., genetics, neurobiological differences) and psychosocial (i.e., temperament, life events) factors involved in their development.

- A thorough diagnostic assessment of pediatric anxiety disorders includes multiple measures, such as multidimensional questionnaires, a semistructured clinical interview, and behavioral observations. Multi-method and multi-informant evaluation is critical in generating a cohesive, accurate diagnostic picture and essential in generating a cognitive-behavioral treatment plan.

- Cognitive-behavioral therapy (CBT) is typically the first-line treatment for pediatric anxiety disorders. A combination of CBT plus medication should be considered for youth with moderate to severe levels of disorder.

- Parents often inadvertently reinforce avoidance and compensate for the child's anxiety. Family involvement in psychotherapy fosters more substantial and lasting gains in treatment.

- The first-line psychopharmacological agents for the treatment of pediatric anxiety disorders are the selective serotonin reuptake inhibitors. Side effects, particularly emerging suicidal ideation or behavior, must be carefully monitored.

References

Albano AM, DiBartolo PM: Stand Up, Speak Out: Therapist Manual for Cognitive Behavioral Therapy for Social Phobia in Adolescents. New York, Oxford University Press, 2007

Albano AM, Pepper L: You and Your Anxious Child: Free Your Child From Fears and Worries and Create a Joyful Family Life. New York, Penguin Group, 2013

Albano AM, Silverman WK: The Anxiety Disorders Interview Schedule for DSM-5, Child and Parent Versions. New York, Oxford University Press, in press

Alfano CA: Are children with "pure" generalized anxiety disorder impaired? A comparison with comorbid and healthy children. J Clin Child Adolesc Psychol 41(6):739–745, 2012 22963176

American Academy of Child and Adolescent Psychiatry: Practice parameter for the assessment and treatment of children and adolescents with anxiety disorders. J Am Acad Child Adolesc Psychiatry 46:267–283, 2007

American Psychiatric Association: Diagnostic and Statistical Manual of Mental Disorders, 4th Edition. Washington, DC, American Psychiatric Association, 1994

American Psychiatric Association: Diagnostic and Statistical Manual of Mental Disorders, 5th Edition. Arlington, VA, American Psychiatric Association, 2013

Angold A, Costello EJ, Farmer EM, et al: Impaired but undiagnosed. J Am Acad Child Adolesc Psychiatry 38(2):129–137, 1999 9951211

Bar-Haim Y, Lamy D, Pergamin L, et al: Threat-related attentional bias in anxious and nonanxious individuals: a meta-analytic study. Psychol Bull 133(1):1–24, 2007 17201568

Becker-Haimes EM, Jensen-Doss A, Birmaher B, et al: Parent-youth informant disagreement: implications for youth anxiety treatment. Clin Child Psychol Psychiatry 23(1):42–56, 2018 28191794

Beesdo K, Bittner A, Pine D, et al: Incidence of social anxiety disorder and the consistent risk for secondary depression in the first three decades of life. Arch Gen Psychiatry 64:903–912, 2007

Birmaher B, Khetarpal S, Brent D, et al: The Screen for Child Anxiety Related Emotional Disorders (SCARED): scale construction and psychometric characteristics. J Am Acad Child Adolesc Psychiatry 36(4):545–553, 1997 9100430

Britton JC, Lissek S, Grillon C, et al: Development of anxiety: the role of threat appraisal and fear learning. Depress Anxiety 28(1):5–17, 2011 20734364

Bufferd SJ, Dougherty LR, Olino TM, et al: Temperament distinguishes persistent/recurrent from remitting anxiety disorders across early childhood. J Clin Child Adolesc Psychol 47(6):1004–1013, 2018 27705002

Chorpita BF, Tracey SA, Brown TA, et al: Assessment of worry in children and adolescents: an adaptation of the Penn State Worry Questionnaire. Behav Res Ther 35(6):569–581, 1997 9159982

Chorpita BF, Yim L, Moffitt C, et al: Assessment of symptoms of DSM-IV anxiety and depression in children: a revised child anxiety and depression scale. Behav Res Ther 38(8):835–855, 2000 10937431

Clark DB, Neighbors B: Adolescent substance abuse and internalizing disorders. Child Adolesc Psychiatr Clin N Am 5:45–55, 1996

Compton S, Walkup J, Albano AM et al: The Child/Adolescent Anxiety Multimodal Study (CAMS): rationale, design and methods. Child Adolesc Psychiatry Ment Health 4:1, 2010 20051130

Costello EJ, Egger HL, Angold A: Developmental epidemiology of anxiety disorders, in Phobic and Anxiety Disorders in Children and Adolescents: A Clinician's Guide to Effective Psychosocial and Pharmacological Interventions. Edited by Ollendick TH, March JS. New York, Oxford University Press, 2004, pp 61–91

Curry JF, March JS, Hervey AS: Comorbidity of childhood and adolescent anxiety disorders: prevalence and implications, in Phobic and Anxiety Disorders in Children and Adolescents: A Clinician's Guide to Effective Psychosocial and Pharmacological Interventions. Edited by Ollendick TH, March JS. New York, Oxford University Press, 2004, pp 116–140

Freidl EK, Hoffman L, Albano AM: Outpatient settings: the collaborative role of psychiatry and psychology, in The Oxford Handbook of Clinical Child and Adolescent Psychology. Edited by Ollendick TH, White SW, White BA. New York, Oxford University Press, 2018, pp 640–653

Ginsburg GS, Becker-Haimes EM, Keeton C, et al: Results from the Child/Adolescent Anxiety Multimodal Extended Long-Term Study (CAMELS): primary anxiety outcomes. J Am Acad Child Adolesc Psychiatry 57(7):471–480, 2018 29960692

Gold AL, Steuber ER, White LK, et al: Cortical thickness and subcortical gray matter volume in pediatric anxiety disorders. Neuropsychopharmacology 42(12):2423–2433, 2017 28436445

Goodman W, Price L, Rasmussen S, et al: Children's Yale-Brown Obsessive-Compulsive Scale (CY-BOCS). New Haven, CT, Yale University School of Medicine, 1991

Gould MS, King R, Greenwald S, et al: Psychopathology associated with suicidal ideation and attempts among children and adolescents. J Am Acad Child Adolesc Psychiatry 37(9):915–923, 1998 9735611

Hill C, Creswell C, Vigerland S, et al: Navigating the development and dissemination of internet cognitive behavioral therapy (iCBT) for anxiety disorders in children and young people: a consensus statement with recommendations from the #iCBTLorentz Workshop Group. Internet Interv 12:1–10, 2018 30135763

Hussain FS, Dobson ET, Strawn JR: Pharmacologic treatment of pediatric anxiety disorders. Curr Treat Options Psychiatry 3(2):151–160, 2016 27648401

Kaufman J, Birmaher B, Brent D, et al: Schedule for affective disorders and schizophrenia for school-age children—present and lifetime version (K-SADS-PL): initial reliability and validity data. J Am Acad Child Adolesc Psychiatry 36(7):980–988, 1997 9204677

Kendall PC: Treating anxiety disorders in children: results of a randomized clinical trial. J Consult Clin Psychol 62(1):100–110, 1994 8034812

Kendall PC, Hedtke K: Cognitive-Behavioral Therapy for Anxious Children: Therapist Manual, 3rd Edition. Ardmore, PA, Workbook Publishing, 2006

Kendall PC, Compton SN, Walkup JT, et al: Clinical characteristics of anxiety disordered youth. J Anxiety Disord 24(3):360–365, 2010 20206470

Khanna MS, Kendall PC: Computer-assisted cognitive behavioral therapy for child anxiety: results of a randomized clinical trial. J Consult Clin Psychol 78(5):737–745, 2010 20873909

Lebowitz ER, Woolston J, Bar-Haim Y, et al: Family accommodation in pediatric anxiety disorders. Depress Anxiety 30(1):47–54, 2013 22965863

Lebowitz ER, Leckman JF, Silverman WK, et al: Cross-generational influences on childhood anxiety disorders: pathways and mechanisms. J Neural Transm (Vienna) 123(9):1053–1067, 2016 27145763

Lebowitz ER, Marin C, Martino A, et al: Parent-based treatment as efficacious as cognitive behavioral therapy for childhood anxiety: a randomized noninferiority study of supportive parenting for anxious childhood emotions. J Am Acad Child Adolesc Psychiatry March 7, 2019 30851397 Epub ahead of print

LeDoux JE: Emotion circuits in the brain. Annu Rev Neurosci 23(1):155–184, 2000 10845062

Li M, D'Arcy C, Meng X: Maltreatment in childhood substantially increases the risk of adult depression and anxiety in prospective cohort studies: systematic review, meta-analysis, and proportional attributable fractions. Psychol Med 46(4):717–730, 2016 26708271

March JS, Mulle K, Stallings P, et al: Organizing an anxiety disorders clinic, in Anxiety Disorders in Children and Adolescents. Edited by March J. New York, Guilford, 1995, pp 420–435

March JS, Parker JD, Sullivan K, et al: The Multidimensional Anxiety Scale for Children (MASC): factor structure, reliability, and validity. J Am Acad Child Adolesc Psychiatry 36(4):554–565, 1997 9100431

Masia-Warner C, Storch EA, Pincus DB, et al: The Liebowitz social anxiety scale for children and adolescents: an initial psychometric investigation. J Am Acad Child Adolesc Psychiatry 42(9):1076–1084, 2003 12960707

McLaughlin KA, Hatzenbuehler ML: Stressful life events, anxiety sensitivity, and internalizing symptoms in adolescents. J Abnorm Psychol 118(3):659–669, 2009 19685962

Merikangas KR, He JP, Burstein M, et al: Lifetime prevalence of mental disorders in U.S. adolescents: results from the National Comorbidity Survey Replication–Adolescent Supplement (NCS-A). J Am Acad Child Adolesc Psychiatry 49(10):980–989, 2010 20855043

Moore PS, March JS, Albano AM, Thienemann M: Anxiety disorders in children and adolescents, in Textbook of Anxiety Disorders, 2nd Edition. Edited by Stein DJ, Hollander E, Rothbaum BO. Washington, DC, American Psychiatric Publishing, 2010, pp 629–651

Muris P, Meesters C, Merckelbach H, et al: Worry in normal children. J Am Acad Child Adolesc Psychiatry 37(7):703–710, 1998 9666625

Muris P, Mannens J, Peters L, et al: The Youth Anxiety Measure for DSM-5 (YAM-5): Correlations with anxiety, fear, and depression scales in non-clinical children. J Anxiety Disord 51:72–78, 2017 28668214

Ollendick TH, King NJ, Frary RB: Fears in children and adolescents: reliability and generalizability across gender, age and nationality. Behav Res Ther 27(1):19–26, 1989 2914001

Ollendick TH, Allen B, Benoit K, et al: The tripartite model of fear in children with specific phobias: assessing concordance and discordance using the behavioral approach test. Behav Res Ther 49(8):459–465, 2011 21596371

Palitz SA, Davis JP, Kendall PC: Treatment of anxiety in children and adolescents, in Treatment of Disorders in Childhood and Adolescence, 4th Edition. Edited by Prinstein M, Youngstrom E, Mash E, et al. New York, Guilford, 2019

Patel DR, Feucht C, Brown K, et al: Pharmacological treatment of anxiety disorders in children and adolescents: a review for practitioners. Transl Pediatr 7(1):23–35, 2018 29441280

Piacentini J, Bennett S, Compton SN, et al: 24- and 36-week outcomes for the Child/Adolescent Anxiety Multimodal Study (CAMS). J Am Acad Child Adolesc Psychiatry 53(3):297–310, 2014 24565357

Pimentel SS, Albano AM: Cognitive behavioral psychotherapy for children and adolescents, in Kaplan and Sadock's Comprehensive Textbook of Psychiatry, 10th Edition. Edited by Sadock B, Sadock V, Ruiz P. Alphen aan den Rijn, The Netherlands, Wolters Kluwer Health, 2017, pp 3749–3760

Pine DS, Cohen P, Gurley D, et al: The risk for early adulthood anxiety and depressive disorders in adolescents with anxiety and depressive disorders. Arch Gen Psychiatry 55(1):56–64, 1998 9435761

Rapp A, Dodds A, Walkup JT, Rynn M: Treatment of pediatric anxiety disorders. Ann N Y Acad Sci 1304:52–61, 2013 24279893

Shaffer D, Fisher P, Lucas CP, et al: NIMH Diagnostic Interview Schedule for Children Version IV (NIMH DISC-IV): description, differences from previous versions, and reliability of some common diagnoses. J Am Acad Child Adol Psychiatry 39:28–38, 2000

Shechner T, Hong M, Britton JC, et al: Fear conditioning and extinction across development: evidence from human studies and animal models. Biol Psychol 100:1–12, 2014 24746848

Shimada-Sugimoto M, Otowa T, Hettema JM: Genetics of anxiety disorders: genetic epidemiological and molecular studies in humans. Psychiatry Clin Neurosci 69(7):388–401, 2015 25762210

Silverman WK: Childhood anxiety disorders: diagnostic issues, empirical support, and future research. J Child Adolesc Psychother 4(3):121–126, 1987

Silverman WK, Ollendick TH: Evidence-based assessment of anxiety and its disorders in children and adolescents. J Clin Child Adolesc Psychol 34(3):380–411, 2005 16026211

Spence SH: A measure of anxiety symptoms among children. Behav Res Ther 36(5):545–566, 1998 9648330

Spence SH: Assessing anxiety disorders in children and adolescents. Child Adolesc Ment Health 23(3):266–282, 2017

Spence SH, Donovan CL, March S, et al: A randomized controlled trial of online versus clinic-based CBT for adolescent anxiety. J Consult Clin Psychol 79(5):629–642, 2011 21744945

Swan AJ, Kendall PC: Fear and missing out: youth anxiety and functional outcomes. Clin Psychol Sci Pract 23(4):417–435, 2016

Walkup J, Albano AM, Piacentini J, et al: Cognitive behavioral therapy, sertraline or a combination in childhood anxiety. N Engl J Med 359:2753–2766, 2008

Weems CF, Silverman WK, La Greca AM: What do youth referred for anxiety problems worry about? Worry and its relation to anxiety and anxiety disorders in children and adolescents. J Abnorm Child Psychol 28(1):63–72, 2000 10772350

Wei C, Kendall PC: Parental involvement: contribution to childhood anxiety and its treatment. Clin Child Fam Psychol Rev 17(4):319–339, 2014 25022818

Recommended Readings

Albano AM, Pepper L: You and Your Anxious Child: Free Your Child from Fears and Worries and Create a Joyful Family Life. New York, Penguin Books, 2013

Chansky T: Freeing Your Child from Anxiety, Revised and Updated Edition: Practical Strategies to Overcome Fears, Worries, and Phobias and Be Prepared for Life—From Toddlers to Teens. New York, Harmony Books, 2014

Kendall PC (ed): Child and Adolescent Therapy, 4th Edition. New York, Guilford, 2011

Whiteside SP, Ollendick T, Biggs B: Exposure Therapy for Child and Adolescent Anxiety and OCD (ABCT Clinical Practice Series), 2nd Edition. New York, Oxford University Press, 2020

CHAPTER 40

Anxiety Disorders in Late Life

Josien Schuurmans, Ph.D.

Gert-Jan Hendriks, Ph.D., M.D.

Claire Van Genugten, M.Sc.

Richard Oude Voshaar, Ph.D., M.D.

Anxiety disorders are a major clinical problem in late life: estimated prevalence rates vary between 6% and 10% (Bryant et al. 2008), with a considerable disease burden comparable to depression. Although research on late-life anxiety has gradually increased in the past two decades, anxiety disorders often remain undetected and untreated in older adults. This discrepancy may be accounted for by a combination of patient variables (e.g., lack of help-seeking behavior and a long duration of illness) and variables related to current clinical practice (e.g., lack of knowledge regarding the appropriate diagnosis and treatment of late-life anxiety as well as "ageism"). This chapter addresses the epidemiology, diagnosis, and treatment of anxiety disorders in older adults to counter any reservations clinicians might still have about appropriately managing these debilitating disorders. Studies of late-life anxiety disorders use an age boundary ranging from 55 to 65 years to distinguish between older and younger adults. This age range is observed in this chapter to be consistent with the international literature. In DSM-5 (American Psychiatric Association 2013), OCD, PTSD, and acute stress disorder have been moved from the anxiety disorders section to two new sections, namely, "Obsessive-Compulsive and Related Disorders" and "Trauma- and Stressor-Related Disorders." This chapter focuses on DSM-5 anxiety disorders that affect older adults, because little to no scientific literature has been published on OCD and PTSD in older adults (save for a few case studies). Anxiety disorders discussed in this chapter are generalized anxiety disorder (GAD), panic disorder, agoraphobia, social phobia, and specific phobia.

Epidemiology

Prevalence

Anxiety disorders are among the most prevalent mental disorders worldwide. Estimates of prevalence rates in both younger and older adults vary widely, but most estimates of current (6-month to 1-year) prevalence rates in older adults fall within the range of 6%–10% (Bryant et al. 2008). Most studies are confined to the Western European and North American populations and are based on DSM-IV criteria (including GAD, phobic disorders, and panic disorder) (American Psychiatric Association 1994). The variations in prevalence rates are probably caused by methodological differences between studies, in particular with regard to the prevalence period, the number of anxiety disorders included, and the diagnostic assessment tools used (Baxter et al. 2013). For individual anxiety disorders, prevalence rates are even more variable, up to a factor of six between studies. An overview is included in Table 40–1. Despite the large variation between studies, epidemiological studies consistently show that, worldwide, anxiety disorders are twice as common in women as in men; furthermore, a higher age (older than 55 years) is associated with a 20% lower anxiety disorder prevalence, and the prevalence of anxiety disorders in late life is comparable with known prevalence rates of late-life depression (Kessler et al. 2005).

Age at Onset

Data from the National Comorbidity Survey Replication show that anxiety disorders have an earlier age at onset compared with mood disorders (Kessler et al. 2005), with a median age at onset of 11 years. Only 1% of lifetime anxiety disorders have an onset after the age of 65. Empirical data suggest that an onset before or after the ages of 25–30 is a reasonable dividing line between early and late-onset disorders (Tibi et al. 2013). Studies of this kind show that later-onset anxiety disorders are generally less severe and have better treatment outcomes. Although in geriatric psychiatry an age around 60 years is traditionally chosen to differentiate between early and late-onset psychiatric disorders, empirical data do not support this boundary for anxiety disorders. The 95th percentile of the age at onset distribution is 51 years for any anxiety disorder (Kessler et al. 2005). This means that only 5% of anxiety disorders have an onset after the age of 51 years. Table 40–1 provides an overview of the age at onset distribution per specific anxiety disorder. Studies choosing an arbitrary cutoff point at 55–65 years to distinguish between early and late-onset anxiety disorder (Ritchie et al. 2013) nevertheless also show that late-onset anxiety disorders are associated with less severe symptoms (Sheikh et al. 2004). Also, patients have a better prognosis after treatment compared with those in whom the anxiety disorder developed at a young age and whose condition is therefore longstanding and chronic (Hendriks et al. 2012).

Course and Disease Burden

That anxiety disorders are chronic conditions is evident from the high prevalence rates in older adults, combined with the fact that most late-life anxiety disorders onset

TABLE 40–1.　Prevalence rates and age at onset of late-life[a] anxiety disorders[b]

Anxiety disorder (DSM-IV[c])	Point prevalence, % (95% CI)	Lifetime prevalence, % (95% CI)	Age at onset (95th percentile[d]), years
Panic disorder	0.88 (0.76–0.99)	2.63 (2.43–2.84)	56
Agoraphobia (with or without panic)	0.53 (0.39–0.66)	1.00 (.54–1.45)	51
Specific phobia	4.52 (4.15–4.89)	6.66 (6.17–7.15)	41
Social anxiety disorder	1.31 (1.18–1.44)	5.07 (4.82–5.32)	34
Generalized anxiety disorder	2.30 (2.03–2.57)	6.36 (5.57–7.14)	66

Note.　[a]Most studies of late-life anxiety disorders use an age boundary ranging from 55 to 65 years to distinguish between older and younger adults.
[b]Source of prevalence rates: meta-analyses by Volkert et al. 2013; source of age at onset rates: Kessler et al. 2005.
[c]DSM-5 data of late-life anxiety prevalence and age at onset were not available.
[d]This means that 5% of the specified anxiety disorder have an onset after the age listed in this column.

in childhood or early adolescence. The burden from anxiety disorders (defined as disability-adjusted life years [DALYs]) is highest in adolescence and young adulthood (peaking between ages 15 and 25 years), with 387 DALYs per 100,000 males and 721 DALYs per 100,000 females, after which it gradually declines (Baxter et al. 2014). However, this does not imply that anxiety disorders are a minor health problem in late life. Compared with healthy older people, those with anxiety disorders report poorer physical health, less feelings of well-being, and lower levels of social and general functioning. Anxiety in late life is also associated with an increased use of health care services (Beekman et al. 2000). The level of impairment in quality of life due to late-life anxiety disorders is similar to that of late-life depression (Wetherell et al. 2004). Furthermore, older people with anxiety disorders often have to contend with mental and physical comorbidity, thus increasing the risk of a chronic course, a higher use of medical care, and even worse quality of life (de Beurs et al. 1999; Mackenzie et al. 2010). Lastly, anxiety disorders in the elderly are associated with a higher risk of vascular disease and related complications (Huffman et al. 2008).

Clinical Features Contributing to Underdiagnosis and Undertreatment

Differences in Presentation and Interpretation in Older Adults

In spite of the high prevalence of late-life anxiety disorders, they often go unrecognized and untreated. Studies show that older adults are more likely to remain untreated for their anxiety symptoms than younger adults (Schuurmans et al. 2005). This section discusses the factors specific to older adults that help explain why recognizing anxiety disorders in advanced age may be more complicated.

Chronic Nature of the Illness

The symptoms of anxiety disorders generally develop at a young age and are characterized by a chronic, fluctuating course. As a result, patients, families, and care professionals alike may consider them to be personality traits or may adopt a resigned or fatalistic attitude, with low expectations for the availability or success of treatment options on all sides.

Comorbidity With Somatic Disorders

Older adults have a higher rate of comorbid medical conditions (Wolitzky-Taylor et al. 2010) and therefore tend to attribute anxiety symptoms to physical impairments and disorders (Wolitzky-Taylor et al. 2010). Many chronic somatic disorders are associated with symptoms of anxiety and depression, in particular illnesses that impair physical fitness, such as cardiovascular disorders, chronic obstructive pulmonary disease, hyperthyroidism, and vestibular problems. Differentiating between "normal" anxiety or concern about having a somatic disorder; anxiety symptoms as a direct result of an underlying somatic disorder, such as hyperthyroidism; and an anxiety disorder warranting adequate psychological or pharmacological treatment can sometimes be quite difficult.

Regarding Avoidance as Consistent With Age

Pathological behavior, such as avoidance in anxiety disorders, may be regarded as "normal" or "realistic" for older adults, a phenomenon known as "ageism" (Fuentes and Cox 2000). Ageism may be displayed not only by health care professionals but also by patients themselves and those around them. Avoiding certain activities, such as walking outside without a companion after a recent fall, may be regarded as an adaptive and appropriate response instead of a sign of a possible comorbid anxiety disorder.

Differences in the Presentation of Anxiety Symptoms

Differences in cognitive symptoms (e.g., worry), emotional symptoms (e.g., feelings of anxiety or fear), and physical symptoms (e.g., palpitations) between younger and older patients with anxiety disorders have been studied mainly in undiagnosed populations with elevated anxiety symptoms or a mixture of anxiety and nervousness (Gould and Edelstein 2010). Although no prospective longitudinal studies have been done on the development of anxiety symptoms within the same individuals as they age, direct comparisons between younger and older adult samples suggest that higher age—especially combined with higher age at symptom onset—is associated with a reduction in both cognitive and emotional anxiety symptoms and physiological arousal. These findings are in line with studies of healthy older adults suggesting that negative feelings and the intensity of emotional reactions decline with age, whereas tolerance for feelings of insecurity increases and coping with stressful events improves (Gould and Edelstein 2010). As a result, anxiety symptoms may be less pronounced or may present in an atypical form. In such subsyndromal cases, it may be more appropriate to step away from the strict DSM criteria when deciding whether symptoms require treatment. The severity of avoidance behavior and other impairments of daily functioning may be more informative in this respect (Grenier et al. 2011).

Clinical Features of Specific Anxiety Disorders in Late Life

The correct appraisal of late-life anxiety disorders may be hampered by the fact that the phenomenology of anxiety in late life can be quite different from anxiety in early adulthood. Older adults may fear different stimuli or situations or may have a different reason for fearing certain stimuli or situations than younger adults. This section describes age-related features of the most common anxiety disorders in later life: panic disorder, (comorbid) agoraphobia, social anxiety disorder, GAD, and specific phobia.

Generalized Anxiety Disorder

On average, elderly patients with GAD are found to have fewer symptoms than younger patients with GAD (Miloyan et al. 2014b), but some specific symptoms, such as difficulty concentrating, dizziness, and gastrointestinal symptoms (nausea and gastric problems) are more common in older patients. The subjects about which they worry also differ: elderly adults worry more about their health and the well-being of loved ones, whereas younger adults worry more about work, money, and social relationships (Miloyan et al. 2014a).

Panic Disorder and Agoraphobia

Phenomenological age-related differences have similarly been studied in older patients with panic disorder and agoraphobia and those with panic attacks as a symptom of another anxiety disorder. Compared with young adults, elderly adults had fewer cognitive, emotional, and physiological anxiety symptoms. For example, the increase in heart rate in older persons during panic attacks was relatively less than in their younger counterparts, and older patients with panic disorder reported fewer and less severe fearful cognitions, such as fear of going crazy or losing control. Panic disorder in the elderly could therefore be regarded as a less severe anxiety disorder (Sheikh et al. 2004). No age-related differences, however, were found in the degree of behavioral avoidance, which can be regarded as a key symptom of panic disorder with comorbid agoraphobia.

Social Anxiety Disorder

Older adult patients with social anxiety disorder similarly demonstrate an age-related reduction in symptoms. The core profile of symptoms and signs of both social anxiety cognitions and related social avoidance behavior remains essentially the same across all age groups, however (Miloyan et al. 2014a). In cases of social anxiety disorder, it may nevertheless be useful to differentiate between early and late age of onset because comorbidity (or overlap) with avoidant personality disorder is much greater in the case of early onset social anxiety disorder (Friborg et al. 2013). In addition, a prospective study demonstrated that although social anxiety decreases with age, the incidence of social anxiety in the elderly is nonetheless substantial (Karlsson et al. 2010).

Specific Phobia and Age-Related Anxiety Problems

The prevalence of specific phobia has been found to decrease with age, especially after the age of 70, halving around the age of 80 (Sigström et al. 2011). This finding is consistent with the lower severity of physiological anxiety symptoms found in older adults as compared with younger cohorts. However, avoidance behavior is similar between age groups.

Fear of falling, in contrast, is a common anxiety problem particularly prevalent among older adults. It occurs among both older adults who have had a recent fall and those who have never had a fall, with reported prevalence as high as 85% and 50%, respectively (for an overview, see Parry et al. 2016). Fear of falling is characterized by anticipatory anxiety cognitions, reduced self-confidence, avoidance of social activities and activities outside the home, increased feelings of dependence, reduced activity, and impaired gait motor function. It requires intervention when the symptoms cause significant distress or impairment in important areas of daily functioning.

Fear of dementia is another type of anxiety related to aging. It is characterized by a strong concern about developing dementia, frequent worrying, and interpreting "normal" forgetfulness as a sign of dementia. In a cohort of subjects older than 50 years, almost 10% were found to have marked and more than 20% moderate concern about developing dementia. The presence of depression reinforces this concern commensurately.

Diagnosis

Differential Diagnosis: Depression

Clinicians initially assumed that anxiety in late life was always comorbid with depression. "Pure" anxiety disorders were thought to be nonexistent. Therefore, it was deemed preferable to use the term "mixed anxiety-depressive syndrome." Indeed, comorbidity between anxiety and depression is high in adult populations, and patients often experience transitions from anxiety to depressive disorders and vice versa (Scholten et al. 2016). However, epidemiological studies show that mixed anxiety-depressive syndrome in the older population is relatively rare, with an estimated prevalence of 1.8% (Schoevers et al. 2003). Comorbidity rates between depression and anxiety are high but no higher than those found in younger populations (Préville et al. 2008). Préville et al.'s (2008) recent epidemiological study of psychiatric disorders in community-dwelling older adults found that among those with a depressive disorder (major and minor), 13.6% had a comorbid anxiety disorder. In those diagnosed with an anxiety disorder, 15.9% met the criteria for a depressive disorder.

Differential Diagnosis: Neurodegenerative Disease

Recently, a growing number of studies have proposed the hypothesis that chronic anxiety and stress contribute to accelerated aging and cognitive decline. This could be the result of various proposed biological mechanisms, such as prolonged stress inducing hypothalamic-pituitary-adrenal axis hyperactivity as well as resulting in reduced telomere length, a marker of cellular aging. According to this hypothesis, anxiety-related cognitive impairment would be partially reversible or preventable by providing adequate treatment. This is supported by recent studies suggesting that anxiety is predictive of cognitive decline (Becker et al. 2018).

However, the evidence so far is inconclusive, and contradictory findings have been reported. For example, anxiety disorders and symptoms were not found to be predictive of cognitive decline in other longitudinal studies (Bierman et al. 2009). As a consequence, some researchers have suggested that advocates of the cognitive decline hypothesis may confuse late-life anxiety disorders with a prodromal phase that is accompanied by anxiety symptoms in the very early stages of a cognitive disorder (Gulpers et al. 2016).

Nevertheless, the higher risk of neurodegenerative disease in older adults warrants the attention of clinicians. Although hardly any studies are available to support this differential diagnosis, the usual age at onset of anxiety disorders earlier in life suggests that we need to be watchful of anxiety disorders that manifest for the first time at an elderly age. Similarly, extra vigilance is advised when late-life anxiety disorders worsen rapidly without an identifiable cause and when diffuse anxiety symptoms present without a specific cognitive focus of worry content. In these types of cases, clinicians can administer a short screening tool, such as the shortened Mini Mental State Examination (Folstein et al. 1975), to assess signs of cognitive decline. Scores of 24 or lower are grounds for a more comprehensive neuropsychological assessment. The Montreal Cognitive Assessment is a suitable alternative reported to be more sensitive in detecting the early stages of a cognitive disorder (Nasreddine et al. 2005). Upon its introduction, a cutoff score of 26 or lower was used to differentiate between normal aging and minimal cognitive impairment. However, a recent meta-analysis revealed that a cutoff score of 23/30 yields a better diagnostic accuracy, with fewer false positives (Carson et al. 2018). In case of a phobic anxiety for dementia or considerable distress caused by a perceived loss of memory function, a full neuropsychological assessment is warranted, even when an initial screening is inconclusive.

Diagnostic Instruments

Interview

The gold standard for diagnosing anxiety disorders is a semistructured interview such as the Anxiety Disorders Interview Schedule or the Structured Clinical Interview for DSM Disorders. These interviews have not been validated for the elderly, however. The examining psychiatrist therefore needs to be properly trained in working with the elderly to be able to weigh the answers correctly and probe further where necessary, because DSM-5 provides hardly any age-specific examples in the notes on disorder-specific criteria, which can differ substantially from those in young adults (see "Clinical Features of Specific Anxiety Disorders in Late Life" earlier in the chapter).

Self-Report Measures

Diagnostic interviews can be supplemented by self-report tools for screening purposes or to assess symptom severity and monitor treatment outcome. Validated questionnaires for the elderly are lacking. One well-validated screening tool for detecting anxiety disorders in the elderly and monitoring the severity of general anxiety symptoms is the 20-item Geriatric Anxiety Inventory (Molde et al. 2019; Therrien and Hunsley 2012). The short form of this measure, with only five items, has been found suitable for use in large-scale epidemiological studies or to screen for anxiety symptoms in the elderly in primary care (Byrne and Pachana 2011). The Penn State Worry

Questionnaire has also been properly validated for use in a geriatric population (Crittendon and Hopko 2006). Unfortunately, both questionnaires focus on GAD-related symptoms, so other questionnaires validated in younger age samples should still be used to assess phobic disorders.

Treatment

In the past, therapists' faith in recovery or alleviation of symptoms appeared to decline with patients' age and the duration of their anxiety disorder (Stanley and Averill 1999). Although this would seem to be a reasonable assumption given the chronicity of late-life anxiety disorders, hardly any empirical support exists for this claim. Various meta-analyses consistently show that both cognitive-behavioral therapy (CBT) and antidepressants (selective serotonin reuptake inhibitors [SSRIs] or tricyclic antidepressants [TCAs]) are effective in treating late-life anxiety disorders (Gonçalves and Byrne 2012; Gould et al. 2012; Hendriks et al. 2008). A direct comparison of the efficacy of CBT for panic disorder found no difference between younger and older patients. In fact, the effect of CBT on avoidance behavior was found to be significantly greater among older compared with younger adults (Hendriks et al. 2014).

Pharmacotherapy

Pharmacotherapy guidelines for late-life anxiety disorder are similar to those in younger adults with an anxiety disorder. In a recent meta-analysis, SSRIs, TCAs, and benzodiazepines have been shown to be equally effective in older and younger adults (Pinquart et al. 2007). However, some adaptations are suggested on the basis of best practices. First, the milder side effect profile of SSRIs and their greater safety with comorbid somatic conditions warrants a slight preference for SSRIs over TCAs as a first line of treatment. Second, it is recommended to start medication at a relatively low dosage and gradually increase the dosage, assessing tolerability and response—the "start low, go slow" principle. However, the optimal therapeutic dosage and the time lag to evaluate treatment response are not different from younger age groups. A third difference is that older people almost always use medication for somatic disorders (e.g., statins, β-blockers, anticoagulants), and the prescribing physician should therefore be vigilant of any possible drug–drug interactions. Fourth, special precaution should be taken with regard to the use of psychotropic medication. A recent meta-analysis showed that all psychotropic medications (i.e., benzodiazepines, SSRIs, TCAs, and antipsychotics) are associated with an increased risk of falls and fractures in older adults (Seppala et al. 2018). Contrary to what is often assumed in clinical practice, the risk profile for falls and fractures is no different for benzodiazepines when compared with SSRIs or other psychotropic agents. However, extra caution is warranted for benzodiazepine prescriptions in older adults because chronic use is also associated with dependence and an increased risk of cognitive impairment and dementia (Lucchetta et al. 2018). Last but not least, it is important to be aware that 75% of mixed-age patients with anxiety have a preference for psychotherapy over drug treatment; the majority of older anxiety patients also prefer nonmedical treatment (McHugh et al. 2013).

Psychotherapy: Cognitive-Behavioral Therapy

It is often claimed that CBT protocols developed for and tested on young adults with an anxiety disorder need to be adapted to the specific needs and preferences of older patients with an anxiety disorder. The proposed adaptations usually involve more psychoeducation, more frequent repetition of the treatment rationale, use of reminders, and homework-support and adherence-promoting interventions. Although the small number of studies in this area have indicated that such adaptations are worthwhile and improve treatment outcomes, they are small-scale studies, and their findings are highly provisional. No critical differences in the treatment of anxiety disorders in the elderly compared with that in younger adults have been found as yet. For the common problem of fear of falling, various types of exercise and postural therapy (e.g., physiotherapy, tai chi) have been studied. Most of these studies suffered from various methodological shortcomings, but the limited evidence suggests a small to moderate effect immediately after the intervention. The evidence for long-term effects is scarce and inconclusive (Kendrick et al. 2014). A CBT program developed for this target group also appears to be effective (Zijlstra et al. 2009). A promising CBT protocol geared specifically to older patients with fear of falling can be easily used by health-care assistants in general practice (Parry et al. 2016).

In an attempt to lower the threshold for older anxiety patients to receive adequate treatment, recent intervention studies have focused on providing care closer to home, in general practice or in the home environment, by means of telephone- or internet-delivered CBT (Brenes et al. 2017; Jones et al. 2016). In general, these studies have shown promising results.

Combination Therapy

Only one study on combined treatment in older adults has been published, in which 12 weeks of escitalopram treatment in older patients with GAD was followed by CBT augmentation. This combination was found to improve outcomes compared with continued medication alone. CBT monotherapy reduced the risk of relapse compared with an SSRI alone, but combination therapy was even better at preventing relapse (Wetherell et al. 2013).

Gaps in the Literature

The amount of research on the treatment of anxiety disorders in those younger than 65 years is in sharp contrast to the small number of randomized clinical trials in older patients with anxiety disorders. The vast majority of studies in older adults focus on GAD; a few studies include a mixed population of elderly patients with GAD, panic disorder, or social anxiety disorder. Only one randomized study on the treatment of panic disorder with comorbid agoraphobia in the elderly is available (Hendriks et al. 2010); no studies at all have been published on the treatment of social anxiety disorder in the elderly.

Another point of concern is the fact that intervention studies to date are primarily based on relatively healthy, cognitively unimpaired, and "young" older adults who do not live in residential facilities. The few available studies in frail or "older old" elderly patients indicate that the features of anxiety disorders in this group tend to be quite different. Therefore, results from the available studies in the field may not be readily extrapolated to this population.

Conclusion

Although anxiety disorders are among the most prevalent psychiatric disorders in the older population and are associated with a substantial disease burden, older people with anxiety disorders often escape the notice of the mental health care system. Because the diagnostic focus of health care providers is generally on physical problems, and patients are reassured to find that they have no underlying physical disorder, the higher use of medical care associated with anxiety disorders often does not lead to correct diagnoses.

The result of this underdiagnosis is a lack of appropriate treatment and a chronically high disease burden. Educational materials and training for the appropriate diagnosis and referral of older adults with anxiety disorders are vital to ensure that these patients receive the help they need.

Key Points

- Despite the high prevalence of anxiety disorders in elderly persons, these disorders still often go unrecognized and untreated.

- Consideration of age-related differences in the presentation of anxiety disorders could help to improve appropriate diagnosis.

- Therapeutic nihilism is unnecessary; studies show that late-life anxiety disorders respond to standard treatment (cognitive-behavioral therapy and selective serotonin reuptake inhibitors).

References

American Psychiatric Association: Diagnostic and Statistical Manual of Mental Disorders, 4th Edition. Washington, DC, American Psychiatric Association, 1994

American Psychiatric Association: Diagnostic and Statistical Manual of Mental Disorders, 5th Edition. Arlington, VA, American Psychiatric Association, 2013

Baxter AJ, Scott KM, Vos T, et al: Global prevalence of anxiety disorders: a systematic review and meta-regression. Psychol Med 43(5):897–910, 2013 22781489

Baxter AJ, Vos T, Scott KM, et al: The global burden of anxiety disorders in 2010. Psychol Med 44(11):2363–2374, 2014 24451993

Becker E, Orellana Rios CL, Lahmann C, et al: Anxiety as a risk factor of Alzheimer's disease and vascular dementia. Br J Psychiatry 213(5):654–660, 2018 30339108

Beekman AT, de Beurs E, van Balkom AJ, et al: Anxiety and depression in later life: co-occurrence and communality of risk factors. Am J Psychiatry 157(1):89–95, 2000 10618018

Bierman EJM, Comijs HC, Jonker C, et al: The effect of anxiety and depression on decline of memory function in Alzheimer's disease. Int Psychogeriatr 21(6):1142–1147, 2009 19615124

Brenes GA, Danhauer SC, Lyles MF, et al: Long-term effects of telephone-delivered psychotherapy for late-life GAD. Am J Geriatr Psychiatry 25(11):1249–1257, 2017 28673741

Bryant C, Jackson H, Ames D: The prevalence of anxiety in older adults: methodological issues and a review of the literature. J Affect Disord 109(3):233–250, 2008 18155775

Byrne GJ, Pachana NA: Development and validation of a short form of the Geriatric Anxiety Inventory—the GAI-SF. Int Psychogeriatr 23(1):125–131, 2011 20561386

Carson N, Leach L, Murphy KJ: A re-examination of Montreal Cognitive Assessment (MoCA) cutoff scores. Int J Geriatr Psychiatry 33(2):379–388, 2018 28731508

Crittendon J, Hopko DR: Assessing worry in older and younger adults: psychometric properties of an abbreviated Penn State Worry Questionnaire (PSWQ-A). J Anxiety Disord 20(8):1036–1054, 2006 16387472

de Beurs E, Beekman AT, van Balkom AJ, et al: Consequences of anxiety in older persons: its effect on disability, well-being and use of health services. Psychol Med 29(3):583–593, 1999 10405079

Folstein MF, Folstein SE, McHugh PR: "Mini-mental state." A practical method for grading the cognitive state of patients for the clinician. J Psychiatr Res 12(3):189–198, 1975 1202204

Friborg O, Martinussen M, Kaiser S, et al: Comorbidity of personality disorders in anxiety disorders: a meta-analysis of 30 years of research. J Affect Disord 145(2):143–155, 2013 22999891

Fuentes K, Cox C: Assessment of anxiety in older adults: a community-based survey and comparison with younger adults. Behav Res Ther 38(3):297–309, 2000

Gonçalves DC, Byrne GJ: Interventions for generalized anxiety disorder in older adults: systematic review and meta-analysis. J Anxiety Disord 26(1):1–11, 2012 21907538

Gould CE, Edelstein BA: Worry, emotion control, and anxiety control in older and young adults. J Anxiety Disord 24(7):759–766, 2010 20708492

Gould RL, Coulson MC, Howard RJ: Efficacy of cognitive behavioral therapy for anxiety disorders in older people: a meta-analysis and meta-regression of randomized controlled trials. J Am Geriatr Soc 60(2):218–229, 2012 22283717

Grenier S, Préville M, Boyer R, et al: The impact of DSM-IV symptom and clinical significance criteria on the prevalence estimates of subthreshold and threshold anxiety in the older adult population. Am J Geriatr Psychiatry 19(4):316–326, 2011 21427640

Gulpers B, Ramakers I, Hamel R, et al: Anxiety as predictor for cognitive decline and dementia: a systematic review and meta-analysis. Am J Geriatr Psychiatry 24(10):823–842, 2016 27591161

Hendriks GJ, Oude Voshaar RC, Keijsers GP, et al: Cognitive-behavioural therapy for late-life anxiety disorders: a systematic review and meta-analysis. Acta Psychiatr Scand 117(6):403–411, 2008 18479316

Hendriks GJ, Keijsers GP, Kampman M, et al: A randomized controlled study of paroxetine and cognitive-behavioural therapy for late-life panic disorder. Acta Psychiatr Scand 122(1):11–19, 2010 19958308

Hendriks GJ, Keijsers GP, Kampman M, et al: Predictors of outcome of pharmacological and psychological treatment of late-life panic disorder with agoraphobia. Int J Geriatr Psychiatry 27(2):146–150, 2012

Hendriks GJ, Kampman M, Keijsers GP, et al: Cognitive-behavioral therapy for panic disorder with agoraphobia in older people: a comparison with younger patients. Depress Anxiety 31(8):669–677, 2014 24867666

Huffman JC, Smith FA, Blais MA, et al: Anxiety, independent of depressive symptoms, is associated with in-hospital cardiac complications after acute myocardial infarction. J Psychosom Res 65(6):557–563, 2008 19027445

Jones SL, Hadjistavropoulos HD, Soucy JN: A randomized controlled trial of guided internet-delivered cognitive behaviour therapy for older adults with generalized anxiety. J Anxiety Disord 37:1–9, 2016 26561733

Karlsson B, Sigström R, Waern M, et al: The prognosis and incidence of social phobia in an elderly population. A 5-year follow-up. Acta Psychiatr Scand 122(1):4–10, 2010 20384601

Kendrick D, Kumar A, Carpenter H, et al: Exercise for reducing fear of falling in older people living in the community. Cochrane Database Syst Rev (11):CD009848, 2014 25432016

Kessler RC, Berglund P, Demler O, et al: Lifetime prevalence and age-of-onset distributions of DSM-IV disorders in the National Comorbidity Survey Replication. Arch Gen Psychiatry 62(6):593–602, 2005 15939837

Lucchetta RC, da Mata BPM, Mastroianni PDC: Association between development of dementia and use of benzodiazepines: a systematic review and meta-analysis. Pharmacotherapy 38(10):1010–1020, 2018 30098211

Mackenzie CS, Pagura J, Sareen J: Correlates of perceived need for and use of mental health services by older adults in the collaborative psychiatric epidemiology surveys. Am J Geriatr Psychiatry 18(12):1103–1115, 2010 20808105

McHugh RK, Whitton SW, Peckham AD, et al: Patient preference for psychological vs pharmacologic treatment of psychiatric disorders: a meta-analytic review. J Clin Psychiatry 74(6):595–602, 2013 23842011

Miloyan B, Bulley A, Pachana NA, et al: Social phobia symptoms across the adult lifespan. J Affect Disord 168:86–90, 2014a 25043319

Miloyan B, Byrne GJ, Pachana NA: Age-related changes in generalized anxiety disorder symptoms. Int Psychogeriatr 26(4):565–572, 2014b 24405581

Molde H, Nordhus IH, Torsheim T, et al: A cross-national analysis of the psychometric properties of the Geriatric Anxiety Inventory (GAI). J Gerontol B Psychol Sci Soc Sci 2019 30624724 Epub ahead of print

Nasreddine ZS, Phillips NA, Bédirian V, et al: The Montreal Cognitive Assessment, MoCA: a brief screening tool for mild cognitive impairment. J Am Geriatr Soc 53(4):695–699, 2005 15817019

Parry SW, Bamford C, Deary V, et al: Cognitive-behavioural therapy-based intervention to reduce fear of falling in older people: therapy development and randomised controlled trial—the Strategies for Increasing Independence, Confidence and Energy (STRIDE) study. Health Technol Assess 20(56):1–206, 2016

Pinquart M, Duberstein PR, Lyness JM: Effects of psychotherapy and other behavioral interventions on clinically depressed older adults: a meta-analysis. Aging Ment Health 11(6):645–657, 2007

Préville M, Boyer R, Grenier S, et al: The epidemiology of psychiatric disorders in Quebec's older adult population. Can J Psychiatry 53(12):822–832, 2008 19087480

Ritchie K, Norton J, Mann A, et al: Late-onset agoraphobia: general population incidence and evidence for a clinical subtype. Am J Psychiatry 170(7):790–798, 2013 23820832

Schoevers RA, Beekman ATF, Deeg DJH, et al: Comorbidity and risk-patterns of depression, generalised anxiety disorder and mixed anxiety-depression in later life: results from the AMSTEL study. Int J Geriatr Psychiatry 18(11):994–1001, 2003

Scholten WD, Batelaan NM, Penninx BWJH, et al: Diagnostic instability of recurrence and the impact on recurrence rates in depressive and anxiety disorders. J Affect Disord 195:185–190, 2016 26896812

Schuurmans J, Comijs HC, Beekman AT, et al: The outcome of anxiety disorders in older people at 6-year follow-up: results from the Longitudinal Aging Study Amsterdam. Acta Psychiatr Scand 111(6):420–428, 2005 15877708

Seppala LJ, Wermelink AMAT, de Vries M, et al: Fall-risk-increasing drugs: a systematic review and meta-analysis: II. Psychotropics. J Am Med Dir Assoc 19(4):371.e11–371.e17, 2018 29402652

Sheikh JI, Swales PJ, Carlson EB, et al: Aging and panic disorder: phenomenology, comorbidity, and risk factors. Am J Geriatr Psychiatry 12(1):102–109, 2004 14729565

Sigström R, Östling S, Karlsson B, et al: A population-based study on phobic fears and DSM-IV specific phobia in 70-year olds. J Anxiety Disord 25(1):148–153, 2011 20869844

Stanley MA, Averill PM: Strategies for treating generalized anxiety in the eldery, in Handbook of Counseling and Psychotherapy With Older Adults. Edited by Duffy M. Chichester, UK, Wiley, 1999, pp 511–525

Therrien Z, Hunsley J: Assessment of anxiety in older adults: a systematic review of commonly used measures. Aging Ment Health 16(1):1–16, 2012 21838650

Tibi L, van Oppen P, Aderka IM, et al: Examining determinants of early and late age at onset in panic disorder: an admixture analysis. J Psychiatr Res 47(12):1870–1875, 2013 24084228

Volkert J, Schulz H, Härter M, et al: The prevalence of mental disorders in older people in Western countries: a meta-analysis. Ageing Res Rev 12(1):339–353, 2013 23000171

Wetherell JL, Kaplan RM, Kallenberg G, et al: Mental health treatment preferences of older and younger primary care patients. Int J Psychiatry Med 34(3):219–233, 2004 15666957

Wetherell JL, Petkus AJ, White KS, et al: Antidepressant medication augmented with cognitive-behavioral therapy for generalized anxiety disorder in older adults. Am J Psychiatry 170(7):782–789, 2013 23680817

Wolitzky-Taylor KB, Castriotta N, Lenze EJ, et al: Anxiety disorders in older adults: a comprehensive review. Depress Anxiety 27(2):190–211, 2010 20099273

Zijlstra GA, van Haastregt JC, Ambergen T, et al: Effects of a multicomponent cognitive behavioral group intervention on fear of falling and activity avoidance in community-dwelling older adults: results of a randomized controlled trial. J Am Geriatr Soc 57(11):2020–2028, 2009 19793161

Index

Page numbers printed in **boldface** type refer to tables or figures.